Encyclopedia of
Feline Clinical
Nutrition

Pascale Pibot

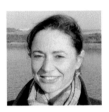

DVM,
Scientific Publishing
Manager, Royal Canin
Communication
Group

Vincent Biourge

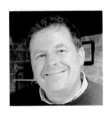

DVM, PhD,
Dipl. ACVN,
Dipl. ECVCN
Scientific Director of
Health-Nutrition,
Royal Canin
Research Center

Denise Elliott

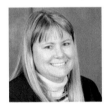

BVSc (Hons), PhD,
Dipl. ACVIM,
Dipl. ACVN
Director of Scientific
Affairs,
Royal Canin USA

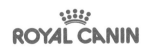

ROYAL CANIN

This encyclopedia is published by Aniwa SAS on behalf of Royal Canin.
Publication: Direction Communication Royal Canin Group/Aimargues – France
Royal Canin coordination: Pascale Pibot
Contact publishing: Sophie Durand-Pomaret
Scientific advisors: Vincent Biourge, Denise Elliott

Production: Diffomédia/Paris
Art director and concept: Élise Langellier, Guy Rolland
Layout: Élise Langellier
© Illustrations: Diffomédia/Élise Langellier, Mickaël Masure
Editorial coordination: Valérie de Leval assisted by Julie Robillard

Foto cover: DR
© 2008 Aniwa SAS

ISBN: 2-7476-0084-X
Copyright: 3d quarter 2008
Printed in EU by Diffo Print Italia

The book is the result of a collaboration with international authors who are specialized in different areas of veterinary medicine. Our warmest thanks to all those who have been involved in producing this Encyclopedia.

Contributors

 Vincent Biourge DVM, PhD, Dipl. ACVN, Dipl ECVCN
Scientific Director of Health-Nutrition,
Royal Canin Research Center (France)

 Nicholas Cave BVSc, MVSc, MACVSc, Dipl. ACVN
Senior lecturer in Small Animal Medicine
and Nutrition, Massey University (New Zealand)

 Valérie Chetboul DVM, Dipl. ECVIM-CA (cardiology)
Professor of Medical Pathology, Alfort National Veterinary
School (Cardiology unit, UMR INSERM-ENVA) (France)

 Fabienne Dethioux MRCVS
Scientific Communication,
International Division of Royal Canin (France)

 Denise Elliott BVSc (Hons), PhD, Dipl. ACVIM, Dipl. ACVN
Director of Scientific Affairs, Royal Canin (USA)

 Jonathan Elliott MA, Vet MB, PhD,
Cert SAC, Dipl. ECVPT, MRCVS
Professor of Veterinary Clinical Pharmacology,
Royal Veterinary College, London (UK)

 Valérie Freiche DVM
Practitioner in a referral practice of Internal Medicine
and Gastroenterology, Bordeaux (France)

 Alex German BVSc (Hons), PhD, Cert SAM,
Dipl. ECVIM-CA, MRCVS
Senior Lecturer in Small Animal Medicine
and Clinical Nutrition, Liverpool University (UK)

 Nicolas Girard DVM
Practicing veterinary dentist and ear,
nose and throat specialist, La Gaude (France)

 Isabelle Goy-Thollot DVM, MSc, PhD
Head of the Critical Care, Anaesthesia and Emergency
Medicine Unit (SIAMU), Lyon National Veterinary
School (France)

 Debra Horwitz DVM, Dipl. ACVB
Practitioner in a private referral practice for Behavior
and consultant for the Veterinary Information
Network (VIN) (USA)

 Doreen Houston DVM, DVSc, Dipl. ACVIM
Clinical Trial Research Director for Medi-Cal
Royal Canin Veterinary Diets (Canada)

 Ariane Junien Eng
Responsible for palatability projects at the Royal Canin
Research Center (France)

 Thomas Lutz DVM, PhD
Professor of Applied Veterinary Physiology,
Zurich University (Switzerland)

 Lucile Martin DVM, PhD
Senior Lecturer at the Nutrition and Endocrinology Unit,
National Veterinary School of Nantes (France)

 Kathryn Michel DVM, Dipl. ACVN
Associate Professor of Nutrition and Chief of the Section
of Medicine, University of Pennsylvania (USA)

 Ralf Mueller DVM, PhD, Dipl. ACVD,
FACVSc, Dipl. ECVD
Chief of the Veterinary Dermatology Service, University
of Munich (Germany)

 Carolien Rutgers DVM, MS, Dipl. ACVIM,
Dipl. ECVIM-CA, DSAM, MRCVS
Independent consultant. Previous Senior Lecturer,
Royal Veterinary College (UK)

 Patricia Schenck DVM, PhD
Professor in the Endocrinology Section of the Diagnostic
Center for Population and Animal Health, Michigan
State University (USA)

 Karin Sorenmo DVM, Dipl. ACVIM, Dipl. ECVIM-CA
Associate Professor of Oncology and Chief
of the Oncology Section, University of Pennsylvania (USA)

Eric Servet Meng
Research Engineer, Royal Canin Research
Center (France)

Jürgen Zentek DMV, Prof, Dipl. ECVCN
Professor of Clinical Nutrition, University
of Berlin (Germany)

Yannick Soulard Eng
Head of Nutritional Research Programs,
Royal Canin Research Center (France)

We would like to express our sincere thanks to all those whose precious help has enabled the production of this Encyclopedia.

Colette Arpaillange DVM
Behaviorist and practitioner in Internal Medicine,
Veterinary Hospital of the National Veterinary School
of Nantes (France)

Robert Backus MS, DVM, PhD, Dipl. ACVN
Director of the Small Animal Nutrition Program,
Department of Veterinary Medicine and Surgery,
University of Missouri-Columbia, Missouri (USA)

Thomas Bissot DVM
Clinical Research Project Manager, Royal Canin
Research Center (France)

Dominique Blanchot DVM,MS, Dipl. ACVD,
Dipl. ACVB
Consultant in Gastroenterology and Endoscopy
(France)

Alexandre Blavier DVM, MSc
Scientific Communication, Royal Canin Research
Center (France)

Luc Chabanne DVM, PhD, MS of Immunology
and Hematology
Head of the Department of Companion Animals and
Manager of the Medicine unit, National Veterinary
School of Lyon (France)

Arnaud Christ DVM
Veterinary Diets Product Manager, Royal Canin
(France)

Larry Cowgill DVM, PhD, Dipl. ACVIM
Professor in the Department of Medicine and
Epidemiology, School of Veterinary Medicine,
University of California-Davis (USA)

Pauline Devlin BSc (Hons), PhD
Veterinary Support Manager, Royal Canin (UK)

Marianne Diez DVM, PhD, Dipl. ECVN
Lecturer, Department of Animal Productions, Faculty
of Veterinary Medicine, Liège University (Belgium)

Linda Fleeman BVSc, MACVSc
Faculty in the School of Veterinary Science, University
of Queensland (Australia)

Pauline de Fornel-Thibaud DVM, DESV of
Internal Medicine for Companion Animals
Veterinary Center of Cancerology
(Maisons-Alfort, France) and faculty position
at the National Veterinary School of Alfort

Marc Gogny DVM, Dipl. ECVPT
Professor of Physiology and Pharmacology, National
Veterinary School of Nantes (France)

Élise Malandain DVM, MSc
Scientific Support and Training Manager, Royal Canin
Research Center (France)

Paul Mandigers DVM, MVM, PhD, Dipl. ECVIM
Department of Clinical Sciences of Companion
Animals, Faculty of Veterinary Medicine, Utrecht
University (The Netherlands)

Andrew Moore MSc
Canadian Veterinary Urolith Center, Analytical
Microscopy Laboratory, Guelph University, Ontario
(Canada)

James Morris PhD, Dipl. ACVN
Professor emeritus, University of California-Davis
(USA)

Mickaël Münster DVM
Specialist for Small Animal Internal Medicine
and Gastroenterology, Köln (Germany)

Paul Pion DVM, Dipl. ACVIM
President and co-founder of the Veterinary
Information Network (VIN)

Brice Reynolds DVM
Associate Professor, National Veterinary School
of Toulouse, Internal Medicine Unit (France)

Christine Rivierre-Archambeaud DVM,
Dipl. ECVD, Dipl. ACVD, MSpVM
Scientific translator

Kenneth Simpson BVM & S, PhD, MRCVS,
Dipl. ACVIM, Dipl. ECVIM-CA
Assistant Professor of Small Animal Medicine, Cornell
University (USA)

Capucine Tournier Eng
Research and Development Engineer, Royal Canin
Research Center (France)

Stéphanie Vidal Eng
Engineer in the Nutrition Research Team, Royal Canin
Research Center (France)

... and of course, the whole team of Diffomédia/Paris
for their wonderful job!

Health and nutrition; more closely related than ever before

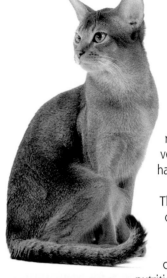

© Y. Lanceau/RC/Abyssin

Feeding a cat may appear ar first glance to be a straightforward exercise. However, this assumption requires some qualification, because cats are strict carnivores with nutritional requirements that differ from those of dogs. In addition, cats generally have very clear dietary preferences that need to be considered. Furthermore, if the cat is ill or has a higher pathological risk, things can sometimes get really complicated.

This Encyclopedia of Feline Clinical Nutrition endeavors to answer the main questions of our time about feline clinical nutrition. The authors were asked first and foremost to summarize the current state of knowledge about cats. When the published data was too succinct, it was sometimes necessary to cite results obtained from other species, while always clarifying where their studies come from and utilizing them in the specific context of feline nutritional characteristics, to avoid incorrect extrapolations.

The following list of questions does not pretend to be an incisive tool to test your knowledge, but you may be interested in how many questions you can answer – without looking at the book.

1. How do you determine the body weight of an obese cat?
2. Which cat breeds are most likely to present dietary sensitivity?
3. What are prebiotics?
4. In the absence of clinical sign of hepatic lipidosis, which blood parameter is used to evaluate hepatic lipid accumulation?
5. What two characteristics should be prioritized in a diet for a diabetic cat?
6. What is the most common cause of hyperlipidemia in cats?
7. Should severe sodium restriction always be recommended in cats with chronic kidney disease?
8. How do you combat both struvite and calcium oxalate stones at the same time?
9. How do you definitively diagnose taurine deficiency?
10. What are the agents active against the development of dental calculus?
11. What are the essential criteria for selecting food for cats with cancer?
12. What is the best feeding route for a cat in intensive care?
13. Why can't cats distinguish sweet taste?
14. What effect is produced by a dramatic increase of omega-3 fatty acids versus omega-6 fatty acids in the diet?

Each of the 14 chapters of the Encyclopedia is filled with information that will enable you to check, correct, refine and perhaps improve your answers.

We hope that during your reading you will find many other subjects of interest and that nutrition will become an even more important aspect of your diagnostic and therapeutic approach.

Pascale Pibot, Denise Elliott, and Vincent Biourge

1. **How do you determine the body weight of an obese cat?**
a. *It's a simple calculation based on the condition of the body*
b. *By bioelectrical impedance analysis*
c. *By indirect calorimetry*

2. **Which cat breeds are most likely to present dietary sensitivity?**
a. *The Persian*
b. *The Maine Coon*
c. *The Siamese and related breeds*

3. **What are prebiotics?**
a. *Non-digestible carbohydrates that are fermented in the gut by bacteria*
b. *Microorganisms that have a beneficial effect on the intestinal flora*
c. *Sources of non-fermentable fiber*

4. **In the absence of clinical sign of hepatic lipidosis, which blood parameter is used to evaluate the lipid accumulation level in the liver?**
a. *Bilirubin*
b. *Cholesterol*
c. *Alkaline phosphatase*

5. **What two characteristics should be prioritized in a diet for a diabetic cat?**
a. *High fiber content and low starch content*
b. *High protein content and low starch content*
c. *Low protein and starch content*

6. **What is the most common cause of hyperlipidemia in cats?**
a. *Primary idiopathic hyperlipidemia*
b. *The animal is not fasted before the sample is taken*
c. *Diabetes mellitus*

7. **Should a severe sodium restriction always be recommended in cats with chronic kidney disease?**
a. *Yes, it helps prevent hypertension*
b. *Yes, it activates the renin-angiotensin-aldosterone system*
c. *No, it can activate the renin-angiotensin-aldosterone system*

8. **How do you combat both struvite and calcium oxalate stones at the same time?**
a. *By encouraging diuresis*
b. *By acidifying the urine pH*
c. *By limiting the dietary consumption of phosphorus*

9. **How do you definitively diagnose taurine deficiency?**
a. *By dosing taurine based on the results of muscle biopsy*
b. *By measuring the taurine level in the plasma*
c. *By measuring the taurine level in the whole blood*

10. **What are the agents active against the development of dental calculus?**
a. *Polyphosphate salts*
b. *Omega-3 fatty acids*
c. *B-group vitamins*

11. **What is the essential criteria for selecting food for cats with cancer?**
a. *High glutamine concentration*
b. *Palatability*
c. *High protein content*

12. **What is the best feeding route for a cat in intensive care?**
a. *The parenteral route*
b. *A combination of parenteral and enteral route*
c. *The enteral route*

13. **Why can't cats distinguish sweet taste?**
a. *Because cats do not have any salivary amylase*
b. *Because the sweet taste receptors are deactivated*
c. *Because cats rarely consume sweet food*

14. **What effect is produced by a dramatic increase of omega-3 fatty acids versus omega-6 fatty acids in the diet?**
a. *Immunostimulant effect*
b. *Immunosuppressant effect*
c. *No effect*

1-a, 2-c, 3-a, 4-c, 5-b, 6-b, 7-c, 8-a, 9-c, 10-a, 11-b, 12-c, 13-b, 14-b

How did you do?
- *More than 10 correct answers: well done, you're going to enjoy this book*
- *7-10 correct answers: not a bad score, but you can do better*
- *Fewer than 7 correct answers: this book could teach you a lot!*

"Let food be thy medicine"

Hippocrates (460-377 BC)

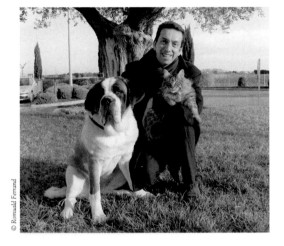

© Romuald Ferrand

It is a long time since cats moved from being the irregular and unwelcome frequenters of farms and alleyways to pampered companions kept for their beauty, gentleness and mystery. With every day that passes their place in western homes becomes more and more assured. Indeed, the cat population now even outstrips the dog population.

Their relationship to humans has developed remarkably and their behavior has adapted to these contacts: this wild animal has become so well adapted to life indoors that its life expectancy has increased significantly, from an average of four years for outdoor cats to 18 years for those that live indoors. This comfortable life does have a downside: obesity for one is a major and growing threat. Nowadays, cat owners are very concerned about the health of their animal. Vaccination, neutering and tattooing or microchipping are all ways to try to extend its life and as such they have become a very important part of the daily routine of veterinarians.

Cats have been the subject of numerous veterinarian studies and in the field of feline nutrition, for one, great – even crucial – advances have been made over the past fifteen years. The range of dedicated food available today makes it easier to control or prevent many diseases (urolithiasis, food allergies, chronic kidney disease to name but a few). For many years Royal Canin has made it a matter of honor to find effective, targeted solutions to the specific problems affecting cats. This species is actually more of a challenge to care for than dogs. They are more demanding and fully capable of starving themselves to death even when they have access to plenty of food, so they demand very precise responses to make up for an 'enzymatic toolbox' that is not really suited to compensating for nutritional deficiencies.

The advancements in knowledge have had a recent but real impact on nutrition courses at veterinary colleges, schools and universities. It is important that clinicians are able to draw on the latest, most complete knowledge on the subject. That is the aim of this encyclopedia, conceived by the Royal Canin research teams, which sets a new standard in feline clinical nutrition.

Twenty-three global specialists have contributed to its 14 chapters, 10 of them are based on a collaboration between a clinician and a nutritionist. I am proud to be able to say that seven of those 23 authors are employees of Royal Canin, which is proof of the commitment of everyone at the company to working as hard as possible and using their know-how to benefit both dogs and cats.

I sincerely hope that this book, like its sister publication about dogs, will prove a useful tool for you and your team and facilitate the employment of nutrition in your daily practice.

Jean Christophe Flatin
Chairman & CEO

Contents

XI   Introduction

XIII   Foreword

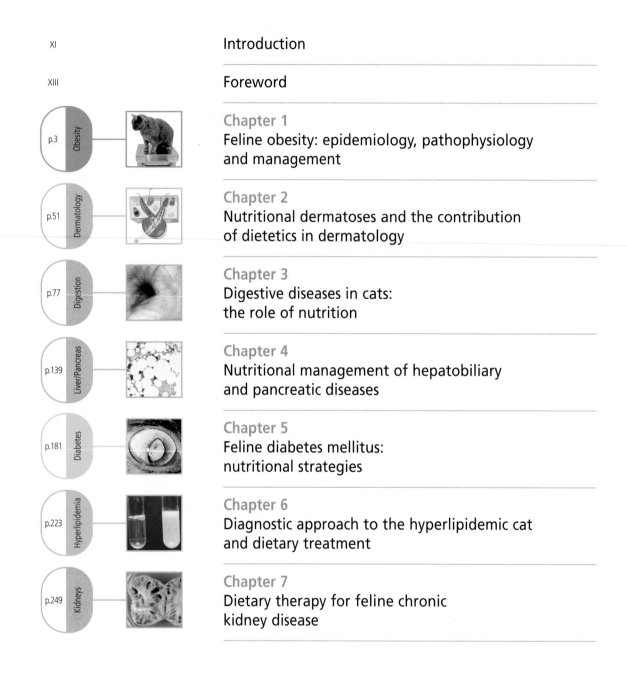

p.3   Obesity

Chapter 1
Feline obesity: epidemiology, pathophysiology
and management

p.51   Dermatology

Chapter 2
Nutritional dermatoses and the contribution
of dietetics in dermatology

p.77   Digestion

Chapter 3
Digestive diseases in cats:
the role of nutrition

p.139   Liver/Pancreas

Chapter 4
Nutritional management of hepatobiliary
and pancreatic diseases

p.181   Diabetes

Chapter 5
Feline diabetes mellitus:
nutritional strategies

p.223   Hyperlipidemia

Chapter 6
Diagnostic approach to the hyperlipidemic cat
and dietary treatment

p.249   Kidneys

Chapter 7
Dietary therapy for feline chronic
kidney disease

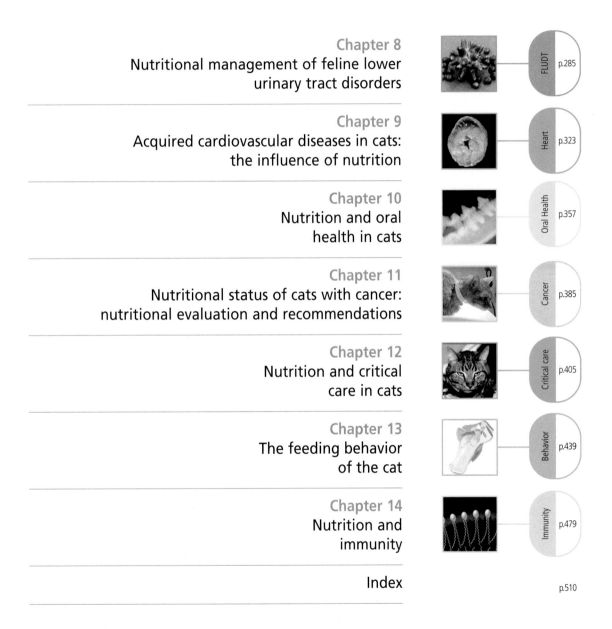

Chapter 8
Nutritional management of feline lower
urinary tract disorders

FLUDT   p.285

Chapter 9
Acquired cardiovascular diseases in cats:
the influence of nutrition

Heart   p.323

Chapter 10
Nutrition and oral
health in cats

Oral Health   p.357

Chapter 11
Nutritional status of cats with cancer:
nutritional evaluation and recommendations

Cancer   p.385

Chapter 12
Nutrition and critical
care in cats

Critical care   p.405

Chapter 13
The feeding behavior
of the cat

Behavior   p.439

Chapter 14
Nutrition and
immunity

Immunity   p.479

Index

p.510

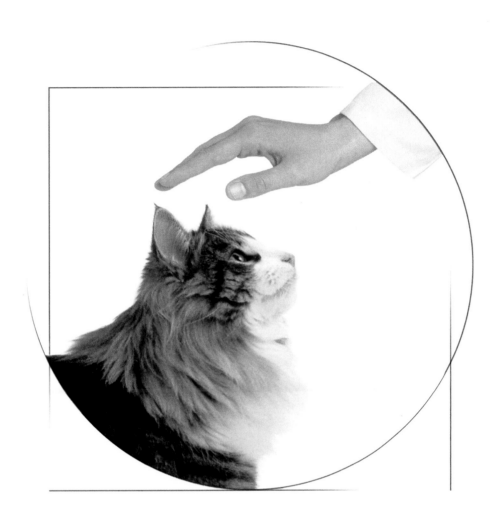

Encyclopedia of
Feline Clinical
Nutrition

Alex GERMAN
BVSc (Hons), PhD,
CertSAM, Dipl.
ECVIM-CA, MRCVS

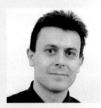

Lucile MARTIN
DVM, PhD

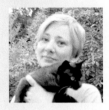

Feline obesity: epidemiology, pathophysiology and management

1 - Definition of obesity 5
2 - Epidemiology of obesity 5
3 - Medical significance of obesity 8
4 - Pathophysiology 12
5 - Clinical evaluation of the obese patient 14
6 - Prevention of feline obesity 20
7 - Five components to a successful weight management strategy for feline obesity 21
8 - Dietary management of pre-existing obesity 27
9 - Composition of the diet 33
Conclusion 39
Frequently asked questions 40
References 41
Royal Canin nutritional information 44

ABBREVIATIONS USED IN THIS CHAPTER

ARA: arachidonic acid
BCM: body cell mass
BCS: body condition score
BMI: body mass index
BMR: basal metabolic rate
BW: body weight
CCK: cholecystokinin
CKD: chronic kidney disease
CLA: conjugated linoleic acid
CP: crude protein
DF: dietary fiber
DEXA: dual energy x-ray absorptiometry
DMB: dry matter basis

DM2: diabetes mellitus type 2
ECW: extracellular water
FFM: fat free mass
FLUTD: feline lower urinary tract disease
FM: fat mass
FBMI™: feline body mass index
GLP (1,2): glucagon-like peptide (1, 2)
GRP: gastrin releasing peptide
HDL: high density lipoprotein
IBW: ideal body weight
ICW: intracellular water
IGF 1: insulin-like growth factor 1
LA: linoleic acid

LBM: lean body mass
LIM: leg index measurement
ME: metabolizable energy
MRI: magnetic resonance imaging
MTPI: triglyceride transfer protein inhibitor
OA: osteoarthritis
PYY: peptide tyrosine-tyrosine
RER: resting energy requirement
SCFA: short chain fatty acid
TBW: total body water

Feline obesity: epidemiology, pathophysiology and management

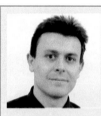

Alex GERMAN
BVSc (Hons), PhD, CertSAM, Dipl. ECVIM-CA, MRCVS

Alex German qualified, with honors, from the University of Bristol in 1994. He then worked for two years in mixed practice before returning to Bristol to undertake a PhD and then residency in small animal internal medicine. He was awarded the RCVS certificate in small animal medicine in August 2001. In October 2002, he moved to Liverpool University, and is currently the Royal Canin Senior Lecturer in Small Animal Medicine and Clinical Nutrition. In September 2004 he became a Diplomate of the European College of Veterinary Internal Medicine. His current research interests include small animal gastroenterology, metabolomics, and obesity biology.

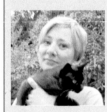

Lucile MARTIN
DVM, PhD

Lucile Martin graduated in 1990 from the National Veterinary School of Nantes (ENVN), where she is now Senior Lecturer at the Nutrition and Endocrinology Unit. After obtaining her PhD in nutrition in 1996, she took charge of a research program on butyrate metabolism and inflammatory bowel diseases at the Human Nutrition and Research Center of Nantes. Since 1999, Lucile has also participated in diagnosis and research with the ENVN LDH (Hormone Assay Laboratory) to study endocrine disorders linked with obesity in domestic carnivores. In January 2001, she was elected to the Board of the AFVAC Dietetic Study Group. In addition to teaching clinical nutrition for pets and horses and acting as a consultant in nutrition and endocrinology at the Veterinary School of Nantes, Lucile is the author of more than 30 publications on research and continuing education.

Obesity is considered to be the most common form of malnutrition in small animal practice. It has been suggested that as many as 40% of pets are obese. The significance of obesity pertains to its role in the pathogenesis of a variety of diseases and the ability to exacerbate pre-existing disease. Obesity has been associated with an increased incidence of osteoarthritis, cardiorespiratory problems, diabetes mellitus, constipation, dermatitis, anesthetic risk, and reduced life-expectancy.

1 - Definition of obesity

Obesity is defined as an accumulation of excessive amounts of body fat *(Bray, 1999)*. In humans, a wealth of epidemiological data demonstrate that morbidity and mortality risk correlates with increasing body fat mass. Criteria are usually based on indirect measures of adiposity such as the body mass index (BMI; weight [kg] divided by height^2 [m]), and definitions exist for "overweight" ($25 < BMI < 30$ kg/m^2) and "obese" (BMI > 30 kg/m^2). A recent large-scale epidemiological study suggested that the optimal BMI for non-smoking 50 year-old adult Caucasians was 20-25 *(Adams et al, 2006)*, and many other studies concur with these findings. In contrast, data on what represents an optimal feline body weight are more limited; cats are classified as being overweight when their body weight is more than 10% above their "optimal body weight", and classified as "obese" when their body weight exceeds 20% of optimal *(Lund et al, 2005)*. In the largest epidemiological studies of their kind, increasing risk of associated diseases is seen with increasing levels of adiposity, as judged by body condition score (BCS) *(Scarlett et al, 1998; Lund et al, 2005)*. This suggests that, like in humans, excessive weight confers a mortality and morbidity risk (see below) and support the need to strive for optimal body condition.

> **OVERWEIGHT OR OBESE?**
> Cats are classified as being overweight when their body weight is more than 10% above their "optimal body weight", and classified as "obese" when their body weight exceeds 20% of optimal.

2 - Epidemiology of obesity

► Prevalence and time trends

Obesity is an escalating global problem in humans *(Kopelman, 2000)*, and current estimates suggest that almost two thirds of adults in the United States are overweight or obese *(Flegal et al, 2002)*. Prevalence studies of companion animal obesity are more limited; reports from various parts of the world, have estimated the prevalence of obesity in the dog population to be between 22% and 50% *(McGreevy et al, 2005; Colliard et al, 2006; Holmes et al, 2007)*. In cats, information is limited to a handful of studies over a time-frame of over thirty years, using a variety of definitions of overweight/obesity and techniques to estimate body condition *(Sloth, 1992; Robertson, 1999; Russell et al, 2000; Harper, 2001; Lund et al, 2005)*. From this work, estimates of obesity prevalence range from 19 to 52% **(Table 1)**.

One of the most recent studies was from the USA, and utilized 1995 records of the National Companion Animal Study *(Lund et al, 2005)*. The results suggested that approximately 35% of adult cats were classed as either overweight or obese (overweight 28.7%; obese 6.4%). However, prevalence of overweight and obesity varies amongst age groups with middle age cats (between 5 and 11 years of age) particularly at risk (overall prevalence 41%; overweight 33.3%, obese 7.7%). Of particular concern was the finding that a clinical diagnosis of obesity was only recorded in 2.2% of cats (despite the BCS findings), suggesting that veterinarians do not consider the condition to be of clinical significance.

Whatever the true figure for feline obesity, it is clear that the condition is one of the most important medical diseases seen by veterinarians, especially for middle-aged adults. Furthermore, studies have reported that owners tend to under-estimate the body condition of their cats, compared with the estimates of their veterinarians *(Kienzle & Bergler, 2006)*; and these individuals may not be presented for assessment.

► Risk factors for feline obesity

Obesity prevalence is influenced by numerous factors. Individual factors that have been identified include gender and neuter status, age, and breed; environmental factors include accommodation, presence of dogs in the household, and the feeding of certain types of diet; additionally, some factors may be the combination of both individual and environmental influences e.g. inactivity. Other studies have implicated owner factors and feeding behavior as risk factors for overweight and obesity in cats *(Kienzle & Bergler, 2006)*.

TABLE 1 - ESTIMATION OF THE PREVALENCE OF FELINE OBESITY

Reference	Country	Incidence rate
Sloth, 1992	UK	40%
Robertson, 1999	Australia	19%
Russel et al, 2000	UK	52%
Lund et al, 2005	USA	35%

FIGURE 1 - PREVALENCE OF FELINE OBESITY ACCORDING TO AGE

(from Scarlett, 1994 and Robertson, 1999; study on 2671 cats)

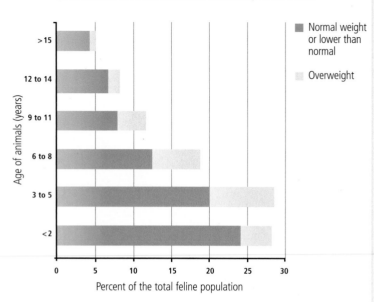

Normal weight or lower than normal

Overweight

Age of animals (years)

Percent of the total feline population

In absolute terms, the highest number of overweight cats is found in the 3-5 years of age category. Relatively speaking, cats aged 6-8 years are most affected: one in three cats in this age group are overweight.

> Age

Middle age is a particular risk factor for overweight and obesity in cats **(Figure 1)**. One study identified that body condition was significantly higher in cats <13 years of age compared with those >13 years *(Russell et al, 2000)*. In another North American study, the prevalence for overweight and obesity was greatest in cats between 5 and 11 years of age *(Lund et al, 2005)*. Such data are critical to veterinarians since they help to identify the population most at risk, and would suggest that prevention strategies, if instigated early (e.g. ~2 years of age) might have the greatest impact on satisfactory management of the condition.

> Neuter status and gender

Neutering is the major cause of obesity in cats with numerous studies confirming the link *(Scarlett et al, 1998; Robertson, 1999; Allan et al, 2000; Russell et al, 2000; Lund et al, 2005; Martin et al, 2001; 2006a)*. Metabolic consequences of neutering will be developed in the pathophysiology section.

Gender itself is also a predisposing factor in some but not all studies, with males over-represented in recent work *(Lund et al, 2005)*. The reasons for such a gender association have not been fully elucidated, not least given that one study has shown that fasting metabolic rate declines in female but not male cats that were neutered *(Fettman et al, 1997)*.

> Endocrine abnormalities

Compared with dogs, obesity in cats is less likely to result from endocrine abnormalities such as hypothyroidism and hyperadrenocorticism. However, the use of progesterones for contraceptive management has been associated with the development of obesity.

In cats, obesity is most of the time associated with increased plasma concentration of prolactin, leptin and insulin-like growth factor (IGF)-1 *(Martin et al, 2006a)*. The hormonal profile is thus completely different from that of the obese dog *(Martin et al, 2006b)*. All these hormones have a direct role in the onset of insulin-resistance *(Melloul et al, 2002)*.

> Breed

A handful of studies have examined the influence of breed on the prevalence of feline obesity. Two studies identified that "crossbred" or mixed-breed cats were approximately twice as likely to be overweight as purebred cats *(Scarlett et al, 1994; Robertson, 1999)*. *Lund et al* (2005) also found mixed breed cats (domestic shorthair, domestic medium hair, domestic longhair) to be at greater risk; Manx cats were also predisposed.

> Environment

Environmental factors reported to influence the prevalence of obesity include the type of accommodation, the number of cats and or the presence of dogs in the household *(Scarlett et al, 1994; Robertson, 1999; Allan et al, 2000)*. With regard to accommodation, both indoor dwelling and living in an apartment have been shown to predispose in some *(Scarlett et al, 1994; Robertson, 1999)* but not all *(Russell et al, 2000)* studies, probably because this type of environment does not respect the normal ethogram of the cat. It is likely that inability to maximally exercise and boredom may play a part.

One study demonstrated that the presence of dogs in the household significantly reduced the odds of developing obesity (*Allan et al, 2000*), possibly due to the behavioral traits of the cats or dogs.

Finally, the type of owner that own exclusively cats might differ from those who own both cats and dogs; in this respect, people who own both might be less inclined to dote upon their cats and less likely to provide premium foods for their pets (see below).

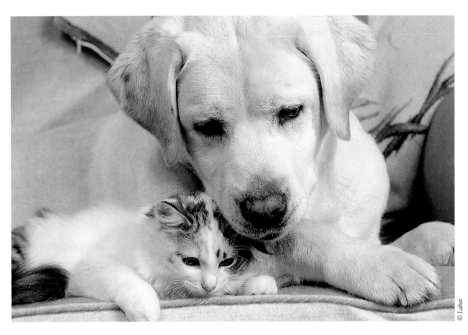

© Lanat

> Activity

Activity is one of the factors influenced both by individual and environmental variables. It is possible that the principle influence of type of accommodation relates to ability to exercise outdoors. Numerous studies have identi- 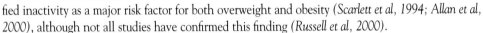 fied inactivity as a major risk factor for both overweight and obesity (*Scarlett et al, 1994; Allan et al, 2000*), although not all studies have confirmed this finding (*Russell et al, 2000*).

> Dietary factors

Some studies have suggested that feeding premium pet foods (*Scarlett et al, 1994*) conveys an increased risk compared with the risk whilst feeding a grocery store diet. The increased palatability may overcome normal appetite control leading to overeating, but in the 1990's, the main reason proposed for such an association was that premium food tended to have a higher fat, and hence energy, content than grocery products; today, many moderate fat-diets (10-14% fat on dry matter basis [DMB]) are available.

Kienzle and Bergler (2006) conducted a study of owner attitudes and compared cats that were overweight with those that were normal weight or thin. The owners of overweight cats tended to offer food on a free-choice basis, but there was no difference in the type of food fed.

Many veterinarians typically feed cats with high-fat diets specifically formulated to prevent FLUTD. These high-fat calorically dense diets are a frequent cause of obesity.

> Owner factors and behavior

Some studies have indicated a number of owner factors in the development of obesity (*Kienzle & Bergler, 2006*) and it is interesting to make comparisons with dogs. For instance, the owners of obese cats tend to "humanize" their cat more, and cats have a potential role as a substitute for human companionship. Over-humanization was also associated with overweight in a dog study, but a close human-dog relationship was not (*Kienzle et al, 1998*). The owners of overweight cats spend less time playing with their pet and tend to use food as a reward rather than extra play. Further, the owners of overweight cats watch their cats during eating more often than owners of cats in normal body condition; this is similar to findings for dog owners. The owners of both overweight cats and dogs have less of an interest in preventive health than those of pets in ideal body condition. Unlike the owners of overweight dogs who tend to have a lower income, there are no demographic differences amongst owners of overweight and normal weight cats. Finally, the percentage of female owners is higher in overweight than in normal weight cats.

Further, many owners misread signals about the behavior of their cat with regard to eating. It is important to remember that:

A cat may eat less when it lives with a dog:
- *it might be intimidated by the presence of a dog, reducing its drive to eat*
- *a dog may drive the cat away from the food bowl*
- *the cat can be stimulated by the dog to play. Its physical activity is thus overall more important than if it only lives alone.*

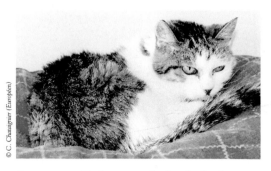
© C. Chataigner (Europen)

For cats, possible factors involved in the development of obesity include anxiety, depression, failure to establish a normal feeding behavior, and failure to develop control of satiety.

- Cats in the wild are designed to be trickle feeders and would typically consume numerous small meals. Despite this, many owners choose to feed their cats in 2-3 large meals per day.
- In contrast to humans and dogs, cats do not have any inherent need for social interaction during feeding times. When the cat initiates contact, owners often assume that they are hungry and are asking for food when they are not. Nevertheless, if food is provided at such times, the cat soon learns that initiating contact results in a food reward. If larger amounts or energy-dense foods are offered, it has the potential of leading to excessive food intake and obesity;
- Play is necessary throughout life **(Figure 2)**. Dog owners are usually conditioned to provide regular exercise through both walks and play; in contrast, most cat owners do not engage in play sessions with their pets.

3 - Medical significance of obesity

It has long been known that dietary restriction can increase longevity in a number of species including dogs *(McCay et al, 1935; Kealy et al, 1992, 1997, 2000, 2002; Lane et al, 1998; Larson et al, 2003; Lawler et al, 2005)*. It is probable that a similar association is present for cats, although data to support such a supposition are lacking.

Whilst it is generally accepted that overweight and obesity increases the risk of suffering from a number of associated diseases in cats **(Table 2)** limited scientific peer-reviewed data are available to support these associations. There have been two large-scale studies assessing disease associations in overweight and obese cats. In a study by *Donoghue and Scarlett* (1998), the major associations recognized were diabetes mellitus, dermatoses, lameness and diarrhea **(Figure 3)**. These authors also noticed that overweight cats have a shorter lifespan.

A subsequent study *(Lund et al, 2005)* assessed disease associations in a population of 8159 cats. For overweight and obesity, the major disease associations included oral cavity disease, urinary tract disease, diabetes mellitus, hepatic lipidosis, dermatopathy and neoplasia.

TABLE 2 - DISEASES ASSOCIATED WITH FELINE OBESITY

Metabolic abnormalities
- Hyperlipidemia/dyslipidemia
- Insulin resistance
- Glucose intolerance
- Hepatic lipidosis

Endocrinopathies
- Hyperadrenocorticism
- Diabetes mellitus

Orthopedic disorders

Dermatologic diseases

Oral cavity disease

Cardiorespiratory disease
- Hypertension

Feline asthma?

Urogenital system
- Feline lower urinary tract disease
- Urolithiasis

Neoplasia

Functional alterations
- Joint disorders
- Respiratory compromise e.g. dyspnea
- Dystocia
- Exercise intolerance
- Heat intolerance/heat stroke
- Decreased immune functions
- Increased anesthetic risk
- Decreased lifespan

FIGURE 2 - A CAT'S LIFE: ETHOGRAM*

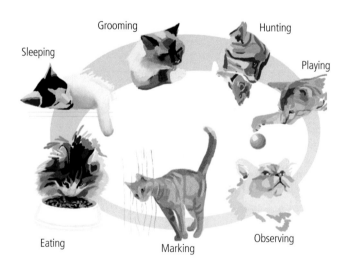

Grooming
Hunting
Sleeping
Playing
Eating
Marking
Observing

Eating represents less than 1hour per day for the cat but sleeping is the most time-demanding activity: 14-18hrs/24hrs, i.e. 60-75% of the time.

FIGURE 3 - INFLUENCE OF FELINE OBESITY ON THE INCIDENCE OF SKIN DISEASES, DIABETES MELLITUS AND LOCOMOTIVE DISORDERS

(from Scarlett & Donoghue, 1998)

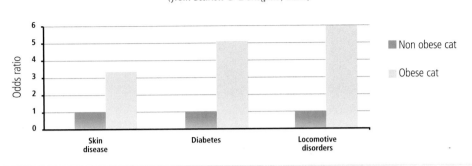

■ Non obese cat

☐ Obese cat

▶ Association between excessive weight, insulin resistance and diabetes mellitus

Insulin secreted by pancreatic β cells controls the uptake and use of glucose in peripheral tissues (see chapter 5).

Cats most often suffer from diabetes mellitus that resembles "type 2" diabetes mellitus in man (DM2), and, therefore, obesity is a major risk factor in this species *(Nelson et al, 1990)*. Of all disease associations, diabetes mellitus is by far and away the most well-known. Indeed, epidemiological studies have confirmed an increased risk of diabetes mellitus in obese cats; in the study by *Lund et al* (2005), an odds ratio of 2.2 was reported for obese cats versus those in ideal body condition. This supports the work of older studies which have also reported an association *(Panciera et al, 1990; Scarlett & Donoghue, 1998)*. Finally, it has been proven that diabetic cats have significantly reduced sensitivity to insulin than cats without DM2 *(Feldhahn et al, 1999)*.

▶ Dermatoses

Both the *Scarlett and Donoghue* (1998) and the *Lund et al* (2005) studies suggested a link between obesity and dermatoses. Diseases represented included feline acne, alopecia, various forms of dermatitis, scale formation, and dermatophytosis. Diffuse scale is commonly observed, most likely due to reduced ability to groom efficiently.

Similar, one of the authors has observed numerous obese cats with fecal soiling; an association with grooming is suggested by the fact that such problems commonly resolve or improve after weight reduction. A single case report has also been published of perivulvular dermatitis associated with obesity; whilst the authors reported that episioplasty was required for resolution of this problem *(Ranen & Zur, 2005)*; unfortunately, there was no mention of an attempt at weight management in this case. Finally, extreme obesity can lead to physical inactivity and to the development of pressure sores **(Figure 4)**.

Figure 4 - 9 year old neutered male Siamese cat with gross obesity (body weight 12.95 kg, condition score 5/5).
The obesity had led to inactivity, inability to groom and pressure sores on the ventral abdomen.

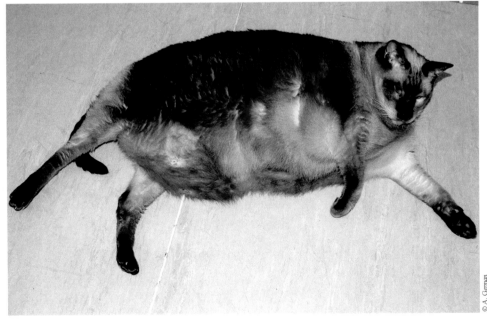

© A. German

9

FIGURE 5A - HIP DYSPLASIA IN A CAT

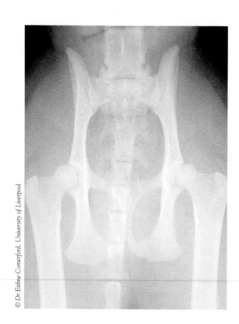

© Dr Eithne Comerford, University of Liverpool

FIGURE 5B - ELBOW OSTEOARTHRITIS IN A CAT

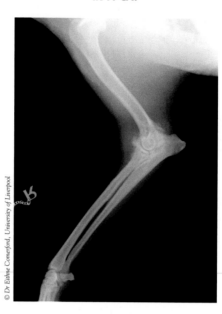

© Dr Eithne Comerford, University of Liverpool

Elbow and coxofemoral joints are commonly affected by osteoarthrosis in obese cats.

► Orthopedic diseases

Similar to dogs, obesity may be a risk factor for orthopedic disease in cats, with one study suggesting that obese cats were five times more likely to limp than cats of normal body condition *(Scarlett & Donoghue, 1998)*. However, not all reports have confirmed this association *(Lund et al, 2005)*. Orthopedic pain may be a reason why obese cats are less likely to groom and hence suffer from dermatoses (see later).

One of the major hurdles with confirming such an association is the fact that the prevalence of orthopedic disease is likely to be under-recognized in this species, compared with dogs. This is likely to be due to differences in behavior between cats and dogs; dogs are commonly taken for walks on a regular basis, such that it will rapidly become evident to the owner if their pet is stiff or lame. In contrast, cats tend to be self-sufficient such that, if orthopedic disease is present, cats rest themselves and it may not be readily evident to the owner that there is a problem. A study examined the prevalence of feline osteoarthritis (OA), by examining radiographs taken to examine other regions (e.g. thorax) *(Godfrey, 2005)*. In this study, there was radiographic evidence of OA in 22% of radiographs from adult cats. These results are particularly concerning in light of the fact that the population examined were not necessarily suspected to have orthopedic disease in the first place. In fact, a recent prospective study of OA in cats has identified the most prominent signs are reduction in the ability to jump and decreased height of jumping *(Clarke and Bennett, 2006)*. This study also demonstrated that the elbow and coxofemoral joints are most commonly affected **(Figure 5)**. In the experience of one of the authors, many cats limp at the time of presentation, and mobility improves markedly after weight loss. Thus, like dogs, weight reduction should be pursued in obese cats who limp.

► Gastrointestinal disease

An association between gastrointestinal disease and feline obesity has been previously reported; *Scarlett and Donoghue* (1998) reported that obese cats were more likely to suffer from diarrhea than those in normal body condition. *Lund et al* (2005) reported gastrointestinal diseases included anal sac disease, inflammatory bowel disease, colitis, megacolon and constipation in overweight or obese cats. However, even if the link between constipation and body weight has been studied in human medicine *(De Carvalho et al, 2006)*, the reasons for such a potential association are not clear and would require further study in cats. Very high fiber diets are suspected to increase the risk of constipation in cats.

► Hepatic lipidosis

The association between feline obesity and hepatic lipidosis is well-known. More information on hepatic lipidosis is presented in chapter 4. Concerns over inducing hepatic lipidosis are often cited

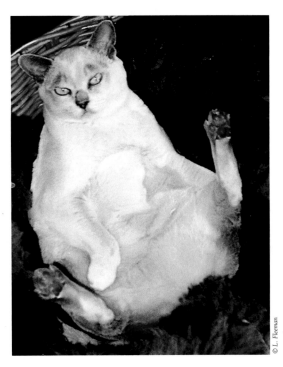

as a reason why veterinarians are reluctant to instigate weight management in obese cats. However, it is not clear how real this concern actually is. In this respect, even marked dietary energy restriction (e.g. 25% [*Biourge et al, 1994*] or 45% [*Watson et al, 1995*] of maintenance energy requirements) did not lead to the development of hepatic lipidosis. Thus, it would appear that for hepatic lipidosis to develop, complete fasting for five to six weeks may be required (*Biourge et al, 1993*). Clinical hepatic lipidosis is probably associated with other inciting factors e.g. concurrent illness.

▶ Neoplasia

A link between obesity and cancer has been widely reported and, if this link is entirely causal, one in seven cancer deaths in both men and women in the USA, might be the direct result of being overweight or obese (*Calle & Thun, 2004*). Similarly, studies in cats have reported an association with neoplasia (*Lund et al, 2005*); reported tumors included adenocarcinoma, basal cell carcinoma, fibrosarcoma, lipoma, lymphoma, mammary tumor, mast cell tumor and squamous cell carcinoma.

Whilst a global association with neoplasia may be present, the risk of developing specific neoplasia would require additional prospective studies. An association between mammary carcinoma and obesity has been reported in some (*Sonnenschein et al, 1991*), but not all (*Perez Alenza et al, 2000a, 2000b*), canine reports. Overweight dogs have also been reported to have an increased risk of developing transitional cell carcinoma of the bladder (*Glickman et al, 1989*), but such a risk has not been reported for cats.

The association between FLUTD and obesity may be a consequence of orthopedic problems: the painful cat may be reluctant to move and position itself for urination. The reduced frequency of urination can be a cause of lower urinary tract disease.

▶ Urinary tract diseases

The *Lund et al.* study (2005) identified that cats which were overweight were more likely to suffer from urinary tract diseases. Diseases reported included acute cystitis, urolithiasis, idiopathic feline lower urinary tract disease, urinary obstruction, and urinary tract infection. As with neoplasia, additional prospective studies are required to determine the exact risk for urinary tract. Of most note is the association with feline lower urinary tract diseases e.g. idiopathic FLUTD and urolithiasis. It is important to remember that obese cats are also most likely to live indoors, which is known as a risk factor for FLUTD.

An association between obesity and diseases of the feline kidney is less clear and, currently, there have been no studies to demonstrate such a link in client-owned cats. However, circumstantial evidence for such a link exists given that there is evidence from dogs that the onset of obesity is associated with histologic changes in the kidney; reported changes include an increase in Bowman's space (as a result of expansion of Bowman's capsule), increased mesangial matrix, thickening of glomerular and tubular basement membranes, and increased number of dividing cells per glomerulus (*Henegar et al, 2001*). Functional changes were noted in the same study, including increases in plasma renin concentrations, insulin concentrations, mean arterial pressure, and plasma renal flow. As a consequence, the authors speculated that these changes, if prolonged, could predispose to more severe glomerular and renal injury.

▶ Oral cavity disease

Obesity was shown to be a risk factor for oral cavity disease in a large scale study of cats in North America (*Lund et al, 2005*), with an odds ratio of 1.4. However, the reasons for such an association are not clear and, to the authors' knowledge, have not been reported in other species. Further work would be required to determine why obesity, per se, is a predisposing factor.

▶ Cardiorespiratory issues

In many species, increased body weight can result in effects on cardiac rhythm, increased left ventricular volume, blood pressure and plasma volume. The effect of obesity on hypertension is controversial since studies have suggested that the effect is only minor (*Bodey et al, 1996; Montoya et al, 2006*). Whilst it could be hypothesised that similar effects may be seen in cats, there are no published scientific studies reporting such a link.

▶ Risks during anesthesia and clinical procedures

Overall, obesity makes clinical evaluation more difficult. Techniques that are more problematic in obese patients include physical examination, thoracic auscultation, palpation and aspiration of peripheral lymph nodes, abdominal palpation, blood sampling, cystocentesis, and diagnostic imaging (especially ultrasonography). Anesthetic risk is reportedly increased in obese dogs, most likely given recognized problems with estimation of anesthetic dose, catheter placement, and prolonged operating time (*Clutton, 1988; Van Goethem et al, 2003*). Although no published data exist, it is likely that similar problems exist in cats. Finally, decreased heat tolerance and stamina have also been reported in obese animals (*Burkholder & Toll, 2000*).

4 - Pathophysiology of obesity

▶ Energy balance: intake versus expenditure

The control of body weight requires the accurate matching of caloric intake to caloric expenditure over time. Despite dramatic fluctuations in caloric intake, normal animals are able to maintain a very stable body weight. Long-term regulation of energy balance is dependent on the coordination and interpretation of peripheral signals indicating the level of energy stores. The best known signals are leptin and insulin. Short-term regulation depends on meal-related signals such as cholecystokinin (CCK) or gastrin related peptide (GRP) (*Strader & Woods, 2005*). Therefore, the central nervous system receives uninterrupted information about body energy stores through metabolic, neural and endocrine factors. Some are from central origin; some originate from the gastrointestinal tract or adipose cells. However, the elementary distinction between central and peripheral mechanisms tends to give way to a more integrated concept. In fact, each peripheral factor acts independently from central control and central factors modulate the secretion of peripheral factors by adjusting the response to ingested nutrients and modifying appetite behavior.

▶ Weight gain and appetite control

A wide range of central neuroendocrine factors have been linked to the control of energy balance. At a mechanistic level, identification of those factors that control appetite remains a challenge and is an important physiological basis to develop new pharmacological treatment strategies. Among new strategies developed against obesity, appetite manipulation is one of the most attractive. The aim is to block endogenous signals that stimulate appetite.

Hunger has cognitive and environmental components, such that the feeling of hunger could develop despite physiological satiety. In this circumstance, there is disruption of the relationship between appetite and food intake and abnormal appetite control is common in obese subjects. Among factors leading a cat to eat in the absence of hunger, there is boredom, availability of palatable food, or emotional stress (*Mattes et al, 2005*).

Many pharmacologic approaches have been considered to control hunger and to modify the secretion of peptides implicated in its regulation (**Table 3**).

One of the most recently identified signals of food intake is the gut peptide ghrelin (*Cummings et al, 2006*). Ghrelin is the unique enteric peptide known to increase food intake. There is a net rise of plasma ghrelin concentration after a period of fasting and it declines in the post-prandial period. In addition, it appears that ghrelin is not only a short-term signal of hunger since, in obesity, its concentration was increased by 24% in a group of subjects who had lost weight (*Cummings et al, 2002*). Thus, the increased concentration of ghrelin, an orexigenic signal, counteracts the effect

Appetite is composed of three phases: **hunger, satiation and satiety**.

Hunger is defined as a biological drive impelling the ingestion of food.

"Satiation" and satiety are defined by some investigators as intra- and inter-meal satiety, respectively:

- **satiation** refers to processes that promote meal termination. A sensation of fullness develops, thus limiting meal size;

- **satiety** refers to postprandial events that affect the interval to the next meal, so regulating meal frequency, which is also influenced by learned habits (*Cummings & Overduin, 2007*). Satiety is considered a motivation not to eat between episodes of eating. The state of satiety delays the onset of a meal and may reduce the amount of food consumed in a forthcoming meal.

of the regimen and tends to promote the regain of lost weight after a period of energy restriction. Future research should focus on dietary interventions that could reduce ghrelin concentration and food intake.

CCK controls satiety. It is released in response to the ingestion of fat and protein in the diet, although its appetite suppression effect is strongly increased by stomach distension (*Kissileff et al, 2003*). Central administration of CCK reduces meal size in animals including humans. However, despite promising results showing that CCK acts to limit energy intake, it appears that long-term chronic administration has no effect on body weight loss. Therefore, the best method to control CCK release seems to be modifying the composition of the diet via protein levels. In cats, it has been demonstrated that dietary protein and amino acids raise plasma CCK concentration (*Backus et al, 1997*). Among amino acids, tryptophan, phenylalanine, leucine and isoleucine were found to be the most effective.

Administration of amylin, bombesin and related-peptides (GRP, neuromedin B, glucagon-like peptide [GLP]-1, glucagon and related peptides (glicentin, GLP-2, oxyntomodulin), peptide tyrosine-tyrosine (PYY) and related peptides (pancreatic polypeptide, neuropeptide Y), gastric leptin and apolipoprotein A-IV reduces food intake. Leptin is an orexigenic factor that leads to glucose intolerance, insulin resistance and hyperinsulinemia; further, chronic hyperleptinemia induces obesity (*Kopelman, 2000*). With the exception of the pancreatic hormones and leptin, all such peptides are synthesized in the brain. This underlines the complexity of the system and shows how difficult it is to understand all the mechanisms implicated in food intake. Therefore, the use of pharmacologic therapies should be extremely cautious and may have strong side effects due to the high complexity of the regulation on a long-term basis.

▶ Neutering and obesity

How neutering leads to weight gain has been the subject of some debate. The main factor seems to be an alteration in feeding behavior leading to increased food intake (*Flynn et al, 1996; Fettman et al, 1997; Harper et al, 2001; Hoenig & Ferguson, 2002; Kanchuk et al, 2003*; see also **Figure 6**), and decreased activity (*Flynn et al, 1996; Harper et al, 2001*).

The metabolic consequences observed after neutering are likely to be secondary to the specific hormonal changes that occur after this procedure. Studies in other species have shown that estrogens can suppress appetite (*Czaja & Goy, 1975*). Thus, removal of the metabolic effects of estrogens and androgens by gonadectomy may lead to increased food consumption. However, the exact mechanism by which this occurs is not known and, in this respect, a recent study has refuted the hypothesis that gonadal hormones may interact with CCK, the gastrointestinal hormone that can

TABLE 3 - GASTROINTESTINAL HORMONES IMPLICATED IN APPETITE REGULATION
(from Strader and Woods, 2005)

Hormone	Effect on food intake
Cholecystokinin	Decreased
Amylin	Decreased
Glucagon like peptide-1 (GLP-1)	Decreased
Peptide tyrosine-tyrosine (3-36) (PYY)	Decreased
Apolipoprotein A_4	Decreased
Enterostatin	Decreased
Bombesin/gastrin releasing peptide (GRP)	Decreased
Glucagon	Decreased
Gastric leptin	Decreased
Ghrelin	Increased

FIGURE 6 - EFFECT OF NEUTERING ON FOOD INTAKE
From Calvert, 2003

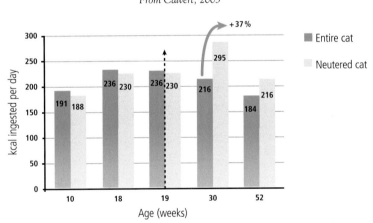

After neutering, cats are less capable of regulating their food intake. This leads to a gain in weight.

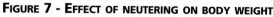

FIGURE 7 - EFFECT OF NEUTERING ON BODY WEIGHT
(from Calvert, 2003)

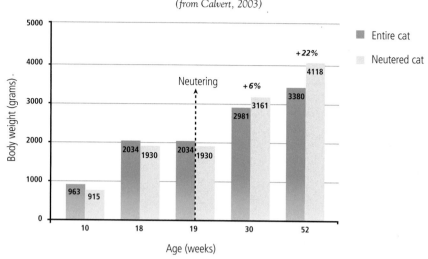

influence appetite *(Backus et al, 2005; Asarian & Geary, 2006)*. Ghrelin is probably implicated in this mechanism.

In studies conducted by one of the authors, plasma concentrations of various hormones were monitored in seven male and six female cats, before and after neutering *(Martin et al, 2004; 2006a)*. All cats were neutered after they had reached sexual maturity, at 11 months of age. By modifying endocrine homeostasis, neutering induces a new state of equilibrium in which the hormones involved in obesity and the dysregulation of glucose metabolism predominate. The earliest hormonal change was a rapid increase in the plasma concentration of IGF-1. This increase was noticeable as soon as the first week after neutering and tended to stabilize over time. Although studies about the regulation of the somatotropic axis in obesity report contradictory results on the secretion of IGF-1, receptors for this molecule have nevertheless been identified in pre-adipocyte and adipocyte cells lines *(Louveau & Gondret, 2004)*. Thus, the increase in IGF-1 secretion following neutering may have a primary role in the onset of obesity in the cat, since it promotes the multiplication and even the growth of adipocytes.

Increase in prolactin concentration varied between the males and females (p <0.0001) *(Martin & Siliart, 2005)*.
- Female cats (with the exception of one cat) demonstrated hyperprolactinemia prior to neutering, that was probably linked to their sexual activity at the time of neutering (heat period). Hyperprolactinemia was maintained over time and by 24 weeks post-neutering, the mean concentration was about 60 ng/mL.
- In male cats, results were markedly different. Prior to castration, the mean plasma concentration was below 20 ng/mL; after 12 weeks it reached about 30 ng/mL.

Two years after castration, the mean prolactin concentration was about 70 ng/mL for both gender. We conclude that neutering induces a persistent hyperprolactinemia, regardless of gender and initial concentrations.

Prolactin has a role in the production and maintenance of adipose tissue *(Flint et al, 2003)*. Additionally, it is possible that an elevated prolactin concentration could also have a deleterious effect on glucose metabolism in the cat in the short or long term.

When energy expenditure is expressed on a lean mass basis, no difference in metabolic rate was noted between entire individuals and individuals that are neutered *(Fettman et al, 1997; Martin et al, 2001; Kanchuk et al, 2003; Nguyen et al, 2004)*. However, neutered cats are more obese than intact ones **(Figure 7)** and they are reported to have resting metabolic rates 20-33% below those of intact cats *(Flynn et al, 1996; Root et al, 1996; Harper et al, 2001; Hoenig & Ferguson, 2002)*. Coupled with reduced physical activity, this lower metabolic rate highlights the necessity to decrease the caloric intake of neutered cats to limit the increase in body weight.

5 - Clinical evaluation of the obese patient

▶ Quantifying obesity in cats

Obesity is defined as an excess accumulation of body fat and all measures of adiposity involve defining body composition. The main conceptual division of importance is between:

TABLE 4 - COMPOSITION OF FAT MASS AND FAT FREE MASS

Body weight	Fat free mass - Heterogenous - Water content 72-74% - Density of 1.1 g/mL	Minerals (Potassium 50-70 mmol/kg)	
		Intracellular water Extracellular water	Water
		Glycogen and proteins from muscles	
	Fat mass - Homogenous - Anhydrous - Potassium free - Density of 0.9 g/mL	Energy	

- fat mass (FM): the adipose tissue
- fat-free mass (FFM) (*Pace & Rathbun, 1945*). The major constituents of the FFM are presumed to be present in fixed ratios and include the intracellular (ICW) and extracellular water (ECW), minerals, and protein. The FFM contains the body cell mass (BCM) which is the metabolically active part of the body responsible for determining most of the resting energy expenditure. BCM encompasses those lean tissues most likely to be affected by nutrition or disease over relatively short periods. Further, since FFM is an index of protein nutrition, changes in FFM likely represent alterations in protein balance.

TABLE 5 - TECHNIQUES AVAILABLE TO MEASURE BODY COMPOSITION

Clinically relevant techniques	Research relevant techniques
Body weight Body condition score Morphometric measurements Feline Body Mass Index Dilutional techniques Bioelectrical impedance analysis Dual energy x-ray absorptiometry	Densitometry Computed tomography Magnetic resonance imaging Total body electrical conductivity Total body potassium Neutron activation analysis

Thus, assessment of FM and FFM provides valuable information about the physical and metabolic status of the individual; the FM represents an energy storage depot, whilst FFM represents the actual health of the animal **(Table 4)**.

Various techniques are available to measure body composition **(Table 5)**, and these differ in applicability to research, referral veterinary practice and first-opinion practice. Broadly speaking, a number of techniques are available to assess the degree of adiposity, including:
- clinical assessments (e.g. morphometric measurements, body condition scoring, sequential body weight measurement, sequential photography)
- experimental procedures (e.g. chemical analysis, dilution techniques (e.g. deuterium determination of total body water), total body potassium, densitometry, total body electrical conductivity, and neutron activation analysis).
- techniques that have potential for application in clinical work (e.g. dual energy x-ray absorptiometry, bioelectrical impedance analysis, computed tomography, magnetic resonance imaging).

Only those of greatest relevance to clinical practice will be discussed in detail.

▶ Established clinical measures of body composition

> Body weight measurement

It is the simplest technique available and should be included in the examination of every patient, especially in very young cats, at the end of the growth period. However, work by one of the authors has suggested that this remains an infrequent part of the routine examination of companion animals (*unpublished observations*). It provides a rough measure of total body energy stores and changes in weight parallel energy and protein balance. In the healthy animal, body weight varies little from day to day.

The body weight recorded at the end of the first year can usually be a good reference of the optimum body weight of the cat during the rest of its life.

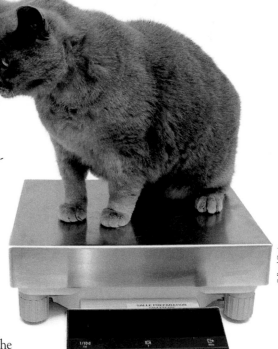

© Royal Canin

FIGURE 8 - INDICATIVE WEIGHT FOR SEVERAL FELINE BREEDS

Source: Royal Canin Encyclopedia of the Cat

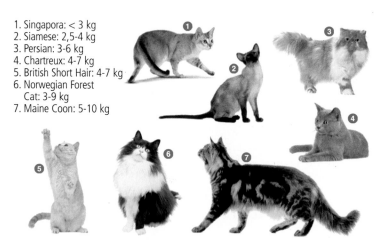

1. Singapora: < 3 kg
2. Siamese: 2,5-4 kg
3. Persian: 3-6 kg
4. Chartreux: 4-7 kg
5. British Short Hair: 4-7 kg
6. Norwegian Forest Cat: 3-9 kg
7. Maine Coon: 5-10 kg

The ratio between the heaviest and the lightest cats of well-known breeds is 1 to 4, which represents a relative homogeneity compared with the canine species where the ratio is 1 to 100.

There can be wide variation between scales though, so it is important to use the same scale for an individual animal each time to avoid inter-scale variation. Body weight can be falsely altered by dehydration or fluid accumulation. Edema and ascites may mask losses in body fat or muscle mass. Likewise, massive tumor growth or organomegaly can mask loss in fat or lean tissues such as skeletal muscle. Further, breed influences can also lead to variability in body weight for cats in similar condition (**Figure 8**). Body weight correlates only moderately with body fat mass (*Burkholder, 2001*).

As a result, sporadic measurements at single time points are of only limited use (if not coupled with concurrent assessment of body condition -**see below**). Nevertheless, sequential body weight measurements (e.g. throughout life in an individual cat, instigated at the time of young adulthood) can provide a sensitive indicator of subtle changes in body composition and could provide a vital tool for the prevention of obesity.

> Body condition scoring

Body condition scoring is a subjective, semi-quantitative method of evaluating body composition that is quick and simple to perform. All systems assess visual and palpable characteristics to assess subcutaneous fat, abdominal fat and superficial musculature (e.g. ribcage, dorsal spinous processes and waist). The technique of body condition scoring does depend on operator interpretation and does not provide any precise quantitative information concerning alterations in fat free or lean body mass relative to fat mass.

Different scoring systems have been described but the most common scoring systems used are the 5-point system (where a BCS of 3 is considered ideal, see **Figure 9**) or the 9-point system (where a BCS of 5 is considered ideal) (*Laflamme, 1997; McGreevy et al, 2005*). Given that half points are often employed in the 5-point system (giving a total of 9 categories), these two systems are virtually equivalent. A 7-point algorithm-based approach (**Figure 10**) is specifically designed to be used by owners to assess their own pets. A study has demonstrated a good correlation between the system and body fat measurements made by Dual Energy X-Ray Absorptiometry (DEXA) with excellent agreement between experienced operators (*German et al, 2006*). Most importantly, good agreement was found between measurements by operators and owners, suggesting that the method may be reliable when used without prior training. However, such data are preliminary and further validation would be required before it is used by owners.

Limitations of the BCS include the subjectivity inherent in the scoring system and inter-observer variation. Finally, like body weight, BCS gives an overall assessment of body condition; it cannot differentiate between body compart-

FIGURE 9 - BODY CONDITION SCORING IN CATS

Grades	Criteria
❶ Emaciated	- Ribcage, spine, shoulder blades and pelvis easily visible (short hair) - Obvious loss of muscle mass - No palpable fat on rib cage
❷ Thin	- Ribcage, spine shoulder blades and pelvis visible - Obvious abdominal tuck (waist) - Minimal abdominal fat
❸ Ideal	- Ribcage, spine not visible but easily palpable - Obvious abdominal tuck (waist) - Little abdominal fat
❹ Overweight	- Ribcage, spine not easily palpable - Abdominal tuck (waist) absent - Obvious abdominal distension
❺ Obese	- Massive thoracic, spinal and abdominal fat deposits - Massive abdominal distension

The BCS in conjunction with body weight gives a clinician a more complete perspective on a patient's body condition and should be recorded at every visit.

FIGURE 10 - WALTHAM S.H.A.P.E.™ GUIDE FOR CATS

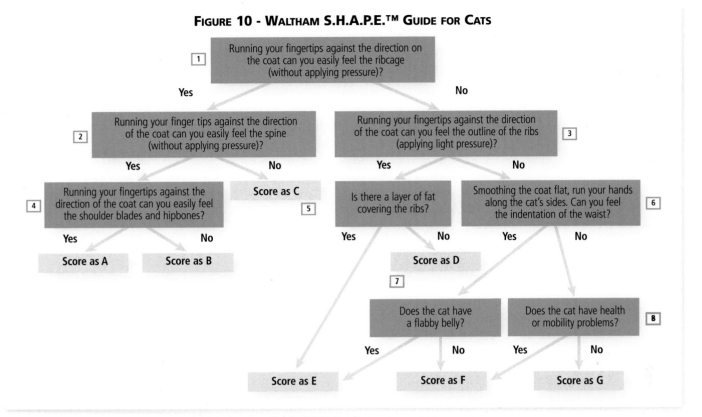

S.H.A.P.E.™ Score	DESCRIPTION
A - Extremely thin	Your cat has a very small amount or no total body fat. > **Recommendation:** seek veterinary advice promptly.
B - Thin	Your cat has only a small amount of total body fat. > **Recommendation:** seek veterinary advice to ensure your cat is offered the appropriate amount of food. Reassess using the S.H.A.P.E.™ chart every 2 weeks.
C - Lean	Your cat is at the low end of the ideal range with less than normal body fat. > **Recommandation:** increase food offered by a small amount. Monitor monthly using the S.H.A.P.E.™ chart and seek veterinary advice if no change.
D - Ideal	Your cat has an ideal amount of total body fat. > **Recommendation:** monitor monthly to ensure your cat remains in this category and have him/her checked by the veterinarian at your next visit.
E - Mildly overweight	Your cat is at the upper end of the ideal range with a small amount of excess body fat. > **Recommendation:** seek veterinary advice to ensure your cat is offered the appropriate amount of food and try to increase activity levels. Avoid excessive treats and monitor monthly using the S.H.A.P.E.™ chart.
F - Moderately overweight	Your cat has an excess of total body fat. > **Recommendation:** seek veterinary advice to implement safety an appropriate weight loss plan including increasing activity levels. Reassess using the S.H.A.P.E.™ chart every 2 weeks.
G - Severely overweight	Your cat has a large amount of excess total body fat that is affecting its health and well being. > **Recommendation:** seek veterinary advice promptly to introduce a weight loss plan to reduce your cat's weight, increase activity levels and improve health.

NB Some breeds and different life-stages may have different ideal S.H.A.P.E.™ scores.

S.H.A.P.E™ (Size, Health And Physical Evaluation) is a new 7-point flow-diagram for measuring body condition, designed to allow owners to assess the body condition of their pets. It correlates well with body fat: all subjects were scanned in dorsal recumbency with a fan-beam DEXA (Lunar Prodigy Advance; GE Lunar; Madison, USA). There is also a good agreement between owner scores and those of experienced operators (German et al, 2006).

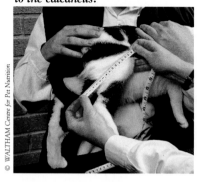

Figure 11A - Measurement of the length of the lower limb (LIM) from the middle of the patella to the calcaneus.

© WALTHAM Centre for Pet Nutrition

Figure 11B - Measurement of the rib cage circumference.

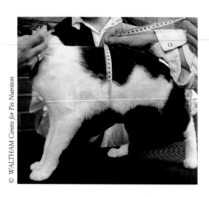

© WALTHAM Centre for Pet Nutrition

ments and does not provide any precise quantitative information concerning alteration in fat free or lean body mass relative to fat mass.

> Morphometric measurements

Morphometry (more appropriately "zoometry" for veterinary species) is defined as the measurement of "form" and, in relation to body composition analysis, refers to a variety of measured parameters that are used to estimate body composition. The three main approaches are:
- dimensional evaluations (where various measures of stature are combined with weight)
- measurement of skin fold thickness
- ultrasound technique.

Dimensional evaluations

Dimensional evaluations are usually performed by tape measure, and a number have been reported in cats. Measurements of "length" (e.g. head, thorax and limb) are correlated with lean body components *(Hawthorne & Butterwick, 2000)*, whilst circumferential measurements have been shown to correlate both with lean body mass (LBM) *(Hawthorne & Butterwick, 2000)*, and body fat *(Burkholder, 1994)*. Segmental limb measures and (likely) truncal length are thought to be better measures of stature and thus correlate best to LBM. By combining more than one measure (usually one that correlates with FM, and one correlating with LBM), equations can be generated to predict different body components.

The best example of such a measure is the feline body mass index (FBMI)™ *(Hawthorne & Butterwick, 2000)*. The FBMI™ is determined by measuring the rib cage circumference at the level of the 9th cranial rib and the leg index measurement (LIM), which is the distance from the patella to the calcaneus **(Figure 11)**.

The percent body fat can be calculated as:
- % fat = (1.54 x ribcage circumference) – (1.58 x leg index measurement) – 8.67 (rib cage circumference and LIM in cm)
- or, more simply: 1.5 (ribcage – LIM)/ 9
- or determined by consulting a reference chart **(Table 6)**.

The FBMI™ is a very simple, yet objective tool to determine the body fat content of the cat. In addition, it is particularly valuable for convincing clients that their cat is indeed overweight and in need of weight loss.

Measurement of skin fold thickness

This technique has been used extensively in people to determine the percent body fat using equations derived for various populations. Unfortunately, these measurements cannot be used in cats because feline skin is easily detached from underlying fat tissue which makes skin-fold measurement impractical and unreliable.

Ultrasound

Another method of measuring the subcutaneous fat layer is by ultrasound. This technique has been used in Beagles and equations have been derived to predict percent body fat from the subcutaneous fat thickness *(Wilkinson & McEwan, 1991)*. These regression equations do not work in other dog breeds but future research may allow investigators to develop new, more accurate equations for this simple technique.

TABLE 6 - FELINE BODY MASS INDEX CHART

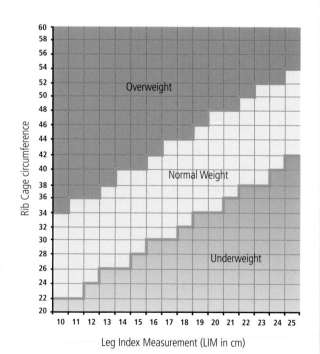

Rib Cage circumference

Overweight

Normal Weight

Underweight

Leg Index Measurement (LIM in cm)

> Bioelectrical impedance analysis (BIA)

Bioelectrical impedance analysis (BIA) is a safe, noninvasive, rapid, portable, and fairly reproducible method of assessing body composition in companion animals. This method has the potential of quantifying total body water (TBW), ECW, ICW, BCM, FFM and FM.

Electrical conductance is used to calculate the composition of the body by measuring the nature of the conductance of an applied electrical current in the patient. Body fluids and electrolytes are responsible for conductance whilst cell membranes produce capacitance. Since adipose tissue is less hydrated than lean body tissues, more adipose tissue results in a smaller conducting volume or path for current and larger impedance to current passage. The FFM contains virtually all the water in the body and thus if bioelectrical impedance is measured a value for FFM can be determined.

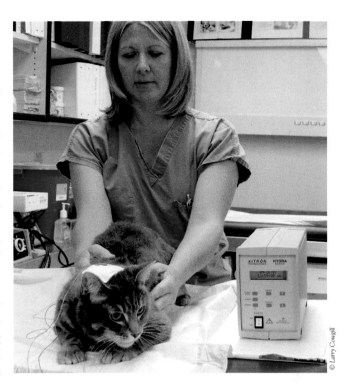

Two types of BIA systems are currently available; single frequency which applies a 50 kHz current, and multi-frequency which utilizes frequencies from 5 kHz to 1000 KHz. A BIA test is performed by placing four small electrodes on the body. The electrical current is introduced into the patient from the distal electrodes. As the current travels through the body it experiences a slight delay due to cells, and the current is then detected by proximal electrodes. The proportion of the current in the ICW and ECW is frequency dependent:

- low frequencies (e.g. 5kHz) pass primarily through the ECW because of high cell membrane capacitance
- in contrast, at higher frequencies the effects of cell membrane capacitance is diminished so the current flows through both the ICW and ECW environments (or TBW).

Bioelectrical impedance analysis (BIA) is a safe, noninvasive, rapid, portable, and reproducible method of assessing body composition in healthy cats.

BIA allows estimation of body composition in healthy dogs, cats, and humans *(Scheltinga et al, 1991; Stanton et al, 1992; Patel et al, 1994)*. However, BIA may be affected by hydration status, consumption of food and water, skin and air temperature, recent physical activity, conductance of the examination table, patient age, size, shape and posture in addition to electrode positioning. Reliable BIA requires standardization and control of these variables. BIA requires further evaluation and validation in disease states, especially those associated with major disturbances in water distribution and states such as sepsis which may alter cell membrane capacitance.

Calculation of ECW-ICW takes approximately 1 minute, hence BIA provides instantaneous on line information of body composition that has never before been available.

> Deuterium (D$_2$O) dilution technique

The water content of the FFM is among the best used techniques for determining body composition due to the relative stability of the FFM hydration between species. Briefly, TBW can be measured by several stable labelled isotopes dilution methods including D$_2$O and the following relationship has been validated:

$$\text{Fat mass} = \text{body mass} - \text{TBW}/0.73$$

The first study on cats was published in 1950 by *Spray and Widdowson.*

In practice, after a 24h fasting period, a sub-cutaneous injection of D$_2$O in an isotonic saline solution is administered (500 mg D$_2$O/kg). The mass of the syringe (and needle) before and after injection should be accurately weighed to determine the exact quantity of labelled-isotope that will dilute in body water. The first blood sample is taken before injection, the second about 3-4 hours after D$_2$O injection. Until recently, this technique was limited due to technological problems but today a new method of analysis has been developed which makes this technique less expensive and more widely available.

> Dual energy X-ray absorptiometry (DEXA)

This technique originally developed for precise measurement of bone mineral content (BMC). However, it is now also used to measure both body fat and non-bone lean tissue. DEXA uses photons of two different energy levels (70 and 140 kVp) to distinguish the type and amount of tissue scanned. The X-ray source is positioned underneath the table supporting the patient, with the detector housed in an arm above the patient.

During a scan the source and detector move together over the patient. The detector measures the amount of X-rays that pass through the subject. The X-rays of the two different energy levels are impeded differently by bone mineral, lipid and lean tissue. Algorithms are used to calculate both the type and quantity of tissue in each pixel scanned. DEXA calculates bone mineral density, bone mineral content, fat mass, and lean body mass.

DEXA's low coefficient of variation for measuring BMC (~1%) makes it a very precise technique but a few constraints have to be noted:
- equipment is still expensive
- short sedation is required
- standardization of the technique is very important *(Raffan et al, 2006)*.

DEXA is safe and quick; with the more modern fan-beam DEXA scanner, it takes under five minutes for a whole body scan in a cat **(Figure 12)**. Similar to other body composition techniques, DEXA relies on the assumption that lean body mass is uniformly hydrated at 0.73 mL water/g.

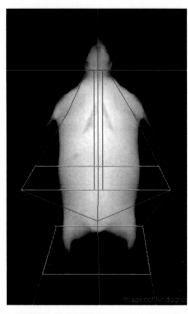

Figure 12 - DEXA examination in an obese cat.
DEXA prior to weight loss shows a body fat content of 54.4% (reference range 18 to 25%).

► Determination of basal metabolic rate (BMR)

Precise knowledge of energy expenditure is important in obese animals to determine the exact amount of energy needed to loose weight. Energy expenditure is the result of internal and external work and of heat yields. Energy originates from nutrients that are converted to various energy forms that can be used by the body. Most chemical reactions in the body need oxygen and produce water and carbon dioxide. So relationships have been established between respiratory and energy expenditure.

Among methods available, indirect calorimetry allows the determination of the basal metabolic rate by measuring only oxygen consumption and carbon dioxide production. In practice, the cat is placed in a specific cage for about 4-h and gas exchanges are measured. The formula used to calculate BMR was validated by *Weir* (1949). An abbreviated Weir formula has also been developed:

$$\text{BMR (kcal/day)} = [3.9 \text{ (kcal/L)} \times V \text{ (O}_2\text{ (L))} + 1.1 \text{ (kcal/L)} \times V \text{ (CO}_2\text{ (L))}]$$

6 - Prevention of feline obesity

The goal of any weight-loss program is to facilitate a progressive decrease of body fat stores without detrimental effects on health. However, success is variable and, since long-term follow-up of weight loss programs is often poor, relapse is frequent. Consequently, it is preferable to prevent obesity occurring in the first place, rather than attempting to cure it once it has developed. As mentioned above, obesity has a number of health and welfare implications, most notably by decreasing both quality and quantity of life.

► Weigh and perform a body condition score on every cat at every consultation

Both of these assessments should form part of a standard physical examination. They enable subtle body composition changes to be noted, and increases in body weight (suggesting over feeding) can therefore be picked up and rectified early on. However, these assessments also have wider health implications, because subtle weight loss might be recognized as the first component of another significant medical disease.

► Communicate the message of obesity prevention early on

Advice on healthy eating and exercise should be included in all kitten consultations and continued for all cats whenever they are seen at the practice.

► Be alert to weight gain in middle-aged cats

Strategies to prevent obesity from developing should be implemented most aggressively in cats between 6 and 10 years of age. Most important is to prevent the onset of obesity in young (adult) cats, since these animals are the ones that will benefit most from avoiding excess adiposity (in terms of effects on longevity and reduced disease risk).

► Be alert to weight gain after neutering

Like with age, neutering is a major predisposing factor for overweight and obesity (**Figures 13 & 14**). It is advisable to schedule 2-3 weight-checks in the first 6-12 months after neutering to identify those cats at risk of weight gain and correct it before it becomes a problem.

► Promote the benefits of a healthy lifestyle for all cats

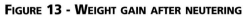

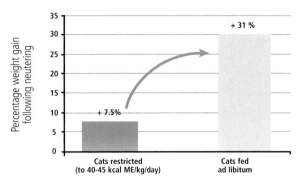

FIGURE 13 - WEIGHT GAIN AFTER NEUTERING
(from Harper, 2001)

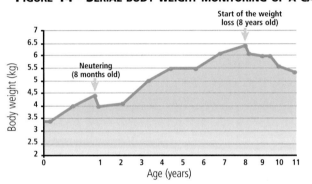

FIGURE 14 - SERIAL BODY WEIGHT MONITORING OF A CAT

The initial body weight was obtained at the time of neutering at 8 months of age. A weight loss program was not implemented until until the cat was 8 years old and 28% overweight.

Encourage responsible feeding behaviors, which utilize many of the strategies discussed for the treatment of obesity (see lifestyle alterations). This includes weighing and recording food intake, avoiding the feeding of extras, and promoting regular physical activity through exercise and play sessions. Ideally, all practice staff should be encouraged to promote these concepts, and waiting room literature and other forms of education and support should be available to all owners.

► Target new pet owners

It goes without saying that people who have only recently taken on a new pet, will have limited experience with pet ownership. Hence, it is important to make sure all new owners have the education and support necessary to prevent obesity problems from developing.

7 - Five components to a successful weight management strategy for feline obesity

It is relatively easy to diagnose obesity and to prescribe a specific diet. The challenge lies in convincing the owner to introduce the necessary changes in the feeding and lifestyle of the animal in order to induce and maintain significant weight loss.
1. Initial assessment
2. Establishing pet owner understanding and commitment
3. Setting and managing owner expectations
4. Intervention
5. Maintenance.

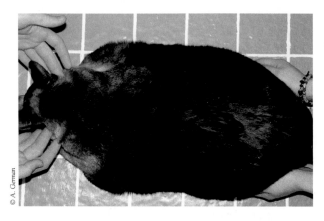

© A. German

When a clinician is presented with an obese cat for the first time, it is essential to perform a thorough assessment of the patient.

► Initial assessment

The aims of the first examination are:
- to quantify the level of obesity. Whilst the language should be positive and constructive, the risk of allowing a cat to continue to be overweight should be firmly stressed. Owners are more likely to want to intervene if the perceived health benefits for their pet are clear;
- to identify predisposing factors for obesity in this cat
- to determine the current health status. This will enable weight loss to be instigated in the safest and most effective manner for the cat:
  - obesity-associated diseases
  - other, potentially unrelated diseases which may affect the way in which the case is investigated and treated.

The recommended components of the initial assessment follow several stages.

History. This should include details of environment, lifestyle, diet and exercise regimes, as well as a complete medical history including previous or current therapy.

Physical examination. The goal is to identify signs of associated diseases (either causing or contributing to weight gain), and any concurrent diseases.

Weight measurement. The use of a single set of electronic weigh scales is recommended which are, ideally, regulated validated for precision and accuracy.

Body condition score. Condition scoring the patient is not only a key diagnostic tool for establishing the degree of obesity but is also an invaluable tool for discussion with owners. Whilst the exact system used is not critical, clinicians should use the same one for all of their patients, since familiarity is likely to lead to more accurate scoring. The 5 or 9-point BCS (discussed earlier) have been validated against body fat measurements made by DEXA, and thus are known to correlate with the degree of adiposity if performed by a trained operator.

General laboratory investigations. Laboratory investigations may be necessary to verify the health status of the cat. These should include routine hematological examination, clinical chemistry, and urinalysis. Additional investigations may be required in some circumstances.

Additional investigations. Additional investigations will depend on the presence or suspicion of any associated disease. Examples include:
- measurement of blood pressure if facilities are available
- fructosamine measurement for diabetes mellitus
- survey radiography for orthopedic and respiratory disease
- hepatic ultrasonography, fine needle aspiration cytology and/or liver biopsy for suspected hepatic lipidosis
- urine culture, ultrasonography, radiographic contrast studies for lower urinary tract diseases.

Exactly what tests are recommended in each circumstance is beyond the scope of these guidelines and are at the discretion of the individual veterinarian. If other conditions are identified, specific therapy should be implemented at an appropriate time (before, during or after the weight management regime). Obviously, weight loss may be a major factor in the treatment of any obesity-associated disease.

► Establishing owner understanding and commitment

Successful treatment of obesity depends above all on the motivation of the owner and their compliance with the weight loss program. Success is most likely when the client understands and accepts the reasons why weight loss is necessary. The clinician must be aware of the reason that the cat was presented for evaluation, as the level of client motivation will vary. There are three main scenarios: presentation for obesity itself, for an obesity-associated disease or for an unrelated reason.

> Presentation for obesity

The owner seeks advice about the weight problem. Client management will be easiest because these owners are already motivated and have accepted the need for intervention. Therefore, they should be most receptive to appropriate veterinary advice. This is the least common presentation.

> Presentation for an obesity-associated disease

The cat presents with a condition that is due to obesity. The clinician can communicate to the client that the obesity is a medical, rather than cosmetic, problem. It is important to explain that the excess weight caused or contributed to the disease, and how it is an essential part of maximizing response. If such arguments are made in a convincing manner, client motivation should not be a problem.

> Presentation for an unrelated reason

The obesity is an incidental observation during a consultation for an unrelated reason. This typically occurs during an annual vaccination or routine health check.

Initiating discussion in these cases is difficult because the reaction of the owner is not predictable. Some may refuse to believe that a problem exists, some may believe that the veterinarian's recommendation is financially-motivated, whilst others believe that they are to be blamed for the problem. An additional problem arises with owners who have obesity or health problems of their own. The approach is to focus on the health of the cat, including any existing morbidity and the potential for future health problems as a result of continuing obesity. The veterinarian should use sensitive language, such that the owner can accept their pet is overweight without being made to feel guilty.

If they believe that their cat is currently healthy and an obvious co-morbidity does not exist, the owner may not be convinced by an argument structured around the potential future health problems that may arise. Instead, it may help to focus on detrimental effects on current quality of life e.g. fitness, physical activity and grooming. Before and after testimonials from previous clients, highlighting the health benefits of weight loss, may help in convincing these owners.

Some owners may still not be convinced of the need for intervention at the initial consultation, and may require several visits before the argument is accepted. Since owner motivation and compliance are essential pre-requisites for successful weight management, there may be little point in embarking upon a weight reduction program without them. However, providing information leaflets for owners to read may help to improve their understanding of the need to intervene.

► Setting and managing owner expectations

Once the veterinarian is happy that the owner is fully committed, treatment of obesity can be started. There are two phases of the program:
- intervention (when the weight loss occurs): this first phase can take many months
- maintenance (when body weight is stabilized and then maintained): the second phase is lifelong. Given that successful weight loss depends mainly on owner commitment, it is vital to ensure that the owner has realistic expectations from the outset.
The timescale of treatment, the level and rate of weight loss, cost of therapy, potential side-effects of treatment, behavioral changes in the pet, time commitment for lifestyle changes (e.g. exercise),

LIPOSUCTION

This common cosmetic surgery technique in humans aims at reducing adipose tissue mass. However, only subcutaneous fat is removed, which carries little metabolic risk, and does not modify dietary behavior. A single canine case study reports the use of liposuction for the treatment of a large subcutaneous lipoma *(Bottcher et al, 2007)* but it is unlikely that this technique will be an ethically justifiable option in companion animals.

BARIATRIC SURGERY

This term is used to describe surgery for the management of obesity through the control of food intake. One of the most successful treatment is the Roux-en-Y gastric bypass *(Strader and Woods, 2005)*, which both reduces the stomach volume and allows a rapid delivery of the stomach contents to the small intestine. Compulsory restriction of meal size, decreased digestibility and changes in endocrine signals of the gut contribute to the weight loss.

behavior of other family members and any other potential pitfalls should be discussed. The aim should be to make sure that the owner is fully informed of all eventualities and has no unexpected surprises. The problems which are most likely to be encountered include:
- difficulty in adapting to the new diet (palatability)
- difficulty in adapting to a reduced amount of food
- behavioral troubles due to permanent hunger with inopportune vocalizing, aggressiveness, stealing food
- very slow loss of weight.

Every step of the way, the veterinarian should remind the owner of the goals of therapy, success so far, future expectations and how long-term success can be achieved. This should help to ensure that the client remains committed to each stage of therapy.

► Intervention

When it comes to management of obesity in any species, there are four potential options:
- surgery
- pharmaceutical intervention
- lifestyle alterations
- dietary management

The usual methods generally lead to a reduction of adipose tissue mass either by reducing energy intake (e.g. dietary management, pharmaceuticals, bariatric surgery) or by increasing energy expenditure (e.g. increasing physical activity through lifestyle changes). In reality, whilst the latter may assist in weight loss, it is rarely successful if used as the sole component. Thus, some form of dietary caloric restriction is usually necessary, although a combination of strategies is likely to be most successful. Finally, for any intervention to be successful, close monitoring is vital. The approach chosen for any one case may vary and, as a result, the following guidelines are deliberately general.

> Surgical procedures

In addition to the ethical concerns, surgical procedures are unlikely to be a viable treatment option for obesity in pets because these procedures are complex, expensive and morbidity is likely to be high (e.g. 23% to 55% of patients have a short- or long-term complication) *(Powers & Pappas,*

PHARMACEUTICAL AGENTS AVAILABLE FOR THE TREATMENT OF OBESITY

Sibutramine

Sibutramine is the only centrally-acting anti-obesity drug approved for use in humans in most countries *(Halford, 2006)*. It works as an inhibitor of the reuptake of serotonin, noradrenaline and dopamine. Sibutramine acts on both satiety and thermogenesis to induce weight loss. The efficacy of sibutramine has been demonstrated in rodents and humans. Numerous side effects may be seen on cardio-vascular function with studies showing increases in both heart rate and blood pressure.

Orlistat, or tetrahydrolipstatin

Orlistat is the saturated derivative of lipstatin (potent inhibitor of pancreatic lipases isolated from *Streptomyces toxytricini*). Its primary function is to prevent intestinal absorption of fat. It is intended for use in conjunction with a supervised low fat calorie diet. Orlistat is minimally absorbed into the systemic circulation and its effect is local. The efficacy of Orlistat has been demonstrated in type 2 human dia-

betes patients. Orlistat induces a significant decrease in blood cholesterol and triglyceride concentrations, and it minimizes cardiovascular risk factors *(Leung et al, 2003)*. Simultaneous administration of soluble dietary fiber (psyllium) significantly reduces the gastrointestinal side effects (steatorrhea and flatulence). Long-term orlistat use may reduce absorption of vitamins A, D, E and beta-carotene and supplementation is necessary.

Microsomal triglyceride transfer protein inhibitors (MTPI)

These drugs are only currently licensed for use in dogs, and block the assembly in the enterocytes and the release of lipoprotein particles into the bloodstream. Dirlotapide can be used as sole therapy for obesity for a maximum period of 12 months. It prevents lipid absorption and it reduces the appetite, the latter effect being the major contributor to weight loss *(Li et al, 2007)*. The most common side effect is vomiting, which can occur in up to 20% of dogs using the drug.

Mitratapide

Mitratapide has recently been approved to aid in weight loss in dogs *(Re, 2006)*. It is designed to be used short-term in conjunction with dietary management and behavioral modification. The drug is given for two 3-week periods punctuated by a 14-day period off the medication. Predominant side effects reported are vomiting and diarrhea. Elevations in liver enzymes can also be seen, although there is no clear evidence of long-term hepatic dysfunction.

1989). Gastric outlet obstruction, vomiting, dumping, gastric leaks and wound infections are common complications. Dietary deficiencies may also result from malabsorption.

> Pharmacologic treatment

For a number of years, pharmaceutical agents have been available for the treatment of obesity in humans. The drugs which are licensed in most countries are sibutramine and orlistat, although other drugs (e.g. rimonabant) are available in some countries. All available agents are successful in producing weight loss in the majority of patients, although the effect is modest at best (~5-10% weight loss). They can reduce obesity-associated diseases but side effects are common and can be problematic. In addition, a predictable rebound effect often occurs when the drug is discontinued.

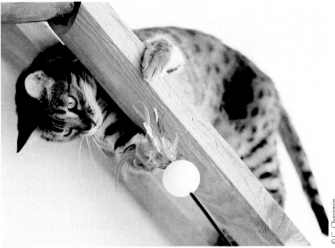

With the ever-increasing global obesity epidemic, pharmaceutical management is a growth area, with many companies investing in the development of newer and more effective pharmaceuticals. Pharmaceutical agents have been recently licensed for treatment of canine obesity: the available agents are from a novel group of drugs, the microsomal triglyceride transfer protein inhibitors (MTPI). At the current time, these pharmaceutical agents are not suitable for use in cats. It is not known whether or not similar drugs will be developed for cats in the future.

Methods to increase physical activity in cats include:
- *increasing play activity*
- *encouraging the cat to exercise itself*
- *increasing movement through the use of food treats.*

> Lifestyle alterations

These changes must be implemented during the intervention phase of the weight loss program but need to be maintained lifelong in order that there is permanent success e.g. a healthy lifestyle has been adopted.

The aim should be to increase the level of activity in gradual steps and to make it a regular feature of the pet's life. In practice, exercise has many advantages:
- it increases energy expenditure during training and in the post-exercise period
- it stimulates fat oxidation
- it protects lean body mass
- it has the potential to reverse the decrease in BMR induced by a low calorie diet.

If possible, cats should be encouraged to spend time outdoors. Activity in cats can also be encouraged by using cat toys. For some cats, encouraging walking activity prior to meal times by moving the feeding bowl can also help. Many obese outdoor cats may voluntarily increase their activity levels once their fitness improves during weight loss. The exact exercise program recommended must be tailored to the individual and take into account medical concerns, existing capabilities, breed and age of the patient, as well as the age, and owner circumstances.

Dangling toys are usually appreciated by cats.

The benefits of exercise go beyond the fact that it burns calories: it builds muscle mass and thus increases the resting metabolic rate, improves mobility, is beneficial for the cardiovascular system in general, enhances the pet/owner bond, provides mental stimulation and generally improves welfare and quality of life. It also enhances compliance and improves the outcome.

In domestic cats, hunting and eating behaviors are independently motivated. Thus, cats have a physiological need to hunt (or perform some alternative to this such as play activity) even when their daily energy requirements are already fulfilled. Although play behavior

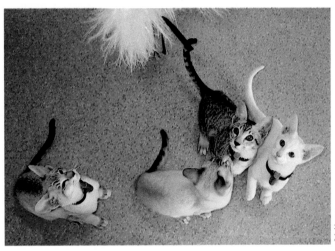

The best-designed stations are those that provide many and varied levels and climbing options (thus making full use of 3-dimensional space), include dangling toys and scratch posts. Scratching is an additional means by which cats can expend energy; posts which allow the cat to stretch at full stretch are best.

Although formulations may vary, most weight loss diets for cats have some or all of the following characteristics:
- **Reduced energy density,** usually through a reduction in fat content and an increased fiber content
- **Increased protein content relative to energy content.** This ensures that protein malnutrition does not occur when energy intake is restricted. This strategy does not increase the rate of weight loss, but minimizes the amount of lean tissue lost during weight management.
- **Increased micronutrient** (vitamins and minerals) contents relative to energy content. This ensures that malnutrition does not occur when energy intake is restricted.
- **L-carnitine supplementation.** This compound is an essential co-factor of lipid oxidation and assists in the transport of long-chain fatty acids into mitochondria. Thus, it facilitates fatty acid oxidation maximizing the amount of fat (and thus minimizing the amount of lean tissue) lost on a weight management program.
- **Fiber supplementation.** Higher dietary fiber content increases the bulk of the diet and may improve satiety.

may be more pronounced in juvenile cats, most owners do not realize that it is necessary throughout life.

When implementing regular play activity, it is best to start with short (~2-3 minutes) sessions each day. This will not overburden the owners, and allow the cat to become accustomed to the activity. Once a regular level of activity is established, and as weight loss progresses, it is possible to increase the duration and intensity of the exercise/play sessions.

A number of toys designed specifically for cats are now available; some features of good cat toys include:
- ability to produce rapid and unpredictable movement
- emission of a high-pitched sound
- small "prey" size
- ability to supply a food reward.

Some home-made objects can work equally well (e.g. rolled up paper, tin foil etc). Feline play stations are another means by which cats can both exercise and fulfill their natural behaviors. These incorporate the opportunity to climb, balance, scratch and hide.

Food can also be a useful motivator for physical activity. Hollow toys can be purchased or constructed, which contain small amounts of kibbles **(Figure 15)**. The cat must then play with the toy (thereby expending energy) to receive the reward. This solution diverts the cat, decreases its boredom when living exclusively indoors, and helps to reduce overall food consumption.

Modifying feeding behavior

Long-term modification of the owners approach to feeding the cat is the second component to a successful program. The following points should be considered.
- Always weigh out food on weigh scales; measuring cups are unreliable.
- Record the amount fed and eaten throughout the weight program.
- Offer the daily food ration in divided meals (2-4 per day) rather than as a single meal.
- Consider methods of slowing food intake at meal times. This can include the use of feeding toys, diets with a larger kibble size (that require more chewing before swallowing), relocating the feed bowl before or during meal times, and activity related rewards e.g. food ration only given after an activity has been performed.
- Avoid feeding additional food in the form of treats or table scraps. Occasional (ideally nutritionally-balanced) treats are acceptable as long as they are factored into the feeding strategy e.g. count towards total daily intake.
- Make certain that all members of the family, friends and neighbors are aware of and are committed to the program.
- If scavenging and begging behavior is seen, do not offer a food reward but encourage another form of positive owner-pet interaction e.g. play session. This will distract the cat from the behavior at the same time as increasing energy expenditure.

> Overview of dietary management

In theory, dietary management can be achieved in three ways:
- using a standard maintenance diet, but reducing the amount of food offered daily
- using a diet which has a lower energy density
- using a food which has low palatability.

It is inadvisable to use a standard maintenance ration and simply restrict the amount of food given. Most nutrients are balanced to the energy content of the ration and, when this is restricted, malnutrition states may develop. For similar reasons, using diets with low palatability are also not an answer; cats will remain hungry, can develop behavioral problems and may become malnourished. Therefore, using diets with a reduced energy density is the key strategy during dietary intervention and additional dietary modifications can help to produce optimal weight reduction with minimal loss of the body fat free mass.

A variety of diets are available, all of which work through caloric energy restriction. Detailed information on the formulation of weight loss diets for cats can be found in future sections. The current information is a summary.

► Maintenance

Although the main medical benefit of a weight reduction program is a long-term reduction in adipose tissue mass, of greater importance is the permanent switch to a healthy lifestyle. As such, success ultimately depends not only on reaching the target, but in avoiding any rebound. In short, a permanent change in the attitude and behavior of the owner is required to ensure so that any weight loss is maintained long term.

The first challenge is to change the cat from a protocol designed for weight loss, to one designed to maintain body weight. The passage to the stabilization diet should be gradual, e.g. the hypoenergetic food should be substituted with a maintenance ration in a step-wise fashion, without provoking any weight gain. The energy level required can be determined in various ways:
- one method is to increase the food intake by 10% every two weeks until no further weight loss occurs. This will enable the veterinarian to set the exactly daily caloric requirement to prevent a rebound;
- alternatively, if food intake was recorded throughout the period of weight loss and, at some point, no weight was lost between consecutive visits, the caloric consumption at this stage may be a suitable estimate of maintenance requirements.

Once target weight has been achieved, regular check-ups should be continued, as well as the support and encouragement for the owner: there should be revisits every 2-4 weeks until the veterinarian is satisfied that weight is being maintained. Thereafter, the interval can gradually be extended but should not be less frequent than once every 3-6 months.

The choice of diet for the maintenance phase is less critical than that used for weight loss. There should be no need to feed a diet specifically formulated for weight loss, long term. However, it may be necessary for the cat to continue on a hypoenergetic diet, albeit consuming larger (i.e. maintenance) quantities. Purpose-formulated diets are available for use in the post-weight loss phase, and contain many desirable characteristics, including reduced energy content and increased fiber level (to promote satiety).

Any strategy that is implemented must aim to put in place a healthier relationship between the cat and the owner. The weight loss program is doomed to failure if no such change is made. For long-term effectiveness, it is essential that the patient does not return to the former situation. The owners should be counseled to the fact that modification of lifestyle is a lifelong (but difficult) process, and that they will need to continue to manage dietary intake for life.

8 - Dietary management of pre-existing obesity

The goal of the treatment is to lose body fat with minimal loss in lean tissue and without negative effects on health. Loss of adipose tissue depends on many factors: the initial body composition, the degree of energy restriction required, the rate of weight loss, the level of protein intake, the metabolic adaptations and the intensity of exercise. Recent work by one of the authors has

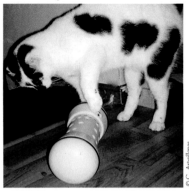

Figure 15 - Examples of good cat toys include devices that encourage the cat to play with the toy to receive its food.

The toy releases a few kibbles when the cat makes it move.

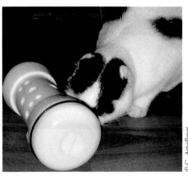

During a play session, cats must be given the opportunity to catch the "prey" object.

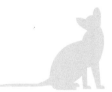

FIGURE 16 - BALANCE BETWEEN ENERGY SUPPLY AND ENERGY EXPENDITURE

Energy supply	Energy expenditure
Food intake through feeding, titbits and any successful hunting expeditions	Short bursts of energy consuming exercise when awake

suggested that cats that lose a higher percentage of body weight overall, tend to lose a greater proportion of lean tissue during weight loss *(German, in press, 2008)*.

In theory, the strategy is simple: in order to achieve weight loss the cat must be fed less energy than it requires **(Figure 16)**. In practice, this means feeding at a level below maintenance energy requirements. This is done by first calculating the energy requirement at ideal body weight and then feeding a proportion of this figure. It is essential to base the calculations on the target body weight and not the current weight.

▶ How do I determine the ideal body weight?

In order to make a correct calculation of maintenance energy requirements for an obese cat, the ideal body weight must already be known or be estimated.

> When ideal body weight is known or can readily be determined

The ideal body weight may have been recorded during a previous visit when the cat was a young adult in ideal body condition (e.g. a condition score of 3/5 or 5/9). It is by far the most accurate guide to optimal body weight in any individual.

> Estimation of ideal body weight from current body weight and body condition*

In the absence of historical information, an estimate of ideal weight can be made from the current body weight and condition. Assuming that each point above 5 (on a 9-integer condition score) or half point above 3 (on a 5-integer condition score) correlates with 10-15% increase in body weight, a simple mathematical equation can then be used to estimate ideal weight e.g.:

> Current weight = 8 kg
> Current condition score = 5/5 or 9/9 (~ 40% overweight)
> Ideal weight = 100/140 x 8 kg = 5.7 kg

▶ Recommending an optimum rate of weight loss

If correct energy restriction is applied, obese cats do lose weight *(Butterwick et al, 1994; Butterwick & Markwell, 1996)*. However, the progress of weight loss must be carefully evaluated. A further question is: what rate of weight loss is best? Is rapid weight loss better than slow weight loss?

Many studies have focused on the ideal rate of weight loss because, for owners, rapid weight loss is more satisfactory. In a study *(Szabo et al, 2000)*, obese cats lost 7 to 10% of their obese body weight (BW) during the first week, 3 to 5% during the second week and 2 to 4% for the remainder of the weight loss period. They were fed 25% of their maintenance energy requirement based on the target ideal body weight. However, at the end of the weight loss period, there was an increase in insulin and glucose concentration suggesting that glucose intolerance may be developing in these cats. Therefore, this level of energy restriction appears to be too strict and the authors concluded that the rapid weight loss might increase risk factors associated with the development of diabetes mellitus.

The recommended rate of weight loss remains a controversial issue in veterinary medicine. The weight loss rate must be consistent with relative sparing of lean tissue. Marked energy restriction (down to 45% of maintenance energy requirement at target weight) leads to more rapid weight loss (~1.3% per week) than moderate energy restriction (60% of maintenance energy requirements leading to ~1% body weight loss per week), but lean tissue loss is greater (18% compared with 8%) *(Butterwick et al, 1994)*. Even if the optimal target rate of weight loss seems to be 1.0 to 1.5% of initial BW per week, the exact rate should be tailored to the exact needs of each individual case and slower rates of weight loss are acceptable if tolerated by the client and veterinarian **(Figures 17 A & B)**.

FIGURE 17A - CLINICAL CASE N°1

Before: 8 kg

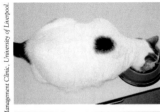

- Breed: DSH
- Age: 8 yrs 10 mths
- Sexual status: neutered male
- Body fat: 40.4%
- BCS: 4.5/5
- Lifestyle: indoor cat

Since body weight has increased, the cat has become far less active. He has problems with grooming behavior, especially in the perineal area. Poor skin and coat condition.

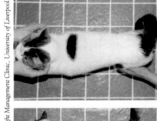

Dr A. German et S. Holden, Weight Management Clinic, University of Liverpool.

Weight loss summary

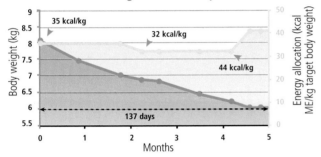

35 kcal/kg
32 kcal/kg
44 kcal/kg
137 days

After: 6 kg

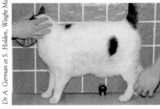

- Weight loss duration: 137 days
- Mean average loss: 1.1%/week
- Average allocation: 36 kcal/kg of target body weight
- Body fat: 18.8%
- BCS: 3/5

The cat has become much more mobile with weight loss: he climbs fences, jumps on kitchen units and initiates play sessions. He is better able to groom, therefore his coat condition has greatly improved.

Dr A. German et S. Holden, Weight Management Clinic, University of Liverpool.

FIGURE 17B - CLINICAL CASE N°2

Before: 8.5 kg

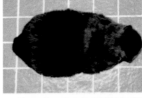

- Breed: DSH
- Age: 13 yrs
- Sexual status: neutered female
- Body fat: 44.5%
- BCS: 5/5
- Lifestyle: indoor cat

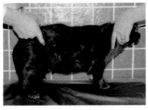

The owners acquired her at approximately 3 years of age and as that time she was already overweight. However, the problem has deteriorated since then. The cat has now decreased mobility, and inability to groom efficiently. She is a very lazy cat. She has a greasy coat, with coarseness to the hair on the caudo-dorsal body.

Weight loss summary

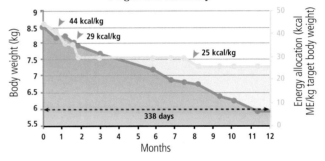

44 kcal/kg
29 kcal/kg
25 kcal/kg
338 days

After: 5.5 kg

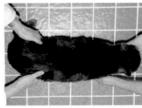

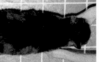

- Weight loss duration: 338 days
- Mean average loss: 0.75%/week
- Average allocation: 30 kcal/kg of target body weight
- Body fat: 31.3%
- BCS: 3/5

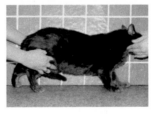

Since her weight loss, the cat can jump up and down off chairs. She follows the owners around the house throughout the day. Her ability to groom has improved. She looks better, her coat condition has improved. According to the owner, she looks definitely happier.

At this rate, the majority of tissue lost is body fat and no adverse metabolic effects were noted in 14 cats (*Center et al, 2000*). Blood glucose and alkaline phosphatase significantly decreased between week 0 and week 18, but cholesterol, alanine aminotransferase and aspartate aminotransferase significantly increased. Nevertheless, absolute changes were small and within reference ranges for all the parameters except blood cholesterol concentrations. Nine cats developed hypercholesterolemia during the weight loss program (*Center et al, 2000*); this effect was also observed in another study (*Szabo et al, 2000*). Further, in a concomitant study (*Ibrahim et al, 2000*), changes in cholesterol concentration were found to be due to increased production of high density lipoproteins (HDL). This study also demonstrated that blood cholesterol concentration could be reduced by a diet containing corn oil, thereby confirming that the type of dietary fat could influence lipoprotein metabolism in cats.

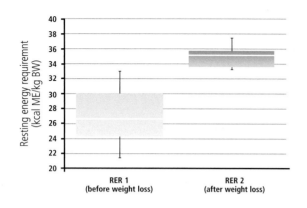

FIGURE 18 - RESTING ENERGY REQUIREMENTS IN CATS BEFORE AND AFTER WEIGHT LOSS

TABLE 7 - RER IN OBESE CATS BEFORE AND AFTER WEIGHT LOSS

	Obese state	After weight loss
Mean BMR (kcal ME/kg BW$^{0.65}$)	58	57
Min	39	49
Max	68	64

TABLE 8 - ENERGY REQUIREMENTS FOR LEAN AND OBESE CATS
according to NRC 2006

Equation	NRC 2006 recommendation
Lean cat (BW* = 4 kg)	100 kcal ME/kg BW$^{0.67}$ = 253 kcal ME/d *(i. e: ≈ 63 kcal/kg BW)*
Obese cat (BW* = 5 kg)	130 kcal ME/kg BW$^{0.4}$ = 247 kcal ME/d *(i. e: ≈ 50 kcal/kg BW)*
According to the experience of the authors, at a maintenance state, this energy allowance is too high for an obese cat who will maintain his body weight. The equation must be based on the ideal body weight and a 40% restriction is necessary to induce weight loss in a obese cat.	
Obese cat (IBW** = 4 kg)	0.6 x 100 kcal ME/kg BW$^{0.67}$ = 152 kcal ME/d *(i. e: ≈ 38 kcal/kg IBW)* 0.6 x 130 kcal ME/kg BW$^{0.4}$ = 136 kcal ME/d *(i. e: ≈ 34 kcal/kg IBW)*

* body weight **ideal body weight

ENERGY INTAKE RECOMMENDED FOR OBESE CATS

Body score	Daily caloric intake per kg of ideal body weight/day
3.5 or 4.0	30 kcal ME
4.5 or 5.0	35 kcal ME

► How do I determine the daily energy allocation to achieve weight loss

> Physiological consequences of energy restriction

Decrease in energy expenditure is a universal response to energy restriction in all species. This adaptation is a survival strategy to protect the organism when the central nervous system detects a state of starvation; therefore, when body weight decreases, BMR decreases. In humans, changes in BMR when in negative energy balance vary between -5% to -25% depending upon the level of energy restriction *(Prentice et al, 1991)*. Such reductions in BMR can make smooth and uniform weight loss difficult.

For humans, there are strong relationships both between the severity of energy restriction and the rate of weight loss, and also between energy restriction and suppression of resting metabolic rate. As a consequence, the greater the level of energy restriction applied, the greater the suppression of BMR. Hence, there may be a threshold below which the perceived advantages of rapid weight loss may, in the longer term, be counterbalanced by a more pronounced physiological defence against weight loss *(Prentice et al, 1991)*. Therefore, the decrease in metabolic rate can be counterbalanced by using either pharmacological approaches or by increasing physical activity.

> Optimum energy intake to achieve weight loss

A study has determined the level of energy intake required to achieve an expected rate of BW loss of 1 to 2% per week in 7 neutered obese cats *(Nguyen et al, 2002)*. In this study, energy expenditure was assessed by indirect calorimetry. The level of energy consumption during the weight loss period to obtain the desirable rate was 40 ± 2 kcal ME/kg ideal body weight e.g. approximately 66% of the energy requirement for an adult cat in optimal BW. Unexpectedly, resting energy requirement (RER) expressed as related to kg BW significantly increased whilst BW and body fat decreased. RER was measured during weight loss **(Figure 18)**. Cats lost 37± 3% of their initial body weight, and the rate of weight loss varied along the study from 0.1 to 3.0% per week and was never linear. Mean RER was 32 kcal ME/kg BW [min 21- max 39] but RER was significantly lower in the obese state (27 ± 2 kcal ME/kg BW) than after weight loss (35 ± 1 kcal ME/kg BW, p=0.028).

According to the current recommendations of the National Research Council (NRC 2006), an allometric coefficient was suggested to calculate the daily energy requirement for cats. The relationship between resting energy expenditure and body weight was best described with a coefficient of 0.65. When RER was expressed as kcal ME/kg BW$^{0.65}$, RER did not statistically differ between the obese and lean state, with a mean value of 58 kcal ME/kg BW$^{0.65}$ **(Table 7)**.

For weight loss, the level of daily energy intake must be adequate to cover the basal metabolic energy expenditure but not the total daily energy expenditure. In practice, the level of energy restriction should not be lower than BMR, e.g. 21 kcal ME/kg BW or 39 kcal ME/kg BW$^{0.65}$ as measured in experimental conditions. The initial energy allowance is estimated at about 60% of calculated energy requirement for the ideal body weight of the cat.

In general, weight loss will be faster at the start of the treatment and will decrease thereafter, but the physiologic response is quite unpredictable **(Figure 19)**. Therefore, it may be necessary to adjust energy intake frequently during the weight loss period to achieve optimal body fat loss and to decrease the risk of hepatic lipidosis and insulin resistance.

The initial allocation is only a starting point; during the weight loss program, the level of allocation has to be adapted to the rate of weight loss. This means a small (e.g. ~5%) reduction of the amount of food fed if the rate is too slow. Measuring cups are an unreliable method of measuring out food; instead, owners should be instructed to weigh the food on kitchen electronic scales which therefore enables small changes to be accurately made.

It is essential to ensure that, if possible, no additional food is given by the owner (or scavenged by the patient). Healthy treats may be allowed as this enables the owner to maintain their bond with the pet. This should, of course, be factored into the overall calorie provision and not on top of it. The caloric value of drinks (e.g. milk) must be also included as part of the overall plan.

FIGURE 19 - VARIOUS WEIGHT LOSS CURVES

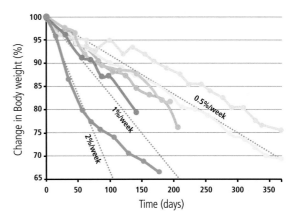

In general, weight loss is faster at the start of the treatment decreases thereafter. It is necessary to adjust energy intake frequently during the weight loss period to achieve optimal body fat loss (adapted from German, et al, 2008, in press).

FIGURE 20 - DURATION OF THE WEIGHT LOSS PROGRAM FOR AN OBESE CAT

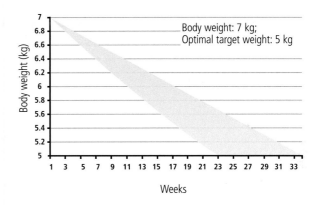

Slower weight loss is acceptable if the owners and clinicians agree with this approach.

Ideal body weight (kg)	Energy allocation (kcal ME/day)	Dry diet (g) (3000 kcal ME/kg)	Canned diet (g) (600 kcal ME/kg)	Dry + canned diets	
				Dry (g)	Canned (g)
3	105	35	175	15	100
3.5	120	40	200	20	100
4	140	45	230	25	100
4.5	160	50	270	35	100
5	175	60	290	40	100
5.5	190	65	320	45	100
6	210	70	350	50	100

TABLE 9 - DAILY AMOUNT OF FOOD ACCORDING TO THE TARGET BODY WEIGHT

Energy allocation based on 35 kcal/kg of ideal body weight (body score ⩾ 4.5)

► How do I evaluate the duration of the weight loss?

Once the clinician knows the target body weight, an estimate of the likely duration of the regimen can be determined (**Figure 20**). Such information has to be clearly explained to the owners, so that they are aware of the time commitment required for success.

► How do I estimate the daily food intake?

Calculation of the starting daily energy allocation is shown in **Table 8**. To ensure compliance of the nutritional treatment, the presentation must look like the usual food: dry food, wet food or a home made diet. More than 2/3 of owners prefer to mix dry and wet foods. It is essential that the exact portion size is accurately measured at each meal time (**Table 9**). Their accuracy can be verified by weighing the first portion of the food at the clinic, and giving it to the owner to weigh on their own scales.

► How do I monitor the weight loss program?

It is essential to follow the progress of patients frequently during any weight management program, particularly during the initial period, when owners need the most support and when problems are most likely to be encountered. It also provides an opportunity to verify compliance, deal with any issues or concerns (e.g. excess begging behavior, problems with implementing play sessions), and to provide feedback, encouragement and support.

> Regular veterinary checks

Owner motivation is the key to a successful outcome. Regular rechecks will help maintain compliance and owner motivation. A check every 2-4 weeks is recommended; if check-ups occur less frequently than every 4 weeks, compliance with the program will slip. It may also lead to a delay before a change is made, meaning that weight loss does not continue at an optimal rate.

> Measurement of the weight loss

At each check-up, the cat should be weighed and a physical examination performed. Owner perspective on progress should be gauged and any problems with the program discussed. If necessary, changes to the dietary plan can be made and any issues identified and resolved.

Body weight is the principal outcome measure of interest and used to decide upon whether changes to the plan are required (reduction in amount of food fed, increase in dose of medication). In order

FIGURE 21 - EVOLUTION OF BODY WEIGHT CHANGE VERSUS MORPHOMETRIC MEASUREMENTS
(Clinical Case n°1)

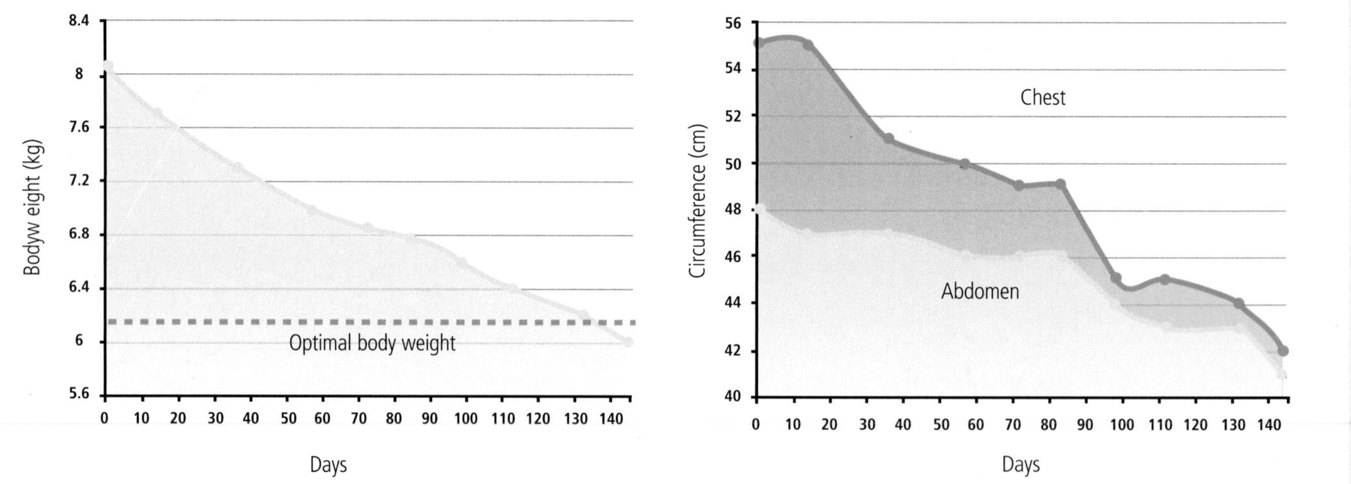

to minimize variability amongst measurement, the same set of electronic weigh scales should be used, and regularly validated. Owners must not be discouraged by the fact that 1% weight loss per week is not very much (e.g. 60g for a 6 kg cat).

The BCS chart can be used as a visual aid for leading discussion and providing owners with positive feedback. However, given that body condition is likely to change gradually, it is not essential to repeat the BCS at every visit.

Morphometric measurements are an additional means of monitoring outcome, and can be used to relay success in terms that the owner will understand (e.g. similar to a decrease in the size of the waist in people) (**Figure 21**).

Periodic photographs provide an excellent visual demonstration of success, but should be taken in a standardized manner to enable comparison between time-points.

All measurements and comments should be recorded and used to provide positive feedback, wherever possible, for the owner. Veterinarians should also encourage owners to record daily food intake in a diary; this information can then be reviewed at each visit.

> Follow-up by phone

A first phone call within 48 hours after starting the regimen might be helpful to ensure the compliance of the owner. Then, regular calls from a technician responsible for overseeing the program, is an excellent means of checking on progress, enhancing compliance and addressing any problems as early as possible. The involvement of other members of the veterinary team is a good way to boost success and make owners appreciate the commitment of the practice.

▶ What should I do at the time of first reassessment?

Regular revisits are made to assess progress throughout the weight loss regimen. Having interim target weights (in addition to the final target) can help maintain the owner's motivation throughout the process. There are three possible scenarios at the time of the first weigh-in.

> Successful outcome

The cat loses weight at a normal rate and the owner is satisfied. One can then renew the regimen and fix the time of the next appointment.

> The cat did not lose weight or even worse, gained weight!

In this situation, it is necessary:
- to verify that the calculation of the daily amount of food is correct. If this is the case and there is no other possible explanation, a reduction (usually 5-10%) in food intake may be necessary.
- to re-evaluate family environment without making the owners feel guilty. How is the motivation of the owner? Are instructions clear enough? Are there any neighbors likely to feed the cat? Verify whether any non-compliance (e.g. feeding additional items) has occurred. If this is the case, it may not be necessary to alter the amount fed.
- to consider additional diagnostic investigations such as to examine for possible hormonal disorders. In cats, hyperprolactinemia and acromegaly are common and alter the ability of the cat to lose weight. Until recently, medical treatment has not been available to correct this situation.

9 - Composition of the diet

Reduction of energy intake is the cornerstone of any dietary intervention. There are many strategies to decrease the energy density of a diet:
- decrease the amount of fat
- increase the dietary fiber content
- increase the water content.

FIGURE 22 - FROM GROSS ENERGY TO NET ENERGY

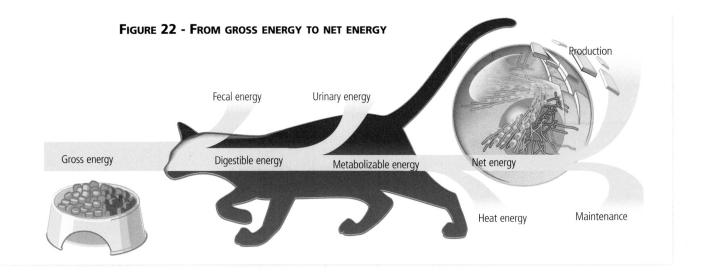

FIGURE 23 - INFLUENCE OF SEX AND ENERGY LEVEL OF THE DIET ON BODY FAT MASS
OF CATS FED AD-LIBITUM FOR ONE-YEAR

From Nguyen et al, 1999b

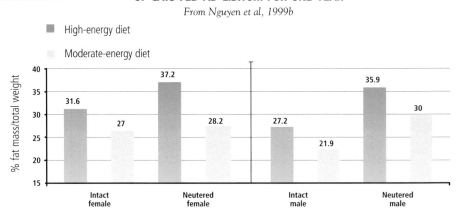

■ High-energy diet

□ Moderate-energy diet

The fat mass increases after neutering because the cat consumes more energy while expending less energy. The phenomenom is especially clear in males that consume a high-energy food. This type of food is not adapted to the needs of a neutered cat.

▶ Influence of energy density on energy consumption

Energy density refers to the amount of energy in a given amount of food. In practice, energy density is expressed as kcal of metabolizable energy per 100 g of food (**Figure 22**). For the same amount of food, a lower quantity of energy is consumed when the diet has a low energy density.

In one study (*Lester et al, 1999*), sedentary entire cats who had previously maintained body weight while consuming ad libitum moist meat-based diets with a constant fat content were able to adapt to a higher-fat meat-based diet by significantly increasing fat oxidation. In addition, along with the increased fat oxidation, the high fat diet did not show any hyperphagic effect. This study underlined the capacity of the cats to maintain their body weight on very high-fat diets in certain conditions. However, the situation is different in neutered animals living indoor and fed ad libitum with very palatable dry food (**Figure 23**).

In these circumstances, feeding low fat dry foods lowers the risk of obesity. In cats, food consumption tends to remain constant and is independent of the calorie content of the food; thus the mass or volume of food consumed appears to be the main factor implicated in the regulation of body weight *(Rolls et al, 2005)*. This suggests that gastric distension is one of the main factors driving satiety in this species. A recent study by one of the authors confirmed that cats tend to eat the same amount of food whatever the energy density of the diet *(Martin et al, 2008)*. Two commercial diets with different levels of energy (diet A: 360 kcal/100g; diet B 415 kcal/100g) were offered to two groups of cats for five weeks (cross-over study). Mean food intake did not differ on the two diets (58±2 g/d/cat with A and 56±2 g/d/cat with B) but the energy intake did vary (44±2 kcal/kg/d for A and 50±2 kcal/kg/d for B). These findings are confirmed by studies which have shown that cats fed high fat dry foods ad libitum are more likely to be obese *(Scarlett et al, 1994)*.

One advantage of feeding a hypoenergetic food to cats undergoing weight loss, is that the volume of food fed is closer to the volume of a maintenance diet fed at maintenance. This can help to improve owner compliance. For example **(Table 9)**, assuming that the same daily energy contribution is required (140 kcal ME); whilst on the weight loss diet the cat will consume 45 g of food per day, which is close to that of cat feed a standard ration at maintenance (50 g). In this example, the cat does not risk a deficiency and has an adequate amount of food per day.

▶ Diet formulation

The main factor that drives weight loss is the level of dietary energy fed, but it should be remembered that diet also provides many essential nutrients. Supplementation of such nutrients (relative to energy content) is usually recommended to prevent deficiency diseases from arising during weight loss. Whatever diet is chosen, the veterinarian has a duty to ensure that the diet is complete and well-balanced.

An additional characteristic of a weight loss diet is palatability since this will maximize compliance with treatment. Thus, there are many factors that must be taken into account when considering the most appropriate meal composition for a cat undergoing weight loss.

> Decreased amount of fat

Fat has a high energy content (9 kcal ME/g) compared to protein and carbohydrates (4 kcal ME/g). Hence, low energy density diets tend to be low fat diets. *Bauer (2006)* has recommended a new classification for dietary lipids.
- A facilitative fat is a saturated fat that increases energy density of the food; it can be stored in adipose tissue for future use, improves palatability and acceptability of the food and promotes fat-soluble vitamins absorption. To decrease energy density, facilitative fats should be limited in the foods.
- Functional fats are usually polyunsaturated fatty acids. They are involved in many biological processes such as growth, reproduction, hormonal synthesis, inflammation and gastrointestinal, skin or brain health. Essential fatty acids must be obligatory found in foods but only small amounts are needed to meet the nutritional requirements.

Cats fed a low fat (9.2% DMB), high protein (33.5% DMB), low fiber diet lose weight safely *(Bouchard et al, 1998)* without signs of hepatic lipidosis or of any deterioration of skin and coat condition.

Minimum fat content of diets designed for obese cats should focus on essential fatty acids. A low fat diet should provide 0.14 g $BW^{0.67}$ linoleic acid (LA) and 0.0005 g $BW^{0.67}$ arachidonic acid (ARA) to meet the maintenance fatty acid requirement of cats *(NRC 2006)*. If we take the example of an obese cat (BW = 6.0 kg, target weight = 4.5 kg), the recommended allowance would be 0.46 g and 0.0016 g for LA and

FIGURE 24 - COMPARATIVE STRUCTURE OF CONJUGATED LINOLEIC ACID AND LINOLEIC ACID

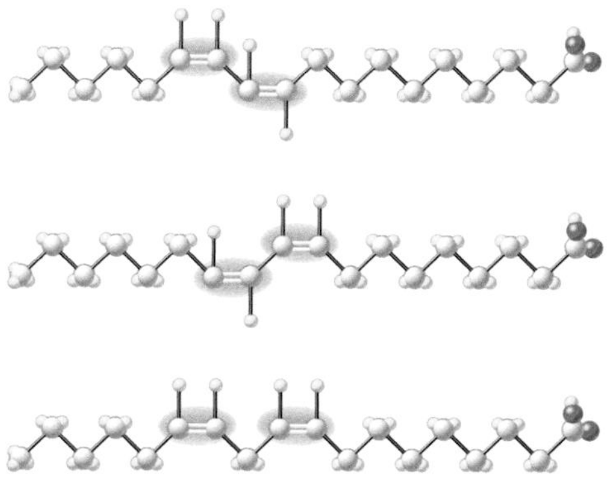

Conjugated linoleic acid: (10-trans, 12-cis)

(9-cis, 11-trans)

Linoleic acid: (9, 12-cis-cis)

The isomers (10-trans, 12-cis) and (9-cis, 11-trans) of linoleic acid are the main components of conjugated linoleic acid. Unlike linoleic acid, the double bonds are not separated by a methyl radical.

for ARA, respectively. This would correspond to a concentration of 5.6 g LA/1000 ME and 0.02 g ARA/1000 ME (These values take into account the fact that the cat may be subjected to a 50% reduction of energy intake.)

Recently, many researchers have focused on the effect of conjugated linoleic acid (CLA) **(Figure 24)** in obesity *(Nagao and Yanagita, 2005)*, because some animal studies have shown promising effects on body weight and fat deposition. The theoretical benefits of CLA are said to include decreased energy and food intake, increased energy expenditure, decreased pre-adipocyte differentiation and proliferation, decreased lipogenesis, and increased lipolysis and fat oxidation. However, recent work in cats has suggested that incorporation of CLA in weight loss diets has no significant effect *(Leray et al, 2006)*.

Obese cats fed high fat diets may present with hyperlipidemia and moderate elevation in serum triglycerides and cholesterol concentrations *(Ginzinger et al, 1997)*. The use of fish oil in the treatment of hyperlipidemia has been extensively studied in a number of other species (see chapter 6). Eicosapentaenoic acid (EPA) and docosahexaenoic acid (DHA) are long-chain omega-3 fatty acids found in fish oil and they are known to decrease the serum concentration of free fatty acids *(Singer et al, 1990)*. A diet high in long-chain omega-3 fatty acids was shown to improve the long-term control of glycemia and lower plasma insulin levels *(Wilkins et al, 2004)*.

> Increased dietary fiber

Fiber is defined as plant components that are resistant to degradation by mammalian digestive enzymes, especially amylase. Indigestible carbohydrates reach the colon and become an available substrate for bacterial fermentation. Substrates for bacterial fermentation mainly include structural polysaccharides (hemicellulose) and non-structural polysaccharides (gums, mucilages) but also resistant starch. Cellulose and pectins are not very good substrates for bacteria in the GIT of cats.

The current classification of dietary fiber is based on their physicochemical properties and their ability to undergo bacterial fermentation. Fermentable fibers yield increased hydrogen, carbon dioxide, ammonia and short chain fatty acids (SCFA). These final end products are of particular interest as they can interact with the host in a variety of ways and are involved in many metabolic processes when reaching the liver or the peripheral blood. Physiological properties include promotion of colonocyte differentiation and proliferation, stimulation of sodium and water reabsorption, inhibition of pathogenic bacterial growth, enhancement of colonic blood flow and colonic longitudinal smooth muscle contraction. As in other species, SCFA concentrations in the feline colon depend on the type of fiber found in the diet *(Sunvold et al, 1995a; 1955b; 1995c)*.

In vitro fermentation techniques using feline colonic bacteria have shown that the greatest total SCFA production occurs when fibers such as locust bean gum, guar gum, and citrus pectin are used, while fibers such as cellulose, gum karaya, or xanthan gum result in production of lower concentrations of SCFA. However, in cats, fibers yielding the largest amount of SCFA produced gastrointestinal side effects, such as increased fecal output and diarrhea *(Sunvold et al, 1995a)*. Beet pulp, which is a fiber source containing a mixture of soluble and insoluble fibers, has been suggested to be a source of choice for cats to optimize both SCFA production and fecal consistency *(Sunvold et al, 1995a)*. Nevertheless, studies on cats are scarce.

High dietary fiber (DF) content allows caloric dilution of the diet which helps to produce a satiety effect and to control body weight in obese cats. Nevertheless, high fiber diets may have unpleasant side effects for owners, such as excessive defecation and/or constipation *(Bouchard et al, 1998)*. When formulating a high fiber diet, the potential impact on nutrient digestibility has also to be considered. However, in practice, no negative impact has been reported with most of the hypoenergetic diets containing large amounts of DF. If high fiber diets present a poor apparent digestibility of the proteins *(Fekete et al, 2001)*, this effect is due to the nitrogen retention by the bacterial flora: excreted biomass increases with the fiber. Apparent and ileal protein digestibility must not be confused.

In deciding on a level of DF to include, it is also necessary to consider the taste preferences of cats. *Houpt & Smith* (1981) noted that cats disliked dilution of their food with a non-caloric solid such as kaolin or cellulose. In practice, according to our clinical experience, high-fiber veterinary foods for obese cats are well tolerated, and for the majority of the animals there is no problem with acceptance.

> Water content

The natural diet of a cat contains about 70-80% water. In addition, high dietary water content can decrease energy intake even on a high fat diet *(Rolls et al, 2005)*. Therefore, using an increased water content to reduce dietary energy density may be a particularly useful method for cats. The amount of food offered with a canned food (about 20% of dry matter) is about three to six times higher than the amount offered with a dry food (90% dry matter) for an equal daily energy allowance **(Table 10)**. It is of particular interest for cats that usually ingest large amount of dry food because the size of the meal could be the main regulator of food intake.

> Avoiding protein deficiency

Given that cats are obligate carnivores, a high level of dietary protein is essential; in wild cats, daily energy is supplied by protein and fat, whilst carbohydrates are not consumed. Nitrogen metabolism is very specific in cats, as hepatic enzymes involved in nitrogen catabolism are not adaptive. Dietary protein provides essential amino acids for protein synthesis and non-essential amino acids as energy substrates. If the amount of protein in the diet is insufficient, the result is

TABLE 10 - AMOUNT OF FOOD OFFERED WITH A COMMERCIAL OBESITY DRY FOOD AND A COMMERCIAL OBESITY CANNED FOOD

Commercial obesity dry food	Commercial obesity canned food
Energy density: 300 kcal/100 g	Energy density: 60 kcal/100 g
Obese cat: body score: 4; ideal body weight (IBW): 5 kg Energy allocation: 30 kcal/kg IBW: 30 x 5 = 150 kcal/day	
Amount 1 ≈ 50 g/d	Amount 2 ≈ 250 g/d

TABLE 11 - ESSENTIAL NUTRIENTS FOR CATS
(from NRC 2006)

	Minimum requirement (g/1000 kcal ME)	Adequate intake (g/1000 kcal ME)	Recommended allowance (g/1000 kcal ME)
Protein	40 (3.97 BW$^{0.67}$)	-	50 (4.96 BW$^{0.67}$)
Fat	-	22.5	22.5
Calcium	0.4	-	22.5
Phosphorus	0.35	-	0.64
Magnesium (mg)	50	-	-
Potassium	-	1.3	-
Taurine	0.08	-	0.1

loss of lean body mass which can then diminish the body's ability to respond to infectious agents and stress.

According to the current NRC requirements (2006), the recommended allowance maintenance requirement of protein for an adult cat is 4.96g crude protein (CP)/ $BW^{0.67}$ **(Table 11)**. Since maintenance protein requirements are expected to be the same in obese adult cats, the protein level of the diet should be supplemented. For example, an obese cat (BW = 6.0kg, target weight = 4.5kg) has a recommended daily protein allowance of 16.5 g CP and should be fed approximately 162 kcal ME/day to achieve weight loss. For a hypoenergetic diet to provide enough protein, it should contain almost 100g CP/1000 kcal ME. Diets with CP concentration less than 85 g CP/1000 kcal ME are not adequate to satisfactorily cover the feline requirement. However, if severe energy restriction is required to induce and maintain weight loss (far lower than expected), even diets supplemented with protein to 100g CP/1000 ME may be deficient.

The reduced energy density of weight loss diets, related to reduced fat content and high fiber and/or water content, can have a negative impact on palatability. Animal proteins are generally considered as attractive for cats. Therefore, providing a diet which is rich in proteins of animal origin may help in maintaining palatability of low energy (low fat) diets.

One potential concern with feeding a high protein diet is that it may be deleterious for health, especially in older animals. In this respect, some clinicians are concerned with a possible negative impact on pre-existing chronic kidney disease (CKD). However, there is no evidence that supports a link between high protein intake and the development of CKD in dogs and cats. Further, the diets are only supplemented in protein relative to energy content, so that when feeding on a weight loss regime, total protein intake is not actually increased.

Two groups of 8 cats were fed two diets designed for weight loss (1% of initial BW per week) *(Laflamme & Hannah, 2005)*; a high protein diet (46% calories from protein - 76 g CP/1000 kcal ME) and a normal diet (36% calories from protein - 60 g CP/1000 kcal ME). During the study, mean energy intake did not differ between the two groups and, neither rate of weight loss or total weight loss differed. However, changes in body composition were observed. Loss of body fat was increased (p<0.001), and loss of lean tissue was reduced (p<0.001) in the high protein group.

In the context of weight loss "high protein diet" does not actually mean increased protein intake, but simply maintaining normal intake whilst energy content is reduced.

> Carbohydrates

Carbohydrates are not essential for cats since this species has specific metabolic adaptations for low carbohydrate intake. Moreover, high dietary carbohydrate content may decrease apparent protein digestibility *(Kienzle, 1994)*. Whilst a limited amount of carbohydrate has no detrimental effect on weight loss in cats, increasing carbohydrate content of a feline weight loss diet may not be beneficial. High carbohydrate diets (> 25% of calories) are not recommended in obese cats as they are commonly insulin-resistant (see chapter 5).

> L-Carnitine

Supplementing a weight loss diet with L-carnitine has been shown to be beneficial in a number of species, including cats. L-carnitine is synthesized in the liver and absorbed in the digestive tract, and is an essential co-factor for lipid oxidation *(Steiber et al, 2004)*. In brief, L-carnitine assists in the transportation of long-chain fatty acids into the mitochondria in various tissues including the liver, the heart and skeletal muscle. It also facilitates α-keto acid oxidation and influences urea cycle function. Stimulation of fatty acid oxidation is beneficial during weight loss, because fatty acid oxidation can affect feeding behavior *(Ronnett et al, 2005)*. In this respect, inhibition of fatty acid oxidation stimulates food intake in animals fed a high fat diet (40% of ME as fat), but is ineffective when fed a low fat diet (7% of ME as fat). Thus, maintaining fatty acid oxidation, by supplementation of L-carnitine, may contribute to the regulation of energy balance and metabolic homeostasis and has an effect on appetite control. In cats, supplementation with L-carnitine has been shown to have a positive effect on weight loss and fatty acid oxidation *(Center et al, 2000; Ibrahim et al, 2003)*. L-carnitine administered at 250 mg PO q12h in cats is safe and has a significant effect on the rate of weight loss in some studies *(Center et al, 2000)*. As this dose is very high and out of economical consideration in petfood, further studies using L-carnitine at a more practical dose are required.

> Antioxidants

An increase in insulin secretion, plasma free fatty acids or plasma glucose leads to an increase in reactive oxygen species (ROS) production and oxidative stress. Moreover, many studies have demonstrated that oxidative stress is associated in both the etiology and complications of diabetes. Many studies conducted *in vitro* or in animal models have shown that antioxidants (mainly α-lipoic acid, vitamin C, vitamin E, glutathione, N-acetyl-L-cysteine, aminoguanine, zinc) improve insulin sensitivity *(Evans et al, 2003)*.

Recently, studies have focused on the benefit of α-lipoic acid on glucose uptake and this antioxidant shows promising results in the prevention and treatment of diabetes mellitus in humans *(Çakatay, 2006)*. Daily dosage ranges in humans were from 600 mg to 1800 mg IV or oral with few to no side effects *(Head, 2006)*. Alpha-lipoic acid is considered safe in humans. Nevertheless, a study in cats *(Hill et al, 2004)* described acute toxicity of α-lipoic acid at a dose of 30 mg/kg. Currently, the maximum tolerated dose (MTD) of LA in cats remains unknown. Additional studies are needed to evaluate the effectiveness of antioxidant treatment in obesity and related diseases and to determine MTD in cats.

Conclusion

It is relatively easy to diagnose obesity in a cat and to prescribe a diet. The challenge lies in convincing the owner to introduce the necessary changes in the feeding and lifestyle of the animal in order to induce and maintain significant weight loss. Every suggested change runs the risk of provoking resistance from the cat-owner system. In order for the weight reduction program to be effective, the owner has to have adequate motivation. To develop this motivation, it is certainly appropriate to use a stage by stage approach and remember that each stage is a stepping stone. Omitting one or more stages will be detrimental to the process.

At the time of every consultation, it is necessary for the veterinarian to recognize where the owner is in relation to these phases. By doing so, he can adjust the arguments used in conversation and can alter recommended treatment approaches in response to the attitude of the client. It is also important to be prepared for resistance on the part of the owner, which can be expressed as doubts and reluctance to comply with the proposed solutions, and to be able to respond appropriately. It may be beneficial to undergo some form of training in order to acquire the ability to motivate clients.

To avoid any nutritional deficit during a weight loss program, specific foods have been formulated. The composition of such diets takes into account the energy restriction such that the relative concentration of nutrients is increased. Therefore, despite the imposed energy restriction, cats on a weight loss program should eat a daily amount of all nutrients (other than fat) which is similar to that of cats fed at maintenance. Therefore, to make a food with a reduced energy value reduce the quantity of the total fat content, increase water and/or fiber and provide enough of the essential nutrients (amino-acids, essential fatty acids, minerals and vitamins) to prevent any deficiency.

Frequently asked questions on feline obesity

Q	A
How do I adapt the cat to the diet?	A weight loss program involves modifying the composition of food (hypoenergetic and high protein) and controlling the quantity of food offered on a daily basis. Since satiety depends primarily on the quantities consumed, many cats have difficulties in consuming a reduced amount of food. Therefore, for some cats it may be necessary to acclimatize them to the reduced intake and new food. In this respect, a ~7-day period of gradual change is usually successful. If a cat refuses a particular food, it may be possible to improve acceptance by temporarily adding a small amount of the previous diet. Alternatively, a different formulation (moist diet) of weight loss diet could be chosen or a home-made devised.
Are there any alternatives to commercial weight loss diets?	It is feasible to develop a home-prepared weight loss diet for cats which is balanced and meets NRC requirements. However, it is the veterinarians duty to advise on such rations and to ensure that the chosen recipe meets nutritional requirements.
Some owners would prefer not to change the food of their cat to avoid behavioral issues or because their cat is a very capricious eater: should this attitude be encouraged?	A maintenance diet meets all nutritional needs when energy requirement is "normal". In the case of a non obese cat weighing 3.5 kg at maintenance, the daily protein contribution will be 16.2 g, 0.4 g of phosphorus and calcium, and 26 mg of taurine. For an obese cat with a target weight of 3.5 kg, the energy restriction imposes an allowance of 126 (36 kcal/kg IBW x 3.5kg) kcal ME per day, instead of 210 kcal ME for maintenance (60 kcal/kg IBW x 3.5 kg). If the same food is fed, the cat will consume 9.4 g of protein per day, 0.2 g of phosphorus and calcium, 15 mg of taurine. Since these amounts are lower than the recommended daily allowance for a cat (NRC, 2006), feeding such a diet over a prolonged period could lead to deficiencies, in particular with regard to nitrogen balance. Moreover, in order to enable such a low level of energy to be consumed, the daily allocation will need to be only 30 g! Most owners would struggle to accept such a proposal. Hence, using a standard maintenance diet is an inappropriate means of treating obesity during a weight loss program. Although concerns over diet palatability are a reason frequently cited by owners for not implementing a weight loss program, lack of diet palatability is rarely a problem for most of the commercial diets on the market if introduced gradually.
How do I manage obesity for a cat in a multi-pet household? © Lucile Martin	Whilst it is difficult enough to instigate an effective weight reduction plan in a cat living alone, multi-cat households represent a particular challenge. One option would be to feed all cats the same (e.g. weight reduction) diet. However, it is likely that group-feeding was one of the factors that allowed the obese cat (s) to become overweight in the first place; in this respect, if food is left out for all cats to share, the tendency is that greedy cats over-eat at the expense of cats with better appetite control. Therefore, in order for an owner to guarantee that all cats maintain their body weight excess food must be left out allowing some of the cats to over-eat. Thus, the only solution is to instigate individual feeding plans for each cat. This can be done in the following ways: - feed the cats in separate rooms or locations - feed the cats in the same locality but supervise them at all times and pick up feed bowls as soon as each cat stops eating - feed cats at different times - put the food for the cat (s) in normal body condition is a location where the obese cat (s) cannot reach. For instance, food could be placed in an elevated position if the obese cat is unable to climb; alternatively, the food could be placed in a box with an opening that only the normal cats can fit through.

References

Adams KF, Schatzkin A, Harris TB, et al. Overweight, obesity, and mortality in a large prospective cohort of persons 50 to 71 years old. N Engl J Med 2006; 355: 763-778.

Allan FJ, Pfeiffer DU, Jones BR, et al. A cross-sectional study of risk factors for obesity in cats in New Zealand. Prev Vet Med 2000; 46:183-196.

Asarian L, Geary N. Modulation of appetite by gonadal steroid hormones. Philos Trans R Soc Lond B Biol Sci 2006; 29: 1251-1263.

Backus RC, Kanchuk ML, Rogers QR. Elevation of plasma cholecystokinin concentration following a meal is increased by gonadectomy in male cats. J Anim Physiol Anim Nutr 2005; 90: 152-158.

Backus RC, Howard KA, Rogers QR. The potency of dietary amino acids in elevating plasma cholecystokinin immunoreactivity in cats is related to amino acid hydrophobicity. Regul Pept 1997; 72: 31-40.

Bauer JE. Metabolic basis for the essential nature of fatty acids and the unique dietary fatty acid requirements of cats. J Am Vet Med Assoc 2006; 229: 1729-32.

Biourge V, Massat B, Roff JM, et al. Effects of protein, lipid or carbohydrate supplementation on hepatic lipid accumulation during weight loss in obese cats. Am J Vet Res 1994; 55: 1406-1415.

Biourge V, Pion P, Lewis J, et al. Spontaneous occurrence of hepatic lipidosis in a group of laboratory cats. J Vet Intern Med 1993; 7: 194-197.

Bodey AR, Mitchell AR. Epidemiological study of blood pressure in domestic dogs. J Small Anim Pract 1996; 37: 116-125.

Bottcher P, Kluter S, Krastel D, et al. Liposuction-removal of giant lipomas for weight loss in a dog with severe hip osteoarthritis. J Small Anim Pract 2007; 48: 46-48.

Bouchard GF, Sunvold GD. Effect of dietary carbohydrate source on postprandial plasma glucose and insulin concentration in cats. In Recent Advances in Canine and Feline Nutrition, volume II, Iams Nutrition Symposium Proceedings. Edited by GA Reinhart, DP Carey, 2000 pp. 91-102.

Bouchard GF, Sunvold GD, Daristotle L. Dietary modification of feline obesity with a low fat, low fiber diet. In Recent Advances in Canine and Feline Nutrition, volume II, Iams Nutrition Symposium Proceedings. Edited by GA Reinhart, DP Carey, 1998 pp. 183-194.

Bray GA. Etiology and pathogenesis of obesity. Clin Cornerstone 1999; 2: 1-15.

Butterwick RF, Markwell PJ. Changes in the body composition of cats during weight reduction by controlled dietary energy restriction. Vet Rec 1996; 138: 354-357.

Butterwick RF, Wills JM, Sloth C, et al. A study of obese cats on a calorie-controlled weight reduction programme. Vet Rec 1994; 134: 372-377.

Burkholder WJ. Body composition of dogs determined by carcass composition analysis, deuterium oxide dilution, subjective and objective morphometry and bioelectrical impedance, Blacksburg, Virginia Polytechnic Institute and State University 1994.

Burkholder WJ. Precision and practicality of methods assessing body composition of dogs and cats. Comp Cont Edu Pract Vet 2001; 23:1-15.

Burkholder WJ, Toll PW. Obesity In: M.S. Hand, C.D. Thatcher, R.L. Reimillard, P. Roudebush, M.L. Morris, B.J. Novotny, eds; Small Animal Clinical Nutrition, 4th ed. Mark Morris Institute, Topeka, KS, USA. 2000; pp 401-430.

Calle EE, Thun MJ. Obesity and cancer. Oncogene 2004;23: 6365-6378.

Calvert E. The effect of diet and hormonal status on growth and body composition in growing kittens. Waltham Centre for Pet Nutrition, 2003, unpublished trial.

Clarke SP, Bennett D. Feline osteoarthritis: a prospective study of 28 cases. J Small Anim Pract 2006; 47:439-445.

Center SA, Harte J, Watrous D, et al. The clinical and metabolic effects of rapid weight loss in obese pet cats and the influence of supplemental oral L-carnitine. J Vet Intern Med 2000; 14: 598-608.

Clutton RE. The medical implications of canine obesity and their relevance to anaesthesia. Br Vet J 1998; 144: 21-28.

Colliard L, Ancel J, Benet JJ, et al. Risk factors for obesity in France. J Nutr 2006; 136:1951S-1954S.

Cummings DE, Weigle DS, Frayo RS, et al. Plasma ghrelin levels after diet-induced weight loss or gastric bypass surgery. N Engl J Med 2002; 346: 1623-1630.

Cummings DE. Ghrelin and the short- and long-term regulation of appetite and body weight. Physiol Behav 2006; 89: 71-84.Cummings DE, Overduin J. Gastrointestinal regulation of food intake. J Clin Invest 2007; 117: 13-23.

Czaja JA, Goy RW. Ovarian hormones and food intake in female guinea pigs and rhesus monkeys. Horm Behav 1975; 6: 329-349.

Çakatay U. Pro-oxidant actions of alpha-lipoic acid and dihydrolipoic acid. Med Hypotheses 2006; 66:110-117.

de Carvalho EB, Vitolo MR, Gama CM, et al. Fiber intake, constipation, and overweight among adolescents living in Sao Paulo City. Nutrition 2006; 22: 744-749.

Donoghue S, Scarlett JM. Diet and feline obesity. J Nutr 1998 ;128(12 Suppl):2776S-2778S.

Evans JL, Goldfine ID, Maddux BA, et al. Are oxidative stress-activated signaling pathways mediators of insulin resistance and β-cell dysfunction? Diabetes 2003; 52: 1-8.

Fekete S, Hullar I, Andrasofszky E, et al. Reduction of the energy density of cat foods by increasing their fibre content with a view to nutrients' digestibility. J Anim Physiol Anim Nutr 2001; 85:200-204.

Feldhahn JR, Rand JS, Martin G. Insulin sensitivity in normal and diabetic cats. J Fel Med Surg 1999; 1: 107-115.

Fettman MJ, Stanton CA, Banks LL. Effects of neutering on body weight metabolic rate and glucose tolerance in domestic cats. Res Vet Sci 1997; 62: 131-136.

Flegal KM, Carroll MD, Ogden CL, et al. Prevalence and trends in obesity among US adults 1999-2000. J Am Med Assoc 2002; 288: 1723-1727.

Flint DJ, Binart N, Kopchick J, et al. Effects of growth hormone and prolactin on adipose tissue development and function. Pituitary 2003; 6: 97-102.

Flynn MF, Hardie EM, Armstrong PJ. Effect of ovariohysterectomy on maintenance energy requirements in cats. J Am Vet Med Assoc 1996; 9:1572-1581.

German AJ, Holden SL, Bissot T, et al. Changes in body composition during weight loss in obese client-owned cats: loss of lean tissue mass correlates with overall percentage of weight loss. J Feline Med Surg, 2008 (in press).

German AJ, Holden SL, Moxham G, et al. A simple reliable tool for owners to assess the body condition of their dog or cat. J Nutr 2006; 136: 2031S-2033S.

Ginzinger DG, Wilson JE, Redenbach D, et al. Diet-induced atherosclerosis in the domestic cat. Lab Invest 1997; 77: 409-419.

Glickman LT, Schofer FS, McKee LJ, et al. Epidemiologic study of insectoside exposure obesity risk of bladder cancer in household dogs. J Toxicol Eviron Health 1989; 28: 407-414.

Godfrey DR. Osteoarthritis in cats: a retrospective radiological study. J Small Anim Pract 2005; 46:425-429.

Halford JC. Pharmacotherapy for obesity. Appetite 2006; 46: 6-10.

Harper EF, Stack DM, Watson TDG, et al. Effects of feeding regimens on body weight, composition and condition score in cats following ovariohysterectomy. J Small Anim Pract 2001; 42: 433-438.

Hawthorne AJ, Butterwick RF. Predicting the body composition of cats: development of a zoometric measurement for estimation of percentage body fat in cats. J Vet Inter Med 2000; 14: 365.

Head KA. Peripheral neuropathy: pathogenic mechanisms and alternative therapies. Alt Med Rev 2006; 11: 294-329.

Henegar JR, Bigler SA, Henegar LK, et al. Functional and structural changes in the kidney in the early stages of obesity. J Am Soc Nephrol 2001; 12: 1211-1217.

Hill AS, Werner JA, Rogers QA, et al. Lipoic acid is 10 time more toxic in cats than reported in humans, dogs or rats. J Anim Physiol Anim Nutr 2004; 88: 150-156.

Hoenig M, Ferguson DC. Effects of neutering on hormonal concentrations and energy requirements in cats. J Am Vet Med Assoc 2002; 63: 634-639.

Holmes KL, Morris PJ, Abdulla Z, et al. Risk factors associated with excess body weight in dogs in the UK. J Anim Physiol Anim Nutr 2007; 91; 166-167.

Houpt KA, Smith SL. Taste preferences and their relation to obesity in dogs and cats. Can Vet J 1981; 22: 77-85.

Ibrahim WH, Szabo J, Sunvold GD, et al. Effect of dietary protein quality and fatty acid composition on plasma lipoprotein concentrations and hepatic triglyceride fatty acid synthesis in obese cats undergoing rapid weight loss. Am J Vet Res 2000; 61: 566-572.

Kanchuk ML, Backus RC, Calvert CC, et al. Weight gain in gonadectomized normal and lipoprotein lipase-deficient male domestic cats results from increased food intake and not decreased energy expenditure. J Nutr 2003; 133: 1866-1874.

Kealy RD, Olsson SE, Monti KL, et al. Effects of limited food consumption on the incidence of hip dysplasia in growing dogs. J Am Vet Med Assoc 1992; 201: 857-863.

Kealy RD, Lawler DF, Ballam JM, et al. Five-year longitudinal study on limited food consumption and development of osteoarthritis in coxofemoral joints of dogs. J Am Vet Med Assoc 1997; 210: 222-225.

Kealy RD, Lawler DF, Ballam JM, et al. Evaluation of the effect of limited food consumption on radiographic evidence of osteoarthritis in dogs. J Am Vet Med Assoc 2000; 217: 1678-1680.

Kealy RD, Lawler DF, Ballam JM, et al. Effects of diet restriction on life span and age-related changes in dogs. J Am Vet Med Assoc 2002; 220: 1315-1320.

Kienzle E, Bergler R. Human-animal relationship of owners of normal and overweight cats. J Nutr 2006; 136:1947S-1950S.

Kienzle E, Bergler R, Mandernach A. Comparison of the feeding behaviour of the man-animal relationship in owners of normal and obese dogs. J Nutr 1998; 128: 2779S-2782S.

Kienzle E. Effect of carbohydrates on digestion in the cat. J Nutr 1994; 124: 2568S-2571S.

Kissileff HR, Carretta JC, Geliebter A, et al. Cholecystokinin and stomach distension combine to reduce food intake in humans. Am J Physiol Regul Integr Comp Physiol 2003; 285: R992-R998.

Kopelman PG. Obesity as a medical problem. Nature 2000; 404: 635-643.

Laflamme DP. Development and validation of a body condition score for cats: a clinical tool. Fel Pract 1997; 25: 13-18.

Laflamme DP, Hannah SS. Increased dietary protein promotes fat loss and reduces loss of lean body mass during weight loss in cats. Intern J Appl Res Vet Med 2005; 3: 62-68.

Lane MA, Black A, Ingram DK, et al. Calorie restriction in nonhuman primates: implications for age-related disease risk. J Anti-aging Med 1998; 1: 315-326.

Larson BT, Lalwer DF, Spitznagel EL, et al. Improved glucose tolerance with lifetime restriction favorably affects disease and survival in dogs. J Nutr 2003; 133: 2887-2892.

Lawler DF, Evans RH, Larson BT, et al. Influence of lifetime food restriction on causes time and predictors of death in dogs. J Am Vet Med Assoc 2005; 226: 225-231.

Leray V, Dumon H, Martin L, et al. No effect of conjugated linoleic acid or garcinia cambogia on body composition and energy expenditure in non-obese cats. J Nutr 2006; 136: 1982S-1984S.

Lester T, Czarnecki-Maulden G, Lewis D. Cats increase fatty acid oxidation when isocalorically fed meat-based diets with increasing fat content. Am J Physiol 1999; 277: R878-R886.

Leung WY, Neil Thomas G, Chan JC, et al. Weight management and current options in pharmacotherapy: orlistat and sibutramine. Clin Ther 2003; 25: 58-80.

Li J, Bronk BS, Dirlam JP, et al. In vitro and in vivo profile of 5-[(4'-trifluoromethyl-biphenyl-2-carbonyl)-amino]-1H-indole-2-carboxylic acid benzylmethyl carbamoylamide (dirlotapide) a novel potent MTP inhibitor for obesity. Bioorg Med Chem Lett 2007; 17: 1996-1999.

Louveau I, Gondret F. Regulation of development and metabolism of adipose tissue by growth hormone and the insulin-like growth factor system. Domest Anim Endocrinol 2004; 27: 241-255.

Lund EM, Armstrong PJ, Kirk CA, et al. Prevalence and risk factors for obesity in adult cats from private US veterinary practices. Intern J Appl Res Vet Med 2005; 3: 88-96.

Martin L, Dumon H, Siliart B, et al. Ghrelin secretion is unrelated to diet composition in cats. In: Proceeding ACVIM forum, San Antonio TX, 2008: 352 (abst).

Martin L, Siliart B, Dumon H, et al. Leptin body fat content and energy expenditure in intact and gonadectomized adult cats: a preliminary study. J Anim Physiol Anim Nutr 2001; 85:195-199.

Martin L, Siliart B, Dumon H, et al. Spontaneous hormonal variations in male cats following gonadectomy. J Fel Med Surg 2006a; 8: 309-314.

Martin L, Siliart B, Dumon H, et al. Hormonal disturbances associated with obesity in dogs. J Anim Physiol Anim Nutr 2006b; 90:355-360.

Martin L, Siliart B. Hormonal consequences of neutering in the cat. Waltham Focus 2005; 15: 32-35.

Mattes RD, Hollis J, Hayes D, et al. Appetite: measurement and manipulation misgivings. J Am Diet Assoc 2005; 105 (5 Suppl 1): S87-97.

McCay CM, Crowell MF, Maynard LA. The effect of retarded growth upon the length of life span and upon the ultimate body size. J Nutr 1935; 10: 63-79.

McGreevy PD, Thomson PC, Pride C, et al. Prevalence of obesity in dogs examined by Australian veterinary practices and the risk factors involved. Vet Rec 2005; 156: 695-707.

Melloul D, Marshak S, Cerasi E. Regulation of insulin gene transcription. Diabetologia 2002; 45: 309-326.

Montoya JA, Morris PJ, Bautisa I, et al. Hypertension: A risk factor associated with weight status in dogs. J Nutr 2006; 136: 2011S-2013S.

National Research Council of the National Academies. Nutrient requirements of dogs and cats. Washington, DC: The National Academies Press, 2006.

Nagao K, Yanagita T. Conjugated fatty acids in food and their health benefits. J Biosci Bioeng 2005; 100:152-157.

Nelson RW, Himsel CA, Feldman EC, et al. Glucose tolerance and insulin response in normal weight and obese cats. Am J Vet Res 1990; 51: 1357-1362.

Nguyen PG, Dumon HJ, Siliart BS, et al. Effects of dietary fat and energy on body weight and composition after gonadectomy in cats. Am J Vet Res 2004; 65: 1708-1713.

Nguyen P, Dumon H, Martin L, et al. Weight loss does not influence energy expenditure or leucine metabolism in obese cats. J Nutr 2002; 132: 1649S-1651S.

Pace N, Rathbun EN. Studies on Body Composition III. The body water and chemically combined nitrogen content in relation to fat content. J Biol Chem 1945; 158: 685-691.

Panciera DL, Thomas CB, Eicker SW, et al. Epizootiologic patterns of diabetes mellitus in cats: 333 cases (1980-1986). J Am Vet Med Assoc 1990; 197: 1504-1508.

Patel RV, Matthie JR, Withers PO, et al. Estimation of total body and extracellular water using single- and multiple-frequency bioimpedance. Ann Pharmacother 1994; 28: 565-569.

Perez Alenza MD, Rutteman GR, Pena L, et al. Relation between habitual diet and canine mammary tumors in a case-control study. J Vet Intern Med 2000a; 12: 132-139.

Perez Alenza MD, Pena L, del Castillo N, et al. Factors influencing the incidence and prognosis of canine mammary tumours. J Small Anim Pract 2000b; 41: 287-291.

Powers MA, Pappas TN - Physiologic approaches to the control of obesity. Ann Surg 1990; 211: 107.

Prentice AM, Goldberg GR, Jebb SA, et al. Physiological responses to slimming. Proc Nutr Soc 1991; 50: 441-58.

Raffan E, Holden SL, Cullingham F, et al. Standardized positioning is essential for precise determination of body-composition using dual-energy X-ray absorptiometry in dogs. J Nutr 2006 136: 1976S-1978S.

Ranen E, Zur G. Perivulvular dermatitis in a cat treated by episioplasty. J Small Anim Pract 2005; 46: 582-584.

Re G, Borghys H, Cuniberti B, et al. Microsomal transfer protein (MTP): a novel anti-obesity target in dogs. Proceedings of the 16th European College of Veterinary Internal Medicine Congress Amsterdam Netherlands 2006; 95-97.

Robertson ID. The influence of diet and other factors on owner-perceived obesity in privately owned cats from metropolitan Perth Western Australia. Prev Vet Med 1999; 40: 75-85.

Rolls BJ, Drewnowski A, Ledikwe JH. Changing the energy density of the diet as a strategy for weight management. J Am Diet Assoc 2005; 105: S98-S103.

Ronnett GV, Kim EK, Landree LE, et al. Fatty acid metabolism as a target for obesity treatment. Physiol Behav 2005; 85: 25-35.

Root MV, Johnston SD, Olson PN. Effect of prepuberal and postpuberal gonadectomy on heat production measured by indirect calorimetry in male and female domestic cats. Am J Vet Res 1996; 57: 371-374.

Russell K, Sabin R, Holt S, et al. Influence of feeding regimen on body condition in the cat. J Small Anim Pract 2000; 41: 12-17.

Scarlett JM, Donoghue S. Associations between body condition and disease in cats. J Am Vet Med Assoc 1998; 212: 1725-1731.

Scarlett JM, Donoghue S, Saidla J, et al. Overweight cats – prevalence and risk factors. Int J Obes Relat Metab Disord 1994; 18: S22-S28.

Scheltinga MR, Helton WS, Rounds J, et al. Impedance electrodes positioned on proximal portions of limbs quantify fluid compartments in dogs. J Appl Physiol 1991; 70: 2039-2044.

Singer P, Wirth M, Berger I. A possible contribution of decrease in free fatty acids to low serum triglyceride levels after diets supplemented with n-6 and n-3 polyunsaturated fatty acids. Atherosclerosis 1990; 83: 167-175.

Sloth C. Practical management of obesity in dogs and cats. J Small Anim Pract 1992; 33: 178-182.

Spray CM, Widdowson EM. The effect of growth and development on the composition of mammals. Br J Nutr 1950; 4: 332-353.

Strader AD, Woods SC. Gastrointestinal hormones and food intake. Gastroenterology 2005; 128: 175-191.

Sonnenschein EG, Glickman LT, Goldschmidt MH, et al. Body conformation diet and risk of breast cancer in pet dogs: a case-control study. Am J Epidemiol 1991; 133: 694-703.

Stanton CA, Hamar DW, Johnson DE, et al. Bioelectrical impedance and zoometry for body composition analysis in domestic cats. Am J Vet Res 1992; 53: 251-257.

Sunvold GD, Fahey GC Jr, Merchen NR, et al. Dietary fiber for cats: in vitro fermentation of selected fiber sources by cat fecal inoculum and in vivo utilization of diets containing selected fiber sources and their blends. J Anim Sci 1995a; 73: 2329-2339.

Sunvold GD, Fahey GC Jr, Merchen NR, et al. In vitro fermentation of selected fibrous substrates by dog and cat fecal inoculum: influence of diet composition on substrate organic matter disappearance and short-chain fatty acid production. J Anim Sci 1995b; 73: 1110-1122.

Sunvold GD, Hussein HS, Fahey GC Jr, et al. In vitro fermentation of cellulose, beet pulp, citrus pulp, and citrus pectin using fecal inoculum from cats, dogs, horses, humans, and pigs and ruminal fluid from cattle. J Anim Sci 1995c; 73: 3639-3648.

Szabo J, Ibrahim WH, Sunvold GD, et al. Influence of dietary protein and lipid on weight loss in obese ovariohysterectomized cats. Am J Vet Res 2000; 61: 559-565.

Van Goethem BE, Rosenweldt KW, Kirpensteijn J. Monopolar versus bipolar electrocoagulation in canine laparoscopic ovariectomy: a nonrandomized prospective clinical trial. Vet Surg 2003; 32: 464-470.

Watson TDG, Butterwick RF, Markwell PJ. Effects of weight reduction on plasma lipid and lipoprotein metabolism in obese cats. J Vet Intern Med 1995; 9: 214.

Weindruch R, Walford RL. The retardation of aging and disease by dietary restriction. Charles C Thomas Publishers Springfield, 1st ed. 1988: 436.

Weir JB. New methods for calculating metabolic rate with special reference to protein metabolism. J Physiol 1949; 109: 1–9.

Wilkins C, Long RC Jr, Waldron M, et al. Assessment of the influence of fatty acids on indices of insulin sensitivity and myocellular lipid content by use of magnetic resonance spectroscopy in cats. Am J Vet Res 2004; 65: 1090-1099.

Wilkinson MJ, McEwan NA - Use of ultrasound in the measurement of subcutaneous fat and prediction of total body fat in dogs. J Nutr 1991; 121: S47-S50.

Royal Canin nutritional information

Focus on:
L-carnitine

Obesity definition and origins

L-carnitine (sometimes know as vitamin B_T) is a water-soluble substance derived from two amino acids, lysine and methionine. It is synthesized in the liver in cats. L-carnitine has a role in energy production in cells.

Dietary sources with the highest content include meat products (50 mg/100 g in beef and 200 mg/100 g in lamb).

Formula

Carnitine exists in two spatial forms – D and L, but only the L form is biologically active. The D form tends to inhibit the action of the L form.

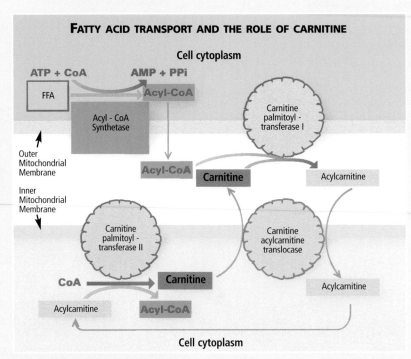

FATTY ACID TRANSPORT AND THE ROLE OF CARNITINE

Cell cytoplasm

ATP + CoA → AMP + PPi

FFA → Acyl-CoA

Acyl - CoA Synthetase

Outer Mitochondrial Membrane

Inner Mitochondrial Membrane

Acyl-CoA   Carnitine   Acylcarnitine

Carnitine palmitoyl - transferase I

Carnitine palmitoyl - transferase II

Carnitine acylcarnitine translocase

CoA → Carnitine

Acylcarnitine   Acyl-CoA   Acylcarnitine

Cell cytoplasm

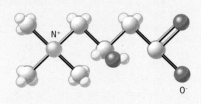

Biological role

L-carnitine is essential to the molecular system that transports long-chain fatty acids inside the mitochondria, where they are oxidized to produce energy.

Benefits of L-carnitine in preventing and treating obesity in cats

In obese cats, supplementation of L-carnitine (250 mg PO/12h), combined with a restricted caloric intake (36 kcal/kg of target weight) helped to accelerate weight loss *(Center et al, 2000)*. Cats receiving L-carnitine lost weight faster than cats in the control group: 23.7% in 18 weeks (1.3% per week) compared with 19.6% in the control group (1.0%/week).

Another study examined the potential role of L-carnitine in fat metabolism during the induction of hepatic lipidosis *(Blanchard et al, 2002)*. Spayed female cats received 40 mg/kg of L-carnitine per kg of food (control group) or 1000 mg/kg (study group). The concentration of L-carnitine increased significantly in the plasma, muscles and liver of cats in the study group. In addition, these cats exhibited better protection against the risk of hepatic lipidosis during fasting following obesity. Therefore, L-carnitine has a favorable impact on hepatic metabolism of obese cats.

References

Blanchard G, Paragon BM, Milliat F, et al. *Dietary L-carnitine supplementation in obese cats alters carnitine metabolism and decreases ketosis during fasting and induced hepatic lipidosis.* J Nutr 2002;132: 204-210.

Center SA, Harte J, Watrous D, et al. *The clinical and metabolic effects of rapid weight loss in obese pet cats and the influence of supplemental oral L-carnitine.* J Vet Intern Med 2000; 14: 598-608.

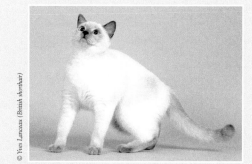

© Yves Lanceau (British shorthair)

Obesity is not generally a reason for the consultation, but rather something that is found during the consultation. Many owners do not want to know that their animal is obese, especially when the owner is also overweight. It can be very difficult to convince owners to maintain the animal's diet if there are no clear visible signs that the cat is losing weight.

Success factors of a weight loss diet for cats

Owner motivation

This is essential. The veterinarian has a very important role to play in convincing owners of the validity of a weight loss diet for overweight cats.

Recommended methods for motivating owners include:
- Getting them to palpate the cat, so they are aware of the fat deposits
- Putting the cat's excess weight into human terms (in equivalent weight); e.g. a cat that is 40% overweight is the same as a 165-pound man actually weighing over 230 pounds!
- Providing information on the following:
  - the health problems caused by excess weight
  - the benefits of a diet in terms of mobility and coat, etc.
  - the importance of the owner's involvement in the success of the animal's diet

NUTRITIONAL PLAN FOR:		
Name of the cat:	Neutered: ☐	Intact: ☐
Age:	Male: ☐	Female: ☐
Date:	Current weight:	

It can be very difficult to convince owners to maintain the animal's diet if there are no clearly visible signs that it is losing weight.

Your cat is overweight
Target body weight:
New diet recommended:

The choice of food and how it is given

Caloric intake will have to be reduced, but there are rules that need to be followed.

• USE ONLY low energy food in the diet

Reducing the daily ration of the typical daily diet will lead to deficiency of essential nutrients such as proteins, vitamins and minerals. This will result in negative consequences: muscle atrophy, poor quality skin and coat, weakening of immune defenses etc.

Furthermore, the choice of a specific food makes it possible to provide adequate meal volume and prevent the cat from developing undesirable behavior, such as agitation, incessant meowing or stealing food.

• DO NOT feed the cat leftovers

• WEIGH the daily ration precisely

Regularly weighing the daily ration is recommended, always with the same scales. Relying on volume measurements (i.e. cups) can result in accuracies and predispose to overfeeding.

• DIVIDE the daily ration

Dividing the daily ration into several servings provided multiple time during the day increases the post-prandial thermogenesis and so increases energy expenditure. Furthermore, it also reduces the feeling of hunger provoked by once daily feeding.

Royal Canin nutritional information

Exercise

Everything that can stimulate the cat to move is potentially beneficial:

- look for games that the cat enjoys
- put the food bowl somewhere else or place the kibbles throughout the home to encourage the cat to move around

Monitoring

Poor follow-up is a major cause of failure. Regular clinical observation makes it very easy to adjust the daily intake to the physiology of the individual cat.

The ideal is to have the owner visit every two weeks to weigh the animal and check that weight loss is advancing at 1-2% per week. If the pace is too slow (< 1%) the results will not be seen and if it is too fast (> 3% per week) there will be a greater risk of relapse and more extensive muscle atrophy at the end of the diet.

It is highly unlikely that the cat will lose weight at the same pace throughout the duration of the diet. Visits every other week will provide an opportunity to adjust the diet and modify the ration based on how weight loss is progressing.

A summary of the results at the end of the consultation provides a convenient way to view how the situation is progressing and how much still has to be done. It is also important to encourage the owner to continue with the dietary therapy.

Initial body weight:			Target body weight:		
Date	Actual body weight (kg)	Weight loss since the last visit (g)	Current diet	Daily food intake (g/day)	Exercise (0/+/++/+++)

Practical pointers for implementing and monitoring a weight loss diet

Weight loss phase

1- Determine the target weight

The target weight is based on the body condition score (BCS) at the first visit.

The BCS enables the estimation of excess weight as a percentage of body weight (see table on the right).

For example a cat weighing 7.2 kg has a BCS of 5/5. Its excess weight is therefore 40% of its actual weight. The target weight is accordingly 7.2/1.4 = 5.14 kg.

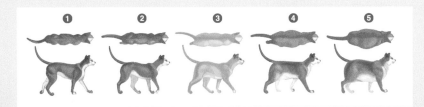

Body condition score	Excess weight
3.0 (ideal body score)	0%
3.5	10%
4.0	20%
4.5	30%
5.0	40%

2- Calculate the caloric intake needed to produce weight loss

Based on the BCS and the ideal body weight, a number of kilocalories per kg of target weight is determined as follows.

Body condition score	Adviced caloric intake
3.5 or 4.0	30 kcal
4.5 or 5.0	35 kcal

This degree of caloric restriction is required to obtain a weight loss of 1-3% per week. For example, the energy needs of a cat with a target weight of 5.14 kg and a BCS 5/5 is 35 x 5.14 = 180 kcal/day.

3- Convert the calorie intake into a daily ration

The daily ration in grams corresponds to the calorie intake as calculated divided by the energy density of the food.

E.g. if the energy density of the diet is 3,500 kcal/kg, the daily ration is 180 kcal/3 500 = 0.051 kg or 51 g/day.

A mixture of dry and wet food is possible, provided precise quantities of each food are prescribed.

4 - Adjust the ration during subsequent visits

The ideal rate of weight loss is 1-2% per week. A diet is generally maintained for several months. Regular visits will provide opportunities to assess the suitability of the energy intake and adjust the pace of weight loss where necessary (if weight loss per week is > 3% or < 1%).

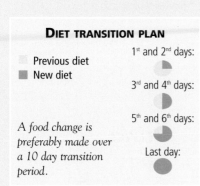

DIET TRANSITION PLAN

☐ Previous diet
■ New diet

1st and 2nd days:

3rd and 4th days:

5th and 6th days:

Last day:

A food change is preferably made over a 10 day transition period.

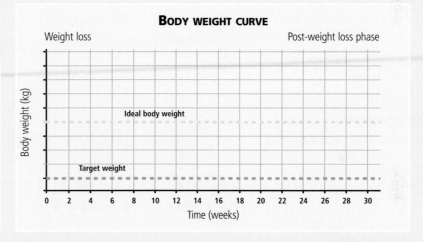

BODY WEIGHT CURVE

Weight loss   Post-weight loss phase

Body weight (kg)

Ideal body weight

Target weight

Time (weeks)

Post-weight loss phase

Once the target weight is achieved, the cat enters the critical weight stabilization phase. Reverting to the cat's original diet without controlling its intake will lead to rapid weight gain (rebound effect), while the final objective of a weight loss diet must be to stabilize the cat's weight long-term.

Changing or keeping the food during the weight loss phase

Keeping the same food makes it easy to see the gradual increase in the ration.

Gradually increasing the daily energy intake

Daily caloric intake must be gradually increased to reach the level at which the optimal weight will be maintained. This is increased by 10% every two weeks.

The cat must be weighed regularly during this phase to verify that the new caloric intake is not causing the cat to gain weight.

Establishing the ultimate ration

Caloric intake should ideally correspond to the cat's maintenance energy requirement (MER), which is easy to find:

MER (kcal/day) = 55 x body weight (kg)

Most cats that are predisposed to obesity stabilize their weight at a level below the theoretical MER. Rather than reverting to the original food, the best option is to select a food that accounts for the animal's risk factors for obesity (e.g. especially, neutering).

Royal Canin nutritional information

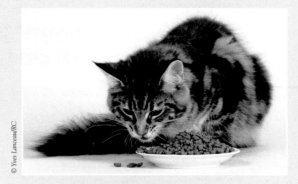

Complete intake of all indispensable nutrients must be achieved when energy consumption is reduced.

Key points
to remember:

Formulating a food that facilitates weight loss in cats

A nutritional food formulated to produce weight loss must obviously be low in energy, but there are other imperatives that need to be addressed.

Nutritional balance adapted to reduced energy consumption

The concept of balance is key. All intake of indispensable nutrients must be envisaged with respect to low consumption. The concentrations of trace elements, vitamins, indispensable amino acids and essential fatty acids must be higher than those in a maintenance food.

When reduced fat intake is necessary, foods with the lowest fat content are not always most effective. More than the fat content, it is vital that the calorie intake is reduced. If the effect of reducing the fat content is also to reduce the energy density of the food, other means are possible to achieve this. These include increasing the fiber and/or the water content, and adapting the physical structure of the food to reduce its density.

Increasing the protein: calorie ratio compared with a maintenance food

During the restriction phase, any deficiency in essential amino acids must be avoided, while any loss of lean mass must be minimized. The protein level must therefore take account of the animal's lower food intake during the weight loss phase.

Conversely, too high a protein level is not advisable, as high-protein foods can easily induce overconsumption when rationing is not strictly observed (see the sidebar).

L-carnitine supplementation

L-carnitine improves nitrogen retention and modifies the body mass in favor of lean mass. In obese animals, limiting the risk of the rebound effect is recommended after the weight loss diet.

Consideration for skin and joint diseases associated with obesity

A weight loss diet generally extends over many months, during which time it is important to consider the cat's general health. Diabetes, joint impairment and poor coat maintenance are the principal risks associated with obesity, so the nutritional approach must take them into account. The available responses include:

- reducing assimilable carbohydrate content and selecting a starch source with a low glycemic index (to reduce the development of insulin resistance)

- incorporating substances like glycosaminoglycans (chondroitin sulfate and glucosamine) to fight premature wear on joint cartilage in overweight animals

- strengthening nutritional intakes of key nutrients vital for optimal skin and hair coat (essential fatty acids, copper, zinc, vitamin A, etc.)

ROYAL CANIN

Dietary strategies to promote the sense of satiety in cats

Obesity introduction

Many low-calorie cat foods designed for weight loss diets are available in the veterinary market.

Unfortunately, these products are not always as successful as the manufacturers hope. The main problem is that the restricted intake changes the cat's behavior. Begging, constant meowing and even aggression may prompt owners to increase the ration, which compromises the success of the diet. The solution is to use a nutritional food that quickly provokes a feeling of satiety in the cat, thus reducing the chances that it will demand more food while keeping to the recommended ration. The aim of this study was to test different dietary strategies for promoting the sense of satiety in cats (reducing food volume and/or energy intake).

Materials and methods

The study was conducted on 16 adult cats of normal weight living in a cattery. These cats had always been fed with dry food. Four different dry foods were assessed in turn:

- a control food (protein: 41%; fat: 10%; TDF: 16%; metabolizable energy (ME): 3200 kcal/kg)

- a similar food but containing fiber with high water binding capacity (HWBC) (ME: 3115 kcal/kg)

- a high-protein food (HP) (protein: 46%; fat: 10%; TDF: 10%; ME: 3365 kcal/kg)

- a moderately high protein food (MHP) (protein: 36%, fat: 10%; TDF: 21%; ME: 3090 kcal/kg).

Four groups of 4 cats consumed these foods for 4 weeks, based on a Latin square protocol. After a 2-day transition, consumption was monitored for 5 days. The cats were fed ad libitum between 2 pm and 8 am next day (18 hours' food availability) with continuous access to water. Each cat was allocated its own bowl, access to which was controlled by means of an electronic collar. The criteria for assessing satiety were: total consumption (ingested energy: kcal/kg weight/day), satiety during feeding (size of meal: g/meal) and inter-meal satiety (time interval between two meals after consumption of at least 1 kcal during the preceding meal (min: sec/1 kcal). The data were expressed as mean ± standard deviation.

Results

The cats consumed all the food. The results are shown in the table below.

Conclusion

Very little information is available on cats (based on rigorously controlled studies). This study was able to demonstrate a "satiety effect" of different nutritional formulations based on the dietary behavior observed (energy consumed, meal size and interval between meals). Contrary to the findings in humans and dogs, high protein content is linked to increased consumption. Restricting protein content (by substituting protein for fiber) is therefore an original strategy for limiting spontaneous food ingestion. The nature of the fiber is important. Insoluble fiber with high water binding capacity has a satiety effect on the stomach.

These observations have been confirmed by recent clinical studies. In the future, they should serve as a basis in the formulation of foods for treating obesity in cats.

Reference

Servet E, Soulard Y, Venet C, et al. Evaluation of diets for their ability to generate "satiety" in cats. J Vet Intern Med 2008; 22: in press.

Criteria	Control	HWBC	MHP	HP
Energy intake (kcal/kg weight/day)	43.8 ± 5.9[ab]	41.9 ± 5.4[a]	39.6 ± 6.3[a]	48.9 ± 6.3[b]
Size of meal (g/meal)	6.5 ± 1.5[ab]	7.3 ± 1.8[bc]	6.1 ± 1.3[a]	7.7 ± 2.1[c]
Interval between 2 meals (min: sec/1 kcal)	07'11" [ab]	10'08" [c]	09'32" [bc]	05'43" [a]

The different letters signify that the data are significantly different (p<0.05).

Prof Ralf S. MUELLER
DMV, PhD,
Dipl. ACVD, FACVSc,
Dipl. ECVD

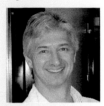

Dr Fabienne DETHIOUX
DMV, MRCVS

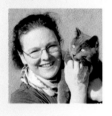

Nutritional dermatoses and the contribution of dietetics in dermatology

1 - Risk factors 53

2 - Nutritional dermatosis 54

3 - Metabolic diseases 64

4 - Nutritional therapy in dermatology 65

Conclusion 68

Frequently asked questions 69

References 70

Royal Canin nutritional information 72

ABBREVIATIONS USED IN THIS CHAPTER

DGLA: dihomo-gamma-linolenic acid
DHA: docosahexaenoic acid
EPA: eicosapentaenoic acid
IgE: immunoglobulin E
ME: metabolizable energy
PUFA: polyunsaturated fatty acid
TEWL: transepidermal water loss

Nutritional dermatoses and the contribution of dietetics in dermatology

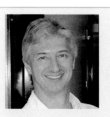

Prof Ralf S. MUELLER

DVM, PhD, Dipl. ACVD, FACVSc, Dipl. ECVD

Ralf Mueller graduated in Munich, Germany in 1985, and worked in several large and small animal practices before completing a residency in veterinary dermatology at the University of California, Davis in 1992. In 1992 he moved to Melbourne, Australia where together with his partner and wife Dr. Sonya Bettenay he was director in a veterinary dermatology specialist practice and consultant at the University of Sydney. In 1999, he became Assistant Professor in Veterinary Dermatology at the College of Veterinary Medicine and Biomedical Sciences, Colorado State University and finished his habilitation thesis at Zurich University, Switzerland. In 2004, he accepted a position as chief of the veterinary dermatology service at the University of Munich, Germany. He has published over 80 studies, articles, book chapters and books.

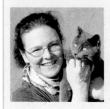

Dr Fabienne DETHIOUX

DVM, MRCVS

Fabienne Dethioux qualified as DVM in 1983 in Belgium, her native country (Université de Liège). In 1984, she started her own practice in Brittany where she stayed 12 years. In 1996, she moved to England and became Clinical Director for a corporate practice. She then worked as a free-lance consultant whilst being an emergency veterinarian in an animal hospital near Windsor. Since 1991, she is also a journalist and writes for several veterinary newspapers both in France and the United Kingdom. She has translated many articles, books and CD-roms. In 2003, she joined the Scientific communication department of Royal Canin. She now works with the International Division of the Group. Her main interest is dermatology.

The skin is a major organ with many different functions. Obviously, it is important for social interactions, giving each individual its characteristic appearance. It also serves as a barrier to maintain a stable internal environment. The skin plays a major role in the immune response to external factors, but also has a distinctive role in metabolism, sensory perception and temperature regulation amongst others. An imbalanced intake of nutrients such as amino acids, fatty acids, vitamins or trace elements disrupts the barrier function and the immune protection provided by the skin. The cat may become more sensitive to infection and may develop allergic reactions more easily. Skin and coat are a mirror of a cat's health and the quality of its food. Nutrition has a special place in feline dermatology, not only as an essential factor in the prevention of skin diseases, but also as a therapy for allergies and metabolic dermatopathies.

1 - Risk factors

► Breed specificities

In contrast to dogs where several skin conditions can be directly related to nutrition, there is little evidence of a link between a breed, nutrient and a specific disease in the feline literature. However, the Siamese seems to have an increased tendency to food allergy (see section on "Dietary hypersensitivities").

► Color of the coat

The color of a cat is a complex feature and influenced by genetics, environment (temperature, UV intensity and humidity all alter the coat's color by degrading the pigmentation) and nutrition (many nutrients play a role in pigment production).

The selection of colors in pure breed cats has become a specialist's hobby. Pigmentation is linked to the distribution of melanin in the hair shaft. Eumelanin (black to brown) and pheomelanin (red to yellow) combine to form the various shades of a cat's coat. The likelihood to produce eumelanin or pheomelanin is genetically determined but the enzyme which catalyzes the conversion from tyrosine can be a limiting factor. Pigment synthesis in the melanocytes depends on the supply of specific amino acids:
- phenylalanine and tyrosine are melanin precursors (**Figure 1**)
- cysteine is needed for the production of pheomelanin. It contains a high proportion of sulphur.

A dietary deficiency in tyrosine (or its precursor, phenylalanine) has been shown to induce a reddish change in the black hair of cats (**Figure 2**). Similarly the deep orange colored cats turned pale orange when experimentally fed a diet lacking tyrosine (*Yu et al, 2001*).

According to the *National Research Council (NRC)* 2006, the adequate intake for an adult cat corresponds to 0.38 g of phenylalanine and tyrosine per kg of metabolic weight i.e. a level of 3.83 g per 1000 kcal of metabolizable energy (ME). In a 4000 kcal ME/kg diet, it represents a minimum level of 15.3 g/kg of dry matter. To maximize black hair color, an equal quantity or greater of tyrosine to that of phenylalanine is required (*NRC, 2006*).

► Environmental factors

White cats are prone to squamous cell carcinoma, especially on the ear pinna and nose. Neoplastic changes are often preceded by solar dermatitis (sun burn). Solar radiation is the most ubiquitous mutagen but except indoor confinement, very little can be done to prevent exposure to sun light and the related free radicals. Research has shown the benefits of antioxidants in preventing UV light induced skin tumors and supplementation of antioxidants in the food may thus be useful (*Liebler & Burr, 2000*).

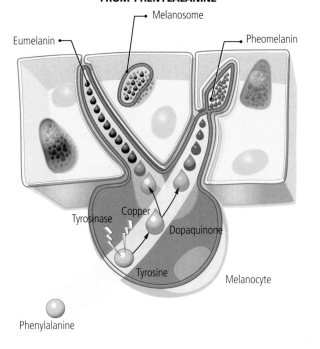

FIGURE 1 - SYNTHESIS OF MELANIN FROM PHENYLALANINE

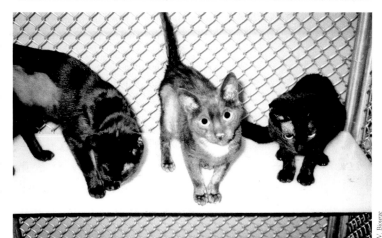

Figure 2 - Influence of dietary tyrosine intake on color intensity in black cats. *Diets that cause the color of hair to change from black to reddish-brown are associated with a reduction in melanin in hair, a decreased total melanin concentration and low concentrations of tyrosine in plasma.*

► Age and physiological states

In health and disease, age and physiological stage can greatly influence the quality of skin and coat. Growth, gestation, lactation, and old age will modify the nutritional requirements and are likely to interfere with the supply of nutrients to the cutaneous structures.

► Obesity

The physical constraints related to excessive weight reduce the ability of the cat to groom. This can lead to skin and/or coat conditions such as matted hair or anal sac impaction. Any other painful factor limiting the range of movement such as arthritis or idiopathic cystitis will have similar consequences.

► Concurrent diseases

The skin is a large organ requiring numerous macro and micro nutrients. Any condition interfering with the absorption of those nutrients will have consequences on the skin and coat (**Table 1**).

► Nutritional balance

There is no published evidence of "generic food skin diseases" in the cat but, usually, when the diet is unbalanced, cutaneous signs often precede weight loss (**Table 2**).

2 - Nutritional dermatosis

Nutritional dermatoses may affect cats in many different ways which are listed in **Table 2**.

► Specific nutritional imbalances

> Protein deficiency

Hair consists of 95% protein, and is rich in sulphur amino acids such as methionine and cystine. The growth of hair and renewal of the skin will absorb 30% of dietary protein (*Scott et al, 2001*). Any situation where protein requirements are not fulfilled will lead to poor coat and skin with generalized scaling, loss of pigment, poor hair growth, easy shedding, thin, dull and brittle hair.

Protein deficiency can either be due to a lack of supply i.e. poor quality diet, unbalanced home prepared food, low protein diet or to protein loss related to a systemic illness such as protein losing gastro-enteropathy, nephropathy, hepatopathy, or chronic bleeding. The reason for the nutritional imbalance needs to be identified and corrected.

TABLE 1 - VARIOUS CONDITIONS INTERFERING WITH THE ABSORPTION OF NUTRIENTS	
Nutrients	**Diseases or diets**
Proteins	Any systemic disease inducing protein loss or impairing protein absorption (i.e: gastroenteropathy, hepatopathy, nephropathy, chronic bleeding)
Fats	Digestive disorders, neoplastic or inflammatory diseases leading to malabsorption or maldigestion Renal or liver diseases
Vitamins and minerals	Polyuria-polydipsia, large consumption of white raw eggs, unbalanced vegetarian diets

TABLE 2 - CUTANEOUS SIGNS OF AN UNBALANCED DIET

- Widespread scaling
- Crusting (non allergic miliary dermatitis)
- Patchy alopecia
- Lack of pigment
- Poor hair growth
- Thin, brittle, dull hair
- Seborrhea oleosa
- Recurring pyoderma
- Impaired wound healing
- Chronic or recurrent otitis

> Essential fatty acid deficiencies

Essential fatty acids are not synthesized by the organism, thus their supplementation in the diet is "essential". They are primarily the precursors of two families of polyunsaturated fatty acids (PUFA), omega-6 fatty acids and omega-3 fatty acids.

PUFA fulfill five main functions:
- incorporation in the structure of the cell membrane, which gives it its flexibility and permeability
- production of eicosanoids (leukotrienes, prostaglandins, etc.)
- maintenance of the skin barrier permeability (especially omega-6 fatty acids)
- cholesterol metabolism and transport
- immunomodulation through an influence on antigen presenting cells and T lymphocytes

PUFA deficiencies are observed in animals suffering from malassimilation or animals fed with poor-quality diets or diets that have been overheated for a lengthy period. The cutaneous signs are xerosis, dull hair and a keratoseborrheic disorder. The response to PUFA supplementation is rapid.

- **Linoleic acid**, a precursor of omega-6 fatty acids, is abundant in most vegetable oils. It represents more than 70% of the fatty acids in evening primrose oil and more than 50% in sunflower oil, corn and soy oils.

DERMATOLOGICAL CONSEQUENCES OF SOME SPECIFIC DEFICIENCIES IN AMINO-ACIDS IN DOMESTIC SHORT HAIR CATS

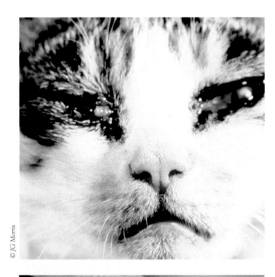

Dermatological consequences of isoleucine deficiency in a short hair cat. Note the crusty material around the eyes, nose pad and mouth. The hair coat is rough. In this kitten, bilateral conjunctivitis and bacterial infection with staphylococci suggest impaired resistance to common dermal bacteria.

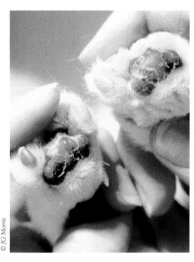

Isoleucine deficiency resulted in desquamation of the outer layer of the epidermis on the pads of the paws with cracking.

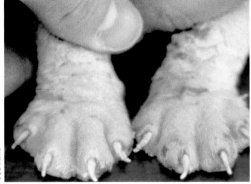

Dermatological consequences of a deficiency of sulphur containing amino-acids in a domestic short hair cat. Note the hyperkeratosis and swelling of the paws.

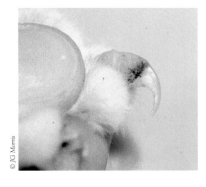

Deficiency of sulphur containing amino-acids. Swelling, reddening and hyperkeratosis of the nail bed.

55

Cats are deficient in Δ-6 desaturase which is the enzyme needed for the first step of the transformation of linoleic acid into arachidonic acid. Thus linoleic acid and arachidonic acid are both essential nutrients for the cat **(Figure 3)**.

- *Alpha linolenic acid*, a member of the omega-3 fatty acids, is found in green vegetables, fruits, grasses and plankton, and in concentrated form in the oil of plants like soy, flax, or linseed. The oils of fish from cold waters contain very high levels of two long-chain fatty acids derived from alpha linolenic acid: eicosapentaenoic acid (EPA) and docosahexaenoic acid (DHA) **(Figure 3)**. These two fatty acids participate in the fluidity of the cell membranes.

In addition to their anti-inflammatory, anti-neoplastic, immuno-stimulant, and cardio-protective properties, omega-3 fatty acids are also often used as anti-pruritic agents. Even in situations of an open wound or post-surgery, the benefit of supplementation still outclasses the mild reduction of perfusion which could potentially impede the healing process *(Scardino et al, 1999)*.

> Zinc deficiency

Zinc is a key element in many cellular mechanisms. Considering the fast turn over of epidermal cells, zinc is particularly necessary for a healthy skin and coat. Zinc is also needed for the biosynthesis of fatty acids, for the metabolism of vitamin A and for the inflammatory and immune response. Absolute dietary deficiency has not been reported in the cat but absorption of zinc can be inhibited by excessive levels of calcium, iron or copper due to competition for the absorption channels. Phytate present in cereals chelates zinc and will reduce its dietary availability. Other conditions preventing the absorption of zinc such as enteritis can also lead to depletion of the metal but usually the symptoms of the protein deficiency will be clinically apparent before signs of zinc deficiency occur.

FIGURE 3 - HEPATIC SYNTHESIS OF LONG-CHAIN OMEGA-6 AND OMEGA-3 FATTY ACIDS FROM THEIR RESPECTIVE PRECURSORS

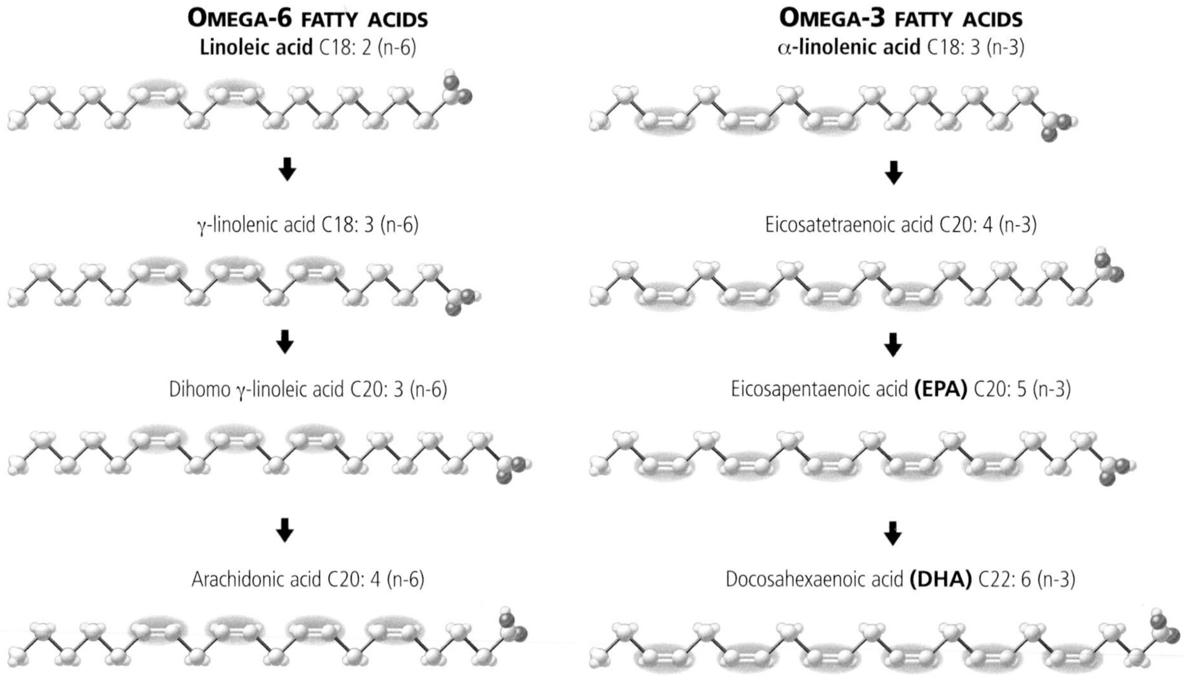

OMEGA-6 FATTY ACIDS
Linoleic acid C18: 2 (n-6)

OMEGA-3 FATTY ACIDS
α-linolenic acid C18: 3 (n-3)

γ-linolenic acid C18: 3 (n-6)

Eicosatetraenoic acid C20: 4 (n-3)

Dihomo γ-linoleic acid C20: 3 (n-6)

Eicosapentaenoic acid **(EPA)** C20: 5 (n-3)

Arachidonic acid C20: 4 (n-6)

Docosahexaenoic acid **(DHA)** C22: 6 (n-3)

> Vitamin E deficiency

Pansteatitis (synonyms: feline vitamin E deficiency, vitamin E deficiency steatitis or yellow fat disease) is characterized by diffuse nodules of fat or fibrous tissue, especially in the groin or on the ventral abdomen. The cat is depressed, febrile, and reluctant to move or jump. Palpation is painful due to inflammation of the subcutaneous fat. Nutritional pansteatitis has been reported in young and obese cats fed a diet containing large amounts of unsaturated fatty acids and/or insufficient vitamin E. Canned red tuna, sardines, herring and cod but also diets based on pig brain have been incriminated. Inactivation of vitamin E can occur during food processing or by fat oxidation. A case of pansteatitis associated with a pancreatic tumor has been described (*Fabbrini et al, 2005*).

Histologically, the subcutaneous fat will exhibit ceroid deposits which are pathognomonic of the condition. In lesions without ceroid, specific staining will have to be performed to differentiate pansteatitis from pancreatic or traumatic panniculitis (*Gross et al, 2005*).

© Renner/RC/Bengal

Cats have high requirements in terms of water-soluble B vitamins and they are unable to convert β-carotene into retinol (active form of vitamin A). These characteristics show that cats are adapted to a carnivorous diet: under natural conditions, they do not lack these vitamins since they are present in large quantities in animal tissues.

> Vitamin A deficiency

Cats are unable to convert β-carotene from plants to vitamin A and thus need to receive preformed vitamin A. Among several functions, vitamin A is required for ocular function but also for skin turn over. With vitamin A deficiency, the cat will exhibit a poor coat, alopecia and generalized scaling. The supply of a balanced, meat containing diet is usually sufficient to cure the condition. Vitamin A supplements are not recommended in the cat when fed a complete food because of the risk of hypervitaminosis A.

> Hypervitaminosis A

This condition was rather common in the past when cats were fed raw liver. It is still seen occasionally when the owner gives large amounts of cod liver oil supplement. The signs are mainly osteo-articular due to the cat's inability to move. As a consequence, the cat will be unable to groom properly, resulting in an unkempt, matted coat.

> Vitamin B deficiency

B complex vitamins are treated as a group. They are water soluble vitamins that cannot be stored. Biotin, riboflavin, niacin, inositol, pantothenic acid and pyridoxine are important for the quality of the skin barrier and deficiencies will lead to dry flaky seborrhoea accompanied by alopecia, anorexia, weight loss and pruritus.

Biotin deficiency sometimes occurs with consumption of numerous uncooked eggs. The avidin in the egg white binds to biotin and blocks its absorption. This will lead to a papulocrustous dermatitis.

A deficiency in riboflavin will lead to head and neck alopecia in cats. Niacin deficiency has also been described in cats fed a low protein high corn diet. Niacin and pyridoxine deficiencies can be produced experimentally. However, appropriately formulated commercial pet food contains high quantities of these vitamins.

Supplementation of B vitamins might be necessary with anorexia or polyuria. Vitamin B complex can be found in brewer's yeast and in balanced commercial food. Certain B vitamins work in synergy with histidine to improve the barrier function of the epidermis and decrease the TEWL (transepidermal water loss) (*Watson et al, 2006*).

TABLE 3 - VARIOUS CLINICAL EXPRESSIONS OF ADVERSE FOOD REACTIONS IN CATS

Cutaneous problems	Miliary dermatitis Self-induced alopecia Head & neck pruritus Eosinophilic granuloma
Gastrointestinal problems	Vomiting Diarrhea Flatulence Weight loss

> Dietary hypersensitivities

The term dietary hypersensitivity or food allergy is used by many veterinarians and owners as a broad term to describe any immunological and non-immunological reactions to ingredients of the diet that result in a clinical adverse reaction in an otherwise healthy cat. This adverse reaction may occur in the form of gastrointestinal problems and/or cutaneous abnormalities typically associated with self trauma due to pruritus (**Table 3**).

In the cat, adverse food reactions are considered to be relatively more common than in the dog (*Scott et al, 2001*). In one search of feline records in a number of veterinary colleges, feline adverse food reaction occurred in 10% of the patients presented with allergic skin disease (*Chalmers & Medleau, 1989*). It was the second most common disorder after flea bite hypersensitivity. However, another more recent report suggested atopic dermatitis to be much more common than adverse food reaction (73 versus 23% of 90 cats) (*Prost, 1998*). This may reflect the different location, different setting of private dermatology referral practice versus veterinary teaching hospitals, the increased awareness of other hypersensitivities besides flea hypersensitivity in the cat, and/or owners increasingly willing to pursue involved diagnostic procedures for their pets. The prevalence of food hypersensitivity in humans is reported to be approximately 10% in infants (*Bock, 1987*) and 2% in adults (*Young et al, 1994*). No such data is available for cats to the authors' knowledge.

> Etiology

In humans, non-immunological food reactions like toxic food reactions (e.g. toxins secreted by *Salmonella spp.*), pharmacologic reactions (e.g. caffeine) and metabolic reactions (e.g. lactase deficiency) comprise the majority of food-related problems (*Sampson, 2003*). The term hypersensitivity is used more stringently only for immunologically mediated reactions to food ingredients. Type I hypersensitivities are most common, although type IV mediated food hypersensitivities and mixed forms have been described (**Figure 4**).

In cats, type I hypersensitivity has been presumed as edema is the predominant clinical sign in some cats (*Walton, 1967*). However, in most clinical cases, the pathophysiological mechanism is not determined and adverse food reaction is diagnosed exclusively by the association between diet and clinical signs.

FIGURE 4 - PATHOGENESIS OF ADVERSE FOOD REACTION

Adverse food reactions (AFR)

Immunological AFR (Hypersensitivities)
- Type I (immediate) hypersensitivity
- Type IV (delayed) hypersensitivity

Non-immunological AFR
- Metabolic food reaction
- Pharmacologic food reaction
- Toxic food reaction

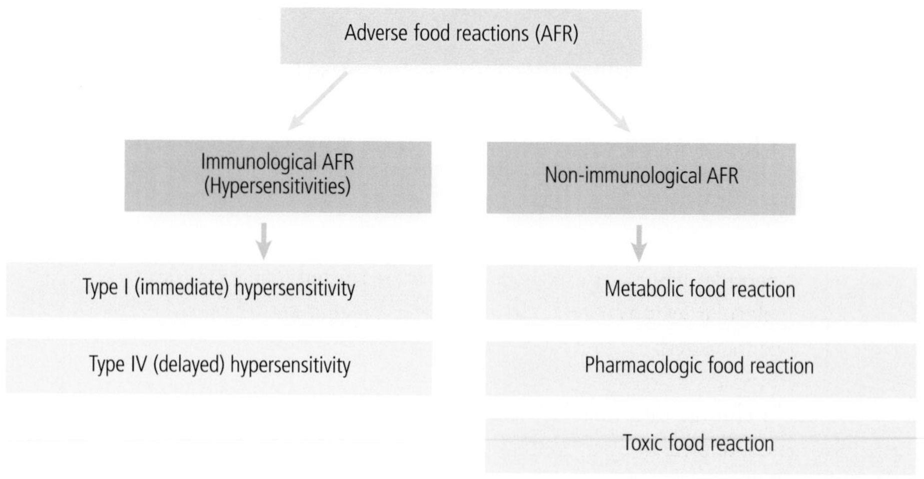

> Break in immune tolerance

In healthy humans, intact food antigens penetrate the gastrointestinal tract and enter the circulation without any clinical signs because most individuals develop tolerance to ingested antigens. This tolerance may be based on the induction of regulatory T cells (*Smith et al, 2000; Zivny et al, 2001*) or T cell anergy (where T cells are stimulated by antigen presenting cells via MHC class II molecules but without appropriate costimulatory signals) (*Chehade & Mayer, 2005*). Maintenance of this immune tolerance depends on a variety of factors listed in **Table 4**.

In humans with a genetic predisposition for atopy, class switching of B cells leads to the production of antigen-specific IgE. A breakdown in oral tolerance and development of hypersensitivity may occur when food allergens penetrate the mucosal barrier and reach IgE antibodies bound to mast cells. Degranulation of these mast cells leads to mediator release, inflammatory cell influx and subsequent clinical signs. In the cat, little is known about the mechanisms underlying oral tolerance and hypersensitivity.

> Dietary allergens

In three studies the most common allergens involved based on provocative challenge were fish, beef and dairy products (*Guaguere, 1993; Walton, 1967; White & Sequoia, 1989*). One third of the cats could not tolerate any commercially prepared diet without recurrence of clinical signs. A list of reported offending allergens is given in **Table 5**.

In one study, almost 30% of 55 cats with chronic gastrointestinal problems showed food hypersensitivity (*Guilford et al, 2001*). Half of these cats reacted to more than one protein. The clinical feature identified to be most sensitive for the diagnosis of adverse food reaction was the concurrent occurrence of gastrointestinal and cutaneous signs.

In humans and dogs, the major food allergens identified so far have been water soluble glycoproteins with molecular weights ranging from 10-70 kD (*Martin et al, 2004; Sampson, 2003*). No such data is available for the feline to the authors' knowledge.

Predisposing factors

Many factors may be involved in the development of feline food hypersensitivity.

Genetic predisposition

In two studies, Siamese or Siamese cross breeds accounted for approximately 30% of the cases and a genetic predisposition for those cats was proposed (*Carlotti et al, 1990; Rosser, 1993*). The relative risk factor of Siamese for food hypersensitivity in one study was 5.0 (*Rosser, 1993*). In the other report, 3 of 10 cats with adverse food reactions were Siamese cats (*Carlotti et al, 1990*).

Maldigestion

Dietary proteins are typically broken down by gastric and intestinal enzymes into amino acids and small peptides which are assimilated by the intestinal mucosa. If digestion is defective, the molecular weight of the proteins is much higher and the risk for break down of tolerance increased.

This explains why chronic intestinal inflammatory disease may be conducive to the development of dietary hypersensitivity. However, if

TABLE 4 - FACTORS INFLUENCING THE MAINTENANCE OF IMMUNE TOLERANCE (Chehade & Mayer, 2005)
Antigen dose High dose: T cell anergy Low dose: activation of regulatory T cells
Antigen form Soluble antigens are tolerated better than particulate antigens
Host genetics **Commensal flora** **Host age** **Gastrointestinal barrier function**

TABLE 5 - ALLERGENS INVOLVED IN FELINE ADVERSE FOOD REACTIONS	
Beef	Eggs
Chicken	Fish
Clam juice	Horse
Cod liver oil	Lamb/Mutton
Commercial foods	Pork
Dairy products	Rabbit

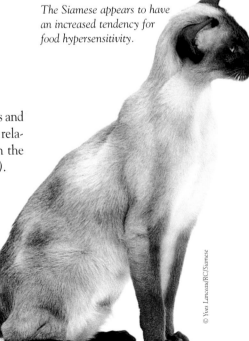

The Siamese appears to have an increased tendency for food hypersensitivity.

© Yves Lanceau/RC/Siamese

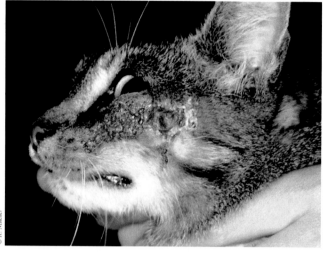

Figure 5 - Consequences of pruritus in a domestic short hair cat. *Face, head, pinnae and neck can all be affected in various combinations.*

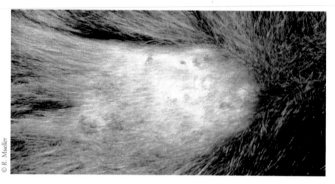

Figure 6 - Characteristic lesion of miliary dermatitis in a domestic short hair cat. *Small papules and crusts on the trunk characteristic of military dermatitis.*

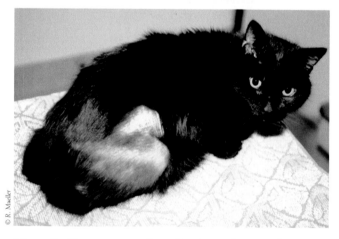

Figure 7 - Consequences of an allergic pruritus in a domestic short hair cat. *Noninflammatory alopecia on the flanks and lateral thighs.*

the gastrointestinal inflammation seen in cats with chronic bowel problems was originally due to other causes and led to food hypersensitivity or if this hypersensitivity is solely responsible for the inflammatory changes is not known at this point.

Other hypersensitivities

Concurrent hypersensitivities such as flea bite hypersensitivity or atopic dermatitis are known in dogs with dietary intolerance and may also be a complicating factor in cats. In one of the first reports studying feline food hypersensitivity, 3 of 14 cats had concurrent hypersensitivities (*White & Sequoia, 1989*). In a recent article, 6 of 16 cats with allergies were diagnosed with a combination of adverse food reaction and atopic dermatitis (*Waisglass et al, 2006*). Another report described 90 allergic cats, 16 cats had an exclusive adverse food reaction, 4 cats had concurrent atopic dermatitis and adverse food reaction and one cat was additionally allergic to fleas (*Prost, 1998*). Thus almost a quarter of cats with an adverse food reaction had concurrent hypersensitivities.

Clinical features

In the cat, clinical signs of adverse food reactions vary from pruritus with associated self trauma, eosinophilic granuloma, respiratory signs to gastrointestinal problems.

Head and neck pruritus

Head and neck pruritus was reported in cats with dietary hypersensitivity (*Guaguere, 1993; Medleau et al, 1986; Stogdale et al, 1982*). Alopecia, crusting, erosions and ulcerations are seen in the affected area as a consequence of self trauma (**Figure 5**). Pruritus is often severe and may be non-responsive to medical therapy. Secondary infections with bacteria or yeast are not uncommon. Pruritus and thus lesions can spread to other body sites and become generalized with time.

Miliary dermatitis

Small papules and crusts either localized (frequently on the head and neck) (**Figure 6**) or generalized are also seen with dietary hypersensitivities (*Mueller, 2000, Scott et al, 2001*). In one study, 21% of the cats with adverse food reaction showed this reaction pattern (*White & Sequoia 1989*). In another study, almost half of the cats with adverse food reactions had military dermatitis (*Carlotti et al, 1990*).

Non-inflammatory alopecia

Self-induced, bilaterally symmetrical alopecia with no macroscopic lesions is also a common reaction pattern associated with feline adverse food reaction (*Mueller, 2000; Scott et al, 2001*). Most commonly affected sites are the ventrum, inguinal area, thighs and flanks (**Figure 7**) Owners may or may not observe excessive grooming as a cause of the alopecia, as some cats do not exhibit that behavior in the presence of humans ("closet groomers"). In one report, 10% of all cats with adverse food reaction showed exclusively alopecia. In another report of 21 cats with presumptive psychogenic alopecia, adverse food reaction was diagnosed in more than half of the cats (*Waisglass et al, 2006*).

Eosinophilic granuloma

Eosinophilic plaques are the most frequently reported lesion of the eosinophilic granuloma complex in cats with adverse food reactions, but other lesions such as linear granuloma have been reported (*Carlotti et al, 1990; White & Sequoia, 1989*). Eosinophilic plaques are well circumscribed, erythematous, severely pruritic and often ulcerated plaques typically on the abdomen or medial thighs (**Figure 8**). Linear granulomas are non pruritic, raised, firm, yellowish plaques, most commonly on the caudal thighs (**Figure 9**).

Gastrointestinal problems

Vomiting, diarrhea and/or flatulence may be clinical signs of feline adverse food reaction (*Guilford et al, 2001; Stogdale et al, 1982*). Vomition may occur within minutes after eating or hours after the meal and often occurs infrequently. In many cats, diarrhea is due to large bowel dysfunction and thus excessive straining to defecate, mucus and/or blood in the feces may be seen. In one study of 55 cats with chronic gastrointestinal problems, almost one third were diagnosed as food sensitive based on resolution of clinical signs with an elimination diet and recurrence of those signs, when challenged with the previous diet. Most of these cats had a history of vomiting (56%) and a quarter of the cats exhibited chronic diarrhea. The remaining 3 cats had both clinical signs (*Guilford et al, 2001*).

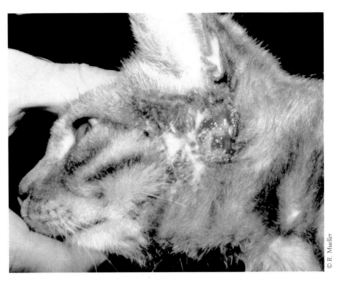

Figure 8 - Facial eosinophilic plaque in a domestic short hair cat.

Diagnosis

Cutaneous signs of feline adverse food reactions usually present themselves as reaction patterns with a number of possible underlying causes, thus a thorough diagnostic work-up is essential in these patients. The list of differential diagnoses depends on the presenting cutaneous reaction pattern and is shown in **Table 6**. Diagnostic tests or trial therapies to rule out differential diagnoses depend on the presenting signs and may include evaluation of cutaneous cytology, superficial and deep skin scrapings, fungal cultures, ectoparasite treatment trials and skin biopsies.

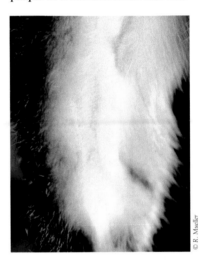

Figure 9 - Linear granuloma on the caudal thigh of a domestic short hair cat.

TABLE 6 - IMPORTANT DIFFERENTIAL DIAGNOSES OF CUTANEOUS REACTION PATTERNS ASSOCIATED WITH FELINE ADVERSE FOOD REACTIONS

Reaction pattern	Differential diagnoses
Miliary dermatitis	• Allergies (flea bite hypersensitivity, atopic dermatitis, adverse food reaction, mosquito-bite hypersensitivity) • Ectoparasites (scabies, cheyletiellosis, ear mites) • Infections (dermatophytosis, bacterial infection) • Immune-mediated diseases (pemphigus foliaceus) • Neoplasia (mast cell tumor)
Self-induced alopecia	• Allergies (flea bite hypersensitivity, atopic dermatitis, adverse food reaction) • Psychogenic alopecia • Drug reaction
Head & neck pruritus	• Allergies (atopic dermatitis, adverse food reaction) • Ectoparasites (scabies, ear mites) • Otitis externa • Neoplasia (epitheliotrophic T cell lymphoma)
Eosinophilic granuloma	• Allergies (flea bite hypersensitivity, atopic dermatitis, adverse food reaction) • Idiopathic eosinophilic granuloma

TABLE 7 - EXAMPLES OF PROTEIN SOURCES FOR ELIMINATION DIETS IN CATS	
• Duck	• Pheasant
• Goat	• Rabbit
• Horse	• Venison
• Ostrich	

Intradermal testing/serum testing for food allergen-specific IgE

It is tempting to measure dietary allergen-specific IgE to identify the offending dietary allergen(s) and to use the results to choose a new diet. Although sometimes recommended by individuals and laboratories offering these tests, at this time there is no evidence available to the authors to justify such tests. In the dog, published data show that these tests are unreliable (*Jackson & Hammerberg, 2002; Jeffers et al, 1991; Kunkle & Horner, 1992; Mueller & Tsohalis, 1998; Wilhelm & Favrot, 2005*). In the cat, only one report evaluated serum antigen-specific IgE in cats with adverse food reactions (*Guilford et al, 2001*). Only half of the cats with confirmed adverse food reaction had a positive test result. The majority of cats either tolerated the food antigen that they had tested positive for or they had never been exposed to it and thus hypersensitivity seemed unlikely. Only 25% of the cats showed results that were consistent with the results of their elimination diet and re-exposures.

Home-prepared elimination diets

The only reliable means to diagnose adverse food reaction in the cat is currently a commercial or a home-prepared elimination diet with a protein source the cat has not been exposed to (*Mueller, 2000; Scott et al, 2001*). Examples of possible protein sources are given in **Table 7**. Such a diet is typically not nutritionally balanced, but may be fed in adult animals for short periods of time (for the trial period, up to 12 weeks) without clinically apparent adverse effects. The protein source should be boiled, grilled or prepared in a microwave. The method of preparation depends on the individual circumstances, owner and cat. Some cats will accept a mixture of a protein and a carbohydrate source, in these cases a combination of both may be fed. However, most cats will prefer a diet based on protein sources only. Although taurine levels in meat are sufficient for cats (*Wills, 1991*), particularly young animals on a home-prepared elimination diet may benefit from vitamin and mineral supplementation without flavors or additives (*Scott et al, 2001; Wills, 1991*).

Commercial elimination diets

As alternative protein sources are sometimes difficult to obtain and require preparation, some owners may only be willing to use a commercial diet. Although numerous hypoallergenic diets are on the market, it is important to remember that the frequency of an adverse reaction to a protein is first and foremost related to the frequency this particular protein is fed to our feline companions. Lamb, fish and chicken, in the past considered first choices for elimination diets, are sometimes reported to be implicated in adverse food reactions of individual cats. These ingredients can still be effective in individual patients but only food with proteins that exclusively come from selected sources that the patient was not exposed to previously are acceptable.

FIGURE 10 – LOWER ALLERGENICITY OF HYDROLYSED PROTEINS VERSUS INTACT PROTEINS

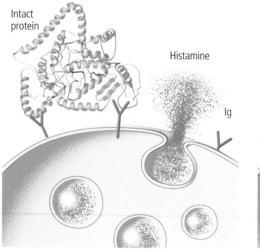

Intact protein

Histamine

Ig

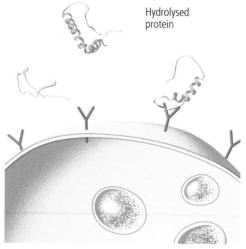

Hydrolysed protein

Degranulation of mast cells (which leads to the release of histamine, responsible for inflammation), results from the binding of two amino acid sequences or epitopes on two immunoglobulins located on the mast cell surface. The lower the molecular weight of the protein, the lower the likelihood of containing these two amino-acid sequences.

Alternatively, hydrolysed diets may be fed. These foods are formulated on the basis of protein hydrolysates. The purpose of the hydrolysation is to fractionate the proteins into small peptides of low molecular weight **(Figure 10)**.

These peptides are less antigenic and more digestible and thus offer less stimulation to the gastrointestinal immune system. Thus, hydrolysed diets are theoretically the most suitable commercial elimination diets. In the dog, studies have documented clinical improvement of allergic patients on hydrolysed diets *(Biourge et al, 2004; Loeffler et al, 2004; Loeffler et al, 2006)*. No such studies have been conducted in cats to the authors' knowledge.

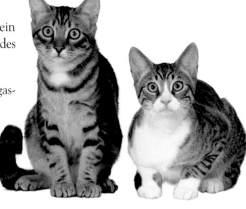

Concomitant treatments

Antipruritic and/or antimicrobial treatment may be indicated during the elimination diet. The cat may also have concurrent disease that requires continuous administration of drugs. In these cases, the prescription of flavored medication must be avoided, as small amounts of offending allergens may lead to clinical signs and prevent remission with the diet. If medication is usually administered with food, any potential protein source previously fed must be avoided.

If there are several cats in the household, either the hypersensitive cat must be prevented from access to the other cats' food, or all the cats must be given the same elimination diet.

© Yves Lanceau/RC/ European shorthair

Special circumstances

Multi-pet households

If more than one animal lives in the same household, then the other animals must be fed separately. This is only possible, if the animals are housed completely separately or if the other animals feed rapidly and thus will empty their food bowl in a very short time when placed into a room without the patient with suspected adverse food reaction. Otherwise it is prudent to feed all the animals in the household the same elimination diet to avoid accidents, where the patient consumes additional food from other pets that will most likely prevent clinical improvement.

Outdoor cats

Many cats either live predominantly outdoors or at least have free and unlimited access to the outside. They may wander into other back yards or houses and help themselves to pet food available there. Thus, ideally these patients need to be kept indoors for the duration of the diet, which can be difficult for the cat and owner.

Cats that typically hunt mice or birds will continue that habit during the dietary trial. Ideally these patients should be kept indoors for the duration of the elimination and challenge dietary trials.

Fussy eaters

Some cats may not like the new food offered to them during the diet trial. Cats can be determined and few owners will tolerate refusal of any given diet for more than a couple of days. With a home-prepared diet, warming up the food, salting it very slightly or preparing it differently may entice the cat to accept it. With commercial diets, a gradual change from the original food to the diet over three or four days may increase the chance of acceptance. If neither of these measures is helpful, a new elimination diet may need to be formulated.

Monitoring the diet

Compliance with the diet can be difficult not only considering the patient, but also the owner. A thorough client education supported by written instructions will increase the chances of success. Every family member and visiting friends must be informed of the need for strict adherence to the agreed diet trial.

A telephone call a few days after instituting the diet will be helpful in identifying possible problems. At that time, any

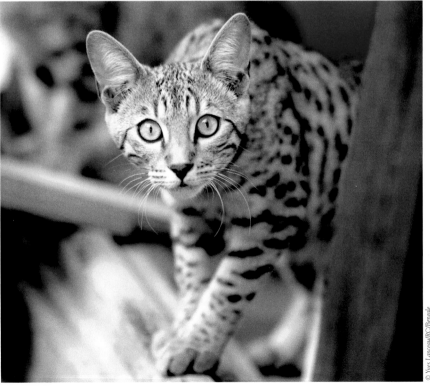

© Yves Lanceau/RC/Bengale

TABLE 8 - EXAMPLE OF PRURITUS SCORES	
Note	**Description**
0	Absence of pruritus
1	Discrete pruritus, not spontaneously described by the owner, less than one hour per day
2	Moderate pruritus, spontaneously described by the owner, one to three hours per day
3	Significant pruritus, three to six hours per day
4	Very significant pruritus, permanent, observed in consultation, sleeping problems

questions the owners may have are answered. Regular appointments after three to four and six to eight weeks are needed to monitor compliance, motivate and emotionally support the owner. Depending on the food and the cat, weight gain or weight loss may ensue. The owner must be instructed to monitor the cat's weight and if there is weight gain, diet intake should be decreased. If the patient loses weight, more food should be offered.

Length of the diet and interpretation of results

A diet trial should be conducted for six to eight weeks. If remission is achieved faster, then of course the diet can be discontinued earlier. After the diet trial, the previous food is fed again and should lead to a recurrence of clinical signs within hours to at the most, two weeks. At this point reinstitution of the elimination diet with subsequent resolution of clinical signs confirms the diagnosis of adverse food reaction. If however after two weeks no deterioration has occurred, then improvement was due to other factors such as treating secondary infections, change of seasons or concurrent ectoparasite treatment trial.

If there is spectacular improvement and complete remission occurs, judgement of success is simple. However, if there is partial improvement, interpretation is more difficult. Scoring systems for pruritus **(Table 8)** and/or lesions or digital photographs may be helpful in these patients. A provocative test is as important in these patients as in the cats with complete remission on the diet to ascertain the diagnosis.

Sequential rechallenge with the introduction of one protein source every one or two weeks allows correct identification of the offending allergen(s). Although many owners are reluctant to perform such a sequential rechallenge due to the associated emotional and organizational efforts, knowledge of the type of allergens involved frequently permits a wider choice of diets likely to be tolerated long term. Alternatively, the elimination diet may be continued long term. With a home-prepared diet, a nutritionist should be consulted to balance the diet and avoid nutritional deficiencies.

3 - Metabolic diseases

► Metabolic epidermal necrosis/necrolytic migratory erythema

Necrolytic migratory erythema is a skin disease in humans, that most commonly occurs secondary to a glucagon-secreting pancreatic tumor (*Tierney & Badger, 2004*). However, liver disease, internal malignancies other than pancreatic tumors and even glucocorticoid administration have been reported as causes of this disease (*Mullans & Cohen, 1998; Tierney & Badger, 2004*).

In the dog and cat, the terms diabetic dermatopathy, hepatocutaneous syndrome, metabolic epidermal necrosis or superficial necrolytic dermatitis have all been used, but a standard nomenclature has not been accepted (*Scott et al, 2001*). In the dog, the most common causes are liver disease, hyperadrenocorticism, diabetes mellitus, pancreatic tumors and phenobarbital administration (*Gross et al, 1993; March et al, 2004; Torres et al, 1997; Yoshida et al, 1996*). Two of the four cats reported in the literature had hepatopathies and the remaining two had pancreatic tumors (*Beardi, 2003; Godfrey & Rest, 2000; Kimmel et al, 2003; Patel et al, 1996*). The exact pathogenesis of metabolic epidermal necrosis has not been elucidated, but a deficiency of amino acids, fatty acids and/or zinc is discussed in the dog (*Outerbridge et al, 2002; Tierney & Badger, 2004*).

Clinical signs in the cat include stomatitis, gingivitis, alopecia, scaling and mild crusting. The skin lesions are bilaterally symmetrical and affect the axillae, ventrum, and inguinal area as well as the tail. Foot pads and mucocutaneous junctions were affected in one cat. Skin biopsies show diagnostic features of severe parakeratosis with underlying severe edema of the upper epidermis, and irregular epidermal hyperplasia with mild to moderate inflammation of the underlying dermis and appendages. Ultrasonography of the liver may reveal a diffusely coarse echotexture with a reticular pattern or a pancreatic mass.

Treatment of human necrolytic migratory erythema involves removal of the pancreatic tumor, skin lesions subsequently resolve without further therapy (*Chastain, 2001; Zhang et al, 2004*). In dogs, removal of a pancreatic tumor has also resulted in complete clinical remission (*Torres et al, 1997*). However, in most patients, advanced liver disease is the cause. In these patients, high quality proteins such as eggs in association with zinc and fatty acid supplementation may be helpful. In severe cases, intravenous amino acid infusion may lead to temporary remission (*Gross et al, 1993, Outerbridge et al, 2002*). However, if the underlying disease cannot be treated successfully, the prognosis is poor. To date, successful treatment of this disease in the cat has not been reported.

► Xanthoma

Feline xanthomas are benign granulomatous lesions with several possible causes (**Table 9**). Hereditary hyperlipoproteinemia is one possible etiology (*Grieshaber, 1991; Johnstone et al, 1990; Jones et al, 1986*). It may be due to congenital deficiency of lipoprotein lipase, an enzyme responsible for hydrolysis of the lipids in the chylomicrons and the release of free fatty acids in the peripheral tissues (*Bauer & Verlander, 1984*). Xanthomas have also been reported in cats with diabetes mellitus (*Jones et al, 1986; Kwochka & Short, 1984*). A case series of 5 cats described frequent high fat treats such as cream, butter and ice cream as possible causes, all of these cats responded to a low fat diet (*Vitale et al, 1998*). Leakage with extra- and intracellular deposition of lipoproteins from the capillaries into the tissue is suspected to occur in humans and may also occur in cats. Idiopathic feline xanthoma may also exist (*Denerolle, 1992*).

Lesions most commonly develop on the head, particularly the preauricular area and pinnae (**Figure 11**). Bony prominences may also be affected.

The diagnosis is confirmed histologically. A nodular to diffuse granulomatous inflammation with foamy macrophages and multinucleated giant cells is characteristic. Diabetes mellitus or excess dietary fat intake should be ruled out as underlying causes.

Treatment consists of addressing the underlying disease and feeding a low fat diet (< 25 % of calories of the diet provided by fat). If diabetes mellitus is treated successfully, the diet may be changed back to normal. In patients with idiopathic or congenital xanthomas, it may be prudent to continue the low-fat diet for the remainder of the pets life.

Lesions due to a specific underlying cause resolve spontaneously once the underlying cause is addressed successfully. A low-fat diet is recommended and will be particularly useful in cats with the idiopathic form of xanthoma.

TABLE 9 - CAUSES OF FELINE XANTHOMAS

- Diabetes mellitus
- Chronic administration of megestrol acetate
- Congenital lipoprotein lipase deficiency
- High dietary fat intake
- Idiopathic

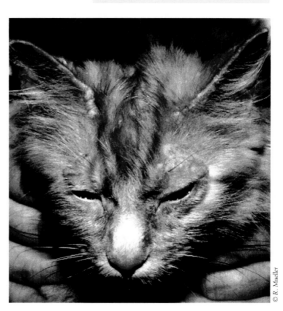

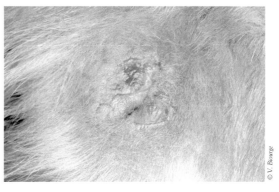

Figure 11 - A DSH cat with facial alopecia, erythema, and papules due to xanthoma. Clinical signs of xanthomas in cats include white to yellowish papules, plaques and nodules that may or may not be ulcerated.

4 - Nutritional therapy in dermatology

► Dull coat, xerosis

The coat's sheen is connected to the composition of sebum secreted by sebaceous gland secretions and stored in the hair follicles. The lipids in the composition of sebum are species and in the dog breed specific (*Dunstan et al, 2000*), but the production and the quality of the sebum is also influenced by food (*Macdonald et al, 1983*). Dryness of the skin (xerosis) is caused by decreased water content. The increased water loss through evaporation may be due to low humidity conditions of the environment or an increased transepidermal water loss. In cats, linoleic acid deficiency has been shown to be a possible cause for the latter (*Macdonald et al, 1983*).

► Color change of black coats to reddish brown

In some black cats, the coat color changes to a reddish brown. This color change is associated with low tyrosine plasma concentrations, has been induced in cats given a tyrosine-deficient diet, and is reversed by diets containing a high concentration of tyrosine or phenylalanine. Current dietary recommendations for dietary tyrosine and phenylalanine for kittens are below those required to support maximal melanin synthesis in black adult cats. The requirement appears to be greater than a combination of 4.5 g tyrosine plus 12 g phenylalanine/kg diet but less than 24 g phenylalanine alone/kg diet (*Yu et al, 2001*).

► Skin wound healing

To maximize wound healing and to be able to formulate appropriate nutritional supplements in the pre- and post-surgery period in humans, nutritionists have studied the stimulation of re-epithelialization and of the immune system to decrease the chance of secondary wound infections. A number of oral preparations are available in human medicine, but similar products for cats are not available to the authors' knowledge.

Protein and zinc deficiencies are associated with delayed wound healing and care should be taken to optimize protein and zinc intake in wounded animals (*Robben et al, 1999*).

Iron and vitamin C are involved in hydroxylation of proline, a major amino acid in the structure of collagen. Iron deficiency affects the quality of the scar tissue.

Omega-3 fatty acids have a positive effect on wound healing in dogs (*Scardino et al, 1999*). A vitamin E supplement helps protect PUFA's from oxidation. Similarly, the positive role of curcumin, aloe vera and bromelaine has been shown in the canine wound healing process (*Fray et al, 2004*). To the authors's knowledge, no such data exists for cats.

► Feline allergic skin disease

Feline atopic dermatitis is a multifactorial disease. However, in contrast to human or canine atopic dermatitis, the cat presents with a number of clinical reaction patterns (*Bettenay, 2000; Rees, 2001*) **(Table 4)**. Additional common causes for these reaction patterns are flea bite hypersensitivity and adverse food reactions (see above). Nutrition may be used in several ways in these feline patients.

A diet that does not contain adequate levels of tyrosine and/or phenylalanine to permit the complete synthesis of melanin induces a coat color change in black cats. The color becomes reddish brown.

> Reduction in inflammation with polyunsaturated fatty acids

Long chain polyunsaturated fatty acids have been shown to alleviate the symptoms of miliary dermatitis (*Harvey, 1993; Harvey, 1991; Lechowski et al, 1998*). The fatty acid profile in plasma of affected cats was different than that of normal cats and omega-3 supplementation increased plasma concentrations of EPA and DHA and decreased dihomo-gamma-linolenic acid (DGLA), corresponding to clinical improvement. A combination of fish oil (omega-3) and evening primrose oil (omega-6) had a higher response rate than fish oil alone (*Harvey, 1993*). Some cats with eosinophilic granuloma, another reaction pattern frequently associated with feline allergies, also respond to fatty acid supplementation (*Scott et al, 2001*).

© V. Biourge

> Prevention or control of dietary hypersensitivities

Up to 40% of cats with atopic dermatitis have concurrent adverse food reactions (*Waisglass et al, 2006*). Such possible dietary hypersensitivities may be addressed by either using food sources avoiding the offending protein allergens or by using a hydrolysed diet where the antigens are of such small size that an allergic reaction may be prevented in many patients.

> Re-establishment of the skin barrier

Defects in intercellular ceramides in canine atopic epidermis have been described and presumably allow increased transepidermal water loss, increased penetration by antigens and increased adherence of staphylococci similar to what is seen in human patients with atopic dermatitis. In vitro studies (keratinocytes cultures) conducted by the Waltham Centre for Pet Nutrition have shown that some nutrients (in particular nicotinamide, pantothenic acid, histidine, inositol and choline) improve the structure and the function of the skin. Others (pyridoxine and proline) stimulate the synthesis of ceramides (*Watson et al, 2006*) **(Figure 12)**.

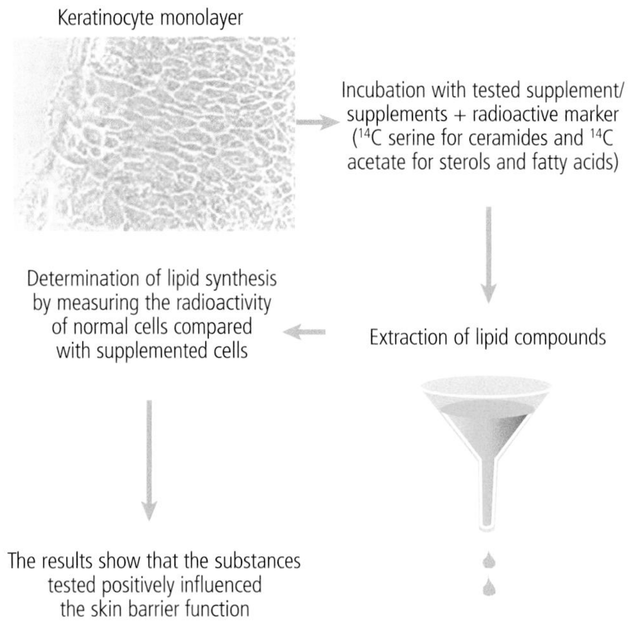

In vivo studies have confirmed this approach. After nine weeks of supplementation with a supplement composed of nicotinamide, pantothenic acid, histidine, inositol and choline, the cutaneous water loss was significantly reduced in atopic dogs. The reduction in water loss and so xerosis can have a positive effect of reducing allergen penetration, and also limit bacterial and fungal colonization, which may cause the development of atopic dermatitis. Unfortunately, no such reports exist for the cat to the authors' knowledge.

FIGURE 12 – MEASURING THE SYNTHESIS OF SKIN LIPIDS
(From Watson, 2003)

Keratinocyte monolayer

Incubation with tested supplement/ supplements + radioactive marker (^{14}C serine for ceramides and ^{14}C acetate for sterols and fatty acids)

Determination of lipid synthesis by measuring the radioactivity of normal cells compared with supplemented cells

Extraction of lipid compounds

The results show that the substances tested positively influenced the skin barrier function

► Miscellaneous skin diseases

> Urticaria pigmentosa

Essential fatty acids were reported to be helpful in the control of exacerbations of feline urticaria pigmentosa, a maculopapular eruption of the ventral trunk with a perivascular to diffuse mastocytic and eosinophilic infiltrate in the dermis (*Noli et al, 2004*).

> Dermatosparaxis/cutaneous asthenia

Dermatosparaxis is an inherited connective tissue disease characterized by excessive fragility and hyperextensibility of the skin. Because vitamin C is necessary in collagen synthesis, it may be useful in the treatment of feline patients with this disease. Although in contrast to dogs, two cats with dermatosparaxis treated with vitamin C did not improve (*Scott et al, 2001*), one of the authors has seen improvement in two cats with this syndrome treated with vitamin C.

> Feline acne

Feline acne is a disorder characterized by comedones and crusts on the chin and lips **(Figure 13)** and the idiopathic form is considered a disorder of follicular keratinization (*Scott et al, 2001*). It responds to a number of topical antimicrobial agents, but cats with recurrent feline acne have been reported to also benefit from fatty acid supplementation (*Rosenkrantz, 1991*).

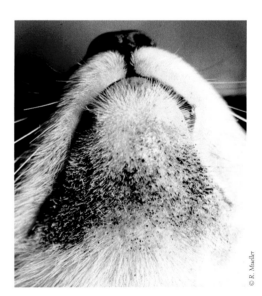

© R. Mueller

*Figure 13 - **Domestic short hair cat with acne.** Comedones and small crusts on the ventral chin.*

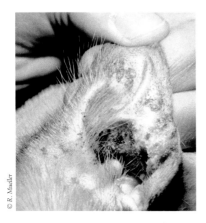

Figure 14 - A cat with pemphigus foliaceus. Crusts on the medial pinnae.

TABLE 10 - EXAMPLES OF NUTRITIONAL RECOMMENDATIONS FOR LIMITING THE RISK OF FOOD ALLERGIES IN CHILDREN
(Sampson, 2004)

- Breastfeeding for three to six months
- Use of hydrolysates if breastfeeding is not possible
- Avoidance of peanuts and seafood during pregnancy and breastfeeding
- Avoidance of high-risk foods (peanuts, hazelnuts, seafood) before three years of age

> Various immune-mediated diseases

Pemphigus foliaceus is a pustular and crusting skin disease **(Figure 14)** characterized by acantholysis of keratinocytes. Typically, immunosuppressive therapy with glucocorticoids or chlorambucil is recommended to treat feline pemphigus foliaceus. However, vitamin E and fatty acid supplementation have been reported to be useful in individual patients *(Scott et al, 2001)*. Similarly, vitamin E and essential fatty acids have been recommended as adjunctive treatment of feline discoid lupus erythematosus *(Scott et al, 2001)*.

► Prophylactic nutrition

In feline dermatology, nutritional interventions have been almost exclusively devoted to therapeutic functions. In human dermatology, nutrition is also used preventively. The problem with preventive nutritional intervention is the identification of the patient at risk. Although most cats kept as pets are domestic short hair cats and most diseases lack clear breed predispositions in the feline, some rare dermatoses show breed predisposition such as adverse food reactions in Siamese and thus may be suited to such interventions. Prospective controlled clinical studies are needed to evaluate the benefit of such an approach.

> Highly digestible foods

In human medicine, hydrolysates are mainly used in the prevention of adverse food reactions for high-risk children or their mothers to reduce the risk that clinical manifestations of atopy will develop **(Table 10)**. If such an approach is useful in feline medicine remains to be elucidated.

> Probiotics

In humans there is a significant difference between the intestinal flora of normal and that of atopic babies *(Bjorksten et al, 2001)*. Similarly, it has been shown, that supplementation of pregnant and breastfeeding mothers with *Lactobacillus rhamnosus* significantly decreases the clinical manifestations in their children *(Kalliomaki et al, 2003)*. In addition, supplementation with lactobacilli has improved the clinical signs of atopic children *(Rosenfeldt et al, 2003)*.

In the cat, the addition of probiotics in food or capsules presents technical problems. In a recent study, none of the probiotic supplements tested contained all the claimed bacteria *(Weese & Arroyo, 2003)*. However, it is possible to include probiotics in dry food and an effect on the feline immune response was observed after supplementation *(Marshall-Jones et al, 2006)*. If these probiotics could be used for the prevention or treatment of atopic disease awaits further study.

Conclusion

Food plays a fundamental role in cutaneous homeostasis and in the treatment of many inflammatory dermatoses. The study of diet is therefore an integral part of the dermatological history. The correction of dietary imbalances (with respect to fatty acids and tyrosine in particular) is a necessary factor in good dermatological therapy.

The treatment of many dermatoses involves the use of nutrients that reinforce the skin barrier function, or modulate the immune system, either as anti-inflammatory or as immunostimulatory agents. In the future, it is likely that more emphasis will be placed on the possible use of food for prophylactic purposes. Furthermore, the exact type and dose of optimal fatty acid supplementations and probiotics will need to be determined to greatly benefit our feline patients.

Frequently asked questions about the contribution of dietetics in dermatology

Q	A
Which nutritional deficiencies are most commonly implicated in feline dermatology?	Essential fatty acid and tyrosine deficiency are possible deficiencies leading to skin disease in cats.
Do cats get zinc deficiency?	In contrast to dogs, zinc deficiency has not been reported in cats.
Are adverse food reactions common?	In cats, adverse food reactions are more frequently seen than in the dog. An adverse food reaction should be considered particularly when head and neck pruritus are observed or there are concurrent gastrointestinal signs associated with the skin disease.
Which foods are the most likely to cause allergic reactions?	Fish, beef and dairy products are the most commonly reported food allergens in the cat. However, this may simply be due to the widespread use of these ingredients in cat food.
Is white meat less allergic than red meat?	This belief is incorrect. The color of the meat does not have any influence on its potential allergenic or hypoallergenic character. The risk increases with the quantity of meat ingested. Red meats such as venison are widely and successfully used as a basis for elimination diets, simply because these foods are not typically found in cat foods.
How do you diagnose atopic dermatitis in a cat?	Atopic dermatitis in the cat may present as a variety of cutaneous reaction patterns. These cutaneous reaction patterns in turn may be caused by many different diseases. Thus, the differential diagnoses for each patient with potential atopic dermatitis need to be ruled out prior to the diagnosis of atopic dermatitis. For example, all cats with potential atopy need to undergo strict flea control and an elimination diet to rule out flea bite hypersensitivity and adverse food reaction.
Can atopic dermatitis be controlled simply with PUFA supplementation?	Yes, but if the response is unsatisfactory after 6-12 weeks of treatment, other therapeutics should be used.
Can diet be the cause of non-inflammatory "endocrine" alopecia in the cat?	Years ago, non-inflammatory alopecia was considered a hormonal disease. However, true endocrine alopecia in cats is very rare. Subsequently, this disease was diagnosed as psychogenic alopecia. Some patients indeed develop psychogenic alopecia and responded to behavioral therapy. However, many of these cats are actually allergic cats; the overgrooming and alopecia is a response to pruritus. An elimination diet to rule out adverse food reaction is an essential diagnostic tool in every cat with non-inflammatory alopecia.

References

Bauer JE, Verlander JW. Congenital lipoprotein lipase deficiency in hyperlipemic kitten siblings. Vet Clin Pathol 1984; 13: 7-11.

Beardi B. Metabolische epidermal Nekrose (MEN) bei einer Katze. Kleintierpraxis 2003; 48: 37-40.

Bettenay SV. Feline Atopy. In: Bonagura JD, ed. Current Veterinary Therapy XIII. Philadelphia: WB Saunders Co., 2000; 564-569.

Biourge VC, Fontaine J, Vroom MW. Diagnosis of adverse reactions to food in dogs: efficacy of a soy-isolate hydrolyzate-based diet. J Nutr 2004; 134: 2062S-2064S.

Bjorksten B, Sepp E, Julge K, et al. Allergy development and the intestinal microflora during the first year of life. J Allergy Clin Immunol 2001; 108: 516-20.

Bock SA. Prospective appraisal of complaints of adverse reactions to foods in children during the first 3 years of life. Pediatrics 1987; 79: 683-688.

Carlotti DN, Remy I, Prost C. Food allergy in dogs and cats. A review and report of 43 cases. Vet Dermatol 1990; 1: 55-62.

Chalmers S, Medleau L. Recognizing the signs of feline allergic dermatoses. Vet Med 1989; 84: 388.

Chastain MA. The glucagonoma syndrome: a review of its features and discussion of new perspectives. Am J Med Sci 2001; 321: 306-20.

Chehade M, Mayer L. Oral tolerance and its relation to food hypersensitivities. J Allergy Clin Immunol 2005; 115: 3-12; quiz 13.

Denerolle P. Three cases of feline cutaneous xanthomas, in Proceedings 2nd World Congress in Vet Dermatol 1992; 84.

Dunstan RW, Herdt TH, Olivier B, et al. Age- and breed-related differences in canine skin surface lipids and pH. In: Thoday KL, Foil CS, Bond R, eds. Advances in Veterinary Dermatology. Oxford: Blackwell Publishing, 2000; 37-42.

Fabbrini F, Anfray P, Viacava P, et al. Feline cutaneous and visceral necrotizing panniculitis and steatitis associated with a pancreatic tumor. Vet Dermatol 2005; 16: 413-419.

Fray TR, Watson AL, Croft JM, et al. A combination of aloe vera, curcumin, vitamin C, and taurine increases canine fibroblast migration and decreases tritiated water diffusion across canine keratinocytes in vitro. J Nutr 2004; 134: 2117S-2119S.

Godfrey DR, Rest JR. Suspected necrolytic migratory erythema associated with chronic hepatopathy in a cat. J Small Anim Pract 2000; 41: 324-328.

Grieshaber T. Spontaneous cutaneous (eruptive) xanthomatosis in two cats. J Am Anim Hosp Assoc 1991; 27: 509.

Gross TL, Ihrke PJ, Walder EJ, et al. Skin Diseases of the Dog and Cat - Clinical and Histopathologic Diagnosis. Philadelphia: WB Saunders Co, 2005.

Gross TL, Song MD, Havel PJ, et al. Superficial necrolytic dermatitis (necrolytic migratory erythema) in dogs. Vet Pathol 1993; 30: 75-81.

Guaguere E. Intolérance alimentaire à manifestations cutanées: À propos de 17 cas chez le chat. Prat Med Chir Anim Comp 1993; 28: 451.

Guilford WG, Jones BR, Markwell PJ, et al. Food sensitivity in cats with chronic idiopathic gastrointestinal problems. J Vet Intern Med 2001; 15: 7-13.

Harvey RG. Management of feline miliary dermatitis by supplementing the diet with essential fatty acids. Vet Rec 1991; 128: 326-329.

Harvey RG. Effect of varying proportions of evening primrose oil and fish oil on cats with crusting dermatosis ("miliary dermatitis"). Vet Rec 1993; 133: 208-211.

Jackson HA & Hammerberg B. Evaluation of a spontaneous canine model of immunoglobulin E-mediated food hypersensitivity: dynamic changes in serum and fecal allergen-specific immunoglobulin E values relative to dietary change. Comp Med 2002; 52: 316-321.

Jeffers JG, Shanley KJ, Meyer EK. Diagnostic testing of dogs for food hypersensitivity. J Am Vet Med Assoc 1991; 198: 245-250.

Johnstone AC, Jones BR, Thompson JC, et al. The pathology of an inherited hyperlipoproteinaemia of cats. J Comp Pathol 1990; 102: 125-137.

Jones BR, Wallace R, Hancock WS, et al. Cutaneous xanthoma associated with diabetes mellitus in a cat. J Small Anim Pract 1986; 26: 33-41.

Kalliomaki M, Salminen S, Poussa T, et al. Probiotics and prevention of atopic disease: 4-year follow-up of a randomised placebo-controlled trial. Lancet 2003; 361: 1869-1871.

Kimmel SE, Christiansen W, Byrne KP. Clinicopathological, ultrasonographic, and histopathological findings of superficial necrolytic dermatitis with hepatopathy in a cat. J Am Anim Hosp Assoc 2003; 39: 23-27.

Kunkle G, Horner S. Validity of skin testing for diagnosis of food allergy in dogs. J Am Vet Med Assoc 1992; 200: 677-680.

Kwochka KW, Short BG. Cutaneous xanthomatosis and diabetes mellitus following long term therapy with megestrol acetate in a cat. Comp Cont Ed Pract Vet 1984; 6: 186-192.

Lechowski R, Sawosz E, Klucinski W. The effect of the addition of oil preparation with increased content of n-3 fatty acids on serum lipid profile and clinical condition of cats with miliary dermatitis. Zentralbl Veterinarmed A 1998; 45: 417-424.

Liebler DC, Burr JA. Effects of UV light and tumor promoters on endogenous vitamin E status in mouse skin. Carcinogenesis 2000; 21: 221-225.

Loeffler A, Lloyd DH, Bond R, et al. Dietary trials with a commercial chicken hydrolysate diet in 63 pruritic dogs. Vet Rec 2004; 154: 519-522.

Loeffler A, Soares-Magalhaes R, Bond R, et al. A retrospective analysis of case series using home-prepared and chicken hydrolysate diets in the diagnosis of adverse food reactions in 181 pruritic dogs. Vet Dermatol 2006; 17: 273-279.

Macdonald ML, Rogers QR, Morris JG. Role of linoleate as an essential fatty acid for the cat independent of arachidonate synthesis. J Nutr 1983; 113: 1422-1433.

March PA, Hillier A, Weisbrode SE, et al. Superficial necrolytic dermatitis in 11 dogs with a history of phenobarbital administration (1995-2002). J Vet Intern Med 2004; 18: 65-74.

Marshall-Jones ZV, Baillon ML, Croft JM, et al. Effects of Lactobacillus acidophilus DSM13241 as a probiotic in healthy adult cats. Am J Vet Res 2006; 67: 1005-1012.

Martin A, Sierra MP, Gonzalez JL, et al. Identification of allergens responsible for canine cutaneous adverse food reactions to lamb, beef and cow's milk. Vet Dermatol 2004; 15: 349-356.

Medleau L, Latimer KS, Duncan JR. Food hypersensitivity in a cat. J Am Vet Med Assoc 1986; 189: 692-693.

Mueller RS. Dermatology for the Small Animal Practitioner. *Jackson: Teton NewMedia, 2000.*

Mueller RS, Tsohalis J. Evaluation of serum allergen-specific IgE for the diagnosis of food adverse reactions in the dog. Vet Dermatol 1998; 9: 167-171.

Mullans EA, Cohen PR. Iatrogenic necrolytic migratory erythema: a case report and review of nonglucagonoma-associated necrolytic migratory erythema. J Am Acad Dermatol 1998; 38: 866-873.

National Research Council of the National Academies. Nutrient requirements of dogs and cats. Washington, DC: The National Academies Press, 2006.

Noli C, Comombo S, Abramo F, et al. Papular eosinophilic/mastocytic dermatitis (feline urticaria pigmentosa) in Devon Rex cats: A distinct disease entity or a histopathological reaction pattern? Vet Dermatol 2004; 15: 253-259.

Outerbridge CA, Marks SL, Rogers QR. Plasma amino acid concentrations in 36 dogs with histologically confirmed superficial necrolytic dermatitis. Vet Dermatol 2002; 13: 177-186.

Patel A, Whitbread TJ, McNeil PE. A case of metabolic epidermal necrosis in a cat. Vet Dermatol 1996; 7: 221-226.

Prost C. Diagnosis of feline allergic diseases: a study of 90 cats In: Kwochka KW, Willemse T, Von Tscharner C, eds. Advances in Veterinary Dermatology. Oxford: Butterworth Heinemann, 1998; 516-517.

Rees CA. Canine and feline atopic dermatitis: a review of the diagnostic options. Clin Tech Small Anim Pract 2001; 16: 230-232.

Robben JH, Zaal MD, Hallebeek JM, et al. Enteral, nutritional support for critically ill patients. Tijdschr Diergeneeskd 1999; 124: 468-471

Rosenfeldt V, Benfeldt E, Nielsen SD, et al. Effect of probiotic Lactobacillus strains in children with atopic dermatitis. J Allergy Clin Immunol 2003; 111: 389-395.

Rosenkrantz WS. The pathogenesis, diagnosis and management of feline acne. Vet Med 1991; 5: 504-512.

Rosser EJ. Food allergy in the cat: A prospective study of 13 cats In: Ihrke PJ, Mason IS. et White SD, eds. Advances in Veterinary Dermatology. Oxford: Pergamon Press, 1993; 33-39.

Sampson HA. Adverse reactions to foods In: Adkinson NF, Yunginger JW, Busse WW, Bochner BS, Holgate ST. et Simons FER, eds. Allergy: Principles and Practice. 6th ed. Philadelphia: Mosby, 2003; 1619-1643.

Scardino MS, Swaim SF, Sartin EA, et al. The effects of omega-3 fatty acid diet enrichment on wound healing. Vet Dermatol 1999; 10: 283-290.

Scott DW, Miller WH, Griffin CE. Small animal dermatology. Philadelphia: WB Saunders Co; 2001.

Smith KM, Eaton AD, Finlayson LM, et al. Oral tolerance. Am J Respir Crit Care Med 2000; 162: S175-S178.

Stogdale L, Bomzon L, Van Den Berg PB. Food allergy in cats. J Am Anim Hosp Assoc 1982; 18: 188-194.

Tierney EP, Badger J. Etiology and pathogenesis of necrolytic migratory erythema: review of the literature. MedGenMed 2004; 6: 4.

Torres SM, Caywood DD, O'Brien TD, et al. Resolution of superficial necrolytic dermatitis following excision of a glucagon-secreting pancreatic neoplasm in a dog. J Am Anim Hosp Assoc 1997; 33: 313-319.

Vitale CB, Ihrke PJ, Gross TL. Diet-induced alterations in lipid metabolism and associated cutaneous xanthoma formation in 5 cats In: Kwochka KW, Willemse T & Von Tscharner C, eds. Advances in Veterinary Dermatology. Oxford: Butterworth Heinemann, 1998; 243-249.

Waisglass SE, Landsberg GM, Yager JA, et al. Underlying medical conditions in cats with presumptive psychogenic alopecia. J Am Vet Med Assoc 2006; 228: 1705-1709.

Walton GS. Skin responses in the dog and cat to ingested allergens. Observations on one hundred confirmed cases. Vet Rec 1967; 81: 709-713.

Watson AL, Fray TR, Bailey J, et al. Dietary constituents are able to play a beneficial role in canine epidermal barrier function. Exp Dermatol 2006; 15: 74-81.

Weese JS, Arroyo L. Bacteriological evaluation of dog and cat diets that claim to contain probiotics. Can Vet J 2003; 44: 212-216.

White SD, Sequoia D. Food hypersensitivity in cats: 14 cases (1982-1987). J Am Vet Med Assoc 1989; 194: 692-695.

Wilhelm S, Favrot C. Food hypersensitivity dermatitis in the dog: diagnostic possibilities. Schweiz Arch Tierheilkd 2005; 147: 165-171.

Wills J. Dietary hypersensitivity in cats. In Practice 1991; 13: 87-93.

Yoshida M, Barata K, Ando-Lu J, et al. A case report of superficial necrolytic dermatitis in a beagle dog with diabetes mellitus. Toxicol Pathol 1996; 24: 498-501.

Young E, Stoneham MD, Petruckevitch A, et al. A population study of food intolerance. Lancet 1994; 343: 1127-1130.

Yu S, Rogers QR, Morris JG. Effect of low levels of dietary tyrosine on the hair colour of cats. J Small Anim Pract 2001; 42: 176-180.

Zhang M, Xu X, ShenY, et al. Clinical experience in diagnosis and treatment of glucagonoma syndrome. Hepatobiliary Pancreat Dis Int 2004; 3: 473-475.

Zivny JH, Moldoveanu Z, Vu HL, et al. Mechanisms of immune tolerance to food antigens in humans. Clin Immunol 2001; 101: 158-168.

Focus on:

Borage oil

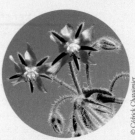

© Cédrick Chataignier

Borage (*Borago officinalis*) is a plant originally from Syria. It is now grown in North Africa and various countries of Europe, including France, Britain, Germany and the Netherlands. The first traces of its use are from the first century AD. Traditionally, the young leaves were consumed in salads or soups and the flowers gave a refreshing flavor to wine.

Borage seeds

Borage blooms over two months, which means that not all the seeds become mature at the same time. It is important to only harvest the mature seeds, which look like grains of pepper, as they have twice the oil content of green seeds (30% vs. 15%).

Harvesting may be done naturally – recovering the seeds as they fall by rolling out a tarp between the rows – or mechanically, using small carts to catch the seeds, which are loosened by vibration.

Borage oil

The seeds dry out naturally somewhere cool in the shade. To avoid mold, they must be used shortly after harvesting. The oil is obtained by grinding and pressing the seeds. The procedure is performed in a cold environment. Above 50 °C (122°F), the fatty acids risk being denatured.

Unparalleled gamma-linolenic acid (GLA) content

The oil is obtained by pressing the borage seeds. Their unsaturated fatty acid content is 80% and they have a large content of a particular fatty acid of the omega-6 family, known as gamma-linolenic acid (GLA). GLA is normally synthesized from linoleic acid.

Most vegetable oils have a very high linoleic acid content, but the only oils that contain a beneficial quantity of GLA are borage oil, the oil of blackcurrant seeds and evening primrose oil.

Linoleic acid undergoes successive transformations to produce all the fatty acids of the omega-6 family. Each step is triggered by a particular enzyme. The metabolism of unsaturated fatty acids in cats remains a controversial subject. Some authors feel that desaturated Δ6 is ineffective in cats (*Sinclair et al., 1979*). More recent studies (*Pawlosky et al., 1994*) show that the conversion of linoleic acid to GLA is possible, with increased efficacy when the animal is deficient. This process however remains limited in the cat. In this study, the authors reported that only 0.06% of the ingested linoleic acid was converted to GLA.

Nutritional benefit of GLA

Borage oil is widely used in nutrition and cosmetology. It is used in products designed to rejuvenate the skin. It is especially indicated for the dry skin of cats that tend towards seborrhea. Cats respond very well to the addition of GLA to the diet.

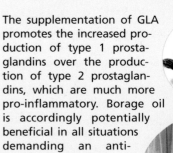

© Roland Hours

The supplementation of GLA promotes the increased production of type 1 prostaglandins over the production of type 2 prostaglandins, which are much more pro-inflammatory. Borage oil is accordingly potentially beneficial in all situations demanding an anti-inflammatory effect.

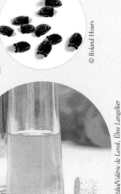

© Roland Hours

© Diffomédia/Valérie de Leval, Elise Langellier

COMPARISON OF THE GLA CONTENT OF DIFFERENT VEGETABLE OILS		
Vegetable sources	Linoleic acid%	Gamma-linolenic acid (GLA)%
Borage	35 to 40	20 to 25
Blackcurrant seeds	45 to 50	15 to 20
Evening primrose	70 to 80	8 to 12
Soy	50 to 55	-
Olive	8 to 10	-

Borage oil has the highest GLA concentration.

The beneficial effects of GLA have been studied most in dermatology. Major alterations to the condition of the skin (dull hair, scaling and skin ulcers that do not heal easily) are observed in cats fed for 18 months with a food containing sunflower seed oil, which is rich in linoleic acid, as the sole source of fat *(Frankel & Rivers, 1980)*. Substituting half the sunflower seed oil with evening primrose oil, which is rich in GLA, helps obtain a fast improvement in the condition of the skin in these animals. Reversion to the original diet results in deterioration of the condition of the skin again. This study therefore confirms the benefit of high GLA oil supplementation to alter linoleic acid desaturation.

Other studies show the benefit of GLA intake in feline dermatology. In cats with papulo-squamous dermatitis, the dietary incorporation of evening primrose oil, helped to obtain better therapeutic results than sunflower oil, *(Harvey, 1993a)*. With feline miliary dermatitis, the efficacy of GLA administration was improved when it was combined with fish oil *(Harvey, 1993b)*.

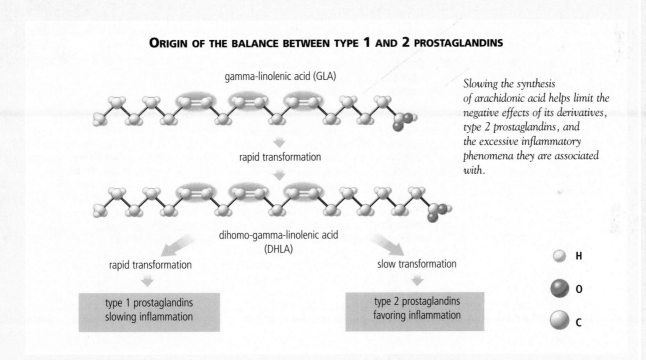

ORIGIN OF THE BALANCE BETWEEN TYPE 1 AND 2 PROSTAGLANDINS

gamma-linolenic acid (GLA)

rapid transformation

dihomo-gamma-linolenic acid (DHLA)

rapid transformation — slow transformation

type 1 prostaglandins slowing inflammation

type 2 prostaglandins favoring inflammation

Slowing the synthesis of arachidonic acid helps limit the negative effects of its derivatives, type 2 prostaglandins, and the excessive inflammatory phenomena they are associated with.

H
O
C

References

Frankel TL, Rivers JPW. The nutritional and metabolic impact of α-linolenic acid on cats deprived on animal lipids. Br J Nutr 1978; 39: 227-231.

Harvey RG. A comparison of evening primrose oil and sunflower oil for the management of papulocrustous dermatitis in cats. Vet Rec 1993a; 133: 571-573.

Harvey RG. Effect of varying proportions of evening primrose oil and fish oil on cats with crusting dermatosis ('miliary dermatitis') Vet Rec 1993b; 133: 208-211.

Pawlosky R, Barnes A, Salem N Jr. Essential fatty acid metabolism in the feline: relationship between liver and brain production of long-chain polyunsaturated fatty acids. J Lipid Res 1994; 35: 2032-2040.

Sinclair AJ, McLean JG, Monger EA. Metabolism of linoleic acid in the cat. Lipids 1979; 14: 932-936.

Protein composition of cat hair

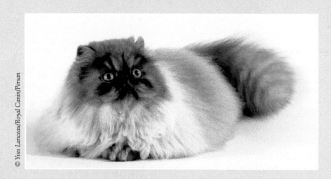

© Yves Lanceau/Royal Canin/Persan

The daily protein requirement to regenerate skin cells and stimulate hair growth is estimated at almost 30% of the daily protein intake (Scott et al, 2001).

There is little data on the amino acid composition of hair. It is determined through hydrolysis with hydrochloric acid for 24 hours. This method may however lead to the degradation of some amino acids or underestimate the content when hydrolysis is incomplete. Studies *(Robel & Crane, 1972; Darragh et al, 1996)* have reported alternative techniques to minimize these inaccuracies. *Hendriks et al* (1998) reported that the color or sex of the animal has no impact on the amino acid composition of the hair.

The total nitrogen content of cat hair is said to be 15.1% *(Hendriks et al, 1998)*. This author also reported that amino acids represent 86% of the hair mass in this species. The remainder is divided between non-nitrogen compounds: minerals, sterols and complex lipids.

The amino acid composition of cat hair is similar to that of dogs, sheep, horses and humans, although the proline content in cats is lower than in the other species. The most abundant amino acids in cat hair protein are cysteine, serine, glutamic acid and glycine **(Table 1)**. Sulphur containing amino acids can account for up to 37% of the total amino acids *(Swift & Smith, 2000)*. They build cysteine bridges, which are essential to hair construction. Cysteine is also involved in the enzymatic production of pheomelanin *(Granholm, 1996)*.

Amino acid	Content (mol/100 mol of residue)				
	Cat	Dog	Horse	Sheep	Human
Cysteine	15.9	16.7	14.4	13.1	17.8
Methionine	0.9	0.9	0.2	0.5	0.6
Aspartate	5.6	5.3	6.0	5.9	4.9
Threonine	6.4	6.2	6.5	6.5	6.8
Serine	10.6	10.5	9.6	10.8	11.7
Glutamate	11.4	11.1	11.3	11.1	11.4
Glycine	9.5	7.8	6.4	8.6	6.4
Alanine	5.1	5.1	5.5	5.2	4.6
Valine	4.9	4.9	5.9	5.7	5.8
Isoleucine	2.5	2.5	3.6	3.0	2.6
Leucine	6.7	6.1	7.5	7.2	5.8
Tyrosine	3.0	2.7	1.9	3.8	2.0
Phenylalanine	2.3	1.7	2.5	2.5	1.6
Histidine	1.2	0.9	1.1	0.8	0.9
Lysine	2.9	3.9	2.9	2.7	2.7
Arginine	6.1	6.3	7.9	6.2	5.8
Proline	4.9	7.3	7.8	6.6	8.4

TABLE 1 - AMINO ACID COMPOSITION OF THE HAIRS OF CATS AND SOME OTHER MAMMALS
(From Hendriks et al, 1998)

Animal color or sex has no impact on the amino acid composition of the hair.

ROYAL CANIN

Key points

for covering protein requirement with respect to hair growth

The quantity of amino acids required for hair growth in a given period of the year can be estimated by multiplying the amino acid concentration in each cat hair by the hair growth rate during that period of the year *(Hendriks et al, 1998)*. The daily protein requirement to regenerate skin cells and stimulate hair growth is estimated at almost 30% of daily protein intake *(Scott et al, 2001)*.

The effects of general protein deficiency:

- Initially, a drop in the diameter of the hair and reduction in the size of the hair bulb

- Subsequently, the hair becomes dull and fragile, growing more slowly and falling out faster.

Isolated deficiency of sulfur amino acids (cysteine, methionine) may lead to the same clinical signs.

Studies show the impact of a deficiency of tyrosine and phenylalanine, a melanin precursor. After a few weeks red hairs begin to appear, especially in black cats. Supplementation reverses this phenomenon. The hairs of reddish cats (which have pheomelanin pigments) also take on a lighter color in response to deficiency *(Morris et al, 2002; Anderson et al, 2002; Yu et al, 2001)*. *Morris et al (2002)* show that around three times as much phenylalanine and tyrosine is needed to obtain optimal coloration of a black coat than is needed for the normal growth of a kitten. These authors recommend a minimum intake of 18 g/kg of dry dietary matter.

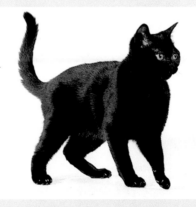

© Yves Lanceau/Royal Canin - Bombay

Around three times as much phenylalanine and tyrosine is needed to obtain optimal coloration of a black coat than is needed for the normal growth of a kitten.

References

Anderson PJ, Rogers QR, Morris JG. Cats require more dietary phenylalanine or tyrosine for melanin deposition in hair than for maximal growth. J Nutr 2002; 132: 2037-2042.

Buffington CA. Nutrition and the skin. In: Proceedings 11ᵗʰ Kal Kan Sympsium 1997: 11-16. Cited in Waltham Focus 9.2 1-7, Lloyd DH, Marsh KA. Optimizing skin and coat condition.

Darragh AJ, Garrick DJ, Moughan PJ, et al. Correction for amino acids loss during acid hydrolysis of a purified protein. Anal Biochem 1996; 236: 199-207.

Granholm DE, Reese RN, Granholm NH. Agouti alleles alter cysteine and glutathione concentrations in hair follicles and serum of mice (A y/a, A wJ/A wJ, and a/a). J Invest Dermatol 1996; 106: 559-563.

Hendriks WH, Tarttelin MF, Moughan PJ. The amino acid composition of cat (Felis Catus) hair. Anim Sci 1998; 67: 165-170.

Morris J, Yu S, Quinton R. Red hair in black cats is reversed by addition of tyrosine to the diet. J Nutr 2002; 132: 1646S-1648S.

Robel EJ, Crane AB. An accurate method for correcting unknown amino acid losses from protein hydrolysates. Anal Biochem 1972; 48: 233-246.

Swift JA, Smith JR. Surface striations of human hair and other mammalian keratin fibres. 10th international wood conference, 2000: http://www.sci.port.ac.uk/spm/HH-1.pdf.

Yu S, Rogers QR, Morris JG. Effect of low levels of dietary tyrosine on the hair colour of cats. J Small Anim Pract 2001; 42: 176-80.

Jürgen ZENTEK
DVM, Prof,
Dipl. ECVCN

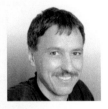

Valérie FREICHE
DVM

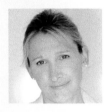

Digestive diseases in cats: the role of nutrition

1. Physiology of the gastrointestinal tract 79

2. Physiology of nutrient digestion 81

3. Microbiology of the digestive tract 83

4. Gastrointestinal mucosal immune system 83

5. Common gastrointestinal syndromes in cats 85

6. Enteral and parenteral nutrition 95

7. Diseases of the esophagus and nutritional approach 96

8. Diseases of the stomach and nutritional approach 103

9. Diseases of the intestines and nutritional approach 107

Conclusion 128

Frequently asked questions 129

References 130

Royal Canin nutritional information 135

ABBREVIATIONS USED IN THIS CHAPTER

BIPS: barium-impregnated polyethylene spheres
IBD: inflammatory bowel disease
Ig (A, G or M): immunoglobulin
IL (6, 10, 12): interleukin
MHC: major histocompatability complex
NSAID: non-steroidal anti-inflammatory drug

PCR: polymerase chain reaction
PEG: percutaneous endoscopic gastrostomy
PLE: protein-losing enteropathy
PPN: partial parenteral nutrition
SCFA: short chain fatty acid
TDF: total dietary fiber

TGF β: transforming growth factor beta
TNF α: tumor necrosis factor alpha
TPN: total parenteral nutrition

Digestive diseases in cats: the role of nutrition

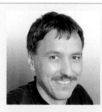

Jürgen ZENTEK

DMV, Prof, specialist degree in animal nutrition, Dipl. ECVCN

Jürgen Zentek graduated from the Faculty of Veterinary Medicine (Tierärzliche Hochschule) in Hanover, Germany in 1985. After employment in a veterinary practice, in 1987 he led a research project at the Department of Animal Nutrition, studying the energy intake and skeletal development in growing Great Danes. He obtained his degree as a specialist in animal nutrition and dietetics in 1993. After a year in Bristol, UK, at the School of Veterinary Science, he took the Chair of Clinical Nutrition at the Veterinary University of Vienna in 2000, becoming the Head of the Institute of Nutrition. Since 2005 he has been a Professor of the University of Berlin. His ongoing research is on clinical dietetics of domesticated animals, the relationship between nutrition, intestinal microflora and immunity of the GI tract.

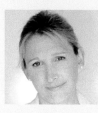

Valérie FREICHE

DVM, Clinique Frégis, Arcueil, France

Valérie Freiche graduated from the National Veterinary School of Alfort in 1988 where she remained as an intern then assistant in the Department of Medicine until 1992. Having developed her own practice in the Paris region Valérie initially worked with dogs and cats before choosing to concentrate on gastroenterology. Between 1992 and 2006, she has been responsible for gastroenterology consultation and gastrointestinal endoscopy at the National Veterinary School of Alfort. She also had the same role in a referral practice, in Paris. Since 2006, she works in a referral practice in Bordeaux, in internal medicine and gastroenterology. Valérie is the President of the Internal Medicine Studies Group (GEMI) of the French Association of Veterinarians for Companion Animals (AFVAC). Valérie regularly participates in conferences and post-university training sessions in gastroenterology.

Nutrition is the cornerstone of the treatment of digestive diseases. However, considering actual pathophysiological knowledge about gastroenterology, it seems obvious that there is no diet adapted to all kinds of digestive cases. The general objectives of the diet are: stimulating dietary consumption, improving digestion and nutrient absorption, maintaining normal digestive motility and intestinal transit, and decrease inflammation when it exists. In addition, the dietetic strategy must plan to provide the right nutrients to optimize the bacterial flora and to protect the mucosal barrier.

1 - Physiology of the gastrointestinal tract

▶ Oral cavity (Figure 1)

Morphologically and physiologically, domestic cats are highly specialized carnivores, as shown by their dentition, nutritional requirements and sense of taste (*Bradshaw, 2006*). The tongue is rough and has multiple hooklike appendages. These filiform or fungiform papillae enable the cat to lick up liquids and to scrape flesh off bones (*Ojima et al, 1997*). There are approximately 250 fungiform papillae on the tongue of an adult cat; they are most numerous on the tip. Their size – and the mean number of taste buds – increases from the tip to the back of the tongue (*Robinson & Winkles, 1990*). A cat's sense of taste – except sweetness – is mediated via taste buds mainly located in the tongue. The cat has specific and unique feeding preferences linked to its ability to smell amino acids and peptides (*Zaghini & Biagi, 2005*). The dentition of cats is typical of carnivores. Cats have 26 milk teeth that are replaced at age five to seven months by 30 permanent teeth. The permanent dentition is made up of 12 incisors, 4 canines, 10 premolars and 4 molars (see chapter 11).

▶ Esophagus (Figure 1)

The esophagus is a tube that transports food from the mouth to the stomach. At body weights of 4-5 kg, the average length is 22-23 cm. The cervical segment of the esophagus accounts for about one third of the whole length and the thoracic segment about two thirds (the abdominal segment is very short in the cat) (*Hegner & Vollmerhaus, 1997*). Coordinated contraction of the longitudinal and circular esophageal musculature is important for the peristaltic transport of a

FIGURE 1 - GENERAL DIGESTIVE TRACT ANATOMY IN THE CAT

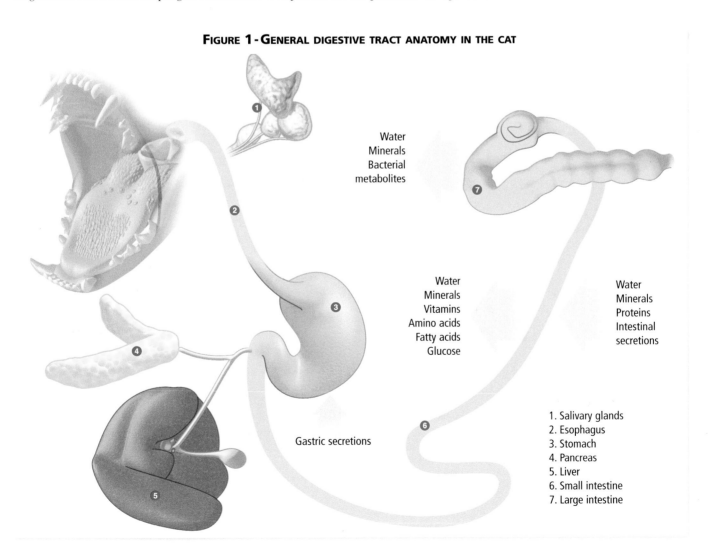

Water
Minerals
Bacterial
metabolites

Water
Minerals
Vitamins
Amino acids
Fatty acids
Glucose

Water
Minerals
Proteins
Intestinal
secretions

Gastric secretions

1. Salivary glands
2. Esophagus
3. Stomach
4. Pancreas
5. Liver
6. Small intestine
7. Large intestine

food bolus through the esophagus (*Dodds et al, 1973*). Motility is subject to a myogenic control system and additional nerve control mechanisms (*Preiksaitis & Diamant, 1999*). The esophageal glands produce a mucinous secretion that helps lubricate the food bolus. Although cats are able to swallow large pieces of food or prey, the esophageal passage of capsules or tablets may be prolonged or tablets may become trapped due to their diameter or surface structure (*Graham et al, 2000*). The possibility of medication-induced esophagitis should be considered when administering ulcerogenic drugs to cats.

▶ Stomach (Figure 1)

The stomach has a comparatively large capacity for prey or food storage. The stomach may be subdivided into several anatomical and functional regions. The cardia is the site of entry, the fundus, body and antrum are the middle parts and the pylorus is the transitional zone to the duodenum. Normally, gastric emptying delivers food to the small intestine at a rate that allows optimal intestinal absorption of nutrients (*Wyse et al, 2003*). The pylorus is surrounded by muscle tissue and regulates food transport into the duodenum. The pyloric muscle prevents the reflux of duodenal contents and bile into the stomach lumen.

Endocrine G-cells are scattered diffusely in the basal part of the mucosa and produce gastrin, a major stimulus of gastric secretory response to meal intake (*Cerny et al, 1991*). In the stomach, hydrochloric acid secretion by the oxytic cells and pepsin, secreted as pepsinogen by the chief cells, initiate protein digestion.

Lipase activity occurs in the surface mucous cells in newborn cats after ingestion of milk (*Knospe & Plendl, 1997*). Lipase is localized as pepsin in the chief cells but is also present in pepsin-free cells, the mucus surface cells of the fundus and the antrum (*Descroix-Vagne et al, 1993*).

Gastric motility and emptying is subject to various regulatory mechanisms, including reflectory, neural and endocrine factors. Diet composition may affect gastric emptying, with fat and large particle size having a delaying effect (*Strombeck, & Guilford 1996a; Hall & Washabau, 1999*). The stomach can retain ingesta for up to 15 hours before it passes to the intestine (*Brugère, 1996*). The gastric transit time, determined from the first exit of barium-impregnated polyethylene spheres (BIPS) from the stomach had a median of 6 h (range 3 to 8) in sedated and a median of 2.5 (range 2 to 6) in unsedated cats. The median of 50% gastric emptying time was 6.4 h (range 2.5 to 10.9), and complete gastric emptying was seen after 12 h with a range 6 to 27 h. The orocecal transit time of BIPS was 6.5 h and the 50% orocecal transit time was 8.8 h (range 4.6 to 12.8) (*Sparkes et al, 1997*).

▶ Small intestine (Figure 1)

The duodenum, jejunum and ileum are the three histologically defined parts of the small intestine. Bile and the pancreatic secretions enter into the duodenum via the common bile duct and are necessary for the solubilization of fat and the enzymatic digestion of the intestinal content.

The small intestinal mucosa has a specific structure with crypts and microvilli covered by a single epithelial layer. The crypts are the location for cell proliferation. The absorptive enterocytes bear a high density of microvilli, which increases the surface area substantially. The paracellular space is closed by different proteins with specific functions that prevent uncontrolled permeation of bacteria or macromolecules through the intestinal wall. A mucous layer, the glycocalix, consisting of carbohydrates and proteins, covers the brush border. The glycocalix has a high enzymatic activity for the breakdown of macromolecules to absorbable units and provides a specific microenvironment for bacteria associated with the gut wall.

Besides its absorptive capacity, the small intestine has a considerable secretory capacity via the crypts and the goblet cells. Endocrine cells contribute to the regulation of the digestive processes.

The duodenal glands are located caudally to the pylorus and produce mucous secretion with neutral, sulphated and carboxylated acid mucosaccharides (*Takehana & Abe, 1983*). The compounds in food that have passed through the small intestine undigested or unabsorbed enter the large intestine and are fermented by microbial enzymes. A sphincter terminates the small intestine and prevents reflux of chyme and bacteria.

► Large intestine (Figure 1)

The cecum, colon and rectum are the three parts of the large intestine where undigested organic matter is fermented and fluid, minerals and bacterial metabolites are absorbed. Due to the carnivorous character of the cat, the size of the large intestine is small (**Table 1**), probably because there was no evolutionary need for a large fermentation chamber (*Chivers & Hladik, 1980*). The large intestine has no microvilli and its surface morphology differs considerably from the small intestine. The crypts of Lieberkuhn contain absorptive and secretory cells. The large intestine of cats is characterized by a dense microbial community with high metabolic activity.

TABLE 1 - RESPECTIVE PROPORTIONS OF THE INTESTINE IN SELECT SPECIES From: *Barone, 1984; **Meyer et al, 1993; ***Dukes, 1984*			
	Dogs	**Cats**	**Humans**
Small intestine*	1.7 - 6 m	1.0 - 1.7 m	6 - 6.5 m
Large intestine*	0.3 - 1 m	0.3 - 0.4 m	1.5 m
Relative weight of the digestive tract/body weight**	2.7% (giant dogs) to 7% (small dogs)	7%	10%
Body length/ intestinal length***	1/6	1/4	1/5

2 - Physiology of nutrient digestion

► Protein digestion (Figure 2)

Protein digestion is located in the upper gastrointestinal tract. Cats are normally very efficient in protein digestion and the apparent digestibility of proteins is similar to dogs (*Zentek et al, 1998; Funaba et al, 2005*). The digestive capacity of the younger cat may be lower than that of adult animals, due either to the physiological development of the gut or diet-induced enzyme modulation (*Harper & Turner, 2000*).

Protein digestion is initiated in the stomach. A sequence of proteolytic enzymes is required to split the dietary proteins. Most important are endopeptidases such as pepsin or trypsin. Proteins are initially digested by pepsins (*Shaw & Wright, 1976*). Pepsins require an acidic environment for their activation: cats produce a highly acidic gastric secretion, the pH in the feline stomach varies from 2-3 (*Hall, 2000*). Pepsin is deactivated as soon as it enters the alkaline milieu of the duodenum and jejunum.

The small intestine has a slightly alkaline pH due to the secretions of the epithelial glands and the bicarbonate-rich pancreatic juice (*Williams, 1996*). This is necessary for the continuation of protein digestion by the proteolytic enzymes of the pancreas and the small intestinal mucosa. Feline trypsin seems to occur in one isoform only and trypsinogen, which is activated to trypsin by the activity of intestinal enterokinase, is closely related to the trypsinogen in other mammalian species (*Steiner et al, 1997*). Luminal protein digestion releases small peptides and amino acids that are transported through the brush border and absorbed by specific active carrier-mediated transport mechanisms through the gut wall.

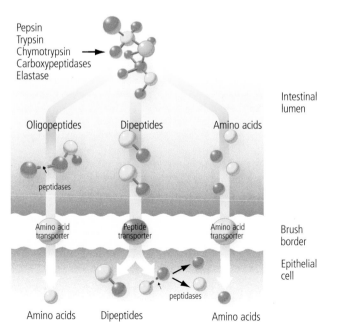

FIGURE 2 - DIGESTION AND ABSORPTION OF PROTEINS

Pepsin
Trypsin
Chymotrypsin
Carboxypeptidases
Elastase

Intestinal lumen

Oligopeptides   Dipeptides   Amino acids

peptidases

Amino acid transporter   Peptide transporter   Amino acid transporter

Brush border

Epithelial cell

peptidases

Amino acids   Dipeptides   Amino acids

FIGURE 3 - DIGESTION AND ABSORPTION OF CARBOHYDRATES

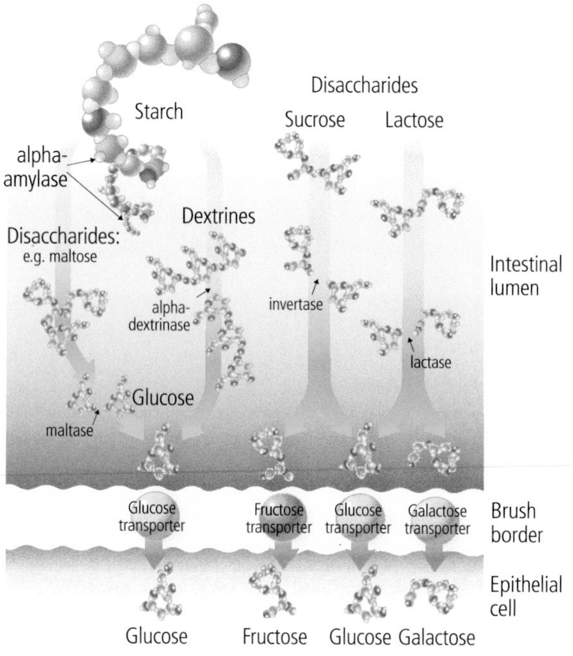

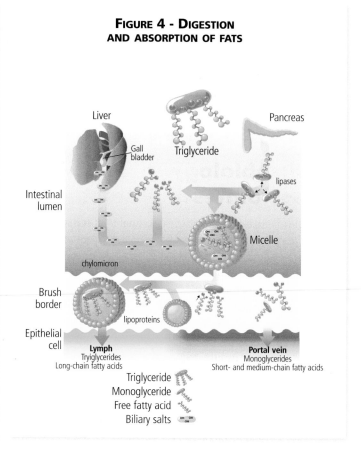

FIGURE 4 - DIGESTION AND ABSORPTION OF FATS

Uptakes of arginine and lysine were high throughout the suckling period and the perinatal intestinal hyperplasia observed in many other mammalian species seems to be absent in cats (*Buddington & Diamond, 1992*).

► Carbohydrate digestion (Figure 3)

The cat's ability to digest and tolerate such complex carbohydrates as starch is very high, although amylase activity in pancreatic tissue and small intestinal content is low compared to most other species (*Kienzle, 1993*). It decreases in the lower gut, probably due to intensive microbial degradation. Dietary carbohydrate levels had no obvious inductive effect on disaccharidase activities.

Maltase, isomaltase and sucrase activity did not depend on age. In contrast, lactase activity decreased from newborn kittens to adult cats and only few adult cats can have significant lactase activity in the jejunum (*Kienzle, 1993*). The tolerance for simple sugars is much more limited due to a limited intermediary capacity for sugar metabolism compared to most other species (*Morris et al, 1977; Kienzle, 1994; Appleton et al, 2004*). Apparent total digestibility of sugars was determined in adult cats and reached almost 100%. However, the prececeal digestibility may be considerably lower depending on the sugar source and the degree that the starch is cooked (*Kienzle, 1993*).

► Fat digestion (Figure 4)

Cats are well adapted to fat digestion. Fats are not only important energy sources but also have additional functional properties (*Bauer, 2006*). Obviously, healthy cats can tolerate high dietary fat levels without a negative impact on digestive function. An age-related reduction in apparent fat digestibility was observed in cats fed on different fat sources with different degrees of saturation. Saturated fatty acids had a slightly lower apparent digestibility in young and senior cats (*Peachey et al, 1999*).

Fat digestion may be severely impaired in cats with exocrine pancreatic insufficiency *(Nicholson et al, 1989)* or in animals with impaired bile secretion. Bile acids are not only important for the solubilization of fatty acids but also for the activation of pancreatic lipase *(Strombeck, 1996b)*. Bile acids are reabsorbed in the ileum and re-circulated to the liver. The absorbed long chain fatty acids are re-esterified in the intestinal epithelium and incorporated into chylomicrons before the release into lymphatics. Medium chain fatty acids can be absorbed directly into the blood, but palatability of medium chain fatty acids is usually low in this species *(MacDonald et al, 1985)*.

3 - Microbiology of the gastrointestinal tract

Microbial colonization of the gastrointestinal tract starts directly after birth, and the composition of the intestinal microflora approaches the spectrum of adult cats during the first weeks of life *(Osbaldiston & Stowe, 1971)*. The development of the microflora in kittens is comparable to other species: *Clostridium perfringens*, *Escherichia coli* and *Streptococci* are among the first organisms to colonize the alimentary tract of kittens. The gut flora of cats is characterized by relatively high numbers of *Clostridium perfringens* and lecithinase negative clostridia, probably reflecting the carnivorous type of diet. Normally, the intestinal microflora maintains a self stabilizing symbiotic balance with the host organism *(Strombeck, 1996a)*. The bacterial concentration in all parts of the gastrointestinal tract of healthy cats is high and bacterial densities of 10^{12}/g feces, mainly anerobic bacteria, are normal.

The intestinal microflora may contribute to the health and well-being of the host, supporting the digestive process, but it may also be a significant factor in the pathogenesis of intestinal diseases. Its composition and metabolic activity is subjected to influences by the individual and interfering diseases. Diet composition, protein quantity and quality, feed processing *(Backus et al, 1994)*, dietary fiber and digestible carbohydrates *(Fahey, 2003)* and feed additives such as probiotics *(Rastall, 2004; Marshall Jones et al, 2006)* also affect the composition of the microbiota.

4 - Gastrointestinal mucosal immune system (Figure 5)

The gastrointestinal tract contains a dense population of immune cells with multiple characteristics and functions. Its main task in healthy animals is to achieve tolerance against dietary and endogenous bacterial antigens. On the other hand, the gastrointestinal immune system must be conditionally reactive against pathogenic bacteria or harmful environmental antigens.

The gut-associated immune system has anatomically defined and diffuse structures. These may act specifically as inductive or effective sites, providing the ability for an adequate immune response. The intestinal mucosa harbors a high density of immune cells that are often organized in cell clusters, either visible as lymph follicles or more prominently as Peyer's patches. Given the antibody secreting cells, IgA+ plasma cells predominate in the small intestine, and IgM+ plasma cells are found in higher concentrations than IgG+ plasma cells *(Waly et al, 2001)*. Plasma cells are found in all regions of the small intestine with greater numbers in the lamina propria and Peyer's patches compared to the epithelium *(Howard et al, 2005)*.

Cats have elevated numbers of intraepithelial lymphocytes a proportion of which express surface IgM, but the significance of this finding is still uncertain. T-cells (CD3+) and T-cell subsets (CD4+ and CD8+) follow a specific distribution pattern with greater numbers in the villous lamina propria than in the lamina adjacent to the crypts. Intra-epithelial lymphocytes are mainly CD8+ T lymphocytes; CD4+ T-cells dominate in the lamina propria. Antigen presenting macrophages and

FIGURE 5 - THE INTESTINAL IMMUNE SYSTEM

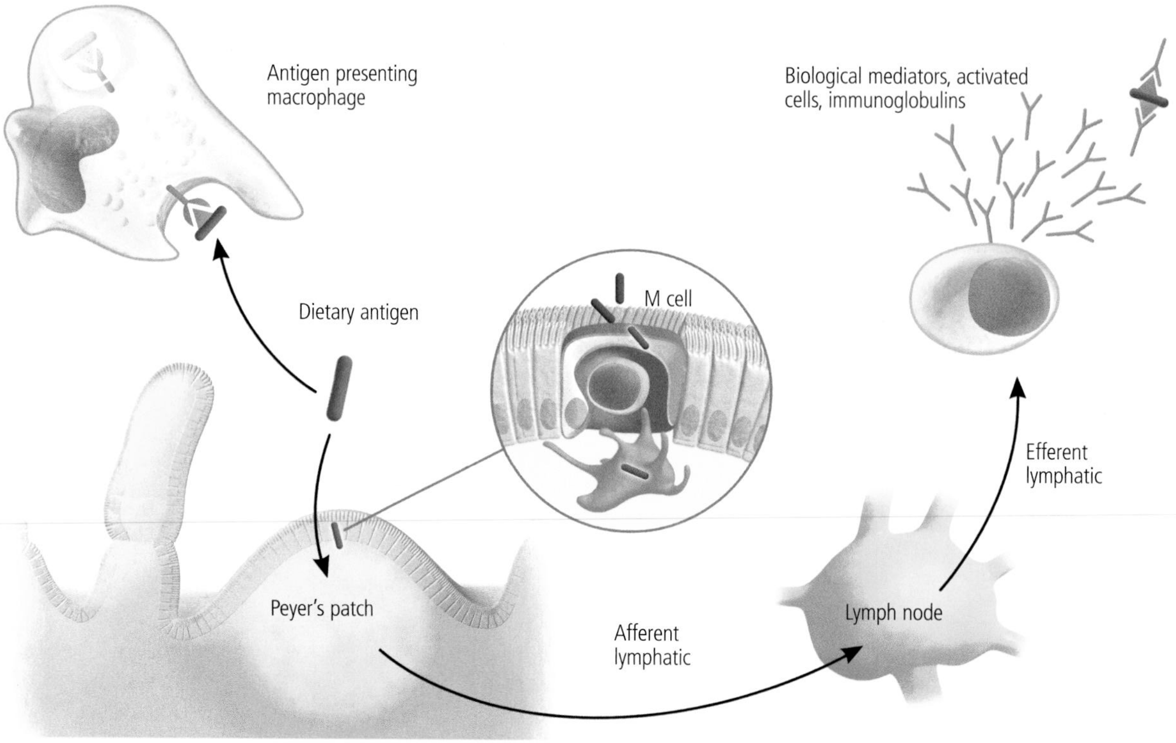

Antigen presenting macrophage

Biological mediators, activated cells, immunoglobulins

Dietary antigen

M cell

Efferent lymphatic

Peyer's patch

Afferent lymphatic

Lymph node

The gastrointestinal immune system of recognition of dietary antigens is mainly due to Peyer's patches and antigen presenting macrophages. The effective mechanisms are dispatched in diffuse intestinal structures.

dendritic cells in the lamina propria express L1 and major histocompatibility complex (MHC) class II. B-cells predominate in Peyer's patches with 40% B-cells, 28% CD4+ T-cells and 20% CD8+ T-cells.

Diseases that are associated with infections or allergic reactions in the gastrointestinal tract involve the local or general immune system (*Day, 2005; Stokes & Waly, 2006*). IgA is the dominant immunoglobulin in intestinal secretions of cats, as in other species. Normally, oral tolerance is induced for short periods after introduction of novel antigens into the diet. In cases of dysregulated immune response, cats may become hypersensitive to the newly introduced dietary antigen prior to the establishment of tolerance.

MHC class II expression by leukocytes with dendritic cell or macrophage morphology in the lamina propria was significantly greater in cats with inflammatory bowel disease compared to healthy cats. MHC class II expression by enterocytes was also more pronounced in diseased cats (*Waly et al, 2004*).

Cytokine expression seems to be important in determining the reaction of the gastrointestinal immune system to antigen challenges. Cats with intestinal inflammation had significantly more transcription of pro-inflammatory and immunoregulatory genes encoding IL-6, IL-10, IL-12, p40, TNF-α and TGF-β than cats with normal histology (*Cave, 2003; Nguyen Van et al, 2006*).

5 - Common gastrointestinal syndromes in cats

► Dysphagia

Dysphagia is a difficulty in swallowing. It may be due to an obstruction, a painful oropharyngeal or esophageal disorder, or it may be a motility problem *(Washabau, 2005)*. The main sign is regurgitation.

Regurgitation is defined as the passive expulsion of saliva or non-digested food. It often occurs very soon after the ingestion of food, although in the event of saliva regurgitation it may occur less rapidly. Contrary to vomiting, regurgitation occurs suddenly, without prodromal signs or abdominal contractions *(Guilford & Strombeck, 1996b)*.

An esophageal disorder produces other clinical signs:
- ptyalism
- halitosis
- dysorexia or anorexia
- odynophagia (painful swallowing)
- polypnea
- coughing and/or discharge in the event of secondary pneumonia.

> Complementary tests

Plain radiography

Physiologically, the esophagus cannot be visualized by radiography. Its appearance on a plain radiograph may be due to localized or generalized dilatation, or to the retention of liquids or solids. These images enable the identification of a radiodense foreign body or suggest the presence of a foreign body based on indirect signs (localized dilatation, localized air densification, pneumomediastinum) *(Konde & Pugh, 2003)*.

Radiography with contrast medium

This confirms any dilatation if the plain radiographs are insufficient. The use of barium is contraindicated if parietal perforation is suspected due to the risk of mediastinitis. The presence of image subtraction suggests a foreign body or an endoluminal mass.

Fluoroscopy

This dynamic test is worthwhile when a functional problem is suspected. It may be beneficial when evaluating the extent of stenosis **(Figure 6)**.

Esophagoscopy

The endoscopic examination **(Figure 7)**, which is conducted under general anesthesia, is the examination of choice to explore all esophageal disorders of anatomical, inflammatory or neoplastic origin. It enables immediate macroscopic evaluation of the surface of the mucosa, biopsies, extraction of foreign bodies or enables dilatation of post-inflammatory or post-traumatic stenosis.

► Vomiting

Vomiting is defined as the active reflexive rejection of the stomach content preceded by prodromal signs (nausea, ptyalism, abdominal contractions). The dietary behavior and lifestyle of carnivores mean that occasional vomiting is not considered alarming. In its more acute and more frequent form however, it is one of the main reasons among cats for a visit to the veterinarian.

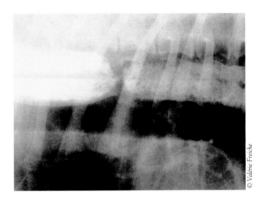

Figure 6 - *Radiograph with contrast medium that indicates esophageal stenosis.*

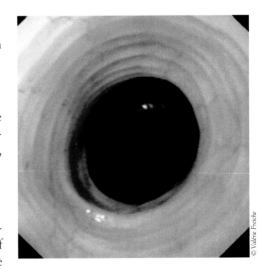

Figure 7 - *Esophagoscopy.*
Normal aspect of the distal esophagus of a cat showing characteristic rings

There are a huge number of disorders that can cause vomiting. Therefore, the etiological diagnosis, when justified, is based on a number of tests, which must be conducted as part of a logical approach. The digestive causes of acute or chronic vomiting are considered after the exclusion of all other potential causes in cats: viral infections, hernias, neoplasia, metabolic diseases, kidney failure, neuroendocrine diseases, intoxication and others (*Moore, 1992; Gaschen & Neiger, 2004; Simpson, 2005*).

Vomiting with a digestive origin may be due to stomach problems. The most common are: inflammatory diseases, neoplasia, the presence of hairballs, pyloric obstruction, ulceration or foreign bodies (**Figure 8**). Primary gastric motility problems may be suspected with chronic vomiting, however, they are more common in dogs than in cats. In the absence of a specific disorder, there may be a problem with stomach emptying (*Hall & Washabau, 1999*).

In cats, vomiting may also be a sign of a more distal disorder, even in the absence of any other sign. This is a peculiarity of the species. Major causes of vomiting not situated in the stomach include pancreatic diseases, inflammatory diseases or cholecystitis (*Strombeck & Guilford, 1996b*).

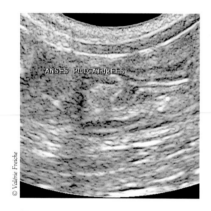

Figure 8 - 5 year old female cat who presented with anorexia.
The abdominal ultrasound shows loops of the small intestine that are abnormally collapsed due to the presence of a linear foreign body.

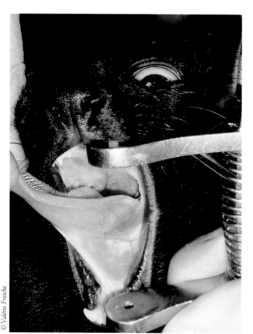

Figure 9 - Foreign body in the oral cavity.
The inspection of the oral cavity is part of the clinical examination. A linear foreign body attached to the base of the tongue can be extracted.

> Signs of vomiting

The aspect or chronology of vomiting with respect to the ingestion of food sometimes provides some pointers. Some criteria are reliable:
- uncontrollable or unpredictable vomiting suggests an occlusive syndrome, peritonitis, pancreatitis, cholangiohepatitis, a metabolic, or a severe viral disorder;
- the presence of undigested food well after meal time suggests a gastric retention syndrome (functional or anatomical in origin) or pancreatitis;
- vomiting in the morning before eating is common with chronic gastritis (or reflux gastritis);
- a large volume is common with an occlusive syndrome or delayed gastric emptying.

However, the nature or time of vomiting with respect to meal time commonly provides no pointers as to the cause:
- the presence of blood may be evidence of an underlying disorder with a very poor prognosis (neoplasia) or conversely an entirely benign and reversible inflammatory state.
- some neoplastic diseases are expressed by crude, non-specific symptoms, that emerge slowly;
- chronic sub-occlusive states are difficult to characterize, especially if they are caused by the ingestion of a linear foreign body.

> Clinical examination

There must be a precise and complete clinical examination as part of an internal medicine approach (*Tams, 1996*). If the cat is not cooperative, moderate sedation will make the examination easier.
- An inspection of the oral cavity (**Figure 9**) must always be conducted. It may reveal the ingestion of a linear foreign body or ulcers caused by uremia.
- Abdominal palpation is likely to provide pointers, such as the identification of a compressive digestive or extra-digestive mass, or palpation of a foreign body. The pressure generated by palpation may reveal induration or the presence of isolated sources of pain. Indirect signs are also seen, such as the accumulation of gas or fluid in front of a digestive lesion.
- If the cat is not obese, the presence of hyperplastic lymph nodes must always be palpated.
- A rectal swab (which generally necessitates tranquilization) enables evaluation of the rectal mucosa and the acquisition of a fecal sample (traces of fresh or digested blood).
- The hydration state of the cat.

TABLE 2 - BENEFITS OF COMPLEMENTARY TESTS USED IN THE DIAGNOSTIC EVALUATION OF VOMITING	
Complementary test	**Diagnostic benefit: specific searches**
Hematological analyses (blood count/CBC)	Anemia – Leucopenia or leucocytosis
Biochemical analyses; basal T_4	Metabolic diseases – Hyperthyroidism – Hypoproteinemia
Serum electrolytes	Dehydration – Addison's Disease (highly unlikely)
Urine analysis	Urine specific gravity – pH
Plain radiography	Radiodense foreign bodies – Digestive mass – Ascites – Ileus
Contrast radiography	Foreign bodies – Parietal modifications
Abdominal ultrasound	Digestive parietal lesions – Foreign bodies – Abdominal lymphadenopathy – Peristalsis – Other abdominal organs
Gastointestinal endoscopy	Gastro-duodenal, distal ileal and colonic parietal lesions – Gastric and duodenal foreign bodies (limits if linear foreign body)

> Diagnosis

Table 2 lists the benefits of complementary tests that may be conducted in the evaluation of a vomiting patient.

▶ Gastric retention syndrome

Gastric retention syndrome is defined as the stomach's incapacity to evacuate its content within the physiological time. This may be due to digestive lesions or functional disorders (primary or secondary digestive motor disturbances). Although more common in dogs, this syndrome has been reported in cats. The clinical signs include vomiting of partially digested food well after mealtime.

> Etiology of gastric retention syndrome

Obstructive digestive or extra-digestive compressive lesions

Some form of pyloric stenosis is the most common cause of gastric retention syndrome in domesticated carnivores. If they are intrinsic, they may be the result of several pathophysiological mechanisms.

- **Congenital pyloric stenosis (Figure 10)**: found in young animals, is due to hypertrophy of the smooth muscle fiber. In cats, it is described in Asiatic breeds, specifically the Siamese (*Strombeck, 1978*)

- **Secondary gastric retention syndrome with hairball (Figure 11)**, which can be lodged chronically and generate repetitive intermittent vomiting.

- **Post-inflammatory pyloric stenosis (Figure 12)**: healed pyloric lesions (old ulcerations, chronic inflammatory lesions causing major parietal fibrosis, foreign bodies trapped in the antral-pyloric mucosa) sometimes cause acquired stenosing lesions.

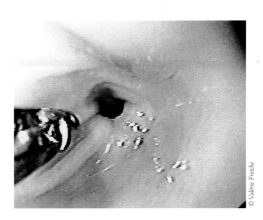

© Valérie Freiche

Figure 10 - Pyloric stenosis in a young European cat a few months of age.
The pyloric diameter compared to biopsy forceps (2.8 mm).

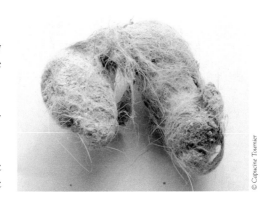

© Capucine Tournier

Figure 11 - Hairball secreted by a Japanese Bobtail (length: 5.5 cm).
Hairballs are the primary cause of gastric retention in cats.

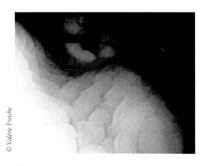

Figure 12 - Post-inflammatory pyloric stenosis in a European cat who historically had gastritis. *Edema is visible in the mucosal antral area.*

© Valérie Freiche

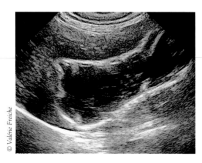

Figure 13 - Male cat, 3 year old, presented for lethargy and vomiting. *The echocardiographic picture shows an abnormal gastric retention.*

© Valérie Freiche

- **Extrinsic digestive compression** (much less common): by adjacent abdominal organs (liver tumor, lymphadenopathy).

Digestive motor disturbances

Digestive motor disturbances leading to slower gastric emptying may be caused by hypomotility or dysregulation of the contraction rhythm. Either primary or secondary in origin, their pathogenesis is thought to be related to dysfunction of the gastric pacemakers. This leads to gastric "arrhythmia", as observed in the event of repetitive hairballs in cats (*Washabau, 2003*). A gastric emptying disorder must be determined by studying the transit of solid food (*Wyse et al, 2003*). This exclusion diagnosis is suspected when other examinations are within normal limits.

There are secondary motor disturbances:
- excessive sympathetic stimulation (stress, pain, deep abdominal lesions: peritonitis, pancreatitis, major parasitism): a very long gastric retention is observed with pancreatitis
- post-surgery iatrogenic trauma
- medical treatment: anticholinergic agents, opiates, non-steroidal anti-inflammatory drugs (NSAID)
- metabolic disorders: acidosis, uremia, hyperkalemia, hypo- or hypercalcemia, endocrinopathies
- neoplastic process or ulceration (pain inhibiting transit by sympathetic stimulation).

> When should the gastric retention syndrome should be suspected?

The characteristic clinical sign of the gastric retention syndrome is vomiting of undigested food well after mealtime. However, owners also often describe vomiting of gastric juice. These signs are due to chronic gastric distension and inflammation of the mucosa, respectively.

Digestive motor disturbances associated with gastric retention syndrome may cause signs of dyspepsia, such as intermittent ptyalism, antalgic gait, gas bloat, very painful spastic crises and yawning. Abdominal palpation confirms the presence of gastric distension. The clinical signs are more alarming when motor disruptions are secondary to metabolic alterations or a septic state (peritonitis, pancreatitis).

> Diagnosis

Table 3 lists the benefits of the complementary tests that may be conducted to assist in the diagnosis of the gastric retention syndrome.

> Treatment

This ensues from the etiology when it can be identified, of the gastric retention syndrome.

Medical treatment

In the event of metabolic problems, treatment includes management of the underlying disorder and administration of prokinetic agents (*Hall & Washabau, 1999*) (metoclopramide, domperidone, ranitidine, etc). The administration of prokinetics entails a potential risk of occlusive syndromes.

Surgical treatment

Depending on the case, pyloroplasty, extraction of a foreign body, excision or the biopsy of polyps or neoplastic lesions may be indicated.

TABLE 3 - BENEFITS OF COMPLEMENTARY TESTS USED IN THE DIAGNOSTIC EVALUATION OF THE GASTRIC RETENTION SYNDROME

Complementary test	Diagnostic benefits
Biochemical analyses	Metabolic diseases – Hyperthyroidism – Hypoproteinemia – Differential diagnosis of vomiting
Serum electrolytes	Rehydration – Differential diagnosis of vomiting
Plain radiography	Gastric dilatation – Radiodense foreign body – Digestive mass – Ileus
Contrast radiography	Gastric distension – Evaluation of gastric emptying time: *the ingestion of barium impregnated polyethylene spheres (BIPS) refines the actual emptying time and calculates the percentage of emptying correlated to time* – Thickening of the stomach wall – Foreign body
Abdominal ultrasound (Figure 13)	Measurement of the stomach wall – Identification of parietal layers – Appearance of the pylorus – Peristaltic waves
Gastrointestinal endoscopy	Stomach lesions – Extraction of foreign bodies – Pyloric lesions and parietal biopsies

Dietary measures

Depending on the etiology, diet can be a significant adjunctive therapy *(Hall & Washabau, 1999)*. Dietary treatment can support gastric emptying. Small meals of a liquid or moist diet are the best recommendation for the initial therapy. If small foreign bodies or trichobezoars (hair balls) have been identified, lubricants such as paraffin that facilitate the propulsion through the gut, maybe beneficial. Bromelain, a cysteine protease contained in pineapple juice, has been suggested as a dietary treatment. In one study, bromelain was able to degrade trichobezoars to a variable extent *(Reed et al, 2004)*. However, more in vivo data are needed for the assessment of efficacy.

Dietary fiber plays an important role in preventing gastric retention. Dietary fiber significantly affects fecal hair excretion in cats and a high-fiber diet (12-15% total dietary fiber [TDF] as fed) is useful in the prevention of hairball formation *(Tournier et al, 2005)* (see Royal Canin Nutritional Information at the end of the chapter).

▶ Diarrhea

Diarrhea is characterized by the increased frequency of evacuation, moisture content and often volume of fecal matter. The owner will not always immediately identify diarrhea if the cat excretes outdoors.

In cats, the moisture content in a normal stool usually varies between 55% and 70%, depending on the food *(internal data from Royal Canin Research Center)*. It can go as low as 40% in constipation and as high as 90% with diarrhea *(Williams & Guilford, 1996)*.

Diarrhea is mainly caused by intestinal diseases, but other systemic diseases may affect intestinal function and can induce hypersecretion or malabsorption *(Battersby & Harvey, 2006)*. It can be due to diseases of the small or large intestine or it may affect both *(Tams, 2004)*. Acute cases can be caused by dietary indiscretion, infections with enteropathogenic viruses, bacteria or parasites. In chronic cases, lymphoplasmacytic or eosinophilic inflammatory bowel disease (IBD), bacterial dysbiosis or dietary allergy or sensitivity can often be the underlying problem. Exocrine pancreatic insufficiency is reported in the cat. It is certainly under-diagnosed in this species *(Williams, 2005)*. Drug intolerance and acute or chronic systemic diseases can induce diarrhea. Digestive tumors are also a common cause of chronic diarrhea in aging cats.

> Origin in the digestive system

There are far fewer clinical criteria to differentiate small intestinal diarrhea from large intestinal diarrhea in cats compared with dogs. This is due to the fact that disorders of the digestive walls are typically diffuse in cats.

Table 4 lists the criteria for differentiating small intestinal diarrhea and large intestinal diarrhea in domesticated carnivores.

> Pathophysiological reminders

Several mechanisms are involved in the increased water content of stools *(Freiche, 2000)*. When the small intestine is injured three types of physiological disturbance may occur separately or collectively to lead to the clinical expression of diarrhea:
- increased secretion of water and electrolytes
- decreased absorption of nutrients (mainly carbohydrates and lipids)
- decreased absorption of water and electrolytes **(Figure 14)**

FIGURE 14 - DIGESTIVE FACTORS THAT MAY AFFECT STOOL CONSISTENCY

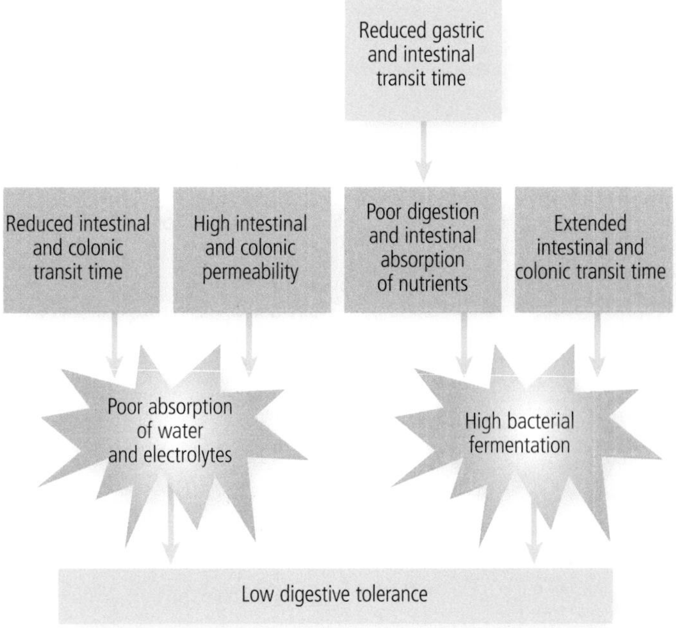

Sign	Small intestinal diarrhea	Large intestinal diarrhea
TABLE 4 - DIFFERENTIATION OF SMALL INTESTINAL AND LARGE INTESTINAL DIARRHEA *(German & Zentek, 2006)*		
Feces		
- Volume	- Markedly increased	- Normal or decreased
- Mucus	- Rarely present	- Common
- Melena	- Rarely present	- Absent
- Hematochezia	- Absent except in acute hemorrhagic diarrhea	- Fairly common
- Steatorrhea	- Present with malabsorption	- Absent
- Undigested food	- May be present	- Absent
- Color	- Color variations occur e.g. creamy brown, green, orange, clay	- Color variations rare; may be hemorrhagic
Defecation		
- Urgency	- Absent except in acute or very severe disease	- Usual but not invariably present
- Tenesmus	- Absent	- Frequent but not invariably present
- Frequency	- 2 to 3 times normal for the patient	- Usually greater than 3 times normal
- Dyschezia	- Absent	- Present with distal colonic or rectal disease
Ancillary signs		
- Weight loss	- May occur in malabsorption	- Rare except in severe colitis and diffuse tumors
- Vomiting	- May be present in inflammatory diseases	- Described in cats with colon disease
- Flatulence and borborygmi	- May occur	- Absent
- Halitosis in the absence of oral cavity disease	- May be present with malabsorption	- Absent unless perianal licking

When the colonic mucosa is responsible, failure of the reabsorption function of the colon and excessive secretory activity of the parietal mucus glands are observed.

> Coherence of diagnosis

Importance of the history and clinical examination

A very large number of diseases may cause chronic diarrhea. There is no general diagnostic plan that can be used in all cases, so the cat's history and a detailed clinical examination are essential.

At the end of these two steps the clinician must attempt to answer two questions that have a significant impact on the choice of treatment:
- does the diarrhea have a strictly digestive origin or could the cause be metabolic?
- is it small intestinal diarrhea or large intestinal diarrhea? **(Table 4)**

Sequence of complementary tests and differential diagnosis

In its specific context, each clinical case demands a logical sequence of complementary examinations. Various tests are possible:

- hemato-biochemical analyses, serological assays
- fecal examination
- biochemical exploration of malassimilation (folate and vitamin B_{12})
- digestive tract imaging: radiography, ultrasound, gastrointestinal endoscopy. These different techniques have radically transformed knowledge of gastroenterology over the past decade.

> Therapeutic consequences

Current therapies

Specific therapeutic plans are provided below for the most common diarrheal disorders in the cat:
- infectious gastroenteritis
- characteristics of diarrhea in kittens
- dietary intolerance
- chronic inflammatory bowel diseases (IBD)
- colonic diseases
- digestive neoplasia.

Dietary treatment

Dietary treatment is more of an adjunctive type of therapy in many cases of chronic small intestinal disease. As undigested food compounds are fermented by the colonic microflora and can have negative effects (such as gas formation and flatulence, and perhaps also promote further diarrhea), the diet should be highly digestible.

• Highly digestible diets

Diets for patients with suspected intestinal dysbiosis, to be characterized either as "small intestinal bacterial overgrowth" or as a disturbed micro-ecology in the upper or lower gastrointestinal tract, should be based on high quality ingredients. They support the patient by providing available carbohydrates and proteins that facilitate nutrient absorption in the small intestine. Highly digestible diets typically present dry matter digestibility values that exceed 85-88% and protein digestibility that exceeds 92%. These diets require less gastric, pancreatic, biliary and intestinal secretions for digestion. This results in almost complete digestion and absorption in the upper small intestine so that minimal residue is presented to the lower bowel (**Figure 15**). Minimal residue reduces bacterial byproducts that may contribute to inflammation and osmotic diarrhea.

The passage of unabsorbed nutrients into the lower gut is reduced, as is the potential load of antigenic material. As long as dietary sensitivity or allergy cannot be excluded, an antigen-limited hypoallergenic diet is advantageous. These diets contain either highly digestible protein sources (e.g. protein hydrolyzates, low-ash poultry, fish) or other meats that are unusual in commercial diets (e.g. venison, duck, rabbit etc).

• Carbohydrates

Mucosal atrophy typically leads to a decreased availability of disaccharidases and carbohydrate malabsorption. Bacterial overgrowth and decreased transport of monosaccharides by malfunctioning enterocytes can also contribute to carbohydrate malabsorption, which in turn contributes to osmotic diarrhea. Therefore, diets formulated for cats with gastrointestinal disease should contain reduced quantities of highly digestible carbohydrate. Rice has long been considered the ideal carbohydrate for gastrointestinal disease. Rice is very highly digestible because it has a limited branched starch structure (amylopectin) and a very low dietary fiber content. Rice does not present any crossed antigenicity with wheat gluten and has rarely been implicated in adverse food reactions.

FIGURE 15 - IMPROVING DIGESTIBILITY TO LIMIT FERMENTATION IN THE COLON

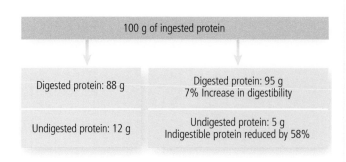

100 g of ingested protein	
Digested protein: 88 g	Digested protein: 95 g 7% Increase in digestibility
Undigested protein: 12 g	Undigested protein: 5 g Indigestible protein reduced by 58%

A very low level of indigestible protein limits fermentation in the intestine and therefore the presence of substances that can promote inflammation and osmotic diarrhea.

TABLE 5 - INFLUENCE OF FERMENTABILITY AND FERMENTATION TIME IN VITRO OF DIFFERENT TYPES OF DIETARY FIBER ON THE DECOMPOSITION OF ORGANIC MATTER AND THE PRODUCTION OF SHORT CHAIN FATTY ACIDS (SCFA) IN CATS

From Sunvold et al (1995b)

Substrates	Soluble fibers	Insoluble fibers	Disappearance of organic matter (OM) (as)			Total production of SCFA (as mmol/g of OM)		
			6h	12h	24h	6h	12h	24h
Fructo-oligo-saccharides	++++		92.5	86.8	86.1	1.35	3.03	4.33
Citrus pectin	++++		49.6	76.6	85.5	2.02	4.2	4.71
Guar gum	+++	+	15.2	44.3	71.5	0.43	2.3	4.99
Beet pulp	+	+++	21.1	24.2	31.5	0.51	1.32	1.93
Cellulose		++++	0.7	0.4	0.6	-0.03	0.08	0.06

Dietary fiber rich in soluble fiber is heavily fermented by the fecal microflora, which leads to an increased production of SCFA.

Furthermore, rice improves the digestibility of dry diets, and contains soluble factors that inhibit secretory diarrhea.

Dietary fiber may benefit from an increased concentration or modified type of dietary fiber despite low-fiber diets (< 10% TDF) often being recommended. When indicated based on the clinical outcome, it can be worthwhile increasing fiber concentration by adding small amounts of insoluble or soluble fiber sources.

- On contact with water, soluble fiber such as pectin forms a gel (gelling capacity) or solution that can be more or less viscous (thickening capacity). Due to this viscosity, such fibers tends to slow down gastrointestinal transit by simply increasing resistance to the flow. Soluble fiber sources are also important regulators of the intestinal microbiota due to their high fermentability (**Table 5**).

- Insoluble fiber such as cellulose increases fecal bulk, fecal water content, absorbs toxins and normalizes both segmental and propulsive motility.

Both insoluble and soluble dietary fiber may be beneficial in the symptomatic treatment of certain large bowel diarrheas. In homemade diets, adequate supplements are 0.5 tablespoons of:
- cellulose or wheat bran when insoluble types of fiber are desired
- psyllium when soluble fiber sources are more promising. In commercial diets designed for intestinal disorders, various sources of fermentable fiber should already be included (e.g. beet pulp, fructo-oligosaccharides [FOS], mannan-oligosaccharides [MOS]).

• **Energy density**
Fat is often regarded critically as a compound in diets for patients with small intestinal disease: when fat digestion is impaired, the bacterial conversion of non-absorbed fatty acids and bile acids into hydroxylated fatty acids and deconjugated bile acids can increase fluid secretion and aggravate clinical signs of diarrhea.

On the other hand, weight loss and poor coat and skin quality can be major problems in cats with small intestinal problems. As high fat diets help provide energy and fat soluble vitamins to debilitated cats, the prescription of high fat diets is advocated. Fat digestibility is generally extremely high (up to 99%). In addition, a high-energy diet (> 20% on DMB) enables a reduction of the volume of the diet and decreases the intestinal load.

Therefore, the level of fat tolerated by cats with small intestinal disorders needs to be individually evaluated when increased dietary fat levels are warranted. It is justified to use increased fat intakes when weight loss is a prominent clinical sign and when a steatorrhea is not present.

• **Probiotics and prebiotics**
Probiotics and prebiotics have been suggested as treatment options for patients with intestinal problems.

Data on the efficacy and the presumed "stabilizing" effect of probiotics on digestive diseases are scarce. Often enough, products have not been evaluated with regards to efficacy or may not be suitable for cats and the specific conditions in the diseased intestinal tract. *L. acidophilus* (DSM 13241 strain) used as a probiotic increased the lactobacilli counts in feces and decreased numbers of *Clostridium spp.* and *Enterococcus faecalis* (*Marshall Jones et al, 2006*).

Prebiotics are non-digestible carbohydrates that are fermented by gut bacteria in the small and large intestine. The basic idea is to offer a substrate to "beneficial" members of the gut flora and to promote a shift in the composition of the gut bacteria in favor of the "healthy" microbiota, such as *lactobacilli* and *bifidobacteria*. Through inhibitory process, these bacteria prevent the proliferation of potentially pathogenic bacteria (*i.e. Clostridium perfringens*). These bacteria produce the short chain fatty acids (SCFA) butyrate, acetate and propionate, which provide fuel for the colonocytes. SCFA enhance sodium and water absorption, increase mucosal blood flow and increase gastrointestinal hormone release. These mechanisms contribute to the trophic effect that SCFA have on the intestinal mucosa, stimulating enterocyte and colonocyte proliferation.

Different prebiotic carbohydrates have been used, mainly inulin and various oligosaccharides (fructo-oligosaccharides, galacto-oligosaccharides, mannan-oligosaccharides). Some gastrointestinal changes can be expected, including pathogen control and reduced putrefactive compound production (*Hesta et al, 2001; Flickinger et al, 2003*). The efficacy of these additives needs to be studied more in clinical patients to evaluate whether such feed additives and feed compounds are beneficial in cats with intestinal disease (*Sparkes et al, 1998*).

> Protein-losing enteropathy

Protein-losing enteropathy (PLE) results from a range of gastrointestinal disorders that lead to non-selective protein loss. They are characterized by a total serum protein content less than 5 g/dL and an albumin concentration lower than 2 g/dL. These values must be interpreted on the basis of the normal reference ranges for the laboratory.

Although lymphangectasia remains the primary cause of PLE, many parietal disorders of the digestive tract are likely to be expressed as hypoproteinemia. Forms of PLE continue to be exceptional in cats, in the event of either IBD or digestive neoplasia. Identification of hypoproteinemia in cats always worsens the prognosis of the underlying disorder.

Disorders involved in PLE are listed in **Table 6.**

Dietary measures

Patients with PLE are often clinically fragile, and careful symptomatic therapy must be integrated with intensive dietary and medical management strategies in most cases (*Peterson & Willard, 2003*). The nutritional management of cats with PLE is mainly based on diets with a low fat concentration. Low fat (≤ 10%, as fed) diets have been proven to be supportive because they counteract the pathophysiological events in PLE.

Long chain fatty acids are transported through the intestinal lymphatics. This may increase lymphatic vessel distension and increase intestinal protein loss and eventually lipid exudation. Linoleic acid and arachidonic acid have to be provided in sufficient amounts to fulfill the requirements. Medium chain triglycerides have some value because of their ability to be absorbed by bypassing the lymphatic system. A general limitation for using this type of fat is its negative effect on palatability and potential

TABLE 6 - ETIOLOGY OF PROTEIN-LOSING ENTEROPATHY IN CATS	
Membrane permeability problems Alterations of the mucosa surface	**Diseases of the lymphatic system**

• Ulcerative stomach lesions
• Lymphoplasmacytic enteritis (IBD)
• Eosinophilic enteritis
• Hemorrhagic gastroenteritis
• Small intestinal bacterial overgrowth (SIBO)
• Gluten intolerance
• Massive digestive parasitism
• Chronic intussusception
• Chronic sub-occlusion (foreign body or tumor)
• Iatrogenic (drugs, toxins)
	• Focal or diffuse congenital lymphangectasia
	
	• Acquired lymphangectasis:
	  - Inflammatory or neoplastic obstruction in the intestine
	  - Obstruction of the peripheral lymphatic vessels (lymphangitis lipogranulomatous – neoplasia)
	  - Lymphatic hypertension (pericarditis, right heart failure, neoplasia)

for inducing vomiting and diarrhea in cats. Higher supplementation with fat-soluble vitamins would be required and there are anecdotal reports of improvement with glutamine supplementation.

▶ Melena

Melena occurs when blood from the stomach or small intestine is passed in the feces. The color is black due to the degradation of hemoglobin. It occurs frequently in combination with coagulation disorders or in those cases when the structure of the gastrointestinal epithelium is severely compromised and if erosions or ulcerations have developed (*Kohn et al, 2003; Dennis et al, 2006*).

▶ Fecal incontinence

Anal, gastrointestinal, neural or muscular disorders can cause fecal incontinence in cats (*Guilford, 1990*). Intervertebral disc disease or tumors can also be associated with the condition (*Munana et al, 2001*).

▶ Flatulence

Gas formation in the intestinal tract is a normal process related to the activity of the intestinal microflora. Around 200 volatile compounds are formed as the bacteria break down the digestive content in the large intestine. The main compounds are alcohols (such as methanol, ethanol etc), sulfur compounds (hydrogen sulfide, methyl/ethyl mercaptans etc), nitrogen compounds (ammonia, indole, phenol, skatole etc), volatile fatty acids (acetic/propionic/butyric/valeric acids etc) and other organic compounds.

Some of the substances produced in the intestinal tract are highly unpleasant (**Figure 16**), such as sulfur compounds, ammonia, biogenic amines, indoles and phenols (*Lowe & Kershaw, 1997*).
- Ammonia is formed mainly from the deamination of amino acids.
- Biogenic amines (cadaverin, histamine, putrescine, tyramine etc) are produced essentially by the decarboxylation of amino acids

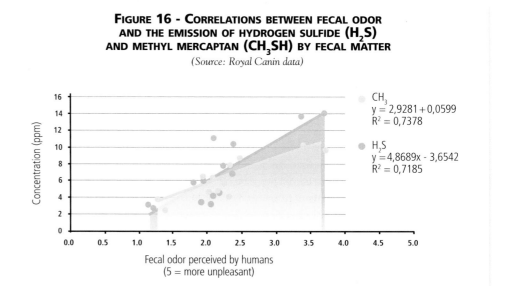

FIGURE 16 - CORRELATIONS BETWEEN FECAL ODOR AND THE EMISSION OF HYDROGEN SULFIDE (H_2S) AND METHYL MERCAPTAN (CH_3SH) BY FECAL MATTER
(*Source: Royal Canin data*)

CH_3
$y = 2,9281 + 0,0599$
$R^2 = 0,7378$

H_2S
$y = 4,8689x - 3,6542$
$R^2 = 0,7185$

Concentration (ppm)

Fecal odor perceived by humans
(5 = more unpleasant)

The hydrogen sulfide (H_2S) content is a good indicator of olfactory emissions, because its concentration is very well correlated with the perception of the human nose. There is also a good correlation between the odor perceived by humans and the methyl mercaptan (CH_3SH) concentration in air.

- Indole and phenolic compounds result from the decomposition of aromatic amino acids (tyrosine and phenylalanine)
- Sulfur compounds (hydrogen sulfide, mercaptans) from that of methionine and cystine.

The different components of an odor can be identified by gas chromatography together with mass spectrometry. It is also possible to judge the intensity of the odor by comparing it with increasing concentrations of 1-butanol (*Sorel et al, 1983*).

Avoidance of dietary ingredients that favor intestinal gaseousness is of primary importance. Many legumes and other vegetable ingredients contain more or less non-digestible and microbially fermentable fractions. Some flatulence cases may be proof either of the poor quality of the food (generally mediocre protein quality) or the existence of a digestive function disorder (*Williams & Guilford, 1996*). Flatulence is common in cases of dietary hypersensitivity. However, the problem is not well understood: some cases respond to dietary changes, and hence dietary treatment has to be adjusted according to the individual case. An eviction diet or an hydrolysed diet can help to manage dietary hypersensitivity cases.

6 - Enteral and parenteral nutrition

(See chapter 12 for more detail)

▶ Assisted feeding and enteral nutrition

For many gastrointestinal diseases, a period of assisted feeding is required. The rapid and thorough attention to the nutritional management of inappetent patients can decrease morbidity and mortality. Diets may be applied either by syringe or as small solid boli depending on the underlying disease or the preference of the patient or owner. Feeding tubes are an accepted way of providing nutritional support to animals unable or unwilling to consume adequate calories on their own (*Wortinger, 2006*).

Enteral feeding is preferred and can be achieved by nasal, pharyngeal, esophageal, gastric or jejunal feeding tubes (*Ireland et al, 2003*). The diameter of the tube should be large enough to permit feeding of the chosen diet, either specific enteral products or blended canned food that may be additionally diluted with water. Percutaneous endoscopic gastrostomy tubes have traditionally been considered to be the best-tolerated feeding device, but they are not without complications (vomiting and stomal site infection) and they require specific equipment and training. Esophagostomy tubes are an alternative and are simpler to place and have lower complication rates. For esophagostomy tubes, vomiting, scratching at the tube and bandage, removal of the tube and mechanical difficulties have been described (*Ireland et al, 2003*).

▶ Parenteral nutrition

Total parenteral nutrition (TPN) is used to fulfill the total nutrient requirements in cats that are anorectic for longer periods and that cannot be maintained on an enteral feeding regime. Although the technique of parenteral nutrition is well established in many veterinary hospitals, it requires some training and equipment to avoid complications. Metabolic (hyperglycemia, hyperkalemia), mechanical (catheter dislodgement, cellulitis), or septic problems may be related to the improper installment of parenteral nutrition in cats (*Crabb et al, 2006*). Often these complications are mild and can be managed without discontinuation of TPN or adjustment of the infusion protocol. A more conservative estimate of energy requirements appears to be associated with a lower risk of hyperglycemia.

Using partial parenteral nutrition (PPN) delivers only a certain part of the required nutrients and energy. The risk of metabolic problems in cats is considerably reduced by this approach, although septic and mechanical complications may also occur (*Chan et al, 2002*). Animals on combined enteral and parenteral nutrition can have a better clinical outcome than those receiving parenteral nutrition exclusively.

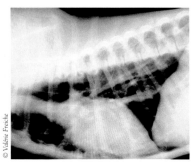

Figure 17 - Thoracic radiograph of a cat consistent with megaesophagus. The esophageal wall, normally not seen, is visible here (two radiodense lines).

7 - Diseases of the esophagus and nutritional approach

► Conformation abnormalities of the esophagus

> Vascular abnormalities

The persistence of some vascular arches in the course of embryogenesis may cause extrinsic compression of the esophagus, leading to the formation of a crop above the stenosis. The most commonly described abnormality is the persistence of the fourth arch of the right aorta (*Twedt, 1994*). The esophagus is clasped in an adhesion formed by the aorta, the non-vascularized residual arterial ligament and the pulmonary artery. The diagnosis is based on radiography (localized proximal esophageal dilatation) and endoscopy, and the treatment is surgical. Other abnormalities have been reported in carnivores (double aortic arch, persistence of subclavian arteries), but these conformation faults remain exceptionally rare in cats.

> Esophageal fistulas

Esophageal fistulas are rare in carnivores. They extend from the esophageal wall to the mediastinum or even the chest cavity. They are congenital, although they can result from trauma. Signs are mostly of a respiratory nature (dyspnea, coughing, fever). The diagnosis is based on radiography with contrast medium or esophagoscopy.

> Megaesophagus: medical aspects

Megaesophagus is a generalized dilation of the esophagus with partial or total loss of peristalsis and motility **(Figure 17)**. The congenital form is distinguished from the acquired form, the origin of which is sometimes identified or remains undetermined (idiopathic megaesophagus) (*Strombeck, 1978*).

Epidemiology and pathophysiology

• Congenital megaesophagus
The congenital form is described in Asiatic breeds, specifically the Siamese (*Tams, 1996*). While it has not been possible to show vagal innervation deficits, modification of the conduction of the afferent reflex arches that generate peristalsis can be suspected. Motility problems are implicated in the pathogenesis of congenital megaesophagus (contractions of ineffective amplitude, alteration of parietal elasticity).

• Acquired megaesophagus
No epidemiological studies have established any breed or sex predisposition for the acquired forms, and no hereditary transmission mechanism is suspected. All disorders entailing parietal lesions of the esophagus or an innervation fault are likely to cause the appearance of megaesophagus.

In the absence of clinical factors suggesting another etiology, acquired megaesophagus in cats should give rise to the hypothesis of dysautonomia. The involved pathogenic mechanisms have not been clearly described. This general disorder of the neurovegative nervous system means that colonic atony is often associated and the clinical signs are much more complex. The appearance of esophageal motility problems – even isolated – may also suggest severe myasthenia (*Moses et al, 2000*).

Clinical signs

In the congenital forms the clinical expression often manifests itself during weaning: ever more frequent regurgitations, stunted growth compared with other kittens in the same litter. In some cases the regurgitations occur well after mealtimes, and owners may interpret them as vomiting, which may cause the clinician to orient towards an incorrect diagnosis.

Other clinical signs described are halitosis, abnormal sounds from the esophagus, coughing secondary to aspiration pneumonia *(Jenkins, 2000)*. However, not all cats with megaesophagus present with respiratory signs. Conversely, respiratory disease is sometimes very important.

Palpation of the esophagus may reveal a perceptible dilatation of the ventral part of the neck. A muco-purulent discharge and audible rales are noted in the event of infectious pulmonary complications. The impairment of the general condition is inconsistent.

Diagnosis

Radiographs of the thorax are used for the diagnosis. In case of doubt radiographs taken after the administration of contrast medium can confirm the esophageal dilatation. Digestive endoscopy is not among the complementary tests that help confirm the diagnosis.

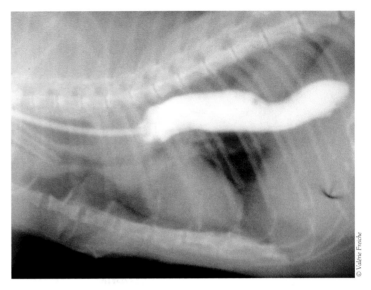

Figure 18 - Extensive esophageal dilatation in a cat who presented for both dysphagia and severe respiratory difficulties.
Thoracic contrast radiography with barium.

• Plain radiography

The esophagus cannot usually be seen on a plain radiograph. Increased esophageal radio transparency is therefore abnormal. The size of the dilatation is variable. It may affect the whole organ or only the thoracic part of it. A radiodense line emphasizes the dorsal wall. These modifications are identifiable on the lateral and ventro-dorsal views. It is important that good quality radiographs are obtained to enable evaluation of the pulmonary tissue for characteristic densities and alveolar infiltrates, which are characteristic of aspiration pneumonia.

• Radiography with contrast medium

The administration of a contrast medium **(Figure 18)** will be necessary if the animal experiences deglutition problems or regurgitations if the plain radiographs are normal or insufficient to establish a definite diagnosis. The contrast medium may be a barium sulfate paste, but this is contraindicated in the event of dysphagia due to the risk of aspiration. Barium is very irritating for the bronchi. In this situation, an iodized product is recommended for contrast enhancement.

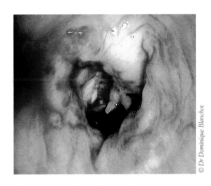

Figure 19 - Esophageal tumor in a 14-year-old European cat.
Histological examination indicated an undifferentiated carcinoma.

• Endoscopy

In the event of megaesophagus, endoscopy can evaluate the integrity of the surface of the mucosa, but it is not the most reliable test for assessing the size of the esophageal lumen. However, in case of doubt in the differential diagnosis, it does help refine the diagnosis and exclude the presence of associated esophagitis.

Differential diagnosis

Owners are often imprecise in describing clinical signs. It is not uncommon for tardy regurgitations to be confused with very early vomiting. The differential diagnosis should include all other disorders that may cause dysphagia or ptyalism:
- pharyngeal disorders: foreign body, laryngeal paralysis (achalasia: very rare in cats)
- other esophageal lesions: foreign body, vascular abnormalities (crop), neoplasia (rare)
  (Figure 19).

Treatment

The treatment of congenital megaesophagus or idiopathic acquired megaesophagus is based on hygienic and palliative measures. It makes great demands on the owner: feeding the animal in a raised position improves the assimilation of the food due to gravity. The consistency of the diet

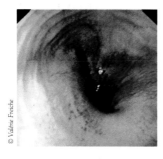

Figure 20 - Endoscopy of the distal esophagus of a cat. *Note the presence of erythematous punctures consistent with an acute inflammatory state.*

© Valérie Freiche

is an important but inconsistent factor: some cats regurgitate less with a liquid food, others have more success with solids.

In the event of bronchopulmonary complications, complementary symptomatic medical treatment can be commenced.
- Prokinetic substances (e.g. cisapride) may enable better esophageal clearance in cats as the distal section of the esophagus is comprised of smooth muscles. Unfortunately, cisapride is no longer readily available in every country.
- Antibiotic therapy is indispensable in the event of secondary bronchopulmonary lesions.
- Mucosal protective agents are indicated if erosive parietal lesions are identified.

However, the prognosis is sometimes so poor (especially in kittens) that euthanasia is ultimately chosen.

► Esophagitis

Inflammation of the esophageal mucosa **(Figure 20)** may be secondary to local trauma (ingestion of toxins, prolonged presence of a foreign body) or to repetitive gastroesophageal reflux (lower esophageal sphincter incompetence, degenerative disorders) *(Lobetti & Leisewitz, 1996; Han et al, 2003)*. General anesthetics (barbiturates) reduce the pressure of the caudal esophageal sphincter, favoring peri-operative reflux *(Freiche, 2006a)*. In rare cases, stenosing parietal lesions appear. The composition and acid pH of the gastric fluid makes it highly irritating for the esophageal mucosa.

> Clinical manifestations and diagnosis

These are not very specific and include pain during deglutition, hypersalivation, and dysphagia. Sometimes, the clinical signs are simply prostration associated with dysorexia.

All inflammatory disorders of the esophagus are likely to be secondary to functional problems due to alteration of motility. These peristaltic problems are very difficult to document in domesticated carnivores. The examinations of choice are fluoroscopy and endoscopy.

> Medical treatment

Nil per os is required to manage highly erosive or diffuse esophageal lesions (see the section on esophageal foreign bodies).

Antacids

The administration of antisecretors and antacids help increase the gastric pH and reduce the risks of parietal erosion in the event of reflux. The most commonly used substances are anti-histamine – 2 agents (cimetidine, ranitidine, famotadine etc) and proton pump inhibitors (omeprazole and derived substances). They must be administered for at least fifteen days. Cimetidine favors augmentation of the caudal esophagus sphincter tone, which is often deficient in esophagitis.

Local topical agents including aluminum-based cytoprotectives, sucralfate, or an association of alginic acid and sodium bicarbonate, are beneficial adjuvant treatments. Administered at the end of the meal, they constitute a protective film on the surface of the mucosa and protect the mucosa from reflux.

Antibiotic therapy

Antibiotic therapy is indispensable in combating local bacterial translocation. It helps prevent more serious lesions. When there are too many lesions on the mucosa or perforation is suspected, the administration of ampicillin is recommended. The association of cephalosporin and metronidazole may be proposed.

Corticosteroids

Their use in the prevention of stenosis is highly controversial. Experimentally, their preventive activity has not been proven. Conversely, they are implicated in the mechanism of perforation during preexisting parietal necrosis. Administered over short periods, they limit pain and present local anti-inflammatory properties.

Inserting a gastrostomy tube

With severe esophagitis, local mechanical trauma in the mucosa can be reduced if no solid or liquid passes through the esophagus for several days. Another advantage of fasting is the reduction in the local fibroblastic reaction, which favors the appearance of a healing stenosis. A gastrostomy tube must be placed at the end of esophagoscopy. An anastomosis is created within a few days between the stomach wall and the abdominal wall. The administration of an energy dense diet and medical treatment is achieved several times a day using syringes connected to a three-way valve attached to the tube. This care can even be provided by the owner following simple instruction. Local tolerance is good *(Ireland et al, 2003)*. Energy density of the enteral diets should be high and fat as energy source is best suited for that purpose. In many cases, blended canned diets can be used. Bolus-feeding techniques can maintain a normal nutritional status in cats.

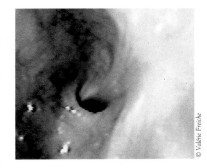

Figure 21 - *Post-operative peptic esophageal stenosis in a 4-year-old female cat*

▶ Esophageal stenosis

The appearance of isolated stenosing lesions of the esophageal wall most commonly follows the ingestion of caustic products or the onset of postoperative gastroesophageal reflux *(Sellon & Willard, 2003; Freiche, 2006a)*. In cats, the oral administration of tetracycline has been implicated in the genesis of severe stenosing esophageal lesions *(McGrotty & Knottenbelt, 2002; German et al, 2005)*. Less commonly, these lesions appear postoperatively **(Figure 21)** or after the extraction of a foreign body.

Esophageal stenosis is predominantly benign in cats. The mucosa loses its elasticity and the affected section becomes fibrotic (simultaneous disorder of the lamina propria and the muscle wall). There does not appear to be any preferred location in the esophagus; lesions can be proximal or distal, or even in multiple locations in the same animal.

> Clinical manifestations

The two clinical signs of stenosis are regurgitation and esophageal dysphagia, the latter of which is a deglutition problem. It may be the consequence of pain or even alteration of the motility inherent to the lesion.

The clinical signs may manifest acutely (dyspnea, often pronounced dysphagia after ingestion of solids but also after ingestion of liquids if the stenosis is pronounced). They are correlated to the severity of the stenosis. The animal may lose weight rapidly. The lesions are incompatible with medium-term survival if the residual diameter of the esophageal lumen is less than 8 mm.

> Diagnosis

Thoracic radiography with or without contrast medium and esophageal endoscopy confirm the diagnosis. The differential diagnosis must exclude other causes of chronic vomiting or regurgitation:
- megaesophagus (rare in cats)
- esophageal crop due to vascular abnormality (rare in cats)
- diverticulum (rare in cats)
- hiatal hernia in the strict sense/gastroesophageal invagination (rare in cats)
- esophageal foreign body (less common in cats than in dogs in this location)

Thoracic radiography

When stenosis is the consequence of parietal fibrosis the plain radiographs do not reveal any abnormalities. Air dilatation may be suspected in front of the lesion, as the esophagus is normally radio-transparent. Food residues may persist and create local contrast that permits diagnostic suspicion. Abnormal images may be seen if there is extrinsic or intrinsic compression by an endoluminal mass.

Radiographs after the ingestion of a contrast medium are often necessary to confirm the diagnosis (introduction of barium under anesthesia using a tube or fluoroscopy): this also helps provide an initial assessment of the scope of the stenosis.

Indications and limitation of esophagoscopy

Endoscopy is the diagnostic test of choice in the exploration of this type of lesion (**Figure 22**). The limit of the examination is the diameter of the lesion, which sometimes limits the passage of the endoscope towards the distal part of the esophagus. Esophagoscopy is complementary to radiography: it can be used to assess the residual diameter of the esophagus. The images obtained in the event of (post-reflux) peptic esophagitis are very characteristic.

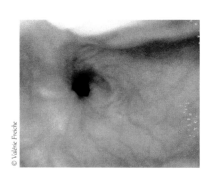

Figure 22a - Esophageal stenosis in a 8-year-old DSH cat.
This serious lesion has a peptic origin and has appeared after a general anesthesia realized for a convenience surgery.

The endoscope examination provides an assessment of the residual diameter of the esophagus (**Figure 23**). It is conducted at the end of the diagnostic radiograph with contrast medium to evaluate the scope of the stenosis. The benefits of endoscopic treatment can also be assessed. If the stenosis is unique and short in length, endoscopic dilatation is indicated. The results are less certain if the stenosis extends for several centimeters or if there are multiple areas of stenosis.

> Treatment of the stenosis: practicalities

The treatment consists of several dilatation appointments using a balloon tube, which can be inflated under manometric control (*Haraï et al, 1995; Adama-Moraitou et al, 2002*). The balloon catheter is introduced in the operator channel of the endoscopy. There is a tube sized to suit every case. The aim is to achieve repetitive parietal dilaceration in the cicatricial zones (*Freiche, 1999; Leib et al, 2001*). However, in the case of annular stenosis with little fibrosis, the mucosa retains sufficient elasticity locally to enable perendoscopic dilatation without local dilaceration being visible at the end of the dilatation maneuvers: in this particular case, a surgical approach must be considered. The aim is to achieve a residual diameter of at least 10 mm at the end of treatment.

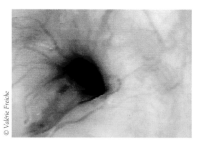

Figure 22b - Esophageal stenosis in a cat, secondary to a thoracic tumor.
In this particular case, due to the origin of the stenosis, endoscopic dilatation is not a therapeutic option.

> Results and complications

The results are generally good when the indication has been properly determined. Endoscopic dilatations do not involve much pain, so they are well tolerated by the animal and lead to general recovery in a few weeks. Extended stenosis may however have a very poor prognosis. The same is true of multiple forms of stenosis or when the stenosis is the consequence of a neoplastic lesion.

Three to five successive appointments every couple of days are suggested for this type of treatment. A reduction in the diameter of the esophagus is systematic between two appointments due to the inevitable partial parietal cicatrisation. The in situ injection of local corticosteroids using an endoscopic catheter helps to limit this complication. This technique should be attempted initially. If such lesions are initially treated surgically, a new stenosis is likely to appear at the surgical site.

Immediate complications

The major risk is parietal rupture during the examination, which is rare. A surgical team must be ready to intervene in the event of complications.

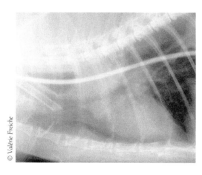

Figure 23 - Insertion of a thoracic labeling tube to measure the extent of esophageal stenosis. *The cat was presented for dysphagia. The esophageal compression was extrinsic.*

Medium-term complications

Esophageal motility is always altered when a lesion is identified in this organ, regardless of the origin. The treatment of stenosis does not guarantee a return to the normal motility activity of the esophagus. For this reason, some cats are euthanized due to the persistence of dysphagia or the appearance of pulmonary complications related to aspiration.

► Esophageal foreign bodies

The rather unselective dietary behavior of carnivores means that the ingestion of foreign bodies is a relatively common reason for consultation. Cats are more "delicate" than dogs, so the incidence of foreign bodies in the esophagus and stomach is much less important in the former.

In cats, linear foreign bodies in the esophagus are often due to a twine or thread becoming trapped under the tongue **(Figure 24)** and lodging in the digestive tract. In this situation, it cannot be extracted by endoscopy. A wide array of objects is ingested, including needles and hooks.

According to studies, foreign bodies tend to lodge where the esophagus contracts, especially at the diaphragmatic hiatus or the entrance to the thorax, although the base of the heart is also possible.

> Clinical diagnosis

The presence of a foreign body in the esophagus can produce alarming clinical signs and demands urgent intervention. Information from the owner is vital as it may provide pointers as to the type of foreign body ingested and especially when it was ingested. These factors impact the choice of the extraction method. On average, the duration between ingestion of the foreign body and presentation to the veterinarian varies from a few hours to a few days.

The severity of the clinical signs depends on the degree of esophageal obstruction and damage to the esophageal wall. If the lumen is only partially obstructed and the esophagus is not perforated, the animal may present in a subnormal clinical state allowing the absorption of liquids without difficulty. This explains why some foreign bodies are not discovered for some time. The differential diagnosis involves all the other causes of esophageal obstruction (neoplasia, congenital anomalies, extrinsic compressions).

> Complementary tests

Plain radiography

This simple and fast procedure will help confirm the diagnosis in more than 85% of cases according to the statistical data described in the literature (*Durand-Viel & Hesse, 2005*). The radiological signs may be:
- direct, when the foreign body is radiodense (bone, metallic)
- indirect, in the event of partial esophageal dilatation or the presence of an abnormal quantity of air or liquid

Radiography with contrast medium

If the images are unable to help confirm the clinical suspicion, radiographs with contrast medium are required. If there is a strong suspicion of a perforated esophagus, an iodized labeling product is preferred over the administration of barium sulfate. Persistence of the contrast agent in front of the lesion or the presence of an image by subtraction, indentified in several consecutive images, is suggestive.

Esophagoscopy

This step is therapeutic. It confirms the nature of the foreign body – after other causes of obstruction or esophageal compression have been excluded – and it helps in the choice of therapy: attempted removal of the foreign body or surgery.

• Practical procedure
The endoscope is used to assess the shape of the foreign body, how tightly it is lodged between the mucosa and how much it can be moved. A foreign body that is initially difficult to move (like a hook) is often more difficult to extract **(Figure 25)**.

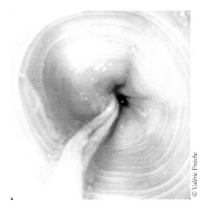

Figure 24 - Twine visible in the esophagus of a one-year-old male Exotic Shorthair. The twine is lodged in the digestive tract.

When a foreign body is lodged in the esophagus, the animal often presents characteristic clinical signs:

- dysphagia
- anorexia
- fever (more inconsistent)
- ptyalism
- lethargy or agitation
- halitosis
- pain
- regurgitation
- breathing difficulties
- weight loss

Cervical palpation is abnormal when the foreign body is lodged in this area (needle).

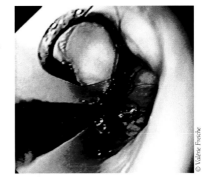

Figure 25 - Close-up of the end of a hook lodged in the esophageal mucosa of a cat. An ulcerative lesion is probably present under the lodgement area.

There are limits to endoscopic extraction:
- suspicion of esophageal perforation,
- highly ulcerated mucosa (risk of esophageal rupture),
- local superinfection in the event of delayed intervention.

Local evaluation of the condition of the mucosa is an important criterion in the decision-making process. If the foreign body has been lodged for more than 72 hours, the risk of perforation is much higher. Generally speaking, it is accepted that all extraction techniques using an endoscope must be attempted before the surgical option is used.

• **Results and complications**
According to the literature, the success rate of this type of intervention varies between 60% and more than 90% (*Durand-Viel & Hesse, 2005*). The latter figure is correlated to the speed of intervention after ingestion of the foreign body, as the condition of the esophageal mucosa deteriorates rapidly when in permanent contact with a foreign body, especially a bone.

If there are clear indications, this procedure has a number of undeniable advantages:
- limits tissue trauma
- speed of functional recovery
- reduces post-surgery care
- timesaving.

The following complications are described:
- massive local hemorrhage (close to the large vessels in the periesophageal area) (*Cohn et al, 2003*)
- tears, perforations of the esophageal mucosa, deep ulcerations produced during the movement of the foreign body.
While the post-intervention lesions in the esophagus or stomach may be large, a tailored medical treatment produces active and rapid healing of the esophageal mucosa **(see Esophagitis)**.

Repeat esophagoscopy is recommended in the event of ulcerative lesions. It must be conducted within four or five hours of extraction. If these lesions are too large, provision of food or water is contraindicated. An enteral feeding tube (PEG) is inserted endoscopically at the end of the examination (*Mark, 2005; Wortinger, 2006*).

► Esophageal neoplasia

> Different histological types encountered

Esophageal tumors are very uncommon in cats, contrary to humans. Esophageal tumors account for less than 0.5% of all cancer cases in domesticated carnivores (*Ettinger & Feldman, 2000*). They usually affect aging animals. The most common histology types are undifferentiated carcinomas, osteosarcomas and fibrosarcomas (*Tams, 1996; Gualtieri et al, 1999; Shinozuka et al, 2001*). In cats, the carcinoma is the most commonly described tumor, although it is much less common than it is in dogs. Benign tumors are rare and often asymptomatic (leiomyomas, papillomas).

In the event of helminthiasis caused by *Spirocerca Lupi* described in Africa, in Réunion and some parts of the United States and Guyana, the migration of larva from the stomach to the thoracic aorta ends in the implantation of an adult parasite in the esophageal wall. This causes the appearance of local nodules, which are likely to undergo neoplastic transformation. The infestation of carnivores mostly occurs after the ingestion of small reptiles or rodents (early treatment of these nodular lesions is with ivermectin). These tumors of parasitic origin generally have a poor prognosis when the diagnosis is established and their metastatic potential is high (*Guilford & Strombeck, 1996c; Freiche, 2005a*). While this larval migration is well described in dogs, its appearance is more anecdotal in cats.

> Clinical signs

The clinical signs are non-specific to the primary lesion, dominated by dysphagia, the intensity of which is related to the degree of esophageal obstruction. The regurgitations are associated with other clinical signs: ptyalism, dysorexia, odynophagia and alteration of general condition. Hematemesis is reported when there is local ulceration. Signs of pneumonia may be secondary to aspiration.

The esophageal wall may also be the site of compressive phenomena of extrinsic origin with thoracic lymphoma, lymphadenopathy, pulmonary neoplasia or thymoma, but they are not primary esophageal tumors.

> Diagnosis

The diagnosis of esophageal tumors is sometimes delayed as the clinical signs manifest themselves at an advanced stage of development. Suspicion is supported by radiographic examination (with or without contrast medium) or ultrasound if the mass is distal. However, the examination of choice to establish a precise diagnosis is esophagoscopy **(Figure 26)**, which enables biopsy, a reliable evaluation of the extent of the lesion, and the surgical options. If the mass is under the mucosa, a tomodensitometric examination is complementary.

Disease staging is based on thoracic radiography. Malignant lesions are aggressive and can metastasize rapidly. In cats, the preferred sites of metastasis of esophageal carcinomas are the lymph nodes in the thorax, the lungs, the kidneys and the spleen.

> Treatment and prognosis

The surgical approach to esophageal tumors is complex because of the risk of local dehiscence of the sutures and the impossibility of wide resection. The prognosis of malignant lesions is often very low in the short term. The chemotherapeutic protocols proposed on the basis of the histological origin of the lesion therefore have only a palliative benefit.

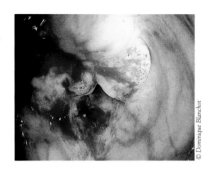

Figure 26 - Malignant esophageal tumor in a 14-year-old European cat.

► Nutritional approach to esophageal diseases

If enteral feeding is not contraindicated and the patient accepts it, food and water bowls should be raised. Cats can be fed "over-the shoulder". Patients can also be held vertical for a short while after feeding. This procedure facilitates the passage of food to stomach. If the patient needs assisted feeding for a longer period, energy and nutrient intakes and fluid volume have to be carefully balanced. The diet should deliver the complete nutrient spectrum in a reasonable volume.

High fat diets are preferred because of their higher energy density. The optimum type of food varies between cases. For some, high-quality liquid diets are best, for others, wet food or moisturized dry food is suitable. Diet viscosity should also be considered.

8 - Diseases of the stomach and nutritional approach

► Gastritis

Chronic gastritis is common in cats of all breeds, ages and sexes. When they are associated with lesions further down the digestive tract, they are considered to be a form of IBD.

> Etiology

The etiology is poorly understood. The inflow of inflammatory cells identified in gastric biopsies – lymphocytes, plasma cells, neutrophilic leukocytes, eosinophilic leukocytes – suggests local

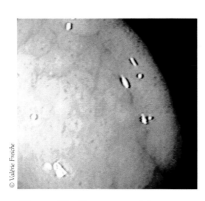

© Valérie Freiche

Figure 27 - Severe gastritis caused by helicobacter identified in a 6-year-old female cat who presented with chronic digestive problems. In low-angled light, compartmentation of the mucosa secondary to a mucosal edema is observable.

immune disturbances in the maintenance of these lesions. Eosinophilic gastritis is often more complex to manage in medical terms. It may be associated with peripheral eosinophilia and the eosinophilic infiltration of other organs. Several publications describe cats infected with toxoplasmosis, presenting gastritis with an eosinophilic component *(McConnel et al, 2007)*. Intracellular parasites are not always found in histopathological analysis.

The incidence of spirochaete *(Helicobacter sp)* is high in domesticated carnivores, but contrary to findings in humans, their pathogenic role remains controversial **(Figure 27)**. However, severe gastritis is associated with high bacterial loads in cats. This is a reason for implementing eradication treatment in this species *(Hwang et al, 2002)*.

Gastritis associated with nematode infestation *(Ollulanus tricuspis)* has been described in the cat *(Cecchi et al, 2006)*. The parasites are identified in endoscopically obtained biopsies.

> Clinical expression

The clinical signs are not very specific dysorexia, intermittent vomiting, alteration of the general condition, developing through crises. The nature of vomiting or its occurrence with respect to meals is not reliable diagnostic information. The presence of blood is not necessarily a poor prognostic indicator, even if it expresses a more extensive alteration of the mucosal surface. This situation can be quickly reversed.

> Complementary tests

Endoscopy with phased biopsies is the examination of choice that produces a final diagnosis. The visual modifications accompanying these lesions include edema of the mucosa, heterogeneous coloration, thickening of some folds, the presence of erosions and multiple small ulcers.

Alterations identified by blood analyses (neutrophilic leukocytes, eosinophilic leukocytes) are not very specific. Radiography or ultrasound images are likely to exclude a number of diseases with similar symptoms. These imaging techniques do not provide an etiological diagnosis.

> Treatment

The medical treatment is specific if a cause can be identified. In most cases the use of corticosteroids is unavoidable. Each case demands individualized treatment based on the scale of the lesions as well as the clinical expression of the disease and the tolerance of the animal. Antacids (anti-H_2 and proton pump inhibitors) are typically indicated in the induction phase. Prokinetics (metoclopramide as cisapride is not available in every country) are beneficial in animals with altered motility. Immunosuppressive agents must be reserved for cases in which the usual treatment is not effective. These substances need a close clinical and hematological follow up and they may induce secondary effects in the cat.

> Specific nutritional approach

Nutritional measures are very important to stabilize the condition of these cats.

Acute gastritis

The patient should be fasted for a short period (less than 24 hours) and subsequently offered small amounts of food. The diet should constitute moist, low-fat food that can be administered in small boli by the owner. If the patient is dehydrated, the fluid, electrolyte and acid base equilibrium should be maintained by parenteral application of adequate solutions *(Remillard, 2000)* and at a later stage by parenteral application of enteral formulas *(Marks, 1998)*. The degree of dehydration determines the amount of fluid that has to be administered. The maintenance requirement for cats is determined by the balance between endogenous water production, water intake and water losses *(Paragon & Mahe, 1994)*. About 50 mL water/day/kg BW is considered as an adequate maintenance requirement. Depending on the degree of dehydration the required amount may be almost doubled if no contraindication is identified.

Chronic gastritis

In chronic cases, it is helpful to feed the animal multiple small meals. The food should be warmed to body temperature and dilution with water often facilitates intake and improves tolerance. This may be explained by the lower osmolality and the faster passage of food through the stomach. Dietary fiber levels should be reduced because many fiber sources increase viscosity of the gastric contents. Diets with a novel protein might be selected if food allergy cannot be excluded. In all other cases highly digestible diets can be chosen.

There are no specific recommendations for the dietary treatment of cats with *Helicobacter* colonization of the gastric mucosa. If gastritis is present, the same dietary measures as given above in the relevant chapter may prove useful.

▶ Gastric foreign bodies

Foreign bodies in the stomach are less common in cats than dogs. Cats accounted for only 9.6% of cases in a study of 146 cases of foreign bodies in the esophagus and stomach *(Durand-Viel & Hesse, 2005)*. The varied nature of foreign bodies (needles, fishhooks, stones, plastic, electric wire) means the intensity of lesions of the mucosa vary also (chronic inflammation, ulceration, laceration if the foreign body is linear and it lodges in the proximal small intestine). In longhaired cats, compacted hairballs lodged in the pyrolic antrum and partially in the proximal small intestine may cause occlusion **(Figure 28)**. In the above study, hairballs accounted for 36% of foreign bodies in the stomach.

> Clinical expression

Vomiting is the most commonly described sign of a foreign body in the stomach. Anorexia, dysorexia and prostration are common. Hematemesis is less common. In the event of gastric laceration subsequent to the presence of a linear foreign body the occlusive signs are more characteristic and a state of shock maybe observed.

> Diagnosis

The diagnosis of a foreign body in the stomach is based on radiograph, ultrasound and endoscope examinations. The ultrasound is the complementary examination of choice. When the foreign body is not linear, endoscopy has the advantage of being therapeutic, enabling extraction with various types of forceps. If endoscopic extraction is not possible, surgery is performed.

▶ Gastric neoplasia

Gastric tumors are much more common than esophageal tumors in domesticated carnivores. The histological and macroscopic characteristics of malignant lesions are different in dogs and cats.

> Different histological types encountered

Benign stomach tumors are uncommon in cats and more common in dogs. They are most often asymptomatic, except when their location or size causes a mechanical problem (exophytic leiomyomas).

The incidence of epithelial tumors in cats varies from 20% to 35% of gastrointestinal neoplasia *(Estrada et al, 1998)* and the stomach is not the most common site. Round cell tumors are common in the stomach of cats. Lymphomas account for the majority of proven neoplasic lesions in cats *(Guilford & Strombeck, 1996c)*. This tumor is considered to be primarily digestive when it is located in the stomach, the intestines and the associated lymph nodes at the time of diagnosis.

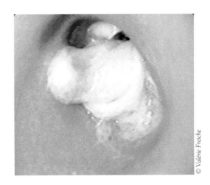

Figure 28 - Hairball identified during gastric endoscopy. The foreign body caused a gastric retention syndrome.

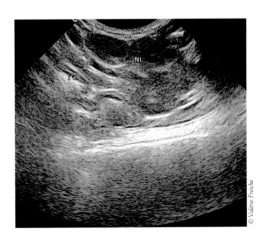

Figure 29 - Ten year old male cat who presented with anorexia and vomiting. The abdominal ultrasound indicated enlarged lymph nodes. Histopathological analysis of biopsies confirmed the diagnosis of lymphoma.

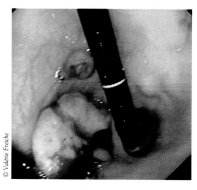

© Valérie Freiche

Figure 30 - 13-year-old female cat who presented for dysorexia, vomiting and weight loss.
Retrovision with the endoscope revealed the presence of parietal mass (es). This appearance is characteristic of one of the forms of lymphoma in the cat.

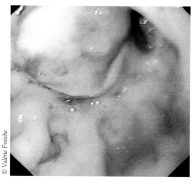

© Valérie Freiche

Figure 31 - Gastroscopy in a 9-year-old Norwegian cat, who presented for gastric retention syndrome.
A large mass is present in the antral area. Enlargement of the abdominal lymph nodes was noted with abdominal ultrasound.

Animals aged ten years or older appear to be most affected (**Figure 29**), but gastric lymphoma may be diagnosed in young animals.

> Etiology

Contrary to findings in humans, the role of inflammatory or dysplastic lesions (follicular gastritis, intestinal metaplasia or lymphoplasmocytic gastritis) has been hypothesized, but a clear role in the development of gastric neoplasia has not been confirmed in the cat.

In cats, Asiatic breeds are affected most often (Siamese) (*Freiche, 2005a*). Predisposing factors include the ingestion of carcinogenic factors (nitrosamines, mycotoxins). The role of these substances in carcinogenesis has not been clearly established.

> Clinical signs

The clinical expression of gastric neoplasia in cats is disconcerting and non-specific. Invasive lesions commonly exist without triggering clinical signs for long periods.

Vomiting – of variable frequency and nature – are commonly observed. Vomiting may become refractory to the prescribed symptomatic treatments. The presence of blood is inconsistent and appears in stages. The time between meals and vomiting does not appear to be a reliable sign for objectifying this serious gastric disorder. The presence of food in the vomitus is not systematic, even if proliferative lesions trigger gastric motility problems.

Other less direct clinical signs that may be observed include:
- dysorexia
- prostration
- weight loss
- antalgic positions (less common in cats than dogs).
- isolation of the animal in unusual places

In some cases there is little or no vomiting and owners note only refractory anorexia and/or ptyalism. Abdominal palpation is not very painful and rarely reveals the presence of a mass.

> Diagnosis of gastric neoplasia

Hemato-biochemical modifications

Few of these modifications are likely to provide pointers for the clinician. Iron deficiency anemia is sometimes identified, expressed as bleeding due to chronic erosion of the mucosa.

Traditional radiography techniques

These are not of great help, especially when lesions are just emerging or they are diffuse through the stomach wall (e.g. lymphoma). Images with contrast medium may reveal abnormalities with gastric filling, abnormal gastric folds or parietal ulcerations associated with suspected thickening of the wall or suggest acquired parietal rigidity. These images are technically difficult to produce in cats and do not provide any evidence of an emerging lymphoma.

Abdominal ultrasound

This complementary examination plays an essential role in the diagnosis of stomach neoplasia. It demands good-quality equipment and special training. The ultrasound examination includes a differential diagnosis of the different histological types of gastric neoplasia (*Penninck, 1998*). Cytological examination by fine needle aspiration may be performed as an alternative to endoscopy, especially for gastric lymphoma (**Figure 30**) if the regional lymph nodes are hyperplastic. Abdominal ultrasound also facilitates disease staging, which is vital prior to medico-surgical treatment (**Figure 31**).

Gastric endoscopy

This is the diagnostic technique of choice when the indications have been rigorously defined. It immediately visualizes the mucosal surfaces and provides multiple parietal biopsies whose histological analysis confirms the diagnosis, especially in this isolated location. This examination also excludes other digestives disorders with the same clinical signs.

Visual appearance of the lesions

- In cats, *gastric lymphoma* may manifest as an infiltrative form that is typically difficult to diagnose visually. Some lesions resemble chronic isolated gastritis or IBD. As a consequence, only the result of histological analyses can be used to confirm the diagnosis. Folds in the stomach are very hyperplastic and edematous, with a cerebroid appearance **(Figure 32)**. Gastric lymphoma may also take an exophytic form, with a less equivocal appearance in endoscopy. The recent advancement in immunolabeling techniques permits a more precise approach to feline lymphoma by localization of membrane antigens *(Fondacaro et al, 1999)*.

- Other gastric tumors are more occasionally found in cats. Leiomyomas or leiomyosarcomas are expressed by the presence of a sometimes large mass projecting from the gastric cavity and if it is located in the antral region, can obstruct stomach emptying. The diagnosis of these lesions relies on visual aspects as endoscopically obtained mucosal biopsies are often negative (tumor of the muscle layers). *Carcinoid tumors* or gastric *fibrosarcomas* are very uncommon.

- *Benign adenomatous tumors* may be responsible for vomiting and weight loss due to their location close to the pylorus, which causes gastric retention syndrome. These lesions cause major mechanical problems. In this case, excision of the tumor mass plays a curative role.

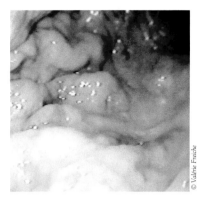

Figure 32 - Gastric lymphoma in a 10-year-old female European cat. Cerebroid-like folding, limited response to insufflation, located in the gastric body: the histological diagnosis confirmed the presence of a gastric lymphoma.

Disease staging

In the event of gastric carcinoma (which is very uncommon in cats) *(Roubardeau & Péchereau, 2006)*, metastasis is initially regional (lymph nodes, liver, spleen, pancreas, peritoneum etc). With lymphoma, regional lymphadenopathy is identifiable at an early stage. Abdominal ultrasound is complementary to endoscopy. Thoracic radiographs rarely reveal pulmonary lesions during the initial diagnosis.

> Prognosis and treatment

The prognosis depends on the histological type of the tumor. In cats with gastric lymphoma, chemotherapy with or without surgery (which is proposed in very specific cases where the lesion is very limited or nodular) produces higher survival rates (often of several months, uncommonly of several years) *(Lanore & Delprat, 2002; Slatter et al, 2003)*.

Leiomyomas, leimyosarcomas and carcinomas should be treated surgically, possibly associated with adjunctive chemotherapy.

9 - Diseases of the intestines and nutritional approach

▶ Diarrhea in kittens

Diarrhea in kittens is a very common consultation that can be difficult for the veterinarian to manage. It may affect a litter or a colony, or a specific kitten in an age range from two to twelve months. Digestive problems in kittens in the perinatal period and up to the age of 2-3 months are the subject of concern for every breeder and they expect urgent, concrete solutions from their

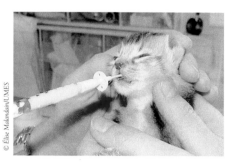

Tube feeding kittens requires skill.
Breeders should be taught by
a veterinarian before attempting
the procedure themselves. If the feeding
tube is not positioned properly (in
the trachea instead of the esophagus)
milk may enter the kitten's lungs
and cause death.

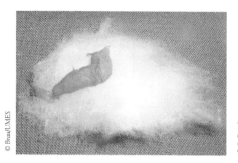

The feces of kittens are usually soft
and yellow.

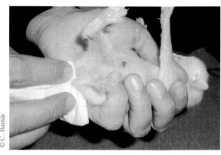

When there is no mother to care for
the kitten, elimination must be stimulated
after each feeding.

Constipation is quite common in the orphan kitten. In the vast majority of cases, it is linked to a lack of perineal stimulation, which stimulates the elimination of stools. For orphaned kittens, large litters and primiparous mothers, the breeder should ensure that defecation and urination is accomplished effectively. Otherwise, the transit of food through the digestive tract will be slower and will promote the reabsorption of water causing constipation to occur. The administration of paraffin oil is not recommended in the kitten. Repeated stimulation of the perineum and soft washing are preferable. In more serious cases, the veterinarian may need to anesthetize the kitten to administer an enema.

veterinarian. A kitten with diarrhea rapidly becomes dehydrated and requires on average 14-16 mL of water/100 g BW (*Malandain et al, 2006*).

When a kitten is presented with diarrhea and its general condition is satisfactory, the two preferred hypotheses are dietary intolerance or parasitism. The prevalence of parasitic diseases in young carnivores is significant and sometimes underestimated, at both the colony and individual level (*Spain et al, 2001*).

> Digestive disorders in orphan kittens

This period of life without maternal assistance is complex. Very young animals are poikilothermic, without a layer of fat. Hypothermia always results in paralytic ileus, so prevention is important. In these circumstances, the living environment requires special attention, and dietary standards need to be fulfilled.
The main causes of diarrhea in this period are:
- over-consumption (*Hoskins, 1995*)
- poorly prepared or poorly conserved milk substitute, given at the wrong temperature.

Factors affecting the successful rearing of an orphan kitten are the quality of mother's milk and hygiene during feeding, thermal regulation, the quality of sleep, nursing, external stimuli and socialization.

> Digestive disorders caused by the diet during weaning

Physiologically, this is a critical phase for the kitten, who has an immature immune and digestive system (**Figure 33**), and is therefore vulnerable when placed in an environment with strong infectious and parasitic pressures. During weaning, a kitten faces several types of stress. The most important are:
- change of diet
- detachment from the mother
- acclimatization to a different environment and microbism

It is difficult to suggest recipe-types of weaning modalities. Every method is respectable if the results are good. Weaning begins the fourth or fifth week and most finish by week 7.

The main causes of diarrhea in this period (not including infectious and parasitic diseases) are:
- poor digestibility of the food
- poor conservation of the food
- over-consumption at mealtimes
- excess starch in the diet (**Figure 34**).

FIGURE 33 - VARIATIONS IN THE DIGESTIBILITY OF DIFFERENT NUTRIENTS DURING KITTEN GROWTH

(from Harper & Turner, 2000)

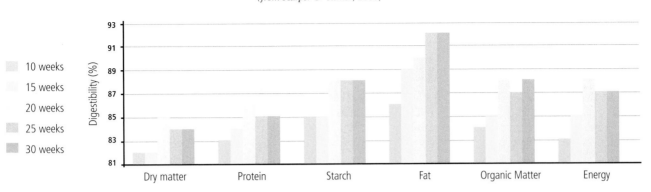

An increase in most parameters is observed from week 20 (n=12).

FIGURE 34 - DEVELOPMENT OF THE KITTEN'S CARBOHYDRATE DIGESTION CAPACITY BEFORE AND AFTER WEANING, COMPARED WITH AN ADULT'S

(from Kienzle, 1993)

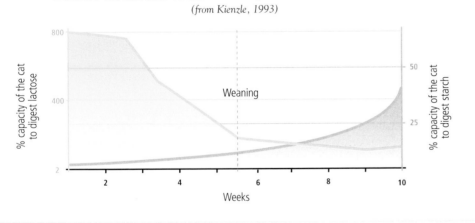

> Idiopathic enteritis in kittens

Kittens aged 6-12 months may present with diarrhea that is refractory to the usual symptomatic treatments, and yet resolves spontaneously in a few months *(Hoskins, 1995)*. These cats present with profuse diarrhea, however, they are in good general condition. The diagnostic tests are all within normal limits. The underlying cause maybe due to improper maturation of the digestive tract's absorption and exchange system, exacerbated by errors in dietary supervision.

> Diagnosis

The clinical signs are not specific to the disease. A methodical approach is necessary to consider the circumstances in which the diarrhea appears, the life context of the animal and the findings of the clinical examination.

A breeder needs to be educated about which clinical signs need to be identified early, the most concerning signs and the criteria for hospitalization. If the kitten is presented by a private individual, a full history (unrestricted access to the outside, contact with sick animals, possibilities that a toxin has been ingested, signs observed) will be needed before the clinical examination can be conducted. The seriousness of the clinical signs is correlated to the origin of the diarrhea.

In practice, weaning can start when the kittens' average daily gain starts to decline. Weaning usually ends around the age of 7 weeks.

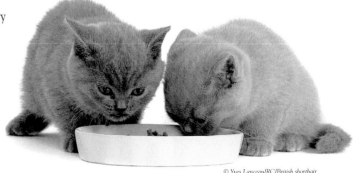

109

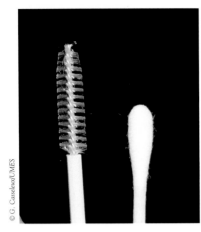

Figure 35 - Cytobrushes used for fecal detection of viral enteritis.
PCR is a laboratory technique for amplifying the genetic material of the virus and detecting its presence even at very low quantities. There are various types of applicators or cytobrushes used to collect samples for coronavirus testing (here per rectum).

© G. Casseleux/UMES

The following hospitalization criteria may be employed for kittens (*Battersby & Harvey, 2006*):
- alteration of the general condition (asthenia, anorexia)
- abnormalities of cardiac rhythm: bradycardia or tachycardia
- hyperthermia or hypothermia
- dehydration
- presence of blood in the feces
- abnormal abdominal palpation (mass, lymph nodes, etc.)
- presence of other clinical signs: frequent vomiting, icterus, etc.

In the event of hospitalization, fluid and electrolyte therapy must be implemented and the kitten placed in isolation, if necessary.

The diagnostic evaluations are adapted to each specific clinical situation and include:
- hemato-biochemical analyses (leucocytosis, anemia, hyper- or hypoproteinemia). Exudative enteropathy is accompanied by hypoproteinemia, while hyperproteinemia is more consistent with feline infectious peritonitis (FIP). The young age of the kitten must not exclude metabolic causes of diarrhea;
- coagulation tests in cases of digestive bleeding
- fecal analyses (fecal cytology, bacteriology, larvae, cysts, protozoans)
- detection of retrovirus (FeLV, FIV)
- PCR on blood and/or rectal sampling (FIV) **(Figure 35)**
- measurement of fTLI, using a specific feline assay.

> Treatment of diarrhea in kittens

A systematic approach is required for acute diarrhea of sudden onset, without alteration of the general condition. Diagnostic examinations must be conducted if the clinical signs persist for longer than a couple of days and a second round of symptomatic treatment should not be started if the first one fails, even if the clinical signs are only a week's duration. Diarrhea is not considered to be chronic until it enters its third or fourth week.

Specific treatment for each disorder must be started. Observance is a limiting factor in cats. It may be difficult for private individuals with many cats or colonies to follow the nutritional instructions. Novel protein diets can be recommended for the dietary treatment of kittens with diarrhea. Low fibre concentrations are probably the best recommendation to start unless there are indications for a large bowel problem. Other helpful supplements are probiotics, that can be helpful in the modulation of the intestinal microbiota (*Guilford & Matz, 2003; Marshall Jones et al, 2006*). The efficacy of prebiotics such as fructo-oligosaccharides has to be evaluated depending on the individual reaction.

► Infectious gastroenteritis

Upon identification of diarrhea in a breeding colony, some practical steps should immediately be implemented: the sick kittens should be isolated, and new kittens, quarantined. Prevention also demands good hygiene and disinfection of the premises.

The term "infectious" is employed liberally here. This section examines forms of viral, parasitic and bacterial gastroenteritis that most commonly affect cats. The exposure of the digestive tract to different pathogenic agents is not always expressed by the appearance of clinical signs (*Guilford & Strombeck, 1996c*). Any disturbance of the physiological mechanisms of homeostasis is however likely to generate an imbalance in the microflora or induce modifications in local antigenicity, causing diarrhea.

> Viral gastroenteritis

The prevalence of all the viruses that infect cats is unknown (*Guilford & Strombeck, 1996c*). These viral infections provoke highly varied clinical signs: discreet alteration of the general condition or

© Yves Lanceau/RC/British shorthair

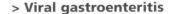

necrosing enteritis in the event of panleukopenia. These diseases propagate themselves quickly and are highly contagious. Their prevention demands a systematic approach comprising rigorous hygiene measures, the quarantine of new individuals and vaccination wherever possible.

Feline enteric coronavirus

Feline coronavirus shares antigenic and morphological characteristics with the one of FIP. Today, it is commonly thought that a mutation of coronavirus can lead to the expression of FIP. Viral replication occurs in the apex of the microvilli. Infected animals develop moderate and transitory digestive problems. Sometimes there are no visible clinical signs.

Feline infectious peritonitis

This disease manifests in a variety of clinical forms. The most commonly described form is the presence of inflammatory effusion in the cavities. The "dry" form is characterized by granulomatous inflammation of the parenchyma (pancreas, liver, digestive wall, lymph nodes). FIP is therefore not expressed as a common chronic or acute gastroenteritis. It often affects young animals, but not exclusively so. Fever is a common sign. Laboratory evaluation (hematology, biochemistry, PCR, etc.) helps to underpin the clinical suspicion.

A last form – more specific and less well known – is atypical isolated granulomatous colitis. The modifications it produces on an ultrasound are equivocal (*Harvey et al, 1996*). The prognosis is invariably poor.

Retroviruses (FeLV – FIV)

The FeLV virus is responsible for superacute mortal enterocolitis and lymphocytic ileitis. The FIV virus is most often implicated in episodes of recurring diarrhea. Cats infected with the FIV virus may survive for long periods, during which time they will intermittently present with digestive disorders of varying intensity. Immunosuppression may favor enteric infection (*Battersby & Harvey, 2006*) and the diarrhea will be secondary to other infectious agents rather than to the presence of the FIV virus.

Feline panleukopenia

Feline panleukopenia is due to a parvovirus with epidemiological, physiopathological and hematological characteristics similar to those of the canine virus (*Squires, 2003*). The pathogenic power of the virus is also expressed on the central nervous system in utero or during the neonatal period (cerebellar hyperplasia) (*Guilford & Strombeck, 1996c*).

The clinical signs manifest themselves 4-7 days after transmission of the virus by the fecal-oral route. The virus is very stable in the exterior environment. Viral replication occurs in tissues that rapidly multiply: bone marrow, lymphoid tissue, intestinal crypts. The jejunum and ileum are the most often affected digestive segments. Viral replication produces leukopenia and necrosis of the intestinal crypts that leads to hemorrhagic enteritis. The clinical signs are dominated by major asthenia, rapid anorexia and weight loss, vomiting and diarrhea. Death may occur before the appearance of the diarrhea in the superacute forms. Massive bacterial translocation is the cause of septic shock. Liver failure is often the cause of death.

Several other viruses cause acute digestive disorders in cats. These include astrovirus (isolated in kittens) rotavirus (which causes neonatal diarrhea), reovirus and calicivirus. Their identification is difficult and their pathogenic role has not been clearly identified.

> Parasitic gastroenteritis

Parasitic infestations

The parasitic infestation must be extensive before clinical signs manifest themselves: bloating, vomiting, diarrhea, skin lesions, coughing during larval migration. The incidence of parasitic enteritis is

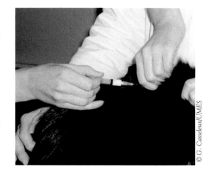

Viral diseases (coronavirus, feline infectious peritonitis, retroviruses, feline panleucopenia) are always likely to appear in a cattery or colony, even when hygiene conditions are good and medical prophylaxis is meticulously observed.

Digestion

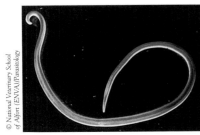

Figure 36 - Adult roundworms.
*Adult roundworms are long
and round, measuring 4-10 cm.*

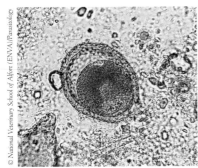

Figure 37 - *Roundworm egg.*

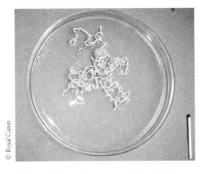

Figure 38 - *Segments of* Dipylidium
caninum.

higher in colonies and in young animals. It is underestimated among individual owners (*Battersby & Harvey, 2006*). Various infestation modes are possible: fecal-oral route, in utero contamination (toxocarosis), transmission through colostrum or milk, ingestion of intermediate hosts (tapeworms).

The location of the parasites is variable. They are often found in the small intestine, but the large intestine is also infested. The presence of these parasites may also cause anemia, melena (hookworm disease), sudden inexplicable deaths in the cattery, stunted growth or fertility problems among breeding stock.

The most commonly encountered parasites are ascarids **(Figures 36 & 37)** (*Toxocara cati, Toxascaris leonina*), tapeworms (mostly *Dipylidium caninum*) **(Figure 38)**, hookworms (*Ancylostoma tubaeformae*) and *Strongyloides tumefaciens* in tropical areas. The diagnosis is based on fecal evaluation (flotation in zinc sulfate).

The treatment of parasitic enteritis uses anthelmintics, which are available in many forms: oral pastes, small caplets adapted to cats, trans-dermal (spot on). The active substances and their spectrum of action are listed in **Table 7**.

Treatment of the mother is recommended two weeks prior to the birth, then during weeks 3, 5 and 7, to stop the parasitic cycle.

Protozoan diseases

The digestive tract of cats may be colonized by protozoans: Giardia, Coccidia and Trichomonas.

Giardia

Less common in cats than dogs, giardiasis is expressed by digestive disorders that may be intermittent (diarrhea does not present a specific aspect) as well as dysorexia episodes or deterioration in the gen-

	Nematodes		Cestodes	
Product	Ringworms	Hookworms	Taenia	Dipylidium
Piperazine	■			
Oxibendazole	■	■		
Pyrantel	■	■		
Milbemycin oxime	■	■		
Selamectin	■	■		
Levamisole; Tetramisole	■	■		
Emodepside	■	■		
Mebendazole 2 days	■	■		
Mebendazole 5 days	■	■	■	
Moxidectin	■	■		
Flubendazole 2 days	■	■		
Flubendazole 3 days	■	■		
Fenbendazole 3 days	■	■		
Niclosamide			■	■
Praziquantel			■	■

TABLE 7 - ANTHELMINTIC SPECTRUM OF COMMONLY AVAILABLE ANTIPARASITIC AGENTS

Note: the use of these compounds in cats can be restricted according to the licence applicable in each country.

eral condition. An immunosuppressive condition favors the clinical expression of giardiasis. Trophozoites are attached to the brush border of the proximal small intestine. They are periodically excreted in the feces, which is why several fecal examinations spaced over intervals of several days are desirable to avoid a false negative diagnosis. An ELISA diagnostic kit is available for practitioners.

The treatment of giardia uses imidazoles: metronidazole, fenbendazole. With resistant strains, the environment should be properly decontaminated (elimination of feces and disinfection with quaternary ammoniums). Animals must be cleaned as recontamination is possible by the ingestion of oocysts **(Figure 39)** deposited on the coat by licking.

Coccidia *(Isospora felis, Isospora rivolta)* **(Figure 40)**
This protozoan disease is common in breeding colonies and its expression is strengthened by an underlying parasitic condition and unfavorable hygiene. The clinical expression may include the following signs:
- stunted growth in kittens
- abdominal pain
- fever
- tenesmus
- mucoid diarrhea.

Hygiene on the premises is important in prevention. Treatment is based on the association of trimethoprim-sulfonamides with clindamycin or toltrazuril for resistant forms.

Trichomonas *(Tritrichomonas fœtus, Pentatrichomonas hominis)*
Trichomoniosis seems to be an under-estimated cause of recurring digestive disorders in young cats, especially in colonies. The pathogenesis of these organisms is multifactorial in interaction with the host's endogenic flora *(Gookin et al, 1999)*. The disease is expressed when hygiene is inadequate: diarrhea predominates with hematochezia and/or mucus, peri-anal inflammation, rectal prolapse. Transmission is directly via the fecal-oral route.

The identification of protozoans by fecal analysis is difficult. They can be easily confused with giardia. Fecal culture tests are commercially available (In Pouch TF©). Their presence in the colon is expressed by an influx of inflammatory cells (lymphoplasmocytes or neutrophilic leukocytes) and sometimes crypt abscesses *(Yaeger & Gookin, 2005)*. Eradication is difficult, as trichomonas are resistant to imidazoles. A recent study mentions the over-representation of purebred cats, especially the Siamese and the Bengal *(Gunn-Moore et al, 2007)*.

> **Bacterial gastroenteritis**

Some pathogenic bacteria may cause episodes of acute or chronic diarrhea. Unlike protozoans, their presence is clearly overestimated. Antibiotic treatment should only be started after isolation of an enteropathogenic bacterial strain. Inappropriate antibiotic treatment may provoke serious imbalances in the intestinal flora, and favor the development of bacterial antibiotic resistance.

The main pathogenic bacteria described in cats and responsible for digestive disorders include *(Henroteaux, 1996)*:
- *Campylobacter* (possible healthy carrier)
- *Salmonella* (possible healthy carrier, septicemic risk if pathogenic)
- *E. coli* (enteropathogenic strains)
- *Clostridium perfringens*
- *Yersinia enterocolitica*.

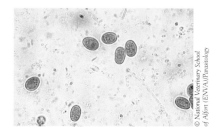

Figure 39 - Oocysts from Giardia. *Oocysts survive in humid environments and some wild animals are reservoirs of this disease.*

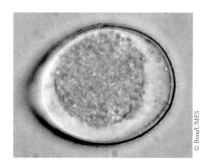

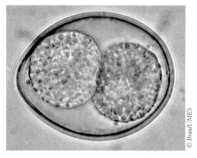

Figure 40 - Oocysts from Isospora felis immature (top) and infectious (lower). *Maturation of the oocysts requires at least 48 hours.*

Clinically, bacterial diarrhea has strong repercussions on the general condition, as well as fever and the regular presence of blood in the feces. A serum electrolyte profile should be conducted to guide fluid and electrolyte rehydration and to correct the frequent hyperkalemia.

The history must probe for sick people that are in contact with the cat. The diagnosis is based on fecal cytology that indicates the presence of leucocytes and bacterial elements. The diagnosis is confirmed by bacterial culture of the feces.

▶ Acute gastrointestinal diseases

> Etiology

In cats, acute gastrointestinal diseases are most commonly caused by diet, parasites or toxins (see above). They are expressed by the association of vomiting and diarrhea with varying characteristics. Cats sometimes tend to defecate outside the litter box when suffering from this type of diarrhea.

Vomiting predominates in the event of occlusion.

> Procedure for diagnostic evaluation

Diagnostic tests are rarely justified initially. Hospitalization should be proposed according to the same criteria as described for diarrhea in kittens:
- alteration of the general condition and dehydration
- tachycardia and bradycardia
- fever
- hematemesis
- abdominal pain or abnormal palpation
- suspicion of peritonitis.

The sequence of diagnostic tests is dictated by the history and tailored to each case. It includes hematological analyses (leukopenia, leukocytosis, anemia), viral tests (FeLV, FIV), fecal analyses, radiograph and ultrasound examinations if occlusion is suspected.

> Nutritional measures

Acute vomiting and diarrhea usually mean that the patient should be fasted (nil per os [NPO]). Oral feeding is not practicable in cats if vomiting persists or diarrhea is profuse. Because of the consequences of vomiting and diarrhea for the electrolyte and acid-base balance, parenteral fluids with electrolytes and buffering substances should be administered. Oral rehydration can be administered when tolerated. If the water losses are high because of vomiting and severe diarrhea, fluid has to be administered by parenteral application. Fluid should be administered as a mandatory measure if there is evidence of dehydration (>5%) or the patient refuses to drink.

If the condition improves and the animal is willing to accept a small amount of food, frequent small meals should be administered for 24-72 hours depending on individual tolerance. Examples of appropriate homemade diets are boiled rice with 2 parts of boiled lean meat (chicken or turkey) or eggs. Milk and milk products such as low fat cottage cheese (low lactose content) can be used, although the high lactose concentration may be a problem. An alternative is a highly digestible commercial diet with a low-fat concentration. During the acute stage it is often recommended to use a protein source that is not part of the normal diet (sacrificial protein) to avoid sensitization or the development of allergies. The fiber content of diets for patients with acute intestinal problems has to be limited to ensure optimal tolerance and digestibility. The levels of potassium, sodium and chloride should be increased because vomiting and diarrhea induce high electrolyte losses. When clinical signs improve, the usual diet can be reintroduced gradually.

► Inflammatory bowel diseases

Inflammatory bowel diseases (IBD) are the main cause of chronic digestive disorders in domesticated carnivores, especially cats. The term covers a group of idiopathic diseases, while certain pathogens have been implicated in their clinical and anatomicopathological expression (food antigens, parasites, bacteria). Many studies implicate complex interactions between the patient's particular predispositions, immunity problems related to the mucosa and the digestive microflora. Knowledge of IBD has progressed over the last fifteen years, with the advent of ultrasound and endoscopic examinations of the cat's digestive tract.

> Definition

IBD is defined in accordance with the histological criteria: infiltration of the mucosa of the small and/or large intestine by a population of inflammatory cells, most often lymphoplasmocytic **(Figure 41)**, although neutrophilic leukocytes, eosinophilic leukocytes and macrophages may also be involved *(Tams et al, 1996a)*.

The most restrictive definition of IBD entails the presence of lesions only in the small and/or large intestine. However, some authors do not exclude IBD in the event of inflammatory gastric lesions *(Guilford, 1996)*. Very often in fact, intestinal lesions are not isolated and the entire digestive mucosa is affected by the influx of inflammatory cells in the *lamina propria*.

> Clinical reminders

No breed or sex predisposition has been recognized and all age groups may be affected, including young adults. The intensity of the clinical signs varies greatly from animal to animal: chronic digestive disorders (diarrhea and/or vomiting), dysorexia and inconsistent alteration of the general condition. These manifestations may develop 'by crises' for months or even years before becoming permanent. These diseases are better documented in cats than in dogs *(Jergens, 2006)*. At the beginning of the disease, vomiting is predominant and may be the expression of intestinal lesions, even distal ones. The vomiting of gastric juice well after mealtime and in the morning on an 'empty stomach' is common.

Diarrhea may be a sign of lesions of the small intestine (profuse, very watery diarrhea) or a colonic disorder (tenesmus, the presence of mucus or blood, minor undermining of the general condition), but this dichotomy is much less specific in cats than dogs. In other cases, episodes of constipation occur before the appearance of diarrhea.

Abdominal palpation may reveal thickening of the intestinal loops and an increase in the size of the associated lymph nodes. In other cases, abdominal palpation may be perfectly normal.

> Diagnosis

The diagnosis of IBD is by exclusion of other diseases that could cause the clinical signs or an inflammatory influx into the digestive mucosa (neoplastic infiltration, bacterial proliferation syndrome, hyperthyroidism, protozoans) *(Krecic, 2001)*.

Endoscopy is conducted after diagnostic tests for other conditions are completed (CBC, biochemical analyses, fecal examination, basal T_4 measurement, abdominal ultrasound) *(Simpson et al, 2001)*.

Abdominal ultrasound

Abdominal ultrasound precedes endoscopy in the exploration of digestive diseases of the cat. The assessment of the parietal layers **(Figure 42)** and the size of the lymph nodes are essential to help eliminate the hypothesis of lymphoma. Ultrasound also confirms whether there are lesions in the pancreas, liver or bile ducts, as cats with IBD often have concurrent cholangitis.

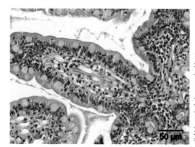

Figure 41 - IBD in a cat: histological examination.

© Valuepath, Laboratory for Veterinary Pathology, Hoensbroek, The Netherlands

41A - Increased number of intra-epithelial lymphocytes in the villus epithelium as well as increased numbers of lymphocytes in the lamina propria of the villus and the basal mucosa between the crypts.

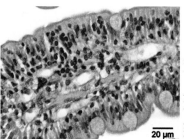

© Valuepath, Laboratory for Veterinary Pathology, Hoensbroek, The Netherlands

41B - High power magnification of a villus with marked presence of intra-epithelial lymphocytes and lymphocytic infiltration of the lamina propria.

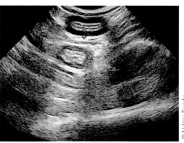

Figure 42 - 3.5 year old female Siamese cross cat, who presented with frequent vomiting.

© Valérie Freiche

Abdominal ultrasound shows an enlargement in the parietal region. Transabdominal biopsies confirmed a diagnosis of severe eosinophilic enteritis.

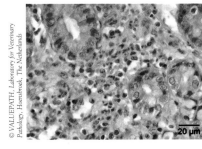

Figure 43 - Eosinophilic colitis in a cat (large intestine).
Marked infiltrate of eosinophilic granulocytes as well as some plasma cells in the lamina propria between the crypts.

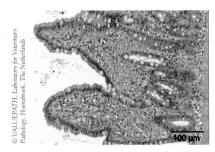

Figure 44 - Chronic eosinophilic enteritis (small intestine).
Villous atrophy with blunted villi, a band of fibrous tissue at the transition between villi and crypts and a moderate infiltrate of eosinophilic granulocytes.

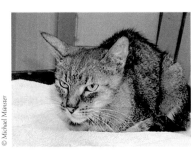

IBD comprises by definition a group of chronic diseases that require protracted treatment. Relapses are common. It is essential to educate the owner about the disease and its management and to set realistic expectations for the care of the cat.

Endoscopy

Both upper and lower gastrointestinal endoscopy is necessary to establish a precise diagnosis. A number of endoscopic biopsies must be obtained from all accessible segments:
- *upper*: stomach, duodenum, proximal part of jejunum
- *lower*: distal part of the ileum, colon.

The histological analysis of biopsies may involve one or more cell types. The most common inflammatory infiltrate is lymphocytic/plasmacytic. The inflammatory infiltration may be polymorphous (the presence of neutrophilic leukocytes, a varied number of eosinophilic leukocytes **(Figure 43)**, histiocytes). Villous atrophy may also be associated with the disease **(Figure 44)**. Its presence often worsens the prognosis.

Visual appearance of the lesions

The visual appearance of the mucosa is never specific. There is poor correlation between the visual appearance and the histological score. In cats, the correlation between the clinical signs and the histological distribution of lesions is unsatisfactory. Visual classification is difficult due to certain subjective parameters that depend on both the operator and the equipment. Endoscopy produces a fairly reliable histological map. It is the fastest exploratory technique and less burdensome for the animal than exploratory laparotomy, which should only be performed in special circumstances. The nature of the inflammatory infiltrate and its distribution along the digestive tract leads to the elaboration of more specific therapeutic protocols *(Strombeck & Guilford, 1991; Sturgess, 2005)*.

Biopsies

Associated parietal fibrosis may be suspected during biopsy (difficulty of taking biopsy fragments of normal size, resistance to traction when the forceps are closed). If this is so, additional biopsies should be performed to obtain samples of sufficient size for reliable histological analysis. This would also permit identification, in the same segment of the digestive tract, of more or less modified sections. Central needle biopsy forceps may also be useful, as they are more effective on a more rigid mucosa surface.

> Management

Medical treatment

Despite the possibility of standardized therapeutic plans, the veterinarian must consider each case as an individual entity. One of the pitfalls of treatment is the lack of observation among cat owners. Treatment comprises the administration of the substances listed below.

- *Digestive flora regulators with immunomodulation properties* (metronidazole) *(Zoran et al, 1999)*.
- *Sulfasalazine* is tolerated less well in cats than dogs and its indications are specific and limited *(see feline colitis)*.
- *Corticosteroids* are proposed in the most severe cases but large doses are not generally essential to ensure clinical stabilization, as refractory cases are uncommon. The minimal effective dose must be established to enable alternate day corticotherapy at the earliest opportunity. Long-acting corticosteroids are used for cats, but they are less effective than prednisolone administered orally.
- *Other immunosuppressive agents* may be proposed if there is no response to corticosteroids, depending on the histology results of biopsies. These include chlorambucil, cyclosporine and azathioprine *(Zoran, 1999)*. Note that cats are extremely sensitive to the toxic side-effects of azathioprine and its administration requires a close monitoring and reevaluation of the treated cat.

Dietary treatment

Patients with inflammatory bowel disease often suffer from malnutrition **(Figure 45)** due to inadequate dietary intake compared to increased requirements, maldigestion and malabsorption, and excessive fecal nutrient losses.

Exclusion diets and hydrolysed protein-based diets are often favorable in IBD cases because they can positively interact with the mucosal inflammation (*Waly et al, 2006*). Inflammation of the gut wall itself can impair the absorption of amino acids, peptides and carbohydrates as well as the transport of minerals and fluid. A highly digestible diet may also be beneficial. Most cats can tolerate a high-fat diet (> 20% DMB in a dry food). Some patients may do better on a low-fat diet ($\simeq$ 10% DMB) because fatty acids can be hydroxylated in the gut by certain bacteria and stimulate secretory diarrhea. Probiotics and prebiotics may be used as feed additives in IBD patients, although there are no controlled clinical trials providing evidence for their efficacy in IBD cases.

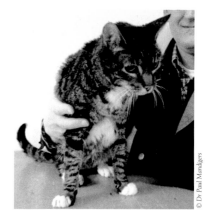

Figure 45 - *Dietary treatment of IBD cases is similar to the management of dietary allergy.*

► Adverse food reactions

Food allergy, intolerance or sensitivities can be summarized under "adverse food reactions". They are often considered to be a cause of chronic gastrointestinal diseases. Commonly, they are divided into:
- non-immunologically mediated reactions
- immunologically mediated reactions, synonymous to "food allergy" (*German & Zentek, 2006*). Clinical signs may affect the gastrointestinal tract or other organs or systems. Dermatological signs are most common in the event of gastrointestinal problems.

> Etiologies

In many cases clinical gastrointestinal signs are caused by food intolerance that is not based on immunological mechanisms. True allergies are difficult to assess in practice and may be less important than commonly assumed. The main compounds in commercial diets that may cause dietary allergy or adverse reactions are protein sources. In principal, all commonly used proteins such as beef, pork, vegetable proteins, and fish have to be considered as potentially problematic.

> Diagnosis

The diagnosis is mainly based on dietary history and clinical investigation. This procedure is subjected to individual influences and the frequency of an "allergy" as a diagnosis is dependent on the investigator.

In all patients that are suspected to have a dietary intolerance, a complete overview of the dietary history of the patient is mandatory, including information on the usual diet, treats or table scraps. In some cases, problematic food compounds can be identified, which is essential for formulating an elimination diet or selecting adequate diets from a commercial source. When it is not possible to identify the offending compound, the choice of an initial elimination diet depends on the history of ingredients used in the individual's diet.

Specific assays for the characterization of adverse reactions to food are not yet available, so first diagnosis is mostly made on the observation that the disease responds to dietary changes (*Hall, 2002*). The gold standard of diagnosis involves the response to the exclusion diet and the subsequent challenge with provocation test (*Allenspach & Roosje, 2004*). A specific diagnosis based on indirect blood allergy tests is questionable and may produce erroneous results.

Common test diets for cats are based on lamb, chicken, rabbit or venison, often in combination with rice or green peas. An improvement in clinical signs is suggestive of food allergy or at least an adverse reaction to food ingredients (*Wills & Harvey, 1994*). The diagnosis should be confirmed by reverting to the original diet. The development of clinical signs can be expected immediately or within one or two weeks of feeding. Therefore, a trial length of 2-3 weeks would appear appropriate in most GI cases. Food provocation trials can be performed to identify the ingredient causing the problem, adding single protein sources sequentially for 7 days at a time. Most owners will not pursue this if the elimination diet has worked successfully. In conclusion, diagnosis requires dietary elimination-challenge trials and clinical signs; routine clinico-pathological data, serum antigen-specific IgE assay, gastroscopic food sensitivity testing, or gastrointestinal biopsy can only be supportive (*Guilford et al, 2001*).

> Dietary treatment

Dietary management of adverse reactions to food follows the same principles as discussed for diagnostic procedures. Unfortunately, the practitioner is dependent on the compliance of the owner. This may become critical, as clinical signs can respond slowly or relapse. Dietary protocols should follow a standard concept. In the long run, a balanced diet composition, high digestibility in the small intestine and a restricted number of ingredients are important (*German & Zentek, 2006*). This facilitates the digestive process, limits the antigenic load in the gut and supports the absorption of nutrients.

Type of diets

Home-prepared diets have a place in the treatment of cats with dietary indiscretions, although commercial diets with limited number of ingredients are often preferred because of the higher safety in application and the greater convenience. Diets with hydrolysed proteins offer an interesting alternative for the treatment of cats with a dietary allergy that is not responsive to "normal" antigen restricted diets.

Dietary change

A dietary change can be helpful regardless of the etiology and can contribute to a better outcome in many cases. A "new" diet may have a beneficial impact on the intestinal digestive processes and it may also influence the composition and metabolic activity of the gut bacteria. A dietary change may limit the growth of undesirable microorganisms and so reduce concentrations of microbial metabolites in the gut. Microbial metabolites like the biogenic amine histamine can have a negative impact on the health of cats.

Once a diet has been selected, it has to be fed as the sole source of food for at least 12 weeks to determine whether the desired response will occur. GI signs will often resolve sooner than dermatological signs.

Protein sources

The choice of the best-suited dietary protein is the key to the outcome of the case.
- **Lamb** has commonly been used, but the widespread use of ovine protein in pet food may make this choice less promising.
- **Fish** is less suitable for cats because many commercial cat foods are fish-based or have fish as a minor ingredient. Fish can be a common cause of adverse food reactions in this species (*Guilford et al, 2001*).
- **Wheat (and barley, oats) gluten** can cause dietary allergy and celiac disease in humans. Their use is probably also critical in cats, which suggests the need to change the carbohydrate source in all cases with suspected food allergy.

Fat sources may also contain small amounts of protein from the basic animal or plant raw material. Although these traces of protein appear to be of minor importance, they could theoritically affect the result of an elimination trial but this potential influence is strongly debated.

Hydrolysed protein sources are often used in commercially available veterinary diets. Protein is treated enzymatically to alter its structure. They are split by enzymatic treatment into small peptides. The enzymatically released peptides are less likely to interact with the immune system due to their low molecular weight. The high digestibility of these diets may be advantageous in patients with gastrointestinal disorders.

Carbohydrate sources

Generally, a single source of carbohydrate is recommended to avoid misinterpretation. Maize, potatoes, rice, green peas, and tapioca may be suitable.

Minerals, trace elements and vitamins

Minerals and trace elements have to be added to make a diet complete and balanced. However, some sources of mineral salt, like bone meal, contain small amounts of protein, which may itself provoke an adverse reaction.

Supplementation of home-prepared diets with vitamins can also be problematic, since some of the commonly used vitamins are protected by encapsulation with gelatin (usually prepared from pork). Although the production process is strict and most potentially antigenic epitopes are destroyed, traces of proteins or peptides may still be introduced into a diet. One option is to use a home-prepared diet, based on a minimum of dietary ingredients. Adult cats will tolerate this for some weeks without developing severe nutrient deficiencies. However, home-prepared diets need to be balanced and complete if they are fed long-term or nutrient deficiencies will develop.

Medical treatment is based on the therapeutic plans implemented for IBD.

▶ Diseases of the colon

> Megacolon

Progressive local or total distension of the colon and the loss of motility lead to fecal retention which is characterized by chronic constipation and aggravates over time. Cats are affected more commonly than dogs.

Physiological reminders

The proximal colon plays an important role in the absorption of water and electrolytes from the luminal content. The mucosal parietal cells actively absorb chloride (Cl^-) and sodium (Na^+) ions by ATP dependent pumps. This mechanism results in passive water absorption.

The distal colon permits the storage and periodical elimination of feces. If peristalsis of the colon is passive (the parasympathetic nervous system generates peristaltic contractions, while the sympathetic nervous system regulates segmentary contractions), defecation is a willful act, under the control of the central nervous system. The colonic transit time is variable in carnivores (forty hours or so).

The longitudinal and circular muscle walls are responsible for motility and colon tone. This motility is regulated by gastrointestinal hormones and intrinsic and extrinsic innervation of the colon. There are movements that mix the contents of the colon (rhythmic segmentary contractions) and retrograde contraction waves in cats (**Figure 46**).

FIGURE 46 - TYPES OF CONTRACTION OBSERVED IN THE COLON

A

B

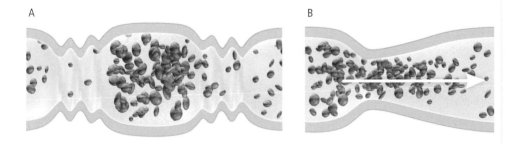

Regular segmentary contractions (A) slow the progress of feces and promote reabsorption of water. Peristaltic contractions (B) favor the advancement of the contents of the colon downstream.

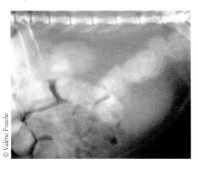
© Valérie Freiche

Figure 47 - Megacolon in a cat who previously suffered from pelvic fractures.

The anaerobic colonic flora participates in a number of reactions: the liberation of medications, and the production of endogenous compounds (volatile fatty acids).

Etiopathogenesis

Congenital megacolon is described in the Siamese. It is said to be due to the absence of ganglion cells in the myenteric and submucosa plexus (aganglionosis).

The acquired forms result from organic lesions (anatomical lesions of the pelvis, neoplasia and intraluminal stricture), metabolic abnormalities (hyperkalemia), neurological disorders (dysautonomia) or are of undetermined origins (idiopathic megacolon, which accounts for around 62% of cases according to *Washabau* (2003)).

Clinical expression

Owners report chronic constipation in cats, associated with vomiting. Painful abdominal palpation is evidence of a highly distended, colon that is hardened throughout its length. A rectal swab without sedative will enable elimination of the cause of distal obstruction and deformations of the pelvic canal.

Low occlusion is observed and demands hospitalization of infused animals (renal biochemical values are often high). The fecalith is evacuated under anesthesia, by colostomy in the most severe cases.

Diagnosis

Radiograph examination suffices to establish the diagnosis **(Figure 47)**. An examination of the front of the pelvis is necessary to exclude any old trauma that may have caused modification of the pelvic canal.

Endoscopy is not useful in establishing a diagnosis, unless an endoluminal lesion is suspected that has caused dilatation proximally in the colon.

Medical treatment

Medical treatment is exclusively palliative. Its success is closely linked to the motivation and availability of the owner, as recurrence is immediate without continuous nursing. In the medium term, surgery or euthanasia may be justified by the owner's lack of motivation.

- *Prokinetics*: cisapride was the drug of choice for treating megacolon, however, it is not available in every country.
- *Laxatives*: lactulose (0.2 mg/kg 3 times per day per os) or appetent medicinal oil sometimes delays the need for surgery. Rectal laxatives empty the rectal ampulla but do not have any effect on transit. Enemas are often poorly tolerated by the animal and are irritating in the medium term.

Dietary treatment of constipation

Many cats with constipation respond positively to an increased fiber level, but the physical and chemical properties of fiber sources differ considerably so they should be selected according to the desired effect.

Insoluble fiber

The gut flora ferments dietary fiber sources with low solubility slowly or not at all. Cellulose is a good example of a dietary fiber source with low degradability by intestinal bacterial fermentative processes. It increases the bulk in the large intestine and the increased gut fill helps stimulate intestinal motility. Depending on the structure and chemical composition, some insoluble fiber sources can trap water *(Robertson & Eastwood, 1981)*. The concentration of insoluble fiber should be limited, as insoluble ingredients tend to lower the digestibility of the diet.

Soluble fiber

Typical examples of soluble fiber sources include beet pulp, psyllium, pectin from carrots or fruits, and gum such as guar gum. Soluble fiber has a higher water-holding capacity than insoluble fiber due to its gel-forming capacity *(Robertson & Eastwood, 1981; Rosado & Diaz, 1995)*.

Soluble fiber is generally easily fermented by intestinal bacteria (except psyllium). The fermentation processes induced by the ingestion of fermentable fiber have a strong impact on the colonic milieu, because bacteria release organic acids as metabolism products that tend to reduce the colonic pH. The SCFA produced by bacteria can be utilized as energy yielding substrates by the colonic mucosa. Butyric acid has beneficial effects on the integrity and function of the gut wall and organic acids may also have some regulatory effects on motility.

Negative effects of higher amounts of soluble dietary fiber include an excessive production of SCFA and a risk of osmotic diarrhea.

In practice, it may be necessary to adjust the amount of fiber according to patient tolerance and the clinical effects. In cases of severe problems due to constipation or fecal impaction, the laxative effects of soluble fibrous sources (e.g. psyllium) are used specifically for treatment. Fermentable carbohydrates like lactulose or lactose may be recommended in constipated cats *(Meyer, 1992)*. The dosage needs to be adjusted on a case by case basis to ensure the patient produces a slightly moist stool with increased acidity. The fecal pH will be around 6.5 when adequate amounts of lactulose are ingested. Liver, milk and milk products are diet ingredients with mild laxative properties.

> Colitis

Colonic diarrhea is the result of failure of the colon's water and electrolyte reabsorption function, which determines the water-content of feces. The colon's reabsorption capacity (colonic reserve) can in fact be saturated. It is the proximal part of the colon that is responsible for this regulatory function.

Inflammatory colonopathies are a group of diseases whose pathophysiology is still largely unknown. Some factors have been clearly identified (e.g. parasitic or bacterial causes), but the origin of the colonization of the colonic mucosa by inflammatory cell populations of different histology types remains obscure. The factors involved are highly varied. They include immune-related, medication (NSAID), diet, hereditary (breed colonopathies) and even behavioral factors. In many cases, the pathogenesis proposed in humans is not transposable to domestic carnivores.

Clinical signs

Most colorectal diseases are clinically expressed by diarrhea or constipation. However, it is uncommon for these clinical expressions to provide information on the etiology of the colon.

The owner of a cat often has difficulty gaining insight in the defecation habits of the animal. Diarrhea is suspected when the cat defecates outside the litter box or in the event of soiled hair around the anus. Diarrhea of the large intestine is generally characterized as follows:
- preserved general condition (except advanced neoplasia)
- frequent emission of soft stools, of normal or increased volume, in a pile, the consistency of which changes in the course of the day (gradual softening)
- regular presence of mucus or blood
- observation of tenesmus, anal pruritus.
In cats, flatulence and vomiting complete the clinical signs.

Diagnosis

The anamnesis provides essential pointers, which sometimes provide information on the duration of the disease's development and whether the diarrhea is acute or chronic, permanent or intermittent. Recurring diarrhea is considered to be chronic.

Abdominal palpation must be done very carefully: thickening of part or the entire colon, hyperplasia of the associated lymph nodes, abnormal rigidity, and abnormal content in one or more segments. A *rectal swab* is difficult to perform on cats without sedation.

Complementary examinations

A parasitic fecal examination should always be performed ahead of any more complex examinations of the colon, even if the animal has been properly dewormed. Evaluation using a fecal float is desirable. Parasites and protozoans most frequently implicated in this location are hookworms (*Uncinaria stenocephala*) and some protozoans: mainly giardia, coccidia.

Fecal culture: few cases of colitis are caused by bacteria (*Campylobacter, Clostridia, Yersinia*). The identification of *Escherichia coli* or *Candida albicans* colonies rarely has pathological significance.

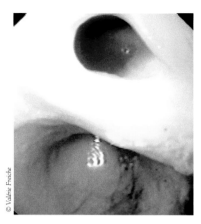

Figure 48 - Normal ileal papilla identified during coloscopy in the cat.
Needle biopsies in the distal segment of the ileus are essential.

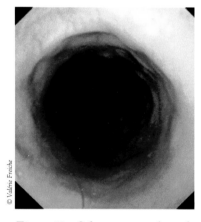

Figure 49 - Colonoscopy performed on an 11-year-old male Persian.
The colonoscopy reveals an irregularity of the surface of the mucosa in the form of small micronodular bands. This is a case of chronic colitis.

Hematological and biochemical examinations are part of the differential diagnosis (e.g. metabolic diseases), but few changes are observed specifically in terms of inflammatory colonopathies (peripheral eosinophilia in case of parasitism or feline hypereosinophilic syndrome).

Radiography: without contrast agent will generally not reveal most parietal colonic diseases, except if the lesions are very large. If an endoluminal mass is suspected, barium contrast studies of the colon should be performed. However, this examination has largely been superseded by ultrasound and endoscopy.

Abdominal ultrasound: the presence of air in the colon adversely affects the quality of the examination. Ultrasound of the colon may be proposed if the animal cannot be anesthetized or the differential diagnosis has been established between an inflammatory lesion and a neoplastic lesion. The presence of abnormal echogenicity or architectural modifications to the colon wall will reveal whether a lesion is isolated or diffuse, or whether there is a parietal tumor.

Coloscopy: Endoscopy is the diagnostic technique of choice when exploring colonic diseases **(Figure 48)**. Endoscopic biopsies are essential. They provide information on the type of cell infiltrate, the treatment and a precise prognosis.

The following visual abnormalities of inflammatory origin maybe observed during colonoscopy:
• congestion and edema of the mucosa
• thickening of the colonic folds
• heterogeneous coloration of the surface of the mucosa: presence of areas of hyperemia, areas of mottled coloration
• dilatation of the parietal glands: grayish punctuations spread across a segment of the colon surface
• abnormal friability of the mucosa as the endoscope passes through
• changes to the surface of the mucosa: presence of more proliferative areas **(Figure 49)**.

Many biopsies samples are performed during the examination. There is variable correlation between the visual aspect of lesions and the results of histological analysis.

Classification of inflammatory colitis

Lymphoplasmocytic colitis (idiopathic chronic colitis)
This is the most common type. The visual signs include the above changes. In cats, they are among the more general clinical signs of IBD.

Eosinophilic colitis
This may be a component of eosinophilia. Eosinophilic cells often predominant in colitis, but they are always associated with a population of lymphocytes, plasmocytes and possibly neutrophilic leukocytes. Hypersensitivity reactions are implicated in the pathogenesis.

Suppurated colitis
This is a relatively rare type, especially in cats. The clinical signs are often acute, sometimes accompanied by superinfected mucoid feces (pus traces). Ulcerative lesions are often associated with it, as are crypt abscesses. The predominant cell population are neutrophils.

Granulomatous colitis
This is considered to be an atypical and rare form of IBD. The segmentary lesions are observed on part of the small intestine and various parts of the large intestine. These lesions have a proliferative aspect and may sometimes lead to massive thickening of the colon wall, producing stenosis. Clinically, diarrhea is profuse, generally hemorrhagic and contains a lot of mucus. An alteration of the general condition is observed.

Medical treatment of inflammatory colitis

Where possible, the treatment should be etiological if the cause can be identified (parasitic, bacterial, viral colitis) (*Zoran, 1999*).

Use of antibiotics

The prescription of antibiotics must be limited to highly precise indications and respond to reasonable use. The clinical and hematological criteria may impose the use of certain wide-spectrum substances of low toxicity.

A regulator effect of metronidazole on the digestive flora in domesticated carnivores has been shown during colonopathies. Metronidazole also has an immunomodulator activity.

Benefit of anti-inflammatory substances

Sulfasalazine is an anti-inflammatory agent with an active substance that is cleaved and released in the colon (5-amino salicylic acid). It regulates local prostaglandin production and reduces the influx of leukocytes.

In cats, the recommended dose is either 10 mg/kg BID or 15 mg/kg SID. Several therapeutic plans are available of varying length. Sulfapyridine, which is released into the colon when the substance is cleaved, is responsible for known side effects: hematological disruptions, skin rashes, hepatic lesions, Sjögren's syndrome. Cats maybe more sensitive to the side-effects of sulfasalazine compared to dogs.

Corticosteroids and immunosuppressors

Corticosteroids are an indispensable part of the treatment of a number of chronic inflammatory colonopathies. A medium-size dose has an anti-inflammatory action (inhibition of prostaglandins and antileukotriene effect), while higher doses have an immunosuppressive effect.

Oral administration is preferred to the parenteral route. Cats tolerate corticosteroids better than dogs. They can be administered in a higher dose in the induction phase. The dose should be adapted on the basis of the clinical response.

In the most serious cases or when corticosteroid therapy is contraindicated, additional immuno-suppressive treatment may be proposed. Several weeks will be needed to judge effectiveness; and there are many side effects (particularly medullary toxicity) and constraining clinical and hema-tological checks will be necessary.

Topical agents and dressings

These are adjuvant substances that provide local protection. Some animals are less likely to be effected a second time if a clay bandage (smectite or zeolithe) is used in the medium term. Zeolite, or sodium silicoaluminate, a tetrahedral clay, is capable of adsorbing bacterial toxins, bile acids, and gases. By forming a protective film over the intestinal mucosa, zeolite helps enhance the intestinal mucosal barrier. Compliance is a limiting factor.

Dietary treatment

Although colitis is most frequently diagnosed in dogs, it is becoming increasingly common in cats (*Simpson, 1998*). Colitis can be beneficially influenced by adequate dietary treatment in cats, although this depends on whether it has mainly an infectious, inflammatory or immune-mediated pathogenesis (*Zentek, 2004*).

Importance of high-quality protein

Unlike fats and well-cooked starches, which are almost totally digested in the small intestine, the digestibility of proteins varies according to source and treatment. The ingestion of low-quality proteins – which therefore are also characterized by poor ileal digestibility – leads to an inflow of indigestible protein matter in the colon. Greater putrefaction of proteins leads to an increase in bacterial biomass and a high secretion of water in the colon – simultaneous phenomena that result in poor stool consistency. High protein putrefaction can disrupt the colonic microflora and orient its profile towards potentially pathogenic strains (*Zentek et al, 1998*). The many aromatic compounds produced (mercaptan, indole, skatole etc) can have a toxic effect on the colonic mucosa in combination with the biogenic amines formed (cadaverin, putrescine, etc) and encourage cancers of the colon and rectum (*MacFarlane & Cummings, 1991*). The high production of ammonia may ultimately affect DNA synthesis, damage the morphology of the colonocytes and shorten their lifespan (*Visek, 1978*).

A good selection of proteins and a controlled manufacturing process makes it possible to considerably improve their digestibility, which is essential to good digestive tolerance in cats. Many cats that suffer from chronic diarrhea as a consequence of colonic inflammation will respond to a novel protein elimination diet or a hydrolysed protein-based diet (*Nelson et al, 1984; Guilford & Matz, 2003*).

Dietary fiber
A hypoallergenic diet can be combined with a fermentable fiber source, such as pectin or guar gum. The addition of fermentable dietary fiber regulates the composition of the colonic microbiota and may reduce the potentially harmful flora.

Soluble fiber is highly fermentable and as such it plays a very important role in the ecosystem of the large intestine. It first acts as a substrate for the bacterial biomass, which provides it with the necessary energy for good growth. The resulting fermentative activity also generates a large quantity of SCFA and lactic acid. Such fermentation products (mainly SCFA) have an extremely important trophic role in maintaining the colonic mucosa in good health. Colon cell atrophy is observed in the complete absence of soluble fiber in food (*Wong & Gibson, 2003*).

Insoluble fiber (cellulose, hemicelluloses, lignin) is not generally decomposed to any great degree by microflora in the colon, which means they remain virtually intact in the stools. Their high hygroscopic capacity (they can absorb up to 25 times their weight) together with their ability to increase the indigestible residuum of feces help improve fecal consistency but also increase the volume of stools (*Sunvold et al, 1995a*).

On the other hand, bearing in mind their high fermentability, an excessive quantity of soluble fiber in food is detrimental to good digestive tolerance. The resulting high moisture content, poor consistency and high volume of stools would appear to be explained mainly by a high proliferation of the bacterial biomass (*Sunvold et al, 1995a*) (**Table 8**).

* In this study, fecal consistency was assessed on a scale from 1 (hard dry stools) to 5 (diarrheic stools), where 2 is considered optimal. Values with different letters for the same parameter (column) are statistically different (p<0.05). A food that is rich in soluble fiber leads to a large quantity of stools, with high moisture content and low consistency. It should also be noted that stools of animals that have eaten a mixture of soluble fiber or beet pulp have a similar water content but very different consistencies. The moisture content of a stool is therefore not always representative of its appearance.

From practical experience, the addition of moderate amounts of insoluble and soluble dietary fiber is common.

TABLE 8 - MOISTURE, CONSISTENCY AND VOLUME OF STOOLS IN CATS (N=5) FED WITH A FOOD ENRICHED (~10%) IN DIFFERENT SOURCES OF DIETARY FIBER
From Sunvold et al (1995a)

Diet	Soluble fiber	Insoluble fiber	Digestive tolerance		
			Moisture (%)	Consistency *	g stools/g fiber ingested
Mixture of soluble fiber	+++		74.9[a]	4.2[a]	13.1[a]
Beet pulp	+++	+	74.7[a]	2.3[b]	7.4[b]
Cellulose		+++	52.6[b]	1.8[b]	3.6[c]

Energy consumption

Cats with enterocolitis often have severe weight loss and anorexia leading to a cachexic body condition (*Hart et al, 1994*). Therefore, the careful adjustment of energy and nutrient intake is a mandatory part of successful dietary management for these patients. The palatability of a food is another very important criterion, as the nutritional treatment is recommended for several months and boredom should be avoided.

▶ Small and large intestinal neoplasia

Small intestinal tumors account for 73% of all intestinal tumors in cats (52% adenocarcinomas, 21% lymphomas). Conversely, colonic tumors are uncommon (10-15% of intestinal tumors in cats) (*Estrada et al, 1998*). The slow appearance of non-specific clinical signs rules out early detection.

Feline intestinal tumors have a better prognosis than esophageal or gastric tumors.

> Small intestinal tumors

Different histological types encountered

The two predominant types of tumor are **adenocarcinomas** (*Kosovsky et al, 1998*) and **lymphomas**. While most cats that present with intestinal lymphoma are FeLV negative, the former presence of the virus is implicated in the neoplastic transformation (*Barr et al, 1995*).

Other tumors are less common: **leiomyomas, leiomyosarcomas, fibrosarcomas**. Benign tumors of the duodenum, of the **adenomatous** polyp type have been described in cats (*Estrada et al, 1998; Freiche et al, 2005b*), especially oriental males without known viral impairment by FIV or FeLV.

Mastocytomas exclusively found in the digestive tract are reported in dogs. Some cases have been described in cats, in the colon of aging animals (*Slawienski et al, 1997*).

Carcinoid tumors (neuroendocrine) are very uncommon. Their clinical expression is generally dominated by the paraneoplastic syndrome (*Guilford & Strombeck, 1996d*).

Relatively undifferentiated **mesenchymatous tumors** in the intestines are described in cats. Biopsies of mesenchymatous lesions may require specific stains and immunolabeling.

Epidemiology

Breed and sex predispositions have been recognized. In cats, the Siamese is commonly implicated, particularly with carcinoma. Generally speaking, the incidence of intestinal lymphomas appears to be higher in males than females. Whatever the nature of the tumor, affected cats are generally at least 10 or 11 years old, although intestinal lymphomas may be identified in much younger cats. Adenomas are less common in the small intestine and are probably under diagnosed.

Clinical signs

The alteration of the wall of the small intestine may lead to digestive transit or nutrient absorption disorders that have clinical consequences and are responsible for signs of the disease. These signs are not very specific: diarrhea, vomiting, melena. Again, they are shared with other gastrointestinal diseases, which means the etiological diagnosis is sometimes made too late.

The clinical expression of small intestinal neoplasia is linked to the location of the lesion in the intestinal wall:
- the more proximal, the more frequent vomiting will be. Melena is a relatively reliable sign, but inconsistent;
- more distal tumors are expressed by diarrheal episodes that worsen over time. The diarrhea is then characteristic of chronic small intestinal diarrhea. The overall condition of the cat is generally altered, with the presence of weight loss, dysorexia and lethargy.

In some much less common cases, the animal presents with occlusion. General loss of body condition is more visible in later stages of development. Weight loss is a sign. Feline intestinal tumors are sometimes very distal (small-large intestine junction) and are expressed in several forms (isolated, multicentric, diffuse). However, in a large proportion of cases, abdominal palpation does not identify a mass, although diffuse or segmentary thickening of the intestinal loops is often suspected.

Diagnosis

The diagnosis is obtained by traditional techniques.

- **Hematobiochemical analyses** provide few pointers. The differential diagnosis must exclude the metabolic causes of chronic diarrhea. Anemia is an important sign to remember (possible in the event of a lymphoma), but many intestinal neoplasias do not produce blood loss on the CBC. However, intestinal mastocytomas do cause mucosal ulcerations that may result in chronic blood loss.

- **Radiography** may be proposed if no other means of investigation is possible **(Figure 50)**. The association of abdominal ultrasound and endoscopy is greatly preferable to a barium study, which is both difficult to perform and to interpret.

- **Abdominal ultrasound** is certainly the investigation of choice when good equipment is available. Precise signs are described for intestinal neoplasia, based on the same types of changes cited for a gastric lesion. These include modification to the parietal layers with localized or diffuse identification faults, variations in echogenicity (hypoechogenicity), abnormal satellite lymph nodes and localized peristaltic problems (*Penninck, 1998; Hittmair et al, 2001*).

- **Endoscopy and histological analysis of biopsies** are proposed when the lesion is accessible (proximal and distal small intestine). They are recommended when an abdominal ultrasound has excluded the presence of an isolated lesion of the small intestine. The histological analysis of endoscopic biopsies obtained from several locations can lead to the diagnosis. This examination has two limitations:
  - isolated lesions of the middle of the small intestine are topographically inaccessible
  - isolated tumor cells under the mucosa or the muscles maybe missed.

- **Laparoscopy** permits a beneficial approach, but it demands more sophisticated equipment.

- Trans-parietal biopsies can be performed during an **exploratory laparotomy** if the above examinations are not possible.

Disease staging

Different types of examination are available to stage the disease: radiology (thoracic imaging), abdominal ultrasound and tomodensitometric examination. These complementary examinations should be used selectively, depending on the case. Metastasis is initially most often regional. Abdominal ultrasound can identify a satellite and/or regional lymphadenopathy, as well as parenchymatous metastasis, while also facilitating fine needle aspiration for an immediate diagnostic approach. The thoracic radiographs can be used to exclude the presence of pulmonary metastasis. The pulmonary tomodensitometric examination is more precise.

Treatment and prognosis

Therapy depends on several factors:
- the animal's general condition and whether medical resuscitation is necessary
- the histopathological nature of the tumor: benign or malignant, risk of metastasis or local recurrence, hematopoietic status

In cats, it may be difficult to differentiate intestinal lymphoma in its diffuse form with severe IBD. The visual aspect of the lesions are similar. When there is no logical correlation between the histological analysis of biopsies and the clinical condition of the animal, the diagnosis must be questioned, because diffuse inflammatory lesions of the digestive tract (often lymphoplasmocytic in nature) are almost always associated with feline gastrointestinal lymphoma.

- local and remote disease staging.

When indicated, diffuse hematopoietic intestinal tumors (lymphoma, mastocytoma), will be treated medically (*Lanore, 2002*). The medical treatment protocols are similar to those for lymphoma and systemic mastocytoma. They vary according to histological type.

Generally speaking, in the event of surgical treatment certain rules need to be observed (*Salwienski et al, 1997*):
- eliminate all tumor cells and include ganglionic excision when possible
- avoid dissemination of neoplastic cells, locally or remotely.

The enterectomy techniques used on healthy tissue are employed, by means of laparotomy for the different segments of the small intestine.

> Colon neoplasia

Different histological types encountered

Tumors of the colon are uncommon in cats. The carcinoma is the most common histological type. It affects aging animals and males more than females. Rectal tumors are more common than colonic tumors.

The isolated colonic form of lymphoma in cats is not common, although it dominates the incidence of carcinomas in this location. In this species, the ileocolic location must always be examined (lymphoma, carcinoma, mastocytoma).

Benign isolated polyps are less common in domesticated carnivores than in humans. They do not appear to particularly precede the appearance of carcinomas, at least not through the same mechanism as in humans.

Clinical signs

All but two of the clinical signs are non-specific. The presence of blood in feces of normal consistency and the presence of abnormally small stools are specific signs. Other clinical signs are identical to those traditionally observed during diarrhea of the large intestine (tenesmus, hematochezia, mucus etc) (*Jergens & Willard, 2000*).

A rectal swab under anesthesia is necessary, as a large proportion of colon lesions caused by a tumor are located in the last few centimeters of the mucosa. There are few benefits to abdominal palpation (the lesions are not always highly exophytic or indurated).

These neoplastic processes may develop slowly and the diagnosis is made in the later stages as described with gastric carcinoma. The alteration of the general state is slow and inconsistent. The deep infiltrative and/or stenosing forms are more pronounced. Tenesmus and pain are generally less marked, except carcinomas located at the colorectal junction, where infiltration is low. The presence of ascites is uncommon at the time of diagnosis.

Diagnostic evaluation

Coloscopy is the diagnostic technique of choice (**Figures 51 & 52**). It does not demand any specific preparation in cats, as the feline colon is short. The administration of a diet without residue exclusively based on white meat or fish without added fiber or fat for the four days prior to the examination, followed by enemas under anesthesia, is sufficient and not very restricting.

Coloscopy is a tool to address part of the disease staging process and to identify whether there is one or more lesions. Colon neoplasia can present several forms: pedunculated, diffuse, in "graps" or scattered along the colonic wall: it is then difficult to macroscopically predict the histological nature of a colorectal mass. Multiple endoscopic biopsy samples must be obtained.

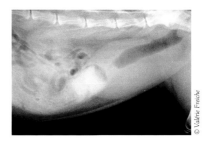

© Valérie Freiche

Figure 50 - Colonic carcinoma revealed by radiography.
The contrast environment generated by distension of the bladder with fluid helps visualize colonic stenosis. The histological diagnosis was achieved by endoscopically obtained biopsy samples. A peripheral lymphadenopathy had been identified during the ultrasound examination.

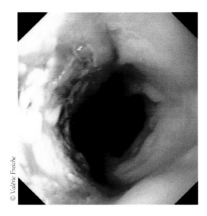

Figure 51 - Coloscopy in an 8-year-old domestic shorthair cat who presented for defecation disorders and hematochezia.
The examination shows a parietal endoluminal mass which is consistent with a non-pedunculated tumor. The histological nature of the tumor cannot be determined during the examination.

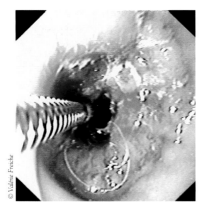

Figure 52 - 16 year old female cat who presented with constipation and marked depression.
Coloscopy shows endoluminal stenosis, which is responsible for distal occlusion. The distal colic stenosis had a post-inflammatory origin.

Disease staging

Abdominal ultrasound is complementary to coloscopy. It allows evaluation of the regional extension of the tumor process, and must be conducted as soon as possible. Liver and lung metastases are seldom observed during the diagnosis.

Treatment and prognosis

Surgery is the treatment of choice for localized malignant tumors. Palliative surgery may extend the animal's life. In the event of carcinoma, the location of the lesion justifies different surgical approaches, the follow-up of which may be difficult to manage.

Radiation therapy is an excellent complementary treatment to the surgical excision of localized distal recto-colic carcinomas.

The administration of corticosteroids alone, without a chemotherapeutic protocol improves or maintains appetite while reducing the cat's inflammation and pain. Local topical drugs such as anti-inflammatory steroids recommended for humans are not particularly beneficial in cats.

Dietary treatment

Dietary treatment is limited to adjusting the diet composition according to the patient's needs. A higher energy density may be efficiently provided by a higher fat diet. Long chain n-3 fatty acids from fish oil have been shown to be beneficial in different models of neoplastic disorders. Therefore, diets with a higher protein concentration, specifically a balanced spectrum of amino acids (arginine) and higher levels of micronutrients (zinc, antioxidant vitamins) may be favorable in these patients. For further information, refer to chapter 11.

Conclusion

Dietary treatment with adequate medication is the key to successful treatment of gastrointestinal disorders in cats. Depending on the suspected disease, the choice is between highly digestible diets in the case of small intestinal and pancreatic diseases, antigen-reduced diets in the case of dietary sensitivity or allergy, and high-fiber diets when the colon is specifically affected or motility disorders occur. In practice, dietary treatment has to be adjusted individually. The response of the patient is not always predictable and good compliance is needed for optimal success.

Frequently asked questions about the role of nutrition in digestive diseases

Q	A
What type of protein is suitable for a cat with dietary sensitivity?	One solution is to feed the cat with sources of protein to which it has not previously been exposed to e.g. capelin, duck, venison, rabbit etc. The term is an elimination diet, as the purpose is to eliminate protein sources that may trigger undesirable reactions. Another alternative is a hydrolysed protein-based diet. Hydrolysed protein is less immunogenic and produces good results in the event of dietary allergy. Cereals are starch sources that also contain protein. The preferred starch sources are rice, tapioca, potatos, and peas.
What type of diet should I choose for a cat with colitis?	Diets formulated with noval proteins and hydrolysed protein-based diets produce very good results in cats with colitis.
How can I overcome palatability problems in cats?	A cat may develop an aversion to the food it is consuming when digestive problems or vomiting manifest themselves. As a consequence, after the cause of these problems has been treated, it may be necessary to change the food or choose another variety in the same range of products. Dietary aversion is connected to the taste and odor of a particular food.
A laboratory reported high numbers of clostridia in a fecal sample of a patient with chronic diarrhea. What can be done and how should the diet be adjusted?	It is not abnormal to observe a high number of *Clostridia* in the feces of a carnivore. Nutritional action should be considered only in the event of chronic digestive problems. A highly digestible diet should be chosen that is not too rich in animal protein so as not to encourage colic fermentation. This diet must also contain fermentable fiber (beet pulp, fructo-oligosaccharides etc).
Can I use digestive enzymes in the treatment of cats with diarrhea?	Digestive enzymes are indicated only if the cat suffers from exocrine pancreatic insufficiency. This pathology is rare in cats but it does exist. It can be revealed by measuring feline trypsin-like immunoreactivity (fTLI), which is different from canine TLI, so the dog test does not work with cats. The enzymes must be mixed into the food. The powder form is preferable (see the chapter on hepatobilary and pancreatic diseases).
How long do I have to perform an elimination trial in a cat with a suspected dietary allergy?	The test must last at least 12 weeks, but improvement is typically observed in most cats after 4 weeks.
Should I prescribe nutritional supplements for cats with chronic diarrhea?	No, it is better to recommend a high-quality, highly digestible food that contains protein sources the animal has not previously encountered or a hydrolysed protein source. The parenteral administration of vitamin B_{12} is indicated in deficient animals.

References

Adamama-Moraitou KK, Rallis TS, Prassinos NN, et al. Benign esophageal stricture in the dog and cat: a retrospective study of 20 cases. Can Vet Res 2002; 66: 55-59.

Allenspach K, Roosje P. Food allergies diagnosis. Proc Aktualitäten aus der Gastroenterologie, Interlaken 2004: 71-78.

Appleton, DJ, Rand JS, Priest J, et al. Dietary carbohydrate source affects glucose concentrations, insulin secretion, and food intake in overweight cats. Nutrition Research 2004; 24: 447-467.

Backus RC, Rogers QR, Morris JG. Microbial degradation of taurine in fecal cultures from cats given commercial and purified diets. J Nutr 1994;124: 2540s-2545s.

Barone R. Anatomie comparée des mammifères domestiques. In: Splanchnologie I, Vol 3, 2e ed. Vigot, 1984: 485-501.

Barr MC, Olsen CW, Scott FW. Feline viral diseases: In: Ettinger S, Feldman E, eds. Textbook of Internal Veterinary Medicine. 4th ed. Philadelphia: WB Saunders Co, 1995; 1: 409-439.

Battersby, I, Harvey A. Differential diagnosis and treatment of acute diarrhoea in the dog and cat. In Practice 2006; 28: 480-488.

Bauer JE. Facilitative and functional fats in diets of cats and dogs. J Am Vet Med Assoc 2006; 229: 680-684.

Bradshaw JWS. The evolutionary basis for the feeding behavior of domestic dogs (Canis familiaris) and cats (Felis catus). J Nutr 2006; 136: 1927s-1931s.

Brugère H. Details of digestion in the cat. Bull Mens Soc Vet Prat Fr 1996; 80: 295-313.

Buddington RK, Diamond J. Ontogenetic development of nutrient transporters in cat intestine. Am J Physiol 1992; 263: G605-G616.

Cave N J. Chronic inflammatory disorders of the gastrointestinal tract of companion animals. N Z Vet J 2003;51: 262-274.

Cecchi R, Wills SJ, Dean R, et al. Demonstration of Ollulanus tricuspis in the stomach of domestics cats by biopsy. J Comp Pathol 2006: 374-377.

Cerny H, Mazanek S, Cerna E. Immunohistochemical localization of endocrine G cells in the epithelium of the pars pylorica mucosa of the cat and mouse stomach. Acta Veterinaria Brno 1991; 60: 317-322.

Chan DL, Freeman LM, Labato MA, et al. Retrospective evaluation of partial parenteral nutrition in dogs and cats. J Veterinary Intern Med 2002; 16: 440-445.

Chivers, DJ, Hladik CM. Morphology of the gastrointestinal tract in primates: comparisons with other mammals in relation to diet. J Morphol 1980; 166 (3): 337-386.

Cohn LA, Stoll MR, Branson KR, et al. Fatal hemothorax following management of an esophageal foreign body. J Am Anim Hosp Assoc 2003; 39: 251-256.

Crabb SE, Freeman LM, Chan DL. Retrospective evaluation of total parenteral nutrition in cats: 40 cases (1991-2003). Crit Care 2006;16: S21-S26.

Day M J. Gastrointestinal immunology. In: Hall E, Simpson J & Williams D, eds. BSAVA Manual of canine and feline gastroenterology. 2nd ed, 2005: 50-56.

Dennis MM, Bennett N, Ehrhart EJ. Gastric adenocarcinoma and chronic gastritis in two related Persian cats. Vet Pathol 2006;43: 358-362.

Descroix-Vagne M, Perret JP, Daoud-el Baba M, et al. Variation of gastric lipase secretion in the Heidenhain pouch of the cat. Arch Int Physiol Biochim Biophys 1993; 101: 79-85.

Dodds WJ, Stewart ET, Hodges D, et al. Movement of the feline esophagus associated with respiration and peristalsis. An evaluation using tantalum markers. J Clin Invest 1973; 52: 1-13.

Dukes' physiology of domestic animals. Melvin J. Swenson, eds. 10th ed. Cornell University Press, 1984.

Durand-Viel M, Hesse C. Place de la vidéo-endoscopie interventionnelle dans l'extraction des corps étrangers oesophagiens, gastriques et duodénaux chez les carnivores domestiques: étude rétrospective sur 146 cas. Th Méd Vét Alfort, 2005.

Estrada M, Dargent F, Freiche V. Tumeurs gastrointestinales chez le chat. Prat Méd Chir Anim Comp 1998; 33: 107-121.

Fahey GC, Flickinger, EA, Grieshop CM, et al. The role of dietary fibre in companion animal nutrition. In: van der Kamp JW, Asp NG, Miller-Jones J, Schaafsma G, eds. Dietary fibre: bio active carbohydrates for food and feed. Wageningen Academic Publishers, The Netherlands, 2003: 295-328.

Flickinger EA, Van Loo J, Fahey GC Jr. Nutritional responses to the presence of inulin and oligofructose in the diets of domesticated animals: a review. Crit Rev Food Sci Nutr 2003; 43: 19-60.

Fondacaro J, Ritcher K, Carpenter J, et al. Feline gastrointestinal lymphoma: 67 cases (1988-1996). Eur J Comp Gastroenterology 1999: 5-11.

Freiche V. Fibroscopie interventionnelle en gastro-entérologie des carnivores domestiques. Point Vet 1999; 30: 9-15.

Freiche V. Diarrhée chez les carnivores domestiques. Gastro-entérologie, Encycl Vét. Éditions scientifiques et Médicales Elsevier SAS, Paris, 2000; 1400: 1-18.

Freiche V. Tumeurs de l'œsophage et de l'estomac. Point Vét (Cancérologie du chien et du chat au quotidien) 2005a; 36: 98-101.

Freiche V. Tumeurs intestinales du chien et du chat. Point Vét (Cancérologie du chien et du chat au quotidien) 2005b; 36: 102-106.

Freiche V. Endoscopie du tractus digestif des carnivores domestiques. Imagerie médicale, Encycl Vét. Editions scientifiques et Médicales Elsevier SAS, Paris, 2006; 3400.

Funaba M, Oka Y, Kobayashi S, et al. Evaluation of meat meal, chicken meal, and corn gluten meal as dietary sources of protein in dry cat food. Can J Vet Res 2005; 69: 299-304.

Gaschen, F, Neiger R. Vomiting in the cat. Proc Aktualitäten aus der Gastroenterologie, Interlaken 2004: 157- 158.

German AJ, Cannon MJ, Dye C, et al. Oesophageal strictures in cats associated with doxycycline therapy. J Feline Med Surg 2005; 7: 33-41.

German, AJ, Zentek J. The most common digestive diseases: the role of nutrition. In: Pibot P, Biourge V and Elliott D, eds. Encyclopedia of canine clinical nutrition. Paris: Diffomédia, 2006: 92-133.

Gookin JL, Breitschwerdt EB, Levy MG, et al. Diarrhea associated with trichomonosis in cats. J Am Vet Med Assoc 1999; 215: 1450-1455.

Graham JP, Lipman AH, Newell SM, et al. Esophageal transit of capsules in clinically normal cats. Am J Vet Res 2000; 61: 655-657.

Gualtieri M, Monzeglio M, D Giancamillo M. *Oesophageal squamous cell carcinoma in two cats.* J Small Anim Pract 1999; 40: 79-83.

Guilford WG. *Fecal incontinence in dogs and cats.* Comp Cont Ed Pract Vet 1990; 12: 313-326

Guilford WG. *Idiopathic inflammatory bowel diseases.* In: Guilford WG, Center S A, Strombeck DR et al, eds. Strombeck's small animal gastroenterology. 3rd ed. Philadelphia: WB Saunders Co, 1996; 24: 451-486.

Guilford WG, Jones BR, Markwell PJ, et al. *Food sensitivity in cats with chronic idiopathic gastrointestinal problems.* J Vet Intern Med 2001; 15: 7-13.

Guilford WG, Matz ME. *The nutritional management of gastrointestinal tract disorders in companion animals.* N Z Vet J 2003; 51: 284-291.

Guilford WG, Strombeck DR. *Diseases of swallowing.* In: Guilford WG, Center S A, Strombeck DR et al, eds. Strombeck's small animal gastroenterology. 3rd ed. Philadelphia: WB Saunders Co, 1996b; 11: 211-238

Guilford WG, Strombeck DR. *Gastrointestinal tract infections, parasites, and toxicoses.* In: Guilford WG, Strombeck DR, Center S A et al, eds. Strombeck's small animal gastroenterology. Philadelphia: WB Saunders Co, 1996c; 21: 411-432.

Guilford WG, Strombeck DR. *Neoplasms of the gastrointestinal tract, APUD tumors, endocrinopathies and the gastrointestinal Tract.* In: Guilford WG, Strombeck DR, Center S A, et al, eds. Strombeck's small animal gastroenterology. WB Saunders Co, 1996d; 27: 519-532.

Gunn-More DA, McCann TM, Reed N, et al. *Prevalence of tritrichomonas foetus infection in cats with diarrhea in the UK.* J Feline Med Surg 2007; 9: 214-218.

Hall JA. *Diseases of the stomach.* In: Textbook of veterinary internal medicine. Diseases of the dog and cat, 5th ed. Vol 1 & 2, 2000: 1154-1182.

Hall JA, Washabau RJ. *Diagnosis and treatment of gastric motility disorders.* Vet Clin North Am Small Anim Pract 1999; 29: 377-395.

Hall E J. *Gastrointestinal adverse food reactions.* Prakt Tierarzt 2002; 83: 30-36.

Han E, Broussard J, Baer KE. *Feline esophagitis secondary to gastroesophageal reflux disease: clinical signs and radiographic, endoscopic, and histopathological findings.* J Am Anim Hosp Assoc 2003; 39:161-167.

Haraï BH, Johnson SE, Sherding RG. *Endoscopically guided balloon dilatation of benign esophageal strictures in 6 cats and 7 dogs.* J Vet Intern Med 1995; 9: 332- 335.

Harper EJ, Turner CL. *Age-related changes in apparent digestibility in growing kittens.* Reprod Nutr Dev 2000; 40: 249-260.

Hart JR, Shaker E, Patnaik AK, et al. *Lymphocytic-plasmacytic enterocolitis in cats: 60 cases (1988-1990).* J Am Anim Hosp Assoc 1994; 30: 505-514.

Harvey CJ, Lopez JW, Hendrick MJ. *An uncommun intestinal manifestation, of feline infectious peritonitis: 26 cases (1986-1993).* J Am Vet Med Assoc 1996; 209: 1117-1121.

Hegner K, Vollmerhaus B. *Applied anatomy of the feline oesophagus. Part III: View, measures, construction, method.* Kleintierpraxis 1997; 42: 621-629.

Henrotaux M. *La diarrhée féline (2ᵉ partie). Forme aigüe.* Ann Med Vet 1996; 140: 225-221.

Hesta M, Janssens GPJ, Debraekeleer J, et al. *The effect of oligofructose and inulin on faecal characteristics and nutrient digestibility in healthy cats.* J Anim Physiol Anim Nutr 2001; 85: 135-141.

Hittmair K, Krebitz-Gressl E, Kübber-Heiss A, et al. *Feline alimentary lymphosarcoma: radiographical, ultrasonographical, histological and virological findings.* J Companion Anim Pract 2001; XI: 119-128.

Hoskins JD. *The digestive system.* In: Hoskins JD, ed. Veterinary Pediatrics: dogs and cats from birth to six months. Philadelphia: WB Saunders Co, 1995: 133-187.

Howard KE, Fisher IL, Dean GA, et al. *Methodology for isolation and phenotypic characterization of feline small intestinal leukocytes.* J Immunol Methods 2005; 302: 36-53.

Hwang CY, Han HR, Youn HY. *Prevalence and clincal characterisation of gastric helicobacter species infection of dogs and cats in Korea.* J Vet Sci 2002: 123-133.

Ireland LM, Hohenhaus AE, Broussard JD, et al. *A comparison of owner management and complications in 67 cats with oesophagostomy and percutaneuous endoscopic gastrotomy feeding tubes.* J Am Anim Hosp Assoc 2003; 39: 241-246.

Jenkins CC. *Dysphagia and regurgitation.* In: Ettinger S, Feldman EC eds Textbook of veterinary internal medicine. Diseases of the dog and cat. 5th ed. Vol 1 & 2, 2000: 114-117.

Jergens AE. *Clinical staging for feline inflammatory bowel disease.* In Proceedings, vol. 20. The North American Veterinary Conference, 2006: 453-454

Jergens A, Willard M. *Diseases of the large intestine.* In: Ettinger S, Feldman EC eds Textbook of veterinary internal medicine. Diseases of the dog and cat. 5th ed. Vol 1 & 2, 2000:1238-1256.

Kienzle, E. *Carbohydrate metabolism of the cat. 3. Digestion of sugars.* J Anim Physiol Anim Nutr 1993; 69: 203- 210.

Konde LJ, Pugh CR. *Radiology and sonography of the digestive system.* In: Tams TR, ed. Handbbok of Small Animal Gastroenterology. 1st ed. Philadelphia: WB Saunders, 2003; 51-96.

Knospe C, Plendl J. *Histochemical demonstration of lipase activity in the gastric mucosa of the cat.* Embryologia (Nagoya) 1997; 26: 303-304.

Kosovsky JE, Matthiesen DT, Patnaïk AK. *Small intestinal adenocarcinoma in cats: 32 cases (1978-1985).* J Am Vet Med Assoc 1988;192: 233-235.

Krecic MR. *Feline inflammatory bowel disease: Pathogenesis, diagnosis and relationship to lymphosarcoma.* Compend Cont Educ Pract Vet 2001: 951-960.

Lanore D, Delprat C. *Chimiothérapie anticancéreuse.* Paris: Masson, 2002.

Leib MS, Dinnel H, Ward DL, et al. *Endoscopic balloon dilatation of benign esophageal strictures in dogs and cats.* J Vet Intern Med 2001; 15: 547-552.

Lobetti R, Leisewitz A. *Gastroeosophageal reflux in two cats.* Feline Pract 1996; 24: 5-12.

Lowe JA, Kershaw SJ. *The ameliorating effect of Yucca schidigera extract on canine and feline faecal aroma.* Res Vet Sci 1997; 63: 61-66.

MacDonald ML, Rogers QR, Morris JG. *Aversion of the cat to dietary medium chain triglycerides and caprylic acid.* Physiol Behav 1985; 35: 371-375.

Malandain E, Little S, Casseleux G, et al. Practical guide of cat breeding. Aniwa SAS, 2006.

Mark SM. Nasooesophageal, esophagostomy, and gastrotomy tube placement techniques. In: Ettinger S, Feldman EC eds Texbook of Internal Medicine. 6th ed. St Louis, Missouri: Elsevier- Saunders 2005; 92: 329-337.

Marks SL. The principles and application of enteral nutrition. Vet Clin North Am Small Anim Pract. 1998; 28: 677-708.

Marshall Jones ZV, Baillon MLA, Croft J M, et al. Effects of Lactobacillus acidophilus DSM13241 as a probiotic in healthy adult cats. Am J Vet Res 2006; 67: 1005-1012.

McConnel JF, Sparkes AH, Blunden AS, et al. Eosinophilic fibrosing gastritis and toxoplasmosis in a cat. J Feline Med Surg 2007; 9: 82-88.

McGrotty YL, Knottenbelt CM.). Oesophageal stricture in a cat due to oral administration of tetracyclines. J Small Anim Pract 2002; 43: 221-223.

Meyer H. Lactose intake in carnivores. Wien Tieraerztl Msschrift 1992; 79: 236-241.

Meyer H, Kienzle E, Zentek J. Body size and relative weight of gastrointestinal tract and liver in dogs. J Vet Nutr 1993; 2: 31-35.

Moore FM. The laboratory and pathologic assessment of vomiting animals. Vet Med 1992; 87: 796, 798-800, 802-805.

Morris, JG, Trudell J, Pencovic T. Carbohydrate digestion by the domestic cat (Felis catus). Br J Nutr 1977; 37: 365-373.

Moses L, Harpster NK, Hartzband L. Esophageal motility dysfunction in cats: a study of 44 cases. J Am Anim Hosp Assoc 2000; 36: 309-312.

Munana KR, Olby NJ, Sharp NJH, et al. Intervertebral disk disease in 10 cats. J Am Anim Hosp Assoc 2001;37: 384-389.

Nelson RW, Dimperio ME, Long GG. Lymphocytic-plasmacytic colitis in the cat. J Am Vet Med Assoc 1984; 184: 1133-1135.

Nguyen Van NK, Taglinger CR, Helps S, et al. Measurement of cytokine mRNA expression in intestinal biopsies of cats with inflammatory enteropathy using quantitative real-time RT-PCR. Vet Immunol Immunopathol 2006;113: 404-414.

Nicholson A, Watson AD, Mercer JR. Fat malassimilation in three cats. Aust Vet J 1989; 66: 110-113.

Ojima, K, Takeda M, Matsumoto S, et al. Functional role of V form distribution seen in microvascular cast specimens of the filiform and fungiform papillae on the posterior central dorsal surface of the cat tongue. Ann Anat 1997; 179: 321-327.

Osbaldiston, GW, Stowe EC. Microflora of alimentary tract of cats. Am J Vet Res 1971; 32: 1399-1405.

Paragon BM, Mahé S. Drinking behaviour and water requirement in the cat. Rec Med Vet Ec Alfort 1994;170: 499-512.

Peachey SE, Dawson JM, Harper EJ. The effect of ageing on nutrient digestibility by cats fed beef tallow-, sunflower oil- or olive oil-enriched diets. Aging (Milano) 1999; 63: 61-70.

Penninck D. Characterization of gastrointestinal tumors. Vet Clin North Am, Small Anim Pract 1998; 28: 777-797.

Peterson PB, Willard MD. Protein losing enteropathies. Vet Clin North Am, Small Anim Pract 2003; 33: 1061-1082.

Preiksaitis HG, Diamant NE. Myogenic mechanism for peristalsis in the cat esophagus. Am J Physiol 1999; 277: G306-G313.

Rastall RA. Bacteria in the gut: friends and foes and how to alter the balance. J Nutr 2004; 134: 2022s-2026s.

Reed EA, Belyea RL, Newcomb MD, et al. Feline trichobezoars: composition and degradation. J Anim Vet Adv 2004; 3: 833-841.

Remillard RL. Parenteral nutrition. In: DiBartola SP, ed. Fluid therapy in small animal practice. 2nd ed, 2000: 465-482.

Robertson JA, Eastwood MA. An examination of factors which may affect the water holding capacity of dietary fibre. Br J Nutr 1981; 45: 83-88.

Robinson PP, Winkles PA. Quantitative study of fungiform papillae and taste buds on the cat's tongue. Anat Rec 1990; 226: 108-111.

Rosado JL, Diaz M. Physico-chemical properties related to gastrointestinal function of 6 sources of dietary fiber. Rev Invest Clin 1995; 47: 283-289.

Roubardeau I, Péchereau D. Adénocarcinome gastrique chez un chat. Prat Méd Chir Anim Comp 2006; 41: 127-130.

Sellon RK, Willard MD. Esophagitis and esophageal strictures. Vet Clin North Am, Small Anim Pract 2003; 33: 945-967.

Shaw B, Wright CL. The pepsinogens of cat gastric mucosa and the pepsins derived from them. Digestion 1976; 14: 142-152.

Shinozuka J, Nakayama H, Suzuki M, et al. Esophageal adenosquamous carcinoma in a cat. J Vet Med Sci 2001; 63: 91-93.

Simpson JW. Diet and large intestinal disease in dogs and cats. J Nutr 1998; 128: 2717S-2722S.

Simpson KW, Fyfe J, Cornetta, et al. Subnormal concentrations of serum cobalamin (Vit B12) in cats with gastrointestinal disease. J Vet Intern Med 2001; 15: 26-32.

Simpson KW. Acute and chronic vomiting. In: Hall E, Simpson J & Williams D, eds. BSAVA Manual of canine and feline gastroenterology. 2nd ed, 2005: 73-77.

Slatter D. Gastric neoplasia. In: Slatter D, ed. Texbook of Small Animall Surgery. 3rd ed. Philadelphia: WB Saunders, 2003: 625-629.

Slawienski MJ, Mauldin GE, Mauldin GN, et al. Malignant colonic neoplasia in cats: 46 cases (1990-1996). J Am Vet Med Assoc 1997; 211: 878-881.

Sorel JE, Gauntt RO, Sweeten JM, et al. Design of 1-butanol scale dynamic olfactometer for ambiant odor measurements. Trans Am Soc Agric Eng 1983; 83: 1201-1205.

Spain CV, Scarlett JP, Wade SE, et al. Prevalence of enteric zoonotic agents in cats less than 1 year old in central New York state. J Vet Intern Med 2001; 15: 33-38.

Sparkes, AH, Papasouliotis K, Barr FJ, et al. Reference ranges for gastrointestinal transit of barium-impregnated polyethylene spheres in healthy cats. J Small Anim Pract 1997; 38: 340-343.

Sparkes AH, Papasouliotis K, Sunvold G, et al. Bacterial flora in the duodenum of healthy cats, and effect of dietary supplementation with fructo-oligosaccharides. Am J Vet Res 1998; 59: 431-435.

Squires RA. *An update on aspects of viral gastrointestinal diseases of dogs and cats.* N Z Vet J 2003; 6: 252-261.

Steiner JM, Medinger TL, Williams DA. *Purification and partial characterization of feline trypsin.* Comp Biochem Physiol B Biochem Mol Biol 1997;116: 87-93.

Stokes, C, Waly N. *Mucosal defence along the gastrointestinal tract of cats and dogs.* Vet Res 2006; 37: 281-293.

Strombeck DR. *Pathophysiology of esophageal motility disorders in the dog and cat: application to management and prognosis.* Vet Clin North Am, Small Anim Pract 1978; 8: 229-244.

Strombeck DR. *Microflora of the gastrointestinal tract and its symbiotic relationship with the host.* In: Guilford WG, Center S A, Strombeck DR et al, eds. Strombeck's small animal gastroenterology. 3rd ed. Philadelphia: WB Saunders Co, 1996a; 2: 14-19.

Strombeck DR. *Small and large intestine: normal structure and function.* In: Guilford WG, Center S A, Strombeck DR et al, eds. Strombeck's small animal gastroenterology. 3rd ed. Philadelphia: WB Saunders Co, 1996b; 17: 318-350.

Strombeck DR, Guilford, WG. *Gastric structure and function.* In: Guilford WG, Strombeck DR, Center S A et al, eds. Strombeck's small animal gastroenterology. Philadelphia: WB Saunders Co, 1996a; 12: 239-274.

Strombeck DR, Guilford WG. *Vomiting: pathophysiology and pharmacologic control.* In: Guilford WG, Strombeck DR, Center S A et al, eds. Strombeck's small animal gastroenterology. Philadelphia: WB Saunders Co, 1996b; 13: 256-260.

Sturgess K. *Diagnosis and management of idiopathic bowel disease in dogs and cats.* In Practice 2005; 27: 293-301.

Sunvold GD, Fahey GC Jr, Merchen NR, et al. *Dietary fiber for cats: in vitro fermentation of selected fiber sources by cat fecal inoculum and in vivo utilization of diets containing selected fiber sources and their blends.* J Anim Sci 1995a; 73: 2329-2339.

Sunvold GD, Fahey GC Jr, Merchen NR, et al. *In vitro fermentation of selected fibrous substrates by dog and cat fecal inoculum: influence of diet composition on substrate organic matter disappearance and short chain fatty acid production.* J Anim Sci 1995b; 73: 1110-1122.

Takehana K, Abe M. *A study of the duodenal glands of the cat.* J College Dairying, Hokkaido, Japan 1983; 10: 205-212.

Tams TR. *Chronic diseases of the small intestine.* In: Handbook of Small Animal Gastroenterology. Philadelphia: WB Saunders Co, 1996a: 267-319.

Tams TR. *Diarrhea in cats: Making the correct diagnosis.* In: Proceedings, 28th Royal Canin/OSU Symposium 2004: 5-8.

Tams TR. *Diseases of the esophagus.* In: Handbook of Small Animal Gastroenterology. Philadelphia: WB Saunders Co, 1996b:163-216.

Tams TR. *Diseases of the pancreas.* In: Handbook of Small Animal Gastroenterology. Philadelphia: WB Saunders Co, 1996c: 472-477.

Tams TR. *Gastrointestinal symptoms.* In: Tams TR, ed. Handbook of Small Animal Gastroenterology. Philadelphia: WB Saunders Co, 1996d: 1-73.

Teske E, Van Straten G, Van Noort R et al. *Chemotherapy with cyclophosphamide, vincristine, and prednisolone (COP) in cats with malignant lymphoma: new results with an old protocol.* J Vet Intern Med 2002; 16: 179-186.

Tournier C, Dumon H, Nguyen P, et al. *Validation d'une stratégie alimentaire innovante pour stimuler l'élimination fécale des poils ingérés par les chats.* In: Proceedings (Poster) 9th ESVCN Turin 2005.

Twedt D. *Diseases of the esophagus.* In: Ettinger S, Feldman EC, eds. Textbook of veterinary internal medicine. 4th ed. Philadelphia: WB Saunders Co, 1994: 1124-1142.

Twedt DC. *Diseases of the esophagus.* In: Ettinger S, Feldman E, eds. Textbook of Internal Veterinary Medicine. 5th ed. Philadelphia: WB Saunders Co, 2000: 1147-1149.

Visek WJ. *Diet and cell growth modulation by ammonia.* Am J Clin Nutr 1978; 31: S216- 220.

Waly NE, Biourge V, Day MJ, et al. *Use of a hydrolysed soya diet in the management of naturally occuring intestinal disease of cats.* In: Proceedings. 49th Annu British Small Animal Veterinary Association Congress 2006, Birmingham, UK: 506.

Waly NE, Gruffydd-Jones TJ, Stokes CR, et al. *Immunohistochemical diagnosis of alimentary lymphomas and severe intestinal inflammation in cats.* J Comp Pathol 2005; 133: 253-260.

Waly NE, Stokes CR Gruffydd Jones TJ, et al. *Immune cell populations in the duodenal mucosa of cats with inflammatory bowel disease.* J Vet Intern Med 2004;18: 816-825.

Washabau RJ. *Dysphagia and regurgitation.* In: Hall E, Simpson J & Williams D, eds. BSAVA Manual of canine and feline gastroenterology. 2nd ed, 2005: 69-72.

Washabau RJ. *Gastrointestinal motility disorders and gastrointestinal prokinetic therapy.* Vet Clin Small Anim 2003; 33: 1007-1028.

Williams DA. *The exocrine pancreas.* In: Kelly NC, Wills JM, eds. Manual of companion animal nutrition and feeding. British Small Animal Veterinary Association, Shurdington, 1996: 161-166.

Williams DA, Guilford WG. *Procedures for the evaluation of pancreatic and gastrointestinal tract diseases.* In: Guilford WG, Strombeck DR, Center S A et al, eds. Strombeck's small animal gastroenterology. Philadelphia: WB Saunders Co, 1996: 6: 77-113.

Williams DA. *Diseases of the exocrine pancreas.* In: Hall E, Simpson J & Williams D, eds. BSAVA Manual of canine and feline gastroenterology. 2nd ed, 2005: 222-239.

Wills J, Harvey R. *Diagnosis and management of food allergy and intolerance in dogs and cats.* Aust Vet J 1994; 71: 322-326.

Wong CS, Gibson PR. *The trophic effect of dietary fiber is not associated with a change in total crypt number in the distal colon of rats.* Carcinogenesis 2003; 24: 343-348.

Wortinger A. *Care and use of feeding tubes in dogs and cats.* J Am Anim Hosp Assoc 2006; 42: 401-406.

Digestion

Wyse CA, McLellan J, Dickie AM, et al. A review of methods for assessment of the rate of gastric emptying in the dog and cat: 1998-2002. J Vet Intern Med 2003; 17: 609-621.

Yaeger Y, Gookin JL. Histologic features associated with tritrichomonas foetus-induced colitis in domestic cats. Vet Pathol 2005;42: 797-804.

Zaghini G, Biagi G. Nutritional peculiarities and diet palatability in the cat. Vet Res Commun 2005; 29: 39-44.

Zentek J. Nutritional aspects in patients with digestion problems. Proc Aktualitäten aus der Gastroenterologie, Interlaken, 2004: 95-108.

Zentek J, Dekeyzer A, Mischke R. Influence of dietary protein quality on nitrogen balance and some blood parameters in cats. J Anim Physiol Anim Nutr 1998; 80: 63-66.

Zentek J, Van der Steen I, Rohde J, et al. Dietary effects of the occurrence and enterotoxin production of clostridium perfringens. J Anim Physiol Anim Nutr 1998; 80: 250-252.

Zoran DL. Diet and drugs: the keys to managing feline colonic disease. Comp Small Anim 1999; 95-108;731-748.

Zoran DL. Is it IBD? Managing inflammatory disease in the feline gastrointestinal tract. Vet Med 2000; 128-140.

Focus on:
Psyllium fiber

Botanical origins

Psyllium is a small annual plant, with low leaves and white flowers, of the plantain genus, which grow in the sandy soils of the Mediterranean basin. One particular variety (*Plantago ovata*), which comes from India and Pakistan, is traditionally used in phytotherapy to treat digestive problems. Psyllium is also known as Ispabgol. The whole plant is used in food, as well as nutrition and therapy. The young leaves may be consumed in salads or with vegetables.

Seeds are rich in fiber

The word psyllium is derived from the Greek *psyllia*, meaning flea, which is what the seeds resemble. They are composed of around 57% total fiber, 25% cellulose and 12% soluble fiber, mucilage, which is made of arabinoxylan, an extremely ramified acid.

The mucilage in psyllium seeds is especially beneficial. Once it has been isolated, the seed coat (tegument) contains a high mucilage concentration of 25-30%.

The particular composition of the tegument means that psyllium seeds can absorb up to ten times their weight in water. When purified psyllium seeds are used, the swelling index is between 70 and 85.

Mucilage regulates digestive transit

Psyllium is renowned for its laxative properties. Mucilage behaves like a sponge, absorbing water to swell up and create a viscous gel. Psyllium has an anti-diarrheic effect, by augmenting the viscosity of the intestinal chyme. In human gastroenterology, psyllium is particularly indicated to:
- relieve gastrointestinal inflammations
- treat irritable bowel syndrome
- help treat constipation.

Digestive transit is sometimes slow in sedentary cats due to the lack of physical activity. They often suffer from constipation and digestive problems caused by hairballs. Psyllium has very positive effects on their digestive transit, regulating the advancement of the content of the small intestine and the colon, and the lubrication induced by the psyllium gel facilitates the elimination of feces. Psyllium fiber is only very partially fermented by the bowel flora in the colon and therefore does not alter the consistency of the feces.

Psyllium seeds are traditionally used as appetite suppressors in weight loss diets. Mucilage absorbs water to form a voluminous gel in the stomach.

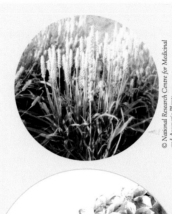

© National Research Centre for Medicinal and Aromatic Plants

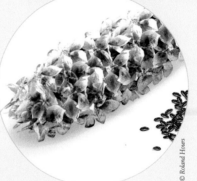

© Roland Hours

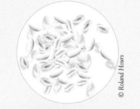

© Roland Hours

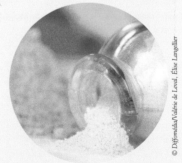

© Diffomédia/Valérie de Leval, Élise Langellier

The fruit of the psyllium is a pod containing two minuscule, flat, oval seeds, that have no odor and scarcely any taste. A thousand seeds weigh less than 2 g.

Digestive problems associated with the formation of hairballs in the cat's digestive tract

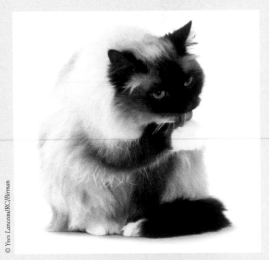

A cat that lives indoors spends around 30% of its time grooming (Benjamin, 1976). It is particularly sensitive to the formation of hairballs.

© Yves Lanceau/RC/Birman

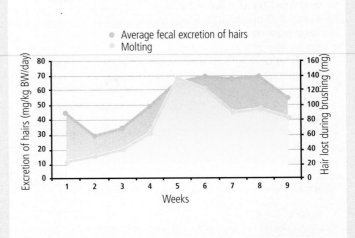

FIGURE 1 - CORRELATION BETWEEN MOLTING AND FECAL EXCRETION OF HAIRS (RESULTS OBTAINED FROM 24 CATS)
(Tournier et al, 2005)

● Average fecal excretion of hairs
● Molting

In cats, licking fulfils many different functions:
- it cleans the coat
- it regulates temperature
- it strengthens a bond between animals in the event of mutual grooming
- it helps reduce stress.

The cat's tongue is carpeted with conical dermal papillae that act like a brush to remove dead hairs and foreign bodies in the coat. When licking itself, the cat ingests hairs that it subsequently eliminates through the bowels. A Royal Canin study shows that fecal excretion varies between 30 mg and 70 mg of hair/kg of body weight/day **(Figure 1)**. In a period of molting, the quantity of hairs excreted in the feces may be up to 100 mg/kg of body weight/day, which is a daily volume of around 10 cm³ for a 4-kg cat *(Tournier et al, 2005)*.

The hairs coalesce in the digestive tract to form a ball (trichobezoar), which is very often regurgitated. In some cases however, they may cause digestive problems *(Barrs et al, 1999)* – vomiting, constipation or intestinal occlusion in the most serious cases. More than half of the veterinarians have had to deal with an intestinal obstruction caused by a hairball and 43% have had to resort to surgery to treat it *(Royal Canin survey, 2004)*.

The formation of hairballs depends on individual factors (connected to the presence of 'retention' pockets in the digestive tract), but mostly on environmental factors. Cats that live indoors are more sensitive than others. When the temperature and lighting are fairly steady, they will molt throughout the year. If they have no access to grass and no opportunity to hunt, they will not

ingest the ballast that naturally stimulates intestinal transit.

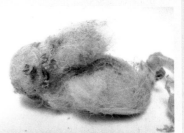

© Capucine Tournier

The hairs swallowed by the cat are regurgitated in the form of balls or eliminated through the feces. In the course of one year, a cat may excrete 60-120g of hairs, representing a volume of 1.5-3 liters.

ROYAL CANIN

Key points
to remember:

Nutritional factors favoring
the natural elimination of hairballs

The natural elimination of hairs may be facilitated by stimulating gastric emptying and intestinal transit. The aim is to prevent the hairs from collecting in the stomach or intestine and forming a ball. This is achieved by increasing the fiber content of the food. This type of diet is especially indicated for cats that live indoors, whose intestinal motility is slowed by the lack of physical activity. Food that activates transit and increases fecal excretion of hairs contains at least 10-15% total dietary fiber **(Figure 2)**.

Fiber constitutes a very heterogeneous material and several types need to be associated to obtain a synergic effect. While the cellulose and other non-fermentable fibers stimulate intestinal transit, some vegetable sources provide fiber with a much more targeted action:

- the fiber in the psyllium tegument favors fecal excretion in constipated cats

- fructo-oligosaccharides provide an energy substrate beneficial to the balance of the digestive flora.

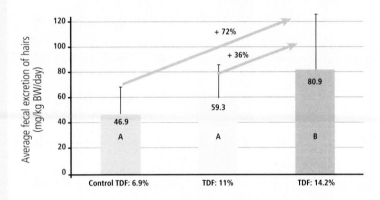

FIGURE 2 - INFLUENCE OF FIBERS ON FECAL EXCRETION OF HAIRS IN A 4-WEEK PERIOD IN 24 CATS
(Tournier et al, 2005)

A specific enrichment with vegetable fiber increases the quantity of hair eliminated through the feces by 72% compared with a control food with a low fiber content. Fecal excretion is measured every week using the method of Hendriks et al. (1998). The results are mean ± SD. ANOVA measurements are used to interpret the results. The letters A and B signify that the results are statistically different (P<0.05).

Beet pulp has a mixed chemical composition that enables the combination of the benefits of fermentable (on flora) and non-fermentable fiber (on transit).

References

Barrs VR, Beatty JA, Tisdall PLC, et al. Intestinal obstruction in five cats. J Feline Med Surg 1999; 1: 199-207.

Hart BL. Feline behavior. Feline Pract 1976, 7: 14-17.

Hendriks WH, Tarttelin MF, Moughan PJ. Seasonal hair loss in adult domestic cats. J Anim Physiol a Anim Nutr 1998; 79: 92-101.

Tournier C, Dumon H, Nguyen P, et al. Validation d'une stratégie alimentaire innovante pour stimuler l'élimination fécale des poils ingérés par les chats. Poster présenté au congrès de l'ESVCN à Turin (22-24 sept. 2005).

H. Carolien RUTGERS
DVM, MS, Dipl. ACVIM,
Dipl. ECVIM-CA,
DSAM, MRCVS

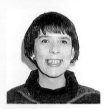

Vincent BIOURGE
DVM, PhD, Dipl. ACVN,
Dipl. ECVCN

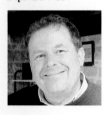

Nutritional management of hepatobiliary and pancreatic diseases

1- Hepatobiliary disease **141**
   Diagnosis 141
   Feline hepatobiliary diseases 144
   Epidemiology 149
   Pathophysiological mechanisms 149
   Nutritional management 153
   Nutritional management of specific feline liver diseases 156
   Frequently asked questions 159
2- Exocrine pancreatic disease **159**
   Pancreatitis 160
   Exocrine pancreatic insufficiency 166
   Conclusion 170
Frequently asked questions 171
References 172
Royal Canin nutritional information 175

ABBREVIATIONS USED IN THIS CHAPTER

AAA: aromatic amino acids
ALP: alkaline phosphatase
ALT: alanine amino transferase
BCAA: branched chain amino acid
CT: computed tomography
DIC: disseminated intravascular coagulation
EPI: exocrine pancreatic insufficiency

FHL: feline hepatic lipidosis
FIP: feline infectious peritonitis
fPLI: feline pancreatic lipase immunoreactivity
fTLI: feline trypsin-like immunoreactivity
γGT: gamma-glutamyl transpeptidase
HE: hepatic encephalopathy
PAA: pancreatic acinar atrophy

PSS: portosystemic shunts
SAMe: S-adenosyl-methionine

Nutritional management of hepatobiliary and pancreatic diseases

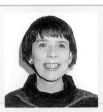

Carolien RUTGERS
DVM, MS, Dipl. ACVIM, Dipl. ACVIM, Dipl. ECVIM-CA, DSAM, MRCVS

Carolien graduated from Utrecht State University and completed an internship at the University of Pennsylvania and a residency and Masters degree at the Ohio State University. In between she worked in referral small animal practice. She joined the University of Liverpool in 1985 as a Lecturer in Small Animal Medicine and moved in 1990 to the Royal Veterinary College, where she later became a Senior Lecturer. She is now an independent consultant. Carolien has published more than 100 scientific papers and book chapters, and has lectured widely in the UK and abroad. Her major research interests are in gastroenterology and liver disease. She is a Diplomate of the American College of Veterinary Internal Medicine (ACVIM), a Foundation Diplomate of the European College of Veterinary Internal Medicine - Companion Animals (ECVIM-CA), and a RCVS Diplomate in Small Animal Medicine. Carolien has been a foundation Board member of the ECVIM-CA and a member of the RCVS Small Animal Medicine and Surgery Board, and a Diploma examiner for both.

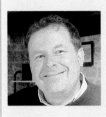

Vincent BIOURGE
DVM, PhD, Dipl. ACVN, Dipl. ECVCN

Vincent Biourge graduated from the Faculty of Veterinary Medicine of the University of Liège (Belgium) in 1985. He stayed as an assistant in the nutrition department for 2 more years before moving to the Veterinary Hospital of the University of Pennsylvania (Philadelphia, USA) and to the Veterinary Medical Teaching Hospital of the University of California (Davis, USA) as a PhD/resident in clinical nutrition. In 1993, he was awarded his PhD in Nutrition from the University of California and became a Diplomate of the American College of Veterinary Nutrition (ACVN). In 1994, he joined the Research Center of Royal Canin in Aimargues (France) as head of scientific communication and then as manager of the nutritional research program. Vincent is now Scientific Director of Health Nutrition at the Research Center of Royal Canin. He has published more than 30 papers, and regularly presents scientific papers as well as guest lectures at International Veterinary Medicine and Nutrition meetings. He is also a Diplomate of the European College of Veterinary Comparative Nutrition (ECVN).

The liver plays a central role in a wide range of metabolic processes and this is reflected in the multitude of pathophysiological derangements that can occur in liver disease. The liver has however a great reserve capacity to perform these functions, and clinical signs occur only when this reserve capacity is exhausted by extensive and progressive disease.

The exocrine pancreas is also essential for the optimal digestion and absorption of nutrients. Conversely to hepatic diseases, disorders of the exocrine pancreas were once believed to be rare in cats, but pancreatitis and exocrine pancreatic insufficiency cases are now recognized with increasing frequency which is likely due to improvements in diagnostic accuracy for this disease. Nutritional support is the keystone in management of cats with liver and pancreatic diseases.

TABLE 1 - MAJOR HEPATOBILIARY FUNCTIONS

Digestive functions
Bile acid synthesis and enterohepatic circulation
- digestion and absorption of lipids
- absorption of vitamins (A, D, E, K)

Detoxification and excretion
Ammonia detoxification (urea cycle)
Drugs and toxins

Storage functions
Glycogen and lipids
Vitamins
Trace elements (copper, iron, zinc, manganese)

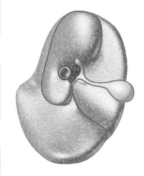

Protein metabolism
- Synthesis of albumin, acute phase proteins, coagulation factors
- Amino acid metabolism (plasma free amino acid homeostasis)

Carbohydrate metabolism
- Glycogen metabolism and storage
- Glucose homeostasis
- Gluconeogenesis

Lipid metabolism
- Synthesis of triglycerides, phospholipids, cholesterol
- Lipid oxidation and ketone production
- Lipoprotein synthesis
- Excretion of cholesterol and bile acids

Vitamin metabolism
- Storage and activation of vitamins B, K
- Activation of vitamin D
- Vitamin C synthesis

Hormone metabolism
- Degradation of polypeptides and steroid hormones

1 - Hepatobiliary disease

Introduction

The liver is essential for the digestion, absorption, metabolism and storage of most nutrients **(Table 1)**. Liver disease often results in malnutrition, which aggravates the disease process and affects outcome (*Center, 1996; LaFlamme, 1999*); it is therefore imperative to maintain nutritional status. Early nutritional intervention can reduce morbidity and mortality. Nutritional support is especially important in anorexic cats, since cats are uniquely predisposed to the development of idiopathic hepatic lipidosis when anorexic.

In acute liver disease, treatment is mainly aimed at supporting the patient during the process of hepatic regeneration, and cats may fully recover provided there has been only a single sublethal insult to the liver. In chronic liver disease, which is the most common form of liver disease in cats, the emphasis is on supporting the limited remaining metabolic capabilities of the liver and to minimize complications.

▶ Diagnosis

> Clinical signs

Cats with liver disease usually do not show any clinical signs until the disease is advanced, and symptoms are vague and variable. Partial or complete anorexia and vomiting are the most common and sometimes the only clinical signs. Other clinical signs include weight loss, depression, vomiting, and occasionally diarrhea **(Table 2)**. Jaundice and abnormal liver size are the physical findings most suggestive of liver disease, but these may also be seen in other diseases not related to the liver. Cats with liver disease tend to have hepatomegaly, but small liver size can be seen in cats with portosystemic shunts or cirrhosis. The only sign specific for liver disease is acholic (grey) feces, found in complete extrahepatic bile duct obstruction, but this is rarely found.

CLINICAL SIGNS

Clinical signs of liver disease in the cat are generally vague and non-specific, and more specific signs such as icterus occur only when the disease is advanced.

TABLE 2 - CLINICAL FINDINGS IN FELINE LIVER DISEASE

Early signs	Common: anorexia; vomiting; depression; weight loss
	Less common: fever (suppurative cholangitis/cholangiohepatitis); ascites (lymphocytic cholangitis)
Severe hepatic insufficiency	Icterus; Hepatic encephalopathy; Coagulopathy
Major bile duct obstruction	* Acholic (pale) feces

* Specific for hepatobiliary disease, but rarely observed.

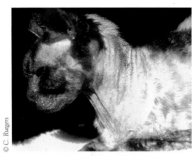

© C. Rutgers

Figure 1 - Jaundice in a Rex cat.

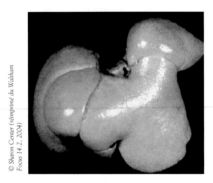

© Sharon Center (réimprimé du Waltham Focus 14.2, 2004)

Figure 2 - Hepatomegaly in a cat.
Enlarged, yellow and friable liver from a cat that died from hepatic lipidosis.

> Differential diagnosis

Jaundice - Jaundice is generally a late sign of liver disease, but tends to occur earlier in the course of feline liver disease than in dogs. It generally signifies severe cholestatic disease, either due to hepatocellular disease or posthepatic causes (extrahepatic bile duct obstruction, biliary rupture) **(Figure 1)**. Hemolytic anemia, which can also cause jaundice, is rare in cats.

Altered liver size - Hepatomegaly **(Figure 2)** is a common finding in cats with both acute and chronic liver diseases, and results from hepatic infiltration with inflammatory cells, fat, neoplastic cells or amyloid. Reduced liver size can however be seen in cats with congenital portosystemic shunts, and in rare end-stage lymphocytic cholangiohepatitis with cirrhosis *(Webster, 2005)*.

Ascites - Cats with liver disease generally do not develop portal hypertension as dogs do, and ascites is therefore an infrequent finding. It may however occur when progressive lymphocytic cholangitis has resulted in cirrhosis, and it then tends to be a modified transudate. The effusion has to be distinguished from that due to protein-losing diseases (transudate), congestive heart failure and neoplasia (modified transudate), and peritonitis, hemorrhage, and ruptured gall bladder (exudates).

> Laboratory testing

Since many of the clinical signs associated with liver disease are non-specific, laboratory assessment is essential to identify and monitor hepatic disease. However, laboratory tests will not recognize specific diseases and may furthermore be influenced by non-hepatic disease (e.g. hyperthyroidism). Baseline tests (hematology, serum biochemistries and urinalysis) are useful in initial screening to look for evidence of hepatic disease as well as other abnormalities.

- *Hematological testing* may reveal anemia or alterations in erythrocyte size and shape, such as microcytosis (e.g. portosystemic shunts), acanthocytes and poikilocytosis. Anemia is usually nonregenerative and most likely associated with chronic disease; a regenerative anemia is uncommon and may reflect infection with blood parasites *(Haemobartonella, Babesia)*, and rarely auto-immune hemolysis. Leukogram changes are inconsistent and depend upon the underlying cause of the disease *(Webster, 2005)*.

- *Serum biochemistries* are usually characterized by increased liver enzyme activities; hyperbilirubinemia is variable. In cats, the half-life of both serum alkaline phosphatase (ALP) and alanine aminotransferase (ALT) is much shorter than in dogs, and liver enzyme induction (e.g. corticosteroids) is uncommon. However, high liver enzymes are frequently seen in hyperthyroid cats. Gamma-glutamyl transpeptidase (γ GT) is a similar enzyme to ALP that increases with cholestasis and is more sensitive for feline inflammatory biliary tract disease than ALP. This may be in part because γ GT arises from predominately bile duct epithelium. Cats affected with idiopathic hepatic lipidosis usually have marked increases in ALP while γ GT concentrations show only mild increases, in contrast to cats with biliary tract disease where there are usually proportionally higher γ GT concentrations than ALP concentrations *(Center, 1996)*.

- *Urinalysis* may show bilirubinuria, which is always abnormal in cats since they have a high renal threshold for bilirubin. Cats with portosystemic shunts may have low urine specific gravity and ammonium biurate crystalluria.

Measurement of fasting and 2-hour post-prandial total serum bile acid concentrations is a sensitive and specific indicator of hepatic function, useful for the diagnosis of subclinical liver diseases and portosystemic shunts. Determination of urine sulfated and nonsulfated bile acids has also been suggested as an alternative diagnostic test for liver disease in cats *(Trainor et al, 2003)*, but this needs further evaluation.

The presence of fasting hyperammonemia can document hepatic encephalopathy (HE), particularly in cats with portosystemic shunts, although not all animals with HE will have abnormal fasting blood ammonia levels. Difficulties in sample handling limit the diagnostic usefulness of this test. Coagulation tests are furthermore indicated in animals with a bleeding tendency and prior to liver aspiration or biopsy (*Lisciandro et al, 1998; Center et al, 2000*).

> Diagnostic imaging

Survey abdominal radiography can be used to assess liver size and shape, and occasionally radiopaque choleliths (**Figure 3**), but ultrasonography gives more specific information about alterations in the liver parenchyma, biliary system, and portal vasculature (*Leveille et al, 1996; Newell et al, 1998*) (**Figure 4**). Ultrasonography performed by an experienced operator has a high accuracy in detecting intrahepatic portosystemic shunts (*Holt et al, 1995*). Color flow and pulse wave Doppler ultrasonography gives the additional advantage of visualization of blood flow direction and measurement of portal blood flow velocity (*d'Anjou et al, 2004*). Ultrasonography can furthermore be used for cholecystocentesis and culture in cats with suspected suppurative cholangiohepatitis, and for precision ultrasound-guided hepatic biopsy. Mesenteric portography can be used before or during surgery to confirm the diagnosis and establish the morphology of the shunting vessel. Suspected portovascular anomalies can also be evaluated by contrast nuclear scintigraphy; this is however limited to research institutions due to the need for radioactivity.

> Biopsy and surgery

The ultimate diagnosis of feline liver disease other than that caused by a congenital portosystemic shunt is usually made by histological examination of a liver biopsy (**Figure 5**), which is essential to clarify the cause of abnormal liver tests and/or size and to develop an appropriate treatment plan (**Figure 6**). Samples can be obtained by fine needle aspiration, percutaneous ultrasound-guided biopsy or surgically. Fine needle aspiration can give useful information in cats with diffuse diseases such as hepatic lymphoma or idiopathic hepatic lipidosis, and may indicate the presence of inflammatory liver disease, but in most cases a biopsy is preferred for assessment of cellular changes and structure of the hepatic parenchyma (*Wang et al, 2004*). Coagulation status must be assessed prior to the procedure, since hemorrhage is the most common complication. Cats with cholestatic disease rapidly develop fat-soluble vitamin deficiencies, and coagulopathies responsive to vitamin K_1 administration can be seen in feline hepatic lipidosis or severe cholangiohepatitis (*Center et al, 2000*).

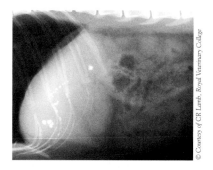

Figure 3 - Lateral abdominal radiograph of a cat with cholelithiasis. Cholelithiasis is visible as multiple radiopaque densities.

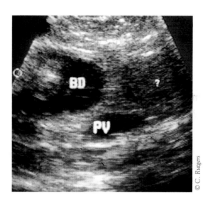

Figure 4 - Ultrasound of a cat with cholestatic jaundice. The ultrasound shows a dilated common bile duct (BD), portal vein (PV), and a hypoechoic hepatic mass.

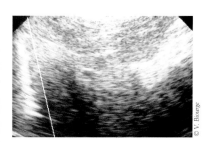

Figure 5 - Liver biopsy. Biopsy is essential to clarify the cause of abnormal liver tests and/or size.

FIGURE 6 - DIAGNOSIS OF LIVER DISEASE

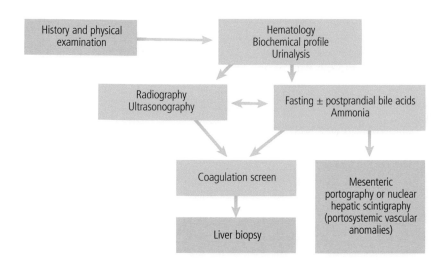

History and physical examination → Hematology Biochemical profile Urinalysis → Radiography Ultrasonography ↔ Fasting ± postprandial bile acids Ammonia → Coagulation screen → Liver biopsy / Mesenteric portography or nuclear hepatic scintigraphy (portosystemic vascular anomalies)

TABLE 3 – HEPATOBILIARY DISEASES IN THE CAT	
Inflammatory	Infectious: - Bacterial (suppurative cholangitis/cholangio-hepatitis complex*, abscess, bartonellosis) - Viral (feline infectious peritonitis) - Protozoal (toxoplasmosis) Non-infectious: - Lymphocytic cholangitis* - Toxic and drug-induced (diazepam, acetaminophen, tetracyclines, stanozolol)
Non-inflammatory	- Metabolic disorders (idiopathic hepatic lipidosis*, amyloidosis) - Congenital portosystemic shunts - Hepatobiliary neoplasia* (primary or metastatic)

* Most common

► Feline hepatobiliary diseases

The incidence of feline liver disease is relatively common. The cholangitis/cholangiohepatitis complex and feline hepatic lipidosis are the major causes of hepatobiliary disease in cats, followed by neoplasia (lymphoma, bile duct). Other inflammatory liver diseases include infectious diseases such as feline infectious peritonitis (FIP) and toxoplasmosis. Hepatotoxicities are uncommon and most often associated with administration of drugs such as acetaminophen, diazepam and tetracyclines. Extrahepatic bile duct obstruction may be related to cholelithiasis or external compression (neoplasia and/or pancreatitis). Hepatic cysts are an infrequent finding and seldom cause problems. Metabolic diseases, like hepatic amyloidosis, are rare (Table 3).

> Cholangiohepatitis/cholangitis complex

The cholangiohepatitis/cholangitis complex is a common but ill-defined inflammatory disorder of the hepatobiliary system in cats. It is distinctly different from dogs, where inflammatory disease is usually centered on the hepatic parenchyma (hepatitis). In cats, the inflammation is almost always centered on the bile ducts. The classification has been complex, but it is now subdivided according to the type of cellular infiltrates into suppurative (neutrophilic) cholangitis/cholangiohepatitis, chronic (mixed inflammatory cell population) and lymphocytic cholangitis (Gagne et al, 1999; Weiss et al, 2001; WSAVA Liver Standardization Group, 2006). Lymphocytic portal hepatitis is furthermore a common finding in older cats, but is now thought to be of questionable clinical significance.

Suppurative cholangiohepatitis/cholangitis may begin as an ascending bacterial infection of the biliary tract, which results in neutrophilic inflammation of the bile ductules and portal triads. It is more common in males. Cats with acute suppurative cholangitis present acutely ill with fever, anorexia, vomiting and lethargy (Caney & Gruffydd-Jones, 2005). They are frequently icteric, and have neutrophilia and raised liver enzymes. Coliforms (E. coli) are the most common bacteria, but there is often a mixed infection including common components of the enteric flora. A positive bacterial culture of the bile or liver of affected cats may help in identifying causative organisms, although the incidence of positive cultures is inconsistent. Complications include sludged (inspissated) bile and cholelithiasis, which can cause partial or complete biliary obstruction and require treatment before the cholangiohepatitis can be controlled or resolved.

Feline **suppurative cholangitis** frequently coexists with other diseases, particularly pancreatitis and inflammatory bowel disease (Weiss et al, 1996). This association has been referred to as triaditis, and may be due to the fact that the pancreatic ducts and bile ducts join before entering the duodenum, allowing bacteria to enter in both. Ascending bacteria initiate the acute disease, and over time it can become chronic. The predominant signs of suppurative cholangiohepatitis are however usually attributable to hepatobiliary disease. It is nevertheless important to look for underlying disease, since these may affect the management and response to treatment (e.g. correction of cobalamin deficiency in cats with concurrent inflammatory bowel disease).

Treatment for cats with suppurative cholangiohepatitis includes fluid and electrolyte therapy as needed, nutritional support, antibiotic and choleretic therapy. In the longer term modified diets formulated for liver support are indicated, but in the early stages maintenance of caloric intake is the priority. Surgical intervention may be indicated for biliary decompression or to remove choleliths. The choice of antibiotics is ideally based upon bile and/or liver culture and sensitivity testing, but effective empirical choices are ampicillin (10-20 mg/kg IV, IM SC q6-8h), amoxicillin (11-22 mg/kg IM, SC or PO q8-12h), and cephalexin (20-20 mg/kg PO q8-12h). Metronidazole (7.5-10 mg/kg PO q12h) can be used in combination with a penicillin, and has a good anaerobic spectrum. Metronidazole is metabolized by the liver, and the dose should be reduced if there is severe hepatic insufficiency. Long-term antibiotic treatment for at least 2 months is recommended, since short duration of therapy may result in reoccurrence of clinical signs.

Choleretic therapy with ursodeoxycholic acid (10-15 mg/kg PO q24h) is of value in restoring bile flow, provided there is no biliary obstruction. Ursodeoxycholic acid also has anti-inflammatory, immunomodulatory and antifibrotic capacities, probably through changing the composition of the bile acid pool by reducing the proportion of hydrophobic bile acids that have toxic effects on hepatocellular membranes (*Nicholson et al, 1996; Webster, 2006*). Antioxidant therapy with vitamin E and S-adenosyl-methionine (SAMe) is furthermore useful to reduce oxidative stress associated with liver disease and cholestasis (*Caney & Gruffydd-Jones, 2005*).

One beneficial effect of S-adenosyl-methionine (SAMe) is believed to be the restoration of hepatic glutathione levels that are reduced in liver disease, leading to increased oxidative damage and exacerbation of liver disease. SAMe is critical in the defence against free oxygen radicals. Other beneficial effects may be due to increasing taurine levels **(Figure 7)**, since taurine is required for bile acid conjugation and has a cytoprotective effect.

Chronic cholangiohepatitis with a mixed inflammatory cell population is thought to be the result of progression of the acute suppurative form. This is generally due to an ascending biliary infection from the gut; liver flukes (*Platynosomum concinnum*) may be a rare contributing factor in endemic tropical areas (*Haney et al, 2006*). Presenting signs are intermittent vomiting, lethargy and anorexia, weight loss, and jaundice. A liver biopsy confirms the diagnosis, but concurrent pancreatitis and inflammatory bowel disease have to be taken into consideration. Treatment is empirical with immunosuppressive therapy (prednisolone, tapering over 2-4 weeks to 0.5-1 mg/kg once daily or every other day), antibiotics if indicated, choleretic therapy with ursodeoxycholic acid, and antioxidants. Liver fluke infestation is diagnosed upon hepatic biopsy or fecal examination, and treated with praziquantel (20 mg/kg/day for 3 days). This disease is slowly progressive, and may eventually result in cirrhosis, which has been compared to human biliary cirrhosis.

Lymphocytic cholangitis is thought to be immune-mediated, and is characterized by lymphocytic infiltration around the bile ducts (*Day, 1996*). Persian cats are predisposed, but there is no sex bias (*Lucke & Davies, 1984*). The condition appears to be very chronic and slowly progressive, and affected cats present with a prolonged history of weight loss, anorexia and variable icterus; in addition, they often have hepatomegaly and a protein rich abdominal effusion. Hypergammaglobulinemia is common and may reflect the chronic nature of the disease, but needs to be differentiated from feline infectious peritonitis (FIP). Treatment is by immunosuppressive therapy with corticosteroids, which have both anti-inflammatory and anti-fibrotic properties. Prednisolone is commonly used at an initial immunosuppressive oral dose (2-4 mg/kg q12h), which is gradually reduced over 6 to 12 weeks according to the patient's response. It should then be tapered to the lowest effective dose. The use of azathioprine should be avoided, since it may have severe adverse effects in cats. Alternative immunosuppressive agents include cyclosporine, chlorambucil, methotrexate and cyclophosphamide, but experience of their use and value is limited. Ursodeoxycholic acid, antioxidant therapy with SAMe and vitamin E, and nutritional support are furthermore important components of the management.

If ascites is severe, particularly if this is causing dyspnea due to pressure on the diaphragm, drainage by abdominal paracentesis may be indicated. Loop diuretics such as furosemide (1-2 mg/kg q12h) combined with restriction of dietary salt may be helpful in mild ascites. Potassium-sparing diuretics (e.g., spironolactone) are alternative agents for treating ascites.

FIGURE 7 - PRODUCTION OF CYSTEINE AND TAURINE FROM S-ADENOSYL-METHIONINE (SAMe)

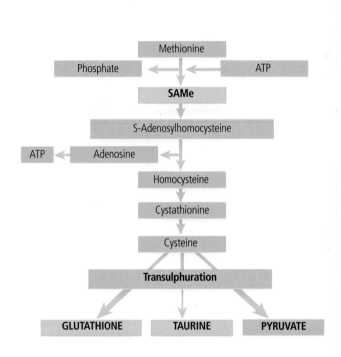

145

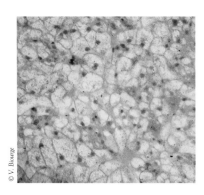

Figure 8 - Liver biopsy of a cat with hepatic lipidosis.
Notice the progressive diffuse lipid vaculolization. The brown areas indicate cholestasis (H&E).

© V. Biourge

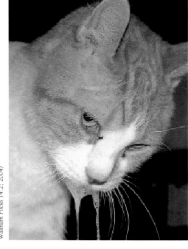

© Sharon Center (reprinted from Waltham Focus 14.2, 2004)

Figure 9 - Ptyalism associated with feline hepatic lipidosis.
Some cats develop remarkable ptyalism, thought to reflect hepatic encephalopathy.

> Feline hepatic lipidosis

Feline hepatic lipidosis (FHL) is a unique syndrome characterized by severe hepatocellular accumulation of triglycerides **(Figure 8)** with resulting intrahepatic cholestasis and liver dysfunction. Cats that were previously overweight and are undergoing rapid weight loss are at increased risk (*Biourge et al, 1994c*); affected animals often have an underlying disorder that causes anorexia and catabolism (*Scherk & Center, 2005*). It occurs primarily in middle-aged to older cats, and there is no breed or sex predisposition.

The etiology is incompletely understood but likely related to metabolic characteristics peculiar to cats, which are obligate carnivores with high requirements for protein, essential amino and fatty acids. Cats also have a high tendency to accumulate triglycerides in their hepatocytes, which is augmented during fasting after weight gain, resulting in progressive hepatocellular vacuolation. In hepatic lipidosis, the rate of peripheral fat mobilization exceeds that of hepatic triglyceride mobilisation and fat oxidation. Hepatic fat accumulation and vacuolation become so severe that it promotes oxidant injury, intrahepatic cholestasis and ultimately liver failure (*Scherk & Center, 2005*).

The cause for the rapid mobilization of peripheral fat is as yet unknown. When anorexic, cats lack essential amino acids that are necessary for mobilization of fat stores as very low-density lipoproteins (*Biourge et al, 1994a*). In addition, several nutritional deficiencies develop including protein malnutrition, which aggravate the liver disease (*Center, 2005*). Cats with liver disease, including hepatic lipidosis, often have reduced hepatocellular levels of the endogenous antioxidants vitamin E and glutathione. This increases oxidative stress and aggravates hepatocellular damage (*Center et al, 2002*). Hepatocellular carnitine deficiency has furthermore been documented and may promote lipid accumulation in the liver; carnitine supplementation has been shown to be helpful to prevent hepatic lipidosis in obese cats during complete fasting (*Blanchard et al, 2002*), but it's role in the management of this disease is still controversial (*Ibrahim et al, 2003*).

Cats with FHL usually present with a history of prolonged anorexia, rapid weight loss and vomiting. There is typically a significant loss of muscle mass while abdominal and inguinal fat stores are spared. On initial presentation, these cats are jaundiced, lethargic and have hepatomegaly. Some cats develop remarkable hypersalivation **(Figure 9)** as a result of hepatic encephalopathy. Hyperbilirubinemia, marked elevations in serum ALP but moderate elevations in serum γGT, and increased serum bile acids are consistent findings. Monitoring of ALP is a useful way to assess liver lipid accumulation: in anorexic cats, SAP is consistently above physiological range three weeks before hyperbilirubinemia and clinical signs appear (*Biourge et al, 1994b*).

Cats with FHL should be investigated for the presence of underlying disease, particularly pancreatitis and inflammatory bowel disease. Nonregenerative anemia, hypokalemia and coagulation abnormalities may be present. Serum vitamin B_{12} level determination is useful to rule out coexistent hypocobalaminemia, which adversely affects liver function.

A definitive diagnosis requires a liver biopsy and hepatic cytology. It is advisable to do this only after administration of at least three doses of vitamin K_1 (0.5-1.5 mg/kg q12h), since fat-soluble vitamins are often deficient in view of the severe cholestasis.

Treatment for idiopathic hepatic lipidosis needs to be aggressive, since otherwise mortality rates are high. Initial therapy requires rehydration with balanced electrolyte solutions; replacement of potassium depletion is important as normokalemia improves survival. Adequate nutrition is however the cornerstone of treatment and prevention of feline hepatic lipidosis (*Center, 2005*). Since these cats are typically profoundly anorexic, tube feeding is usually initially necessary to provide the essential nutrients. Oral force-feeding is generally contra-indicated, since this can lead to further food aversion. Initially, a nasoesophageal tube may be used **(Figure 10)**, and once the patient is more stable an esophageal or gastrostomy (PEG) tube can be inserted for longer-term use. Feeding a high quality diet for 2-6 weeks, or until the cat begins to eat on its own again, is the most important aspect of treatment. Dietary protein content is important since it helps hepatic regeneration. For most cats with hepatic lipidosis, proteins can represent 35-50% of dietary calories. If a cat exhibits signs of hepatic encephalopathy, the dietary protein content can then be progressively lowered to the minimum level of 25%.

Other supportive measures aim at controlling vomiting and providing nutritional supplements:
- L-carnitine supplementation (250 mg/cat/day) to improve lipid metabolism
- antioxidant therapy with SAMe (200 mg/day; 20 mg/kg q12h when given with food) and vitamin E (20-100 IU daily PO)
- B vitamins are advised since these cats will have depleted hepatic stores, and it will improve appetite and cellular metabolism. Parenteral vitamin B_{12} supplementation (1 mg IM) is suggested because of the multifactorial causes of FHL, many of which lead to vitamin B_{12} deficiency.

> Toxic hepatopathies

The liver is uniquely susceptible to toxicities, since it detoxifies all agents coming from the portal blood. Acute toxic hepatopathies are however rare in cats and usually due to administration of certain therapeutic agents, such as diazepam, tetracyclines, acetaminophen, stanozolol, and methimazole (*Harkin et al, 2000, Hooser, 2000*). Signs appear within a few days or weeks following administration and are characterized by anorexia, increased liver enzymes, hyperbilirubinemia, and may progress to acute hepatic failure unless the drug is discontinued at the first sign of increases in serum ALT levels. Histopathology mainly reveals hepatic lobular necrosis. Discontinuing the drug is essential for recovery, coupled with fluid, electrolyte and nutritional support, and antioxidant therapy. The cat's susceptibility to adverse drug reactions may be partially due to its inability to glucuronidate some metabolites in combination with its tendency for accelerated depletion of glutathione stores; however, some drug reactions are idiosyncratic.

Hepatic copper accumulation is very rare in cats, in contrast to dogs. Liver disease associated with periacinar copper accumulation has been described in a small number of Siamese cats, and some cats with chronic lymphocytic cholangitis were reported to have copper positive granules within portal hepatocytes (*Haynes & Wade 1995; Fuentealba & Aburto 2003*). There are no reports of treatment.

> Portosystemic shunts

Feline portosystemic shunts (PSS) are less common in cats than in dogs. They are usually congenital, single and extrahepatic **(Figure 11)**, and are in most cases found in cats less than 2 years of age. Cats very rarely develop acquired portosystemic shunts due to portal hypertension (*Langdon et al, 2002*).

Most cats with PSS are domestic shorthairs, but in purebreds there may be a breed predisposition in Persians and Himalayans (*Levy et al, 1995*). The history most commonly includes failure to thrive or weight loss, and variable signs of hepatic encephalopathy (lethargy and depression, ataxia, seizures, behavioral changes, blindness; intermittent hypersalivation can furthermore be a symptom of HE in cats) and occasionally ammonium biurate urolithiasis. There may also be a history of tranquilizer or anesthetic intolerance. Affected cats sometimes have copper colored irises, but this is not specific for shunts.

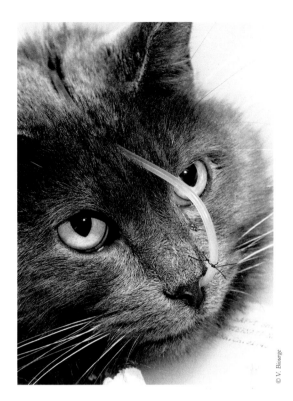

© V. Biourge

Figure 10 - *Nasoesophageal tube as a supportive measure for anorexic cats.*

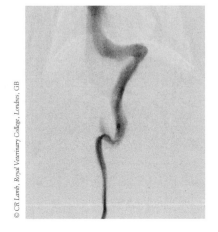

© CR Lamb, Royal Veterinary College, Londres, GB

Figure 11 - Digital subtraction angiogram of cat with congenital extrahepatic PSS.
Before ligation: the perfusion of the liver is altered.

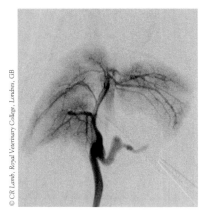

Figure 12 - Digital subtraction angiogram of cat with congenital extrahepatic PSS after ligation. *Satisfactory perfusion of the liver.*

Hematological and biochemical abnormalities may include anemia, red cell microcytosis, increased ALT, and decreases in serum glucose and cholesterol. Cats with PSS can have normal albumin concentrations. Urinalysis abnormalities include low urine specific gravity and ammonium biurate crystalluria. Because of increased urinary excretion of ammonia and uric acid, dogs and cats may also develop uroliths. Urate uroliths are often radiolucent and therefore may not be detectable on survey radiographs unless they are combined with struvite. Elevations of both pre- and postprandial serum ammonia concentrations, or marked elevation of the postprandial values in relationship to the preprandial ones are common. Radiography usually shows small liver size, and ultrasonography is useful to detect the presence and location of a shunt.

Medical management of HE with lactulose, oral antibiotics and a protein-restricted diet stabilizes cats in anticipation of surgery and is also used for those patients in which surgical correction is not possible. Surgical options for PSS occlusion are shunt ligation, or attenuation and slow vessel occlusion using ameroid constrictors or cellophane banding (*Kyles et al, 2002; Hunt et al, 2004*). Complete ligation of the shunt **(Figure 12)** in a single procedure is possible in less than half of the cases. Partial ligation however commonly results in recurrence of clinical signs (*Schunk, 1997*). Repeated staged surgeries to completely ligate the shunt vessel may be more effective in these cases (*Tillson et al, 2002*), with a good long-term prognosis if complete ligation eventually is achieved.

> Hepatic amyloidosis

Hepatic amyloidosis has been described as an uncommon familial disorder in young adult Oriental shorthair and Abyssinian cats.

Systemic amyloidosis also involving the liver is generally secondary to chronic systemic inflammatory responses. However, predominant hepatic amyloidosis has been described as an uncommon familial disorder in young adult Siamese and Oriental shorthair cats, and as sporadic cases in other breeds (*van der Linde-Sipman et al, 1997*). Hepatic involvement has also been described in familial amyloidosis of Abyssinian cats, but signs of renal disease predominate in this breed. Clinical signs may be vague and suggestive of liver disease, but accumulation of hepatic amyloid sometimes results in spontaneous hepatic rupture and acute hemorrhagic abdominal effusion (*Beatty et al, 2002*). Diagnosis is based on cytology of a liver aspirate or a biopsy, which have been stained with Congored. There is currently no treatment for this condition in cats.

> Hepatobiliary neoplasia

Hemolymphatic neoplasia, mainly including lymphoma, is the most common form of hepatobiliary neoplasia in the cats. Primary hepatobiliary neoplasms occur uncommonly. Clinical signs are often vague and nonspecific, and cats may also be asymptomatic. Finding a cranial abdominal mass or hepatomegaly is the most frequent physical abnormality. Diagnosis is by ultrasound and confirmatory biopsy. Lymphoma may be amenable to chemotherapy protocols, some smaller primary tumors could be explored surgically to see whether they can be excised.

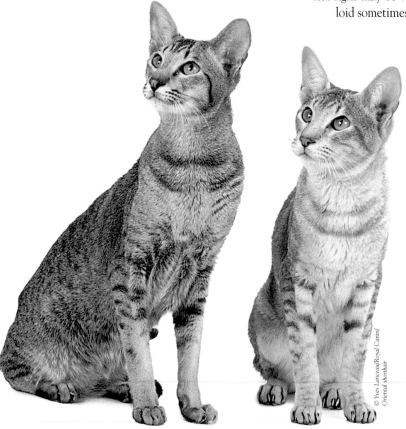

TABLE 4 - PUREBRED BREED PREDISPOSITION IN FELINE LIVER DISEASES

Cholangiohepatitis	Congenital portosystemic shunts	Hepatic amyloidosis
Lymphocytic cholangitis is more commonly seen in Europe, with a predisposition in **Persian cats**.	Congenital portosystemic shunts are most frequently seen in domestic shorthair cats, but two related breeds, **Himalayans and Persians**, are at increased risk *(Levy et al, 1995)*.	This is a familial disorder in **Siamese, Oriental and Abyssinian cats**. The amyloid protein in Siamese cats differs from that in Abyssinian cats, which suggests that the Siamese has a unique isotype *(van der Linde-Sipman et al, 1997)*.

► Epidemiology

> Breed predisposition

In general, breed predisposition to the development of hepatic disease is difficult to ascertain in cats, due to the high numbers of domestic shorthair cats that are of mixed breeding. Increased incidence in specific breeds may be significant, although numbers are often small **(Table 4)**.

> Risk factors

Feline hepatic lipidosis

It is well established that there are two predisposing factors for most cases of idiopathic lipidosis: **obesity and anorexia**. Regardless of the cause of anorexia, an anorectic obese cat **(Figure 13)** is likely to develop hepatic lipidosis. The process may begin after only a few days of anorexia, but it usually does not become clinically significant until at least a few weeks.

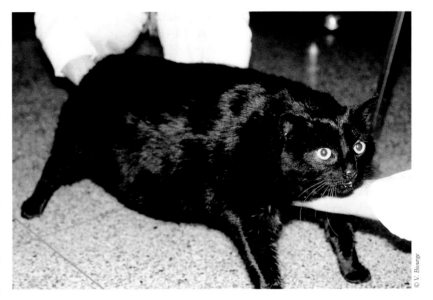
© V. Biourge

Figure 13 - Obesity is a major predisposing factor for feline hepatic lipidosis.

Drugs

Certain drugs may provide a risk factor for development of acute liver disease in cats, with acetaminophen, diazepam and tetracyclines the best recognized *(Center et al, 1996; Hooser, 2000)*.

► Pathophysiological mechanisms

Hepatocellular dysfunction is associated with a number of metabolic disturbances that alter the utilization of nutrients **(Table 5)**. These are compounded by cats' nutritional peculiarities, which are due to their development as strict carnivores. Cats have very high daily protein requirements and they utilize protein for gluconeogenesis and energy production, even when the diet is high in carbohydrates. They have very limited ability to down-regulate this continuous protein catabolism *(Zoran, 2002)*. Hepatic glycogen stores are relatively small in cats, and blood glucose concentrations are maintained through gluconeogenesis from amino-acids.

Anorexia and malnutrition therefore rapidly result in augmented protein catabolism and peripheral lipolysis, and progressive loss of fat and muscle. The major consequences of malnutrition are decreased immunocompetence, decreased tissue synthesis and repair, and altered intermediary drug metabolism.

Cats are obligate carnivores with high daily dietary requirements for protein and certain amino acids (arginine, taurine), and a limited ability to digest, absorb and metabolize carbohydrates. Other nutrients considered essential in feline diets are vitamins A, D, niacin and arachidonic acid.

Hepatocellular dysfunction often causes metabolic disturbances that are compounded by malnutrition, which is a common complication of liver disease. Anorexia and malnutrition furthermore predispose cats to the development of idiopathic hepatic lipidosis.

149

TABLE 5 - NUTRITIONAL CONSEQUENCES OF FELINE HEPATOBILIARY DISEASE

Substrate	Clinical effect
Protein metabolism	
Increased catabolism	Malnutrition, weight loss, HE
Impaired urea cycle (decreased urea production)	HE
Decreased synthesis of coagulation factors	Coagulopathy
Decreased albumin synthesis	Hypoalbuminemia
Fat metabolism	
Increased lipolysis	Malnutrition, hepatic lipidosis
Decreased excretion of bile acids	Malabsorption of fat and fat-soluble vitamins; steatorrhea, coagulopathy
Carbohydrate metabolism	
Decreased hepatic glycogen storage	Hypoglycemia (acute disease)
Increased gluconeogenesis	Loss of muscle, malnutrition
Glucose intolerance and insulin resistance	Hyperglycemia (chronic disease)
Vitamin metabolism	
Decreased storage	Vitamin B deficiency
Decreased absorption of vitamins A, D, E, K	Oxidant damage
Minerals and trace elements	
Decreased zinc levels	Decreased antioxidant protection
Detoxification and excretion	
Decreased excretion bilirubin	Jaundice
Decreased detoxification (drugs, ammonia)	Toxic hepatopathies, HE

HE = hepatic encephalopathy

> Protein, fat and carbohydrate metabolism

Protein

The liver has an essential role in protein synthesis and degradation. It controls serum concentrations of most amino acids, with the exception of branched chain amino acids (BCAA), which are regulated by skeletal muscle. The liver synthesizes the majority of circulating plasma proteins and is the only site of albumin synthesis (*Center, 2000a*). Albumin has a relative priority for synthesis, although hypoalbuminemia is relatively uncommon in feline liver disease; it does not occur until the disease is chronic and is compounded by malnutrition.

The liver furthermore synthesizes the majority of the coagulation factors. Lack of synthesis in liver failure may lead to prolonged coagulation times, but only when factors are reduced to less than 30% of normal. Disseminated intravascular coagulation (DIC) is yet the most common coagulopathy associated with liver disease, and the most likely to cause spontaneous hemorrhage. Decreased absorption of vitamin K in chronic cholestasis may also lead to prolonged clotting times, but these can be corrected by parenteral administration of vitamin K_1 (*Bauer, 1996*).

The liver has a large functional reserve and is able to preserve homeostasis and minimize catabolism for a long time, despite extensive damage. Cats are expert in hiding signs of disease, and appearance of metabolic alterations and clinical signs of liver dysfunction signify advanced disease.

In acute disease, functional proteins in skeletal muscle and other tissues are catabolized to meet the demands for the synthesis of host defense proteins. In chronic liver disease, the etiology of the catabolic state is multifactorial (Bauer 1996; Krahenbuhl & Reichen 1997). Plasma concentrations of aromatic amino acids (AAA) increase in liver disease due to increased peripheral release and decreased hepatic clearance, but BCAA levels decrease because of enhanced utilization as an energy source by muscle. This imbalance between AAA and BCAA has been implicated in the pathogenesis of HE, although its clinical significance in the cat is unknown.

Deficiency of specific amino acids may furthermore play a role in feline liver disease. Cats have a relatively high dietary requirement for arginine (recommended allowance: 1.93g/1,000 kcal ME: NRC 2006) because they lack alternative synthetic pathways, and thus rely on dietary arginine to drive the urea cycle. Arginine-free diets will result in hyperammonemia and HE within hours, whereas diets low in arginine will propagate HE in a later stage. Cats also need dietary taurine, (recommended allowance: 0.1g/1,000 kcal ME: NRC 2006) which is essential to conjugate bile acids and promote choleresis; in addition, it has a mild antioxidant function. Dietary requirements are higher when cats are fed canned diets, since these promote increased growth of enteric flora, deconjugation of bile acids and degradation of taurine (Kim et al, 1996). NRC 2006 recommends an allowance of 1.0g of taurine/kg dry diet, whereas the allowance for canned diets is 1.7g/kg diet.

Cats may furthermore develop L-carnitine deficiency in liver disease, due to insufficient intake of L-carnitine or its precursors, reduced hepatic synthesis, or increased turnover. L-carnitine supplementation may be protective against the development of hepatic lipidosis in obese and anorexic cats, although this is still unproven (Biourge, 1997).

Carbohydrate

The liver is responsible for the maintenance of blood glucose levels because it is the primary organ for glycogen storage and glycogenolysis. In liver disease, serum concentrations of glucagon and insulin are increased due to reduced hepatic degradation, with the effects of hyperglucagonemia generally predominating (Marks et al, 1994; Center 2000a). Liver disease results in more rapid depletion of hepatic glycogen stores, and glucose needs are then supplied through catabolism of muscle proteins to amino acids. This causes muscle wasting and increases the nitrogen load, which may potentiate hyperammonemia and HE. Fasting hypoglycemia may occur in severe acute liver disease and portosystemic shunts due to inadequate glycogen storage and gluconeogenesis. In contrast, a mild hyperglycemia can occur in chronic liver disease (esp. cirrhosis) due to peripheral insulin resistance related to an increase in glucagon levels.

Fat

The liver has an important function in the synthesis, oxidation and transport of lipids. Liver disease causes an increase in peripheral lipolysis in order to generate fatty acids for energy production, resulting in fat depletion, while the rate of hepatic fatty acid oxidation increases (Bauer, 1994; Marks et al, 1996).

Through its synthesis of bile acids and secretion of bile the liver plays an important role in the digestion and absorption of fat and fat-soluble vitamins (A, D, E, K). Fat malabsorption is nevertheless not common in liver disorders, since some dietary triglycerides can still be absorbed in the complete absence of bile acids. However, in severe cholestatic liver disease the reduced availability of enteric bile acids can cause malabsorption of fats, fat-soluble vitamins (especially vitamins E and K) and some minerals.

The liver is the only site of cholesterol synthesis. Hypocholesterolemia may occur in acute liver failure and portosystemic shunts, whereas hypercholesterolemia is seen in obstructive jaundice (Center, 2000a).

Protein catabolism is increased in all liver diseases. Protein breakdown is augmented in patients with infections or gastrointestinal hemorrhage, which can precipitate HE due to increased ammonia production.

> Micronutrient metabolism

Vitamins

The liver stores many vitamins and converts them to metabolically active forms. Liver disease can therefore result in deficiency of vitamins stored in the liver, such as B-complex vitamins. Vitamin deficiencies are augmented by increased demands for hepatocyte regeneration, reduced metabolic activation and increased urinary losses *(Center, 1998)*. Vitamin C can be synthesized in cats but is not stored. Its synthesis may be affected by liver disease *(Center, 2000a; Marks et al, 1994)*.

Deficiencies of the fat-soluble vitamins A, D, E and K can occur in any condition that impairs the enterohepatic circulation of bile acids or fat absorption; vitamin E deficiency is particularly common in chronic liver disease *(Center, 1996)*. Deficiencies of vitamins E and K are most significant.

- Vitamin E is an important antioxidant that protects lipoproteins and cell membranes from lipid peroxidation. Vitamin E deficiency is important since it causes an increased susceptibility to oxidative stress, which perpetuates ongoing liver injury *(Sokol, 1994)*.
- Vitamin K deficiency is less common but more easily recognized since it develops rapidly and results in a clinically detectable bleeding tendency.

Minerals and trace elements

Iron, zinc and copper are the main trace elements stored in the liver. Both iron and copper can be hepatotoxic in high levels, but only copper appears to be a potential hepatotoxin in companion animals. The liver is central to the maintenance of copper homeostasis, since it takes up most of the absorbed copper and regulates the amount retained by controlling excretion through the biliary tract. Hepatic copper accumulation is rare in cats, but it has been reported in cats with cholestatic liver disease *(Fuentealba & Aburto, 2003)* and as a possible primary copper hepatotoxocosis *(Meertens et al, 2005)*. In physiological hepatic concentration, copper is complexed by proteins but excessive hepatic accumulation of copper results in mitochondrial injury, generation of reactive oxygen species and free radicals*, and hepatocellular damage *(Sokol et al, 1994)*.

$$* \ Cu^3 + O_2^- + H_2O_2 \ > \ Cu^{2+} + OH^- + OH^\bullet$$

Zinc is an essential cofactor in many biological processes; it has an antioxidant role, anti-fibrotic properties, and enhances ureagenesis *(Marchesini et al, 1996)*.

Antioxidants

Free radicals are generated in many types of liver disease, and play an important role in perpetuating hepatic pathology. They damage cellular macromolecules via lipid peroxidation and other mechanisms, and can initiate and perpetuate liver injury. Their production is increased in inflammation, cholestasis, immunological events, and exposure to heavy metals and toxins *(Sokol et al, 1994; Feher et al, 1998)*. Endogenous enzymatic antioxidant defense systems that hold the generation of free radicals in check may become deficient during liver disease **(Table 6)**. All antioxidant systems work synergistically to prevent cellular damage. A disruption in these natural defense systems results in oxidant stress **(Figure 14)**. Nutritional antioxidants include vitamins E and C as well as SAMe whereas taurine and zinc have also a weak antioxidant effect.

Detoxification and excretion

The liver is the primary site of detoxification of both endogenous by-products of intermediary metabolism (e.g. ammonia) and exogenous substances absorbed from the gastrointestinal tract. All of these may play a role in the etiology of HE. The precise pathogenesis is likely to be multifactorial, and may be based on inter-related changes in reduced hepatic clearance of gut-derived substances such as ammonia, altered amino acid neurotransmission and endogenous benzodiazepines. Ammonia is the substance most commonly linked with HE, although serum ammonia

---

Zinc deficiency is common in chronic liver disease, due to poor dietary intake, reduced intestinal absorption and increased urinary loss. Deficiency results in low resistance to oxidative stress and reduces ammonia detoxification in the urea cycle, thus promoting HE.

TABLE 6 - HEPATIC ANTIOXIDANT DEFENSES

Dietary antioxidants	Endogenous antioxidants
Vitamin E Vitamin C Taurine Glutamine S-adenosyl-methionine (SAMe)	Glutathione Superoxide dismutase Catalase

FIGURE 14 - ETIOLOGY OF OXIDANT STRESS IN LIVER DISEASE

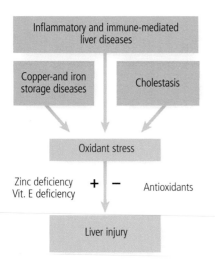

FIGURE 15 - AMMONIA METABOLISM

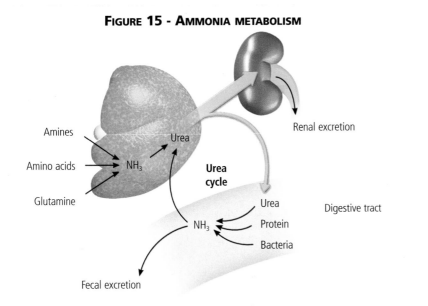

levels correlate poorly with the degree of HE (*Maddison, 2000*). A large part of this ammonia is produced in the gastrointestinal tract by urease-producing bacteria **(Figure 15)**.

▶ Nutritional management

> Nutritional goals

Effective management of hepatobiliary disease requires both treatment of the underlying disease and nutritional support. Nutrient requirements of cats with liver disease are the same if not higher of those of normal animals, with those for protein and micronutrients even greater (*Michel, 1995*). The diet must be highly palatable and provide adequate energy, protein, fat, and all essential micronutrients. Care must be taken to avoid overwhelming the remaining metabolic capacities of the diseased liver. It is furthermore becoming increasingly evident that it is possible to modulate metabolic and pathological processes through the use of specific nutrients and metabolites (*Remillard & Saker, 2005*).

Malnutrition is common in cats with hepatobiliary disease, due to decreased intake and the metabolic consequences of the disease **(Figure 16)**. Negative protein and energy balance have a harmful influence on hepatocellular regeneration and repair, reduce immune response, alter intermediary metabolism, promote HE, and increase mortality (*Biourge, 1997; Center, 1998*). Correction and prevention of malnutrition are essential in management. Maintaining adequate nutritional intake is furthermore the only effective treatment in cats with hepatic lipidosis. Providing several small and palatable meals throughout the day will help to promote food intake and nitrogen balance. Cats that are anorexic for more than 3-5 days require tube feeding, whereas immediate tube feeding is usually recommended in cats with hepatic lipidosis. Force feeding and appetite stimulants are not recommended in cats in order to avoid learned food aversions (*Remillard & Saker, 2005; Delaney, 2006*).

The aims of dietary management of feline liver disease are:
- to supply adequate energy and nutrients to fulfill basic energy requirements and prevent/correct malnutrition
- to limit further hepatocellular damage by reducing oxidative stress
- to support hepatocellular regeneration by providing limiting nutrients, especially protein
- to prevent or minimize metabolic complications such as HE.

ENERGY

Cats with liver disease are usually catabolic and have increased energy requirements.

FIGURE 16 - ETIOLOGY OF MALNUTRITION IN LIVER DISEASE

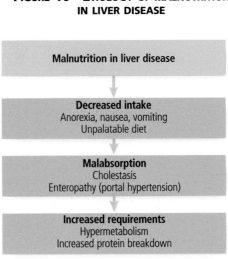

Malnutrition in liver disease

Decreased intake
Anorexia, nausea, vomiting
Unpalatable diet

Malabsorption
Cholestasis
Enteropathy (portal hypertension)

Increased requirements
Hypermetabolism
Increased protein breakdown

PROTEIN

- Provision of adequate high-quality protein as well as calories is essential to ensure a positive protein balance and enable hepatic regeneration.
- Cats have high dietary protein requirements which are often increased in liver disease. Dietary protein should not be restricted unless there is clear evidence of hepatic encephalopathy and hyperammonemia.

The diet should have a high palatability and energy density, since cats with liver disease usually have reduced appetites. An adequate supply of energy (50-60 kcal/kg/day) and protein is essential to prevent catabolism and manutrition (*Biourge, 2004; Remillard & Saker, 2005*). The use of nonprotein calories is important to prevent the use of amino acids for energy and reduce the need for gluconeogenesis. In cats, nonprotein calories should mainly come from fat sources and include some highly digestible carbohydrates (e.g. rice).

Fat is a highly palatable and concentrated source of energy, and the diet's caloric density is proportional to its fat content. Cats with liver disease can tolerate larger quantities of fat in the diet (30-50% of calories) than previously assumed. Fat restriction should only be considered in cats with severe cholestatic liver disease and suspected fat malabsorption, although adequate essential fatty acids must be provided. Incorporation of medium chain triglycerides in the diet is not recommended, since they may decrease palatability.

Altered carbohydrate metabolism in feline liver disease usually presents as a problem in maintaining euglycemia. Cats have a limited ability to digest, absorb and metabolize carbohydrates, and are often glucose intolerant in chronic liver disease. Carbohydrates should not represent more than 35% of the calories of the diet. Boiled white rice is useful because of its high digestibility, providing non-encephalopathogenic energy (*Center, 1998*). Complex carbohydrates such as soluble fiber can be useful in cats with cirrhosis and a tendency to hyperglycemia, because they smooth the postprandial glycemic response and prolong glucose delivery to the liver.

Incorrect protein restriction in cats with liver disease causes further catabolism of endogenous proteins and loss of muscle mass, both of which increase the potential for HE. Feeding of excessive and/or poor quality protein should also be avoided since this may aggravate hepatic encephalopathy (*Laflamme, 1999*). The aim is to gradually increase the amount of protein in the diet, keeping the protein intake as close to normal as can be tolerated without precipitating signs of HE. As protein deficiency appears to be important in the pathogenesis of hepatic lipidosis, clinicians should provide patients the highest level of protein they will tolerate as soon as possible (*Biourge, 1997*). Protein digestibility and amino acid content are important. Although vegetable, soy or dairy proteins may be better tolerated than meat proteins in HE.

BCAA (branched chain amino acid) supplementation has been advocated in people with advanced liver disease and HE, since a decreased plasma ratio of BCAA to AAA (aromatic amino acids) has been considered an important pathogenic factor in its pathogenesis. The use of BCAA supplementation is expensive and controversial, and has not been investigated in cats.

Deficiencies of specific amino acids have furthermore been speculated to occur in feline liver disease, but study results have been conflicting and speculative. However, there is evidence that L-carnitine supplementation may protect cats against hepatic lipid accumulation and thus may be an useful dietary supplement for patients with liver disease (*Ibrahim et al, 2003*). A suggested dose is 250-300 mg/day. L-carnitine is a quaternary ammonium compound, and is an essential cofactor for the transport of long chain fatty acids into the mitochondria for subsequent oxidation and energy production (*Remillard & Saker, 2005*). It is normally synthesized in the liver from the amino acids lysine and methionine.

Fiber

Moderate quantities of dietary fiber can have several beneficial effects in liver disease. Soluble fiber is of benefit in managing HE. Colonic fermentation of soluble fiber (e.g. fructo-oligosaccharides) lowers the intraluminal pH and thus reduces the production and absorption of ammonia, the effects of which are similar to that of lactulose. Colonic fermentation also favors the growth of acidophilic bacteria (e.g. *Lactobacillus spp*) that produce less ammonia and promote incorporation and excretion of ammonia in fecal bacteria.

Fiber (both soluble and insoluble) binds bile acids in the intestinal lumen and promotes their excretion. Insoluble fibers (lignin, cellulose) act by increasing transit time, preventing constipation and adsorbing toxins. Diets high in soluble fiber and with some insoluble fiber should therefore be useful in the long-term dietary management of cats with HE (*Center, 1998*). Foods low in fiber can be supplemented with psyllium (1/2 tsp per 2.5 kg body weight per meal).

Minerals

Potassium and zinc deficiencies are most frequent. Hypokalemia **(Figure 17)** is a common precipitating cause of HE in cats with liver disease (*Center, 1998*), and may be corrected by fluid therapy and dietary supplements. It usually occurs due to a combination of anorexia, vomiting or diarrhea, or excessive use of diuretics in the management of ascites. Zinc deficiency is related to reduced intake and is aggravated by the liver disease.

Zinc benefits the urea cycle and central nervous system neurotransmission, has hepatoprotective effects against a variety of hepatotoxic agents and has antioxidant functions (*Feher et al, 1998, Marchesini et al, 1996*). Zinc supplementation is furthermore useful to prevent hepatic copper accumulation in copper hepatotoxicosis, since zinc inhibits the absorption of copper from the gastrointestinal tract by causing induction of the intestinal copper-binding protein metallothionein. Dietary supplementation with zinc in cats with liver disease is done empirically, including zinc acetate (2 mg/kg per day), gluconate (3 mg/kg per day) or sulphate (2 mg/kg per day) divided into two or three daily doses. Zinc acetate is preferred because it is less irritating to the stomach; it should be given 1-2 hours before or after feeding. Serum zinc concentrations should be determined before and regularly after treatment is started in order to prevent iatrogenic zinc toxicity. Diets high in zinc (58 mg/1000 kcal) are furthermore useful for all patients with liver disease.

Vitamins

Vitamin deficiency is common in chronic feline liver disease. Water-soluble vitamins, especially B vitamins, which are essential for hepatic metabolism of nutrients; may be lost through vomiting or urinary losses or can become deficient as a result of anorexia, intestinal malabsorption, or decreased hepatic metabolism (*Remillard & Saker, 2005*). High daily B vitamin intakes are recommended for cats with chronic liver disease; this is safe since excesses are excreted in the urine. The diet should furthermore contain adequate levels of vitamin C in order to take advantage of its antioxidant properties.

Fat-soluble vitamins (vitamins A, D, E, and K) may become deficient in cholestatic liver disease, because their absorption depends on the availability of bile salts. Vitamin E is an important endogenous free radical scavenger that protects against oxidative injury. Supplementation (400-600 IU/day) is particularly indicated in cholestatic liver disease, but is likely also important in other forms of chronic liver disease. In severe cholestatic disease parenteral administration or an oral water-soluble form are preferred, since a certain level of enteric bile acids are required for its absorption.

Vitamin K deficiency is mostly relevant in cholestatic disorders, although it also may become depleted in severe chronic liver disease. Deficiency is documented by demonstration of prolonged coagulation times and normalization after parenteral administration of vitamin K_1. Coagulopathies secondary to vitamin K deficiency should be treated with two or three doses of vitamin K_1 (0.5-1.0mg/kg intramuscular or subcutaneously every 12 hours). The same dose can be given biweekly or monthly in chronic disorders in which continued repletion of vitamin K is required.

Antioxidants

Liver disease is associated with increased generation of free radicals **(Figure 18)**. Supplementation with antioxidants such as vitamins E and C, as well as taurine, is essential in order to minimize oxidative injury. A combination of dietary antioxidants is better than a single one, since they

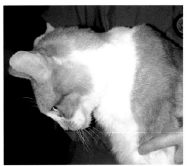

Figure 17 - Head/neck ventroflexion in a cat with severe hypokalemia associated with hepatic lipidosis. A cat with feline hepatic lipidosis demonstrating severe head/neck ventroflexion (this is a very rare clinical sign). This cat had severe hypokalemia and hypophosphatemia; correction of the electrolyte imbalances resolved these clinical signs.

Zinc supplementation may reduce lipid peroxidation, has antifibrotic properties, prevents hepatic copper accumulation, and can reduce the severity of hepatic encephalopathy.

FIGURE 18 - ANTIOXIDANT ACTION SITES IN THE CELL

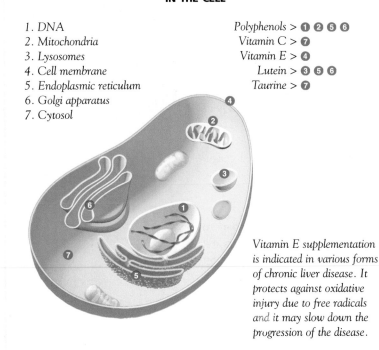

1. DNA
2. Mitochondria
3. Lysosomes
4. Cell membrane
5. Endoplasmic reticulum
6. Golgi apparatus
7. Cytosol

Polyphenols > ❶ ❷ ❺ ❻
Vitamin C > ❼
Vitamin E > ❹
Lutein > ❸ ❺ ❻
Taurine > ❼

Vitamin E supplementation is indicated in various forms of chronic liver disease. It protects against oxidative injury due to free radicals and it may slow down the progression of the disease.

act synergistically. A good balanced diet should also contain nutrients such as zinc, manganese and selenium, which are normally incorporated in enzymatic antioxidant systems.

SAMe is a nutraceutical that may be helpful in reducing hepatic oxidative injury. It is a precursor of glutathione, an important hepatic antioxidant enzyme that is often reduced in liver disease (*Center et al, 2002*). Oral supplementation helps to replenish hepatic glutathione stores and may thus improve antioxidant function. In addition, SAMe has anti-inflammatory properties. It is given as an enteric-coated tablet at 20 mg/kg/day. Side effects of the drug are rare.

► Nutritional management of specific feline liver diseases

> Acute liver disease

Cats are more likely to have chronic liver disease, since they are good at hiding early signs of any disease. Acute liver disease is mostly caused by hepatotoxins, and its management includes removal of the toxin (if known), and supportive treatment with fluids and antioxidants (vitamin E, SAMe). Tube-feeding may be necessary if the cat remains anorexic, since anorexia may predispose it to the development of hepatic lipidosis.

> Chronic liver disease

Dietary management is particularly important in chronic liver disease. Treatment is essential in restoring the energy balance, especially by providing protein. The amount fed should at first be based on an estimation of the cat's energy requirements. Every effort should be made to get the cat to eat voluntarily, although force-feeding should be avoided in order not to create food aversion. Food should be palatable and fed in small portions several times daily. Cats that refuse to eat or consume insufficient amounts to meet minimum requirements require tube feeding, usually initially via an indwelling nasoesophageal tube, in order to halt the vicious cycle of excessive muscle catabolism and worsening signs of liver dysfunction. Protein restriction should only be instituted when there are signs of HE. It is also essential that the diet contains increased zinc levels and a mixture of antioxidants including vitamin E and C. Zinc supplementation is useful because it is an antioxidant, and also has antifibrotic properties and can reduce the severity of HE.

> Hepatic lipidosis

The key to treatment is for the cat to receive adequate protein and fat calories via tube feeding to correct the nutritional imbalance that has been created by the disease **(Figure 19)**. Since these cats are usually profoundly anorexic, tube feeding is indicated as an initial treatment. An esophagostomy or a gastrostomy feeding tube should be placed as soon as the cat is stabilized. Ideally, a moderate to high protein (30-40% of calories), complete and balanced diet that has been specifically formulated for cats should be utilized unless the cat has or develops signs of HE. The energy requirements of cats with hepatic lipidosis are presumed to be similar to healthy cats (50–60 kcal/kg/day), divided into equal sized portions. In addition, a predisposing condition (e.g. stress, pancreatitis, cholangiohepatitis) should be investigated and managed. Attention should also be given to appropriate protein intake, at least 3.8-4.4 g/kg/day. The goal is to restore the energy balance and supplement amino acid deficiencies, especially arginine and taurine. L-carnitine may also be an important nutritional factor because as it may help the beta oxidation of fatty acids by the hepatocytes.

Cats should derive their caloric intake via the feeding tube for the first 7–10 days of therapy. At this time, the cat can be offered food orally. If the cat remains anorexic, tube feeding should continue for another 5–7 days prior to offering food again. The feeding tube can be removed after the cat has has started eating voluntarily and is maintaining its caloric intake and body weight. Several dietary supplements have been recommended, but not critically evaluated by various authors. These include L-carnitine (250–500 mg/cat/day), taurine (250–500 mg/cat/day), vitamin B complex, zinc (7–10 mg/kg elemental zinc/day), and vitamin E (20–100 mg/cat/day). Weekly parenteral vitamin K_1 (0.5–1.5 mg/kg SQ) is indicated for those cats with documented coagulopathies.

Hepatic encephalopathy

HE is a metabolic disorder affecting the central nervous system, which develops secondary to hepatic disease (Michel, 1995). In cats, it is usually a result of congenital portosystemic shunts and less commonly due to severe hepatocellular disease. Signs are typically intermittent, may be precipitated by a high-protein meal, and vary from anorexia, vomiting, diarrhea and polyuria/polydipsia to disorientation, apparent blindness and seizures. Stunted growth or failure to gain weight may occur in young cats with congenital shunts. A high index of clinical suspicion is important, since appropriate management of HE will greatly improve the patient's demeanor and may restore appetite.

Cats with signs of HE are initially offered a protein-restricted diet (<20-25% of calories) in combination with medication aimed at reducing colonic absorption of ammonia (lactulose, oral antibiotics) **(Figure 20)**. Protein quantity is gradually increased at weekly or biweekly intervals when the cat becomes neurologically asymptomatic. Serum protein should be monitored to prevent hypoalbuminemia, in which case dietary protein content should be increased in association with more aggressive adjunct treatment. Maintenance of a positive nitrogen balance is essential in reducing the risk of HE.

The source of proteins is important in the management of HE, since ammonia production and absorption can be minimized by providing highly digestible sources of protein. When hepatic encepalopathy persists despite a protein-restricted diet and adjunct medication, it may be helpful to replace meat proteins with highly digestible vegetables (e.g. soy hydrolysate) and/or milk proteins (e.g. casein, cottage cheese). Milk and vegetable proteins are better tolerated in human patients with hepatic encephalopathy. Soy and milk protein diets are low in nitrogen compared to meat diets, which could contribute to their beneficial effects.

The addition of soluble fiber (psyllium 1-3 tsp mixed with food daily) adds bulk to the stool and prevents constipation.

Homemade versus commercial diets

Commercial diets are preferred above homemade ones because they are nutritionally complete. It is difficult to create homemade diets that are balanced enough to be used for prolonged periods.

Conclusion

Diets for cats with liver disease should be highly digestible with a high energy density provided by fat and carbohydrates **(Table 7)**. Protein restriction should be avoided as much as possible, especially in cats with acute inflammatory hepatic disease or necrosis. Moderate protein restriction may be necessary in cats with clinically evident HE, but in general, it is important to feed cats the highest level of protein they can tolerate without precipitating signs of encephalopathy.

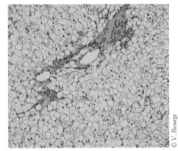

At the end of the fasting period (severe hepatic lipidosis).

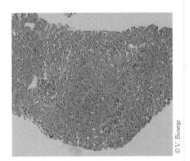

After 5 weeks of adequate nutritional support.

FIGURE 20 - OVERVIEW OF NUTRITIONAL MANAGEMENT OF CATS WITH LIVER DISEASE

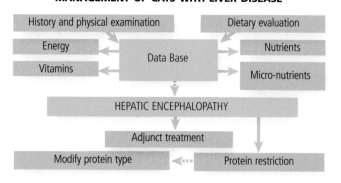

Protein quality should be very high. In addition, the diet should contain high normal to increased levels of water-soluble vitamins, enhanced zinc (>43 mg/1000kcal), restricted sodium (<0.5 g Na/1000 kcal) in case of ascites, and a moderate amount of predominantly soluble fiber.

Correction of enteric bleeding, constipation, infection, alkalosis, hypokalemia and azotemia is important in reducing the risk of hepatic encephalopathy. Maintenance of a positive nitrogen balance (muscle mass) is essential.

TABLE 7 - DIETARY RECOMMENDATIONS FOR THE MANAGEMENT OF LIVER DISEASE IN CATS

• Individualize management per cat and type of liver disease

Energy
• High palatability and high energy density
• Small meals fed frequently
• Prolonged anorexia necessitates placement of an enteral feeding tube, BUT cats with confirmed hepatic lipidosis should be tube fed immediately

Provide adequate protein – AVOID negative nitrogen balance
• Protein should be of high quality and digestibility
• Do not restrict protein unless encephalopathic
• Provide essential amino acids

Fat
• Normal levels (30-50%) of dietary calories
• Restrict only with severe cholestasis and/or steatorrhea

Carbohydrates
• In glucose intolerance: avoid simple sugars, increase complex carbohydrates

Fiber
• Moderate amounts, predominantly soluble fiber

Provide adequate vitamins and minerals
• Increased vitamins B and E
• Moderate restriction of sodium
• Restricted copper
• Increased zinc (>43 mg/1000kcal)

Include additional antioxidants
• Zinc, vitamin E, vitamin C, taurine

Management of complications
• Hepatic encephalopathy:
  - restrict dietary protein if necessary to control HE
  - increase dietary protein tolerance with adjunctive treatment (lactulose, metronidazole, neomycin, soluble fiber)
  - ± vegetable or dairy proteins
  - correct precipitating factors (e.g. hypokalemia)
• Ascites
  - dietary sodium restriction (<0.5 g Na/1000kcal)
  - adjunctive treatment (spironolactone, furosemide)

Frequently asked questions about the dietary treatment of feline hepatobiliary diseases

Q	A
Cats with liver disease often have a decreased appetite or are anorexic. How can they be stimulated to eat?	The diet must be highly palatable and high in energy, and provide adequate protein, fat, and all essential micronutrients. Slightly warming the food, and feeding small amounts frequently can increase palatability. Force-feeding is in most cases contraindicated since it can lead to learned food aversion. Tube feeding, initially via a nasoesophageal tube, may be required in cats that are anorexic, since correction and prevention of malnutrition are essential to provide the building stones for hepatic repair and regeneration, and to prevent or treat hepatic lipidosis.
How do you feed a cat diagnosed with idiopathic hepatic lipidosis?	The key to treatment of cats with hepatic lipidosis is to supply adequate nutrients in order to reverse increased peripheral fat metabolism and metabolic derangements. Since these cats are typically profoundly anorexic, this is done usually through a feeding tube (esophagostomy or gastrostomy tube) until their metabolism normalizes. Feeding a high quality, moderate to high protein diet until the cat begins to eat on its own again, in general after 2-6 weeks, is the most important aspect of treatment.
What is the role of antioxidants in the diet of a cat with liver disease?	There is mounting evidence that free radical production is increased in many liver diseases and that it can play an important role in initiating and perpetuating liver injury. Cats with liver disease, especially hepatic lipidosis, also appear to have decreased liver concentrations of the endogenous antioxidant glutathione, and thus may be at greater risk of oxidant damage to hepatocytes. The diet should therefore contain adequate to increased amounts of antioxidants such as vitamin E and S-adenosyl-methionine. A combination of dietary antioxidants is better than a single one, since they appear to act synergistically.
Do cats with liver disease need additional vitamins?	Stores of B-vitamins are often depleted in liver disease, and supplementation of B vitamins is suggested to improve appetite and cellular metabolism. Some cats with severe cholestatic liver disease will develop malabsorption of fat-soluble vitamins, and added vitamin E and K may be necessary as well.

2- Exocrine pancreatic disease

Introduction

The exocrine pancreas is essential for the optimal digestion and absorption of nutrients (**Table 8**). Pancreatic acini synthesize and secrete digestive enzymes such as trypsin, lipase and amylase, which break down proteins, lipids and carbohydrates in the proximal duodenum. Bicarbonate rich secretions are released with pancreatic enzymes to maintain an optimal pH for enzyme activity, and secretion of pancreatic intrinsic factor enables the absorption of cobalamin (vitamin B_{12}). In addition, the exocrine pancreas produces bacteriostatic peptides that regulate the upper gastrointestinal flora, and has a role in maintaining the integrity of the intestinal mucosa. The pancreas also has an inbuilt mechanism to prevent it from premature intrapancreatic activation of digestive enzymes and autodigestion.

TABLE 8 - FUNCTIONS OF THE EXOCRINE PANCREAS	
Secretion of digestive enzymes	Trypsin, lipase, amylase
Secretion of bicarbonate	Neutralizes gastric acid emptied into the duodenum, creating a neutral pH for optimal digestive enzyme absorption
Facilitation of cobalamin absorption	Secretion of pancreatic intrinsic factor that enables absorption of cobalamin (Vitamin B_{12})
Secretion of antibacterial factors	Production of bacteriostatic peptidases (pancreatic secretory trypsin inhibitor) and defensins that regulate the upper GI flora
Modulation of intestinal mucosal function	

Pancreatitis is the most common feline exocrine pancreatic disorder, followed by exocrine pancreatic insufficiency; exocrine pancreatic neoplasia and other miscellaneous conditions are less commonly seen in cats.

▶ Pancreatitis

Feline pancreatitis can be difficult to diagnose as clinical signs, laboratory findings and imaging results are often nonspecific (*Ferreri et al, 2003*). However, pancreatitis has now emerged as a significant disease in cats. It may be acute or chronic and of variable severity. The etiology of most cases of feline pancreatitis is idiopathic. Chronic pancreatitis is the most common form of the disease in cats (*De Cock et al, 2007*). It is usually mild, and may be only recognized by the development of secondary diabetes mellitus or exocrine pancreatic insufficiency (*Steiner & Williams, 2005*).

Pancreatitis is sometimes only diagnosed when related conditions, such as hepatic lipidosis, are being investigated. Severe acute pancreatitis (necrotizing, hemorrhagic) can result in extensive pancreatic necrosis and multisystemic complications; however, fulminating pancreatitis associated with severe systemic complications is rare in cats.

> Diagnosis

History and physical examination

Clinical signs vary depending on the severity of the disease. The most common signs are lethargy, anorexia and dehydration, which are symptoms seen in many feline diseases (*Mansfield & Jones, 2001b*). Vomiting and cranial abdominal pain are far less common than in dogs with pancreatitis. Cats diagnosed with acute pancreatitis and with concurrent hepatic lipidosis are more likely to be cachectic and have coagulation abnormalities. Some cats with acute pancreatitis are presented because of icterus due to extrahepatic bile duct compression (*Zoran, 2006*). Severe acute pancreatitis may infrequently result in systemic vasodilatation leading to hypotension and sometimes renal failure. Because cats display less commonly key clinical signs observed in dogs, the diagnosis of pancreatitis is much more difficult and a high index of clinical suspicion is warranted.

Chronic pancreatitis may be subclinical and may cause anorexia and weight loss.

> Clinical signs of pancreatitis in cats are nonspecific, including anorexia, lethargy and weight loss. Diagnosis can therefore be difficult, and requires a combination of clinical suspicion, appropriate physical examination findings, elevations in pancreas-specific enzymes and abdominal ultrasonography.

> Diagnostic tests

Hematology, biochemistries and urinalysis
(Table 9)

Routine laboratory findings are generally nonspecific and cannot distinguish between acute and chronic pancreatitis (*Ferreri et al, 2003*). Leukocytosis and neutrophilia are more common in acute pancreatitis, and nonregenerative anemia can be found in both acute and chronic disease. Serum biochemical abnormalities are highly variable; most common are elevations in serum liver enzyme activities (alanine amino-transferase [ALT], alkaline phosphatase [ALP]). Severe acute pancreatitis can cause hyperbilirubinemia due to extrahepatic bile duct compression. Azotemia is variably present, and may be pre-renal or renal, either due to dehydration or rarely due to acute renal failure secondary to pancreatitis.

TABLE 9 - LABORATORY FINDINGS IN FELINE PANCREATITIS

Hematology and serum biochemistries	- Inconsistent anemia and leukocytosis - Hypoalbuminemia - Hyperglycemia / glucosuria - Increased liver enzymes - Hyperbilirubinemia - Azotemia (prerenal most common) - Hypokalemia - Hypocalcemia
Serum vitamin concentrations	Decreased serum cobalamin (vitamin B$_{12}$) concentration
Pancreas-specific enzymes	Increased serum fPLI concentration (most specific) Increased serum fTLI concentration

fPLI – feline pancreatic lipase immunoreactivity
fTLI – feline trypsin-like immunoreactivity

Electrolyte abnormalities (hypokalemia, hypocalcaemia) are frequently seen in severe cases. Hypocalcemia (total and serum ionized) appears to be a more frequent finding in cats than in dogs; it may result from several mechanisms, including peripancreatic formation of calcium salts with fatty acids (fat saponification), and is associated with a worse prognosis (*Kimmel et al, 2001*). Other abnormalities may include hypoalbuminemia, hypercholesterolemia and hyperglycemia.

Urinalysis often reveals an elevated urine specific gravity secondary to dehydration. In severe cases acute renal failure may ensue, resulting in reduced urine specific gravity and casts in the sediment.

None of these findings are specific, but the tests are nonetheless important because they serve to rule out disorders other than pancreatitis and to assess the overall status of the patient.

Pancreas specific enzymes

Measurement of serum lipase and amylase activities is very insensitive and of no clinical value in the diagnosis of feline pancreatitis. Determination of serum feline trypsin-like immunoreactivity (fTLI), which is specific for exocrine pancreatic function, is more helpful but its sensitivity for detection of pancreatitis in cats is less than 50%, making it a suboptimal diagnostic test (*Swift et al, 2000; Steiner, 2003; Forman et al, 2004*).

Recently, a serum feline pancreatic lipase immunoreactivity (fPLI) test has been validated, which appears to be a more sensitive and specific test for the diagnosis of feline pancreatitis, more so for acute than chronic pancreatitis (*Forman et al, 2004; Steiner, 2004*).

Diagnostic imaging

Radiography – The sensitivity of abdominal radiography is generally low for the diagnosis of feline pancreatitis, and especially for chronic pancreatitis. Radiographic abnormalities in acute pancreatitis may include a generalized or focal loss of serosal detail (suggesting peritonitis or peritoneal effusion), increased opacity or the presence of a mass in the area of the pancreas, displacement of the duodenum and/or a dilated and hypomotile duodenum. Cats with concurrent hepatic lipidosis often have hepatomegaly. These changes occur much less commonly than in canine acute pancreatitis, and are not specific (*Whittemore & Campbell, 2005*).

Ultrasonography – Abdominal ultrasonography is more specific and sensitive for detecting pancreatic abnormalities, and is currently one of the most commonly used tools for the diagnosis of pancreatitis in cats. It also allows the evaluation of concurrent disease, e.g. liver disease or biliary obstruction. Ultrasound is widely available today, although sonographic examination of the pancreas requires a high level of operator expertise. Changes identified include pancreatic swelling, changes in echogenicity of the pancreas (hypoechogenicity in acute pancreatitis and hyperechogenicity in chronic pancreatitis and fibrosis) **(Figures 21 & 22)**, hyperechoic peripancreatic fat and mesentery, abdominal effusion, a dilated common bile duct, and less frequently a mass effect in the area of the pancreas **(Figure 23)**. Cavities of the pancreas are generally due to abscesses or pseudocyst formation, and appear as anechoic or hypoechoic cavities, possibly with a thickened wall **(Figure 24)**. Mild pancreatitis may however be more difficult to diagnose via abdominal ultrasound.

Computed tomography (CT) – Other imaging modalities, such as CT-scanning, are more expensive and thought to be less helpful than abdominal ultrasonography (*Gerhardt et al, 2001; Forman et al, 2004*).

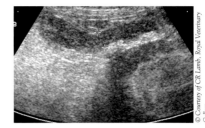

Figure 21 - Ultrasound image of a cat with acute pancreatitis. *The cat had a serum fTLI concentration >400 mg/L. Ultrasound shows a diffusely hypoechoic parenchyma. The pancreas is not enlarged.*

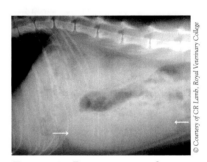

Figure 22 - Chronic active pancreatic necrosis in a diabetic cat. *Ultrasound shows a diffusely hypoechoic, enlarged pancreas.*

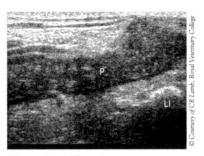

Figure 23 - Pancreatic pseudocyst in a cat. *The lateral abdominal radiograph indicates an oblong soft tissue opacity along the ventral abdomen.*

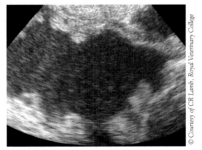

Figure 24 - Ultrasound scan of a cat with a pancreatic pseudocyst. *The ultrasound scan shows a cavitary mass with thick irregular walls.*

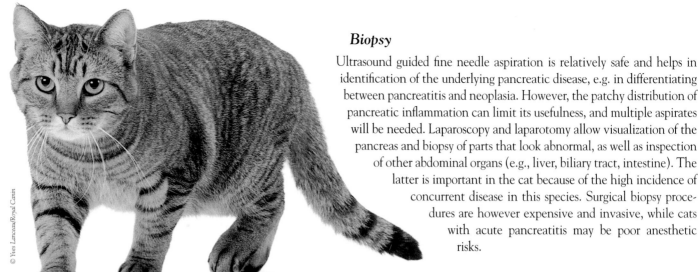

© Yves Lanceau/Royal Canin

Most cases of pancreatitis are seen in domestic short-hair cats. There is no breed or sex predisposition.

Biopsy

Ultrasound guided fine needle aspiration is relatively safe and helps in identification of the underlying pancreatic disease, e.g. in differentiating between pancreatitis and neoplasia. However, the patchy distribution of pancreatic inflammation can limit its usefulness, and multiple aspirates will be needed. Laparoscopy and laparotomy allow visualization of the pancreas and biopsy of parts that look abnormal, as well as inspection of other abdominal organs (e.g., liver, biliary tract, intestine). The latter is important in the cat because of the high incidence of concurrent disease in this species. Surgical biopsy procedures are however expensive and invasive, while cats with acute pancreatitis may be poor anesthetic risks.

Differential diagnosis

The clinical signs of feline pancreatitis are nonspecific, but this disease should however be suspected in any cat with evidence of hepatic, biliary or inflammatory bowel disease.

Pancreatic neoplasia is much less common than pancreatitis, but signs and ultrasonographic findings can be similar in cats (*Seaman, 2004; Hecht et al, 2007*). Identification of a pancreatic mass and lymphadenopathy upon ultrasonography may be helpful, but fine-needle aspiration or surgical biopsy is needed for definitive diagnosis.

> Epidemiology

Etiology

Most feline pancreatitis cases are idiopathic, and causes and risk factors have been described in only a small number of cases. Traumatic pancreatitis associated with road traffic accidents or falls from a great height ("high rise syndrome") has been reported in some cases. Several infectious agents have been implicated, although a cause-and-effect relationship has only been established for *Toxoplasma gondii* and in very rare cases aberrant migration of the feline liver fluke (*Amphimerus pseudofelineus*). Feline herpesvirus, coronavirus (feline infectious peritonitis -FIP-) and panleukopenia virus are putative causative factors for pancreatitis in cats, but there is little or no scientific evidence to support this (*Steiner & Williams, 1999; Mansfield & Jones, 2001a*). Drugs have been implicated as causing pancreatitis in humans and dogs, but this is poorly documented in cats. Pancreatitis was reported in two cats following topical administration of the organophosphate fenthion (*Hill & Van Winkle, 1993*).

Risk factors

There are few known risk factors for the development of pancreatitis in cats. Many cats with chronic pancreatitis have concurrent biliary tract and/or gastrointestinal tract disease ("triad disease"), but the cause-and-effect relationship remains unclear. The incidence of chronic pancreatitis is however significantly correlated with increasing age (*De Cock et al, 2007*). In contrast to dogs, there is no evidence that overweight body condition, nutritional factors (ingestion of high-fat meals) or endocrine diseases (hyperadrenocorticism) play a role in the etiology of feline pancreatitis. Pancreatitis may occur in cats of any breeds. An older report suggesting that Siamese cats were at increased risk has not been confirmed in recent studies. There is no sex predisposition.

> Pathophysiological mechanisms

Regardless of the initiating cause, pancreatitis is thought to be due to premature intrapancreatic activation of trypsinogen which, when activated to trypsin, activates other digestive proenzymes resulting in a local and systemic inflammatory response. Under normal conditions this does not happen due to a number of protective mechanisms, which include:
1) synthesis, storage and secretion of pancreatic enzymes as zymogens (inactive proenzymes) that must be activated by trypsin within the gut prior to being functional
2) strict segregation between lysosomes and zymogens
3) secretion of pancreatic secretory trypsin inhibitor.

Pancreatitis develops when all these protective mechanisms are overwhelmed, resulting in fusion between lysosomes and zymogens, and intrapancreatic activation of digestive enzymes (*Steiner & Williams, 1999*).

Acute mild pancreatitis can be self-limiting, and usually has few symptoms. Severe acute pancreatitis is uncommon in cats, but can have serious local and systemic complications. Activated digestive enzymes cause local effects, such as inflammation, hemorrhage, acinar cell necrosis, and peripancreatic fat necrosis **(Figure 25)**. Cytokines released into the blood stream may cause systemic effects, including systemic inflammatory changes, vasodilatation leading to hypotension, pulmonary edema, disseminated intravascular coagulation (DIC), central neurological deficits, and multi-organ failure. Depletion of pancreatic acinar glutathione can furthermore stimulate oxidative stress that contributes to tissue injury. However, the exact pathophysiology of spontaneous pancreatitis in cats remains speculative.

> Treatment

Medical management

Acute pancreatitis

Treatment for feline acute pancreatitis is mainly supportive and aimed at restoring and maintaining fluid and electrolyte balance, inhibiting inflammatory mediators and pancreatic enzymes, controlling pain and vomiting, and management of complications and/or concurrent diseases (*Simpson, 2005*). Initial fluid therapy is usually with Lactated Ringers solution; potassium and glucose should be added where necessary based upon the results of serum biochemistries. The type of fluid should then be adjusted based upon measurements of electrolyte levels and pH. Efforts should also be made to identify and remove an underlying cause; however, more than 90% of cases are idiopathic.

In severe acute pancreatitis, other therapeutic strategies may furthermore involve plasma administration (20 mL/kg IV) to replenish α2-macroglobulin, a scavenger protein for activated proteases in serum. However, although it has been reported to be of value in dogs with pancreatitis, little is known about its usefulness in cats.

Abdominal pain is commonly recognized in humans and dogs but not in cats with pancreatitis, likely because many cats do not show clear signs of abdominal discomfort. They may however benefit significantly from analgesic therapy, and the presence of abdominal pain should be suspected. Treatment with analgesic drugs e.g. (buprenorphine 0.005-0.1 mg/kg SC q 6-12 hrs) can help cats with acute pancreatitis to feel better and promote eating (*Whittemore & Campbell, 2005*).

It is common practice to give parenteral antibiotics during this supportive period, but cats with pancreatitis seldom have infectious complications. Antibiotic administration is best avoided unless the cat is febrile and/or has toxic changes on the white blood cell count.

The goals of management are removal of the inciting cause if possible, provision of supportive and symptomatic therapy, and monitoring for and treatment of complications. Nutritional support is especially important in cats since anorexia predisposes them to hepatic lipidosis.

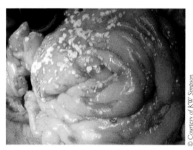

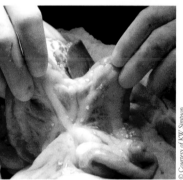

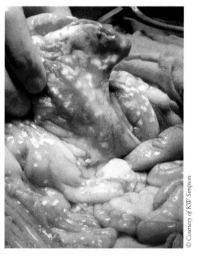

Figure 25 - Peripancreatic fat necrosis. Exploratory laparotomy and histopathology confirm severe multifocal fat necrosis in a cat with fatal acute pancreatitis.

Concurrent diseases are common in feline pancreatitis, and need to be addressed to improve response to therapy (*Simpson, 2005*). Associated diseases include inflammatory bowel disease, cholangiohepatitis and interstitial nephritis (*Weiss et al, 1996*). Concurrent hepatic lipidosis is common (*Akol et al, 2001*), which emphasizes the need for early nutritional support.

Chronic pancreatitis

Medical management is supportive and mostly focuses on treatment of secondary diabetes mellitus and/or exocrine pancreatic insufficiency. Whenever possible the underlying cause should be removed. Exposure to unnecessary drugs should be avoided, and consideration should be given to the treatment of pancreatic flukes, especially in areas where they are known to be prevalent. Concurrent diseases, notably inflammatory bowel disease, cholangiohepatitis and interstitial nephritis, are common in cats with chronic pancreatitis, but little is known about how to best treat these in conjunction with managing the pancreatitis (*Ferreri et al, 2003*).

Abdominal pain is frequent in people with chronic pancreatitis and is likely to occur in cats as well, although it is generally poorly recognized. Meperidine or butorphanol can be used parenterally. This has not been documented in cats, but trial therapy with pancreatic enzymes should be considered in patients with chronic pancreatitis that show either abdominal pain or anorexia attributable to abdominal discomfort (*Steiner & Williams, 2005*). Supplementation with pancreatic enzymes may be helpful to reduce abdominal pain by a negative feedback on endogenous pancreatic enzyme secretion.

> Nutritional support is essential in cats with acute pancreatitis, since they are generally anorexic and often have concurrent hepatic lipidosis. Nutrition furthermore helps tissue repair and recovery, and can modulate the inflammatory response.

TABLE 10 - RECOMMENDATIONS FOR MANAGEMENT OF EXOCRINE PANCREATIC DISEASE IN CATS

Provide adequate energy	- High diet palatability and energy density - Small meals fed frequently - Moderate fat intake
Provide adequate protein	- Protein should be of high quality and digestibility - Do not restrict protein
Fiber	- Moderate amounts, predominantly soluble fiber
Provide adequate vitamins and minerals	- Increase vitamin B and E - Parenteral cobalamin supplementation
Include additional antioxidants	- Vitamins E and C, taurine

Management of complications	• Persistent anorexia
	  - Enteral tube feeding
	  - (Parenteral nutrition)
	• Exocrine pancreatic insufficiency
	  - Exogenous pancreatic enzyme supplementation mixed within each meal
	• Diabetes mellitus
	  - Exogenous insulin

Nutritional management (Table 10)

To feed or not to feed

The traditional recommendation for patients with acute pancreatitis is not to feed orally for three to four days in order to prevent further pancreatic stimulation ("rest the pancreas"). This recommendation is justified in patients that vomit, but most cats with acute pancreatitis do not vomit. The issue is complicated further in cats by the fact that cats with severe pancreatitis are anorexic and often develop hepatic lipidosis, which worsens their prognosis (*Akol et al, 2001*). Pancreatitis is a catabolic state in which metabolic and energy demands can be very high. Starvation will only serve to compound malnutrition and will also adversely affect immune response and bowel mucosal integrity. Cats with pancreatitis should therefore receive nutritional support at an early stage. There is no clinical impression that such enteral nutrition exacerbates the course of pancreatitis, and in fact cats clearly do better overall when nutritional support is given.

If the cat is not eating on its own within three days, nutritional support via a feeding tube is indicated to prevent or treat hepatic lipidosis, protein/calorie malnutrition and immunosuppression.

How to feed

Oral force feeding is not recommended since it is difficult to achieve the appropriate levels of caloric intake by this method, and also because it can induce food aversion. The choice is then between enteral or parenteral nutrition. There is increasing evidence in humans and animals that enteral nutrition is superior to parenteral nutrition in the treatment of acute pancreatitis (*Marik & Zaloga, 2005; Simpson, 2005; Makola et al, 2007*). Enteral nutrition prevents intestinal mucosal atrophy and bacterial translocation which accompany parenteral nutrition. It is also more economical, has less risk of septic complications and is far less complicated to use. The simplest and most widely used methods of enteral feeding are via a nasoesphageal, esophagostomy or percutaneous endoscopic gastrostomy (PEG) tube **(see chapter 12)**. Postpyloric feeding via a jejunostomy tube (distal to the site of pancreatic stimulation) has the theoretical advantage of minimizing pancreatic stimulation, but there are now several studies in human patients that the nasogastric route may be just as effective and safer. Jejunostomy tube placement historically required invasive surgery, but recently a percutaneous endoscopic transpyloric placement technique has been described (*Jergens et al, 2007*). It remains however open whether cats with acute pancreatitis really require jejunal feeding.

Parenteral nutrition may be necessary for cats in which persistent vomiting cannot be controlled by anti-emetic treatment; it is however expensive, difficult to administer in practice, and may cause complications such as sepsis.

What diet to feed

The diet for patients with pancreatitis should be highly digestible. Dietary fat restriction is recommended for human and canine patients with pancreatitis in order to reduce pancreatic stimulation, but is less applicable to felines. Cats are obligate carnivores and require fairly high dietary fat levels, and in contrast to dogs there is little clinical evidence to suggest that dietary fat restriction influences the outcome of feline pancreatitis. In addition, low-fat diets are energy restricted and not a good choice for sick cats with poor appetites. The best compromise is to select a palatable, complete and balanced diet formulated for maintenance with a moderate fat content (10-12% on a dry matter basis). The important thing is to stay away from a high fat diet (> 16 % fat on a dry matter basis), especially in those cats that have both pancreatitis and diabetes mellitus (*Steiner J, personal communication 2007*).

Dietary protein should be of good quality and meet the cat's requirements for maintenance and tissue repair. However, diets excessively high in protein should be avoided in order to minimize pancreatic stimulation by peptides. Novel antigen diets may be useful in cats with pancreatitis and concurrent inflammatory bowel disease (*Biourge & Fontaine, 2004*).

Dietary supplements

Antioxidants – Oxidative stress caused by inflammatory mediators can aggravate severe acute pancreatitis in humans (*Schulz et al, 2003*), although the role of antioxidant treatment in its management is controversial (*Johnson, 2007*). There are no data about the role of antioxidants in the management of feline pancreatitis.

Fatty acids – Supplementation with n-3 polyunsaturated fatty acids (fish oil) can ameliorate inflammation through modulation of eicosanoid synthesis. A clinical trial in human patients with acute pancreatitis suggested a clinical benefit based upon shortened time of hospital stay and jejunal feeding *(Lasztity et al, 2005)*. Its use in cats with exocrine pancreatic disease has not yet been evaluated.

Cobalamin – Cobalamin malabsorption is common, because intrinsic factor (IF), a cobalamin binding protein that promotes cobalamin absorption in the ileum, is produced only by the pancreas in cats (as opposed to the stomach and pancreas in dogs). Cobalamin deficiency is even greater in cats with concurrent small intestinal disease. Cats with subnormal serum cobalamin concentrations should be supplemented parenterally (SQ or IM, 250 µg once a week for six weeks and then monthly) *(Simpson et al, 2001)*. The necessity for further treatments should be assessed by regular measurement of serum cobalamin concentrations.

Vitamin K – Coagulation abnormalities should be treated with parenteral vitamin K; in cats with severe necrotizing pancreatitis, the possibility of disseminated intravascular coagulation should be assessed, which may require administration of fresh frozen plasma (10-20 mL/kg).

► Exocrine pancreatic insufficiency

> Introduction

The exocrine pancreas plays a central role in the digestion and absorption of nutrients. Pancreatic acinar cells synthesize and secrete enzymes that digest proteins, fats and carbohydrates (protease, lipase and amylase). Pancreatic duct cells furthermore secrete bicarbonate to maintain an optimal pH for digestive and absorptive function, as well as intrinsic factor to facilitate cobalamin absorption.

Exocrine pancreatic insufficiency (EPI) results from deficient synthesis and secretion of pancreatic digestive enzymes. The lack of digestive enzymes in the duodenum leads to maldigestion and malabsorption of intestinal contents. The exocrine pancreas has a large functional reserve capacity and clinical signs of maldigestion do not occur until 90% of secretory capacity is lost.

> Diagnosis

Overview

EPI is an uncommon cause of chronic diarrhea in cats; however, in the past it has been under diagnosed due to the lack of specific clinical and laboratory findings. Diagnostic accuracy has now been facilitated by the fTLI test, which is a species specific radioimmunoassay.

Clinical signs

Clinical signs in affected cats are not specific for EPI: the most commonly reported clinical signs in cats with EPI are weight loss and soft voluminous feces *(Steiner & Williams, 2005)*. Polyphagia despite weight loss is not as commonly seen as in dogs. Many cats also develop a greasy, unkempt hair coat, especially in the perianal and tail regions, resulting from the high fat content of their feces. Some cats have watery diarrhea secondary to intestinal disease. Affected cats may also have a previous history of recurring bouts of acute pancreatitis (e.g., anorexia, lethargy, vomiting) that resulted in chronic pancreatitis and EPI. Concurrent disease of the small intestine, hepatobiliary system and endocrine pancreas may be present.

Differential diagnosis

The main differential diagnoses for a cat presented with diarrhea, weight loss and changes in appetite are hyperthyroidism, diabetes mellitus and chronic small intestinal disease (most commonly inflammatory bowel disease). Physical examination may help in differentiating these, e.g. by palpating a thyroid nodule or thickened intestinal loops. However, these diseases may be coexisting, especially in older cats, and laboratory testing and imaging (particularly ultrasound) are mandatory.

Laboratory testing

Routine laboratory tests

Results of hematology and serum biochemistries are generally within normal limits or show nonspecific changes. Older cats may have evidence of concurrent renal disease, whereas cats with hyperthyroidism often have increased serum liver enzyme concentrations. Microscopic examination of feces will demonstrate steatorrhea and undigested fat, but this is not pathognomonic for EPI.

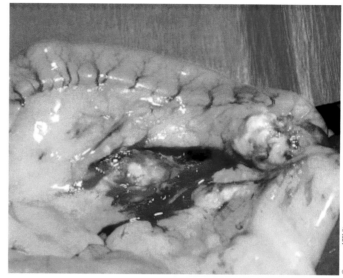

Figure 26 - *Chronic pancreatitis is the most common cause of EPI in cats.*

Serum concentrations of cobalamin and folate should also be determined in all cats with suspected EPI, because of the common occurrence of low levels (especially for cobalamin) (*Steiner & Williams, 1999*).

Pancreas-specific tests

A feline-specific radioimmunoassay for trypsin-like immunoreactivity (fTLI) has now been developed and validated, it is sensitive and the test of choice to diagnose EPI in cats. Fasting serum fTLI concentrations less than 8 µg/L (reference range = 17-49 µg/L) are diagnostic for feline EPI (*Steiner & Williams, 2000*). When the fTLI concentration is between 8-17 µg/L, the test should be repeated ensuring adequate fasting; it is also possible the cat has partial EPI that in time may progress to complete EPI. The TLI test is a simple and reliable way of confirming the diagnosis of EPI; however; it is essential to use an assay specific for feline TLI since there is no cross reactivity between canine and feline TLI.

Diagnostic imaging

Imaging findings are inconsistent; abdominal radiography and ultrasonography generally do not show any abnormalities.

> Epidemiology

Risk factors

Chronic pancreatitis is the most common cause of feline EPI **(Figure 26)**, occurring mainly in mature and older cats. In most cases, it is idiopathic. Rare causes of feline EPI without chronic pancreatitis are pancreatic duct obstruction by liver flukes or pancreatic neoplasia (adenocarcinoma), leading to acinar atrophy. Fecal examination can help in the diagnosis of a fluke infestation, whereas abdominal ultrasonography is essential in detecting a pancreatic mass.

Pancreatic acinar atrophy (PAA) similar to the disease commonly observed in dogs has not been documented in cats.

Breed and sex predisposition

There is no breed or sex predisposition for the development of EPI in cats.

> Pathophysiology

Cats with EPI have an extensive and chronic disease, which is usually due to chronic and irreversible pancreatitis.

The typical signs of EPI (diarrhea, weight loss and polyphagia) are due to decreased intraduodenal concentrations of pancreatic digestive enzymes and bicarbonate with resultant malassimilation of fats, carbohydrates and proteins. This leads to malabsorption, osmotic diarrhea and steatorrhea, and malnutrition. In addition, there are secondary disturbances of intestinal mucosal growth and transport mechanisms that aggravate malabsorption. Cats normally have high numbers of anerobic organisms in their proximal small bowel (*Johnston et al, 1993*) and it is not known whether they develop changes in the nature and number of small intestinal flora, which is common in dogs with EPI.

Fat malabsorption may result in deficiencies of the fat-soluble vitamins (esp. vitamins K and E). Vitamin K-dependent coagulopathy has been reported in a cat with EPI (*Perry et al, 1991*) and may occur in other cases as well. Vitamin E deficiency could aggravate oxidative stress, but there are no reports documenting this in feline EPI.

Many cats with EPI have low serum cobalamin concentrations, which impairs their response to treatment. Cobalamin is absorbed in the distal small intestine after it has formed a complex with intrinsic factor, a protein that in cats is exclusively secreted in the pancreatic juice (*Fyfe, 1993*). The lack of pancreatic intrinsic factor in EPI impacts severely the ability to absorb cobalamin. In addition, concurrent small intestinal disease (*Weiss et al, 1996*) may further impair cobalamin absorption in cats. Cats seem predisposed to develop markedly reduced serum cobalamin levels under those circumstances (*Simpson et al, 2001*). Uncorrected cobalamin deficiency may lead to villous atrophy, intestinal inflammation and worsening malabsorption, with resultant failure to respond to pancreatic enzymes alone.

Serum folate concentrations may be decreased in the case of concurrent small intestinal disease resulting in malabsorption of folate. This differs from the situation in canine EPI, where folate levels are often increased due to secondary small intestinal bacterial overgrowth. Cats have however normally high levels of bacteria in their small intestine and bacterial overgrowth is not a recognized syndrome in this species (*Johnston et al, 1993; 2001*).

> Treatment

Enzyme supplementation

Addition of exogenous pancreatic enzymes to the food is essential for resolution of clinical signs.

Synthetic dried pancreatic extracts are available in several forms.
Powdered pancreatic extracts are most commonly used due to their effectiveness and ease of use. Tablets, capsules and enteric-coated tablets are not recommended since they are usually less effective (*Steiner & Williams, 2005*). The powdered extract should be mixed within the food immediately prior to feeding (0.5 to 1 tsp per meal twice daily); pre-incubating the enzymes with the food or concurrent antacid therapy are unnecessary (*Steiner & Williams, 1999*). The amount should be adjusted based on its efficacy in resolving clinical signs; it is common practice to start with the higher dosage, after which it can be gradually decreased to the smallest dose that maintains remission.

Raw chopped pancreas (30-90 g per meal twice daily) may be used as an alternative and can be very effective. It can be stored frozen for at least three months, but is generally less convenient to use and has the potential for causing gastrointestinal infections (e.g., *Salmonella, Campylobacter*). Bovine pancreas is safest, since there is always a risk of transmitting Aujeszky's disease when using

> EPI in cats is usually due to chronic pancreatitis, and many cats have concurrent diseases (inflammatory bowel disease, cholangiohepatitis, and diabetes mellitus) that may require additional treatment.

> Adequate management of cats with clinical EPI depends on long term enzyme replacement and dietary manipulation.

> It is important that dietary management and enzyme supplementation are kept constant, since variation and especially the consumption of a non-supplemented meal can cause a return of the diarrhea.

porcine extracts. Raw chopped pancreas can however be a solution when the cat develops aversion to the powdered extract.

Vitamin supplementation

Cats with EPI almost always have marked depletion of body cobalamin stores and severely decreased serum cobalamin concentrations. In addition, many cats with EPI have concurrent small intestinal disease which further impairs cobalamin absorption. Supplementation is by parenteral cobalamin (250-500 µg/kg subcutaneously every two or three weeks) to maintain normal serum concentrations of cobalamin (*Ruaux et al, 2005*).

Cats with EPI with or without concurrent small intestinal disease may also have low serum folate concentrations and should be treated with oral folate at 400 µg once daily for 2-4 weeks or longer, until serum levels have normalized.

Malabsorption of fat-soluble vitamins (vitamin A, D, E and K) may occur in EPI, although the clinical importance in cats is unknown. Cats with evidence of a coagulopathy should be supplemented with vitamin K. It may also be helpful to increase dietary vitamin E levels because of its antioxidant function, especially in cats that do not respond to enzymes and supportive management alone and especially in cats with concurrent diseases.

Management of concurrent diabetes mellitus

Cats with chronic pancreatitis resulting in EPI as well as diabetes mellitus will need insulin treatment in addition to management of the EPI.

> Nutritional management (Table 10)

High digestibility is a mainstay of dietary management, since it requires less gastric, pancreatic, biliary and intestinal secretions for digestion, and thus facilitates absorption in the upper small intestine. Dietary modification may be required in cats that present with severe weight loss and protein-calorie malnutrition, and also in cats that do not respond adequately to this management.

Protein

The diet during early refeeding should contain higher protein levels, since many patients with EPI suffer from protein-calorie malnutrition. If response to treatment is poor, concurrent intestinal disease has to be investigated further, e.g. by a dietary trial with an antigen restricted diet. A diet based on rice and soy protein hydrolysate proved to be beneficial in the management of canine EPI (*Biourge & Fontaine, 2004*). This strategy remains to be validated in cats.

Fat

Fat malabsorption and steatorrhea are major signs in patients with EPI (*Williams, 2005*). However, fat restriction is of questionable benefit for cats, especially since this species needs a relatively high-fat diet. In addition, there is evidence that higher fat diets promote better digestibility (*Suzuki et al, 1999*). The cause is unclear, but it may be related to improved preservation of exogenous pancreatic enzymes, particularly lipase. Furthermore, a higher fat and thus more energy dense diet will help an animal in poor body condition to regain its optimal body weight faster. Dietary fat levels can therefore be within the normal range, but high digestibility is essential.

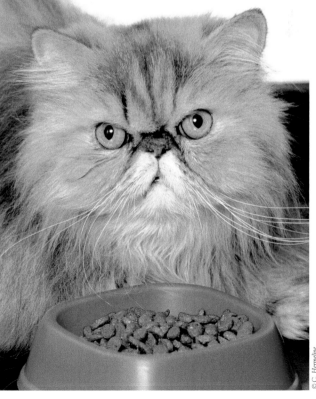

Cats with EPI should be fed a highly digestible, good quality and energy dense diet, with an appropriate pancreatic enzyme supplement mixed into it (Simpson, 2005).

©C. Hermeline

Fiber

Diets containing moderate amounts of fermentable fiber will help to improve GI health by its positive actions upon the mucosal barrier.

Carbohydrate

Cats are poorly adapted to handling carbohydrates, so excessive amounts should be avoided.

Trace elements and vitamins

The diet should contain high-normal concentrations of B-vitamins, since body stores are often depleted.

> Treatment failures

Reconfirm EPI

- Make sure the diagnosis is correct, and resubmit an fTLI.
- One should also ensure that serum cobalamin and folate concentrations are managed appropriately.

Inadequate enzyme supplementation

Ensure that the enzyme supplement being fed is appropriate (non-enteric coated powder), not out-of-date, and fed at the right dose with each meal.

Small intestinal disease

Concurrent small intestinal disease may cause continued malabsorption despite adequate enzyme supplementation. Dietary modifications, e.g. to an antigen-restricted or protein hydrolysate diet, can help to evaluate for dietary intolerance/sensitivity. The diet should be fed exclusively, with added enzyme supplementation, for at least two to three weeks. If gastrointestinal signs resolve after the dietary trial, the cat should be challenged with components of its former diet in order to confirm a diagnosis of dietary intolerance/sensitivity.

If dietary modification is not effective, the cat should be investigated for structural intestinal disease (e.g. inflammatory bowel disease) with abdominal ultrasound and endoscopy with intestinal biopsy. Cats with concurrent inflammatory bowel disease usually can be successfully managed with oral prednisolone (*Steiner & Williams, 2005*).

Conclusion

Feline exocrine pancreatic disease, particularly acute pancreatitis, is more common than previously thought. It however requires a high level of clinical suspicion. Assay of serum fPLI combined with abdominal ultrasound is recommended for the diagnosis of pancreatitis, whereas a severely decreased serum fTLI concentration is diagnostic for EPI in the cat. In both pancreatitis and EPI, concurrent diseases should be assessed and addressed as necessary.

Provision of adequate calories and nutrients is essential in the management of cats with exocrine pancreatic disease. Supportive therapy is important to prevent complications and decrease mortality in acute pancreatitis, and early enteral feeding may be required in order to prevent secondary hepatic lipidosis. Cats with EPI will at least require dietary supplementation with pancreatic enzymes for resolution of clinical signs, and additional treatment with parenteral cobalamin is necessary in many cases.

Frequently asked questions about the dietary treatment of feline pancreatic diseases

Q	A
How should I feed a cat with acute pancreatitis?	Most cats with acute pancreatitis are anorexic, which puts them at risk of developing hepatic lipidosis. It is therefore important that they receive nutritional support at an early stage, provided they are not vomiting. In most cases this is done via an enteral feeding tube. Cats with intractable vomiting that do not respond to anti-emetic treatment may need parenteral nutrition.
Should cats with pancreatic disease be fed a fat-restricted diet?	There is no evidence that dietary fat levels play a role in feline pancreatic disease, nor that fat restriction improves the cat's response to treatment. In addition, cats require a relatively high-fat diet and need the calories from fat to improve their often poor body condition.
What are the dietary recommendations for cats with EPI?	It is best to divide daily intake in at least two or three meals to reduce dietary overload and osmotic diarrhea. Ensure you add the enzyme supplementation to each meal and mix thoroughly. The diet should have high diet palatability and energy density, contain normal levels of fat (which protects the enzymes, provides energy as well as palatability), adequate levels of high quality protein and contain some fermentable fiber.
Do I have to pre-incubate the food with the pancreatic enzymes before feeding it to a cat with EPI?	No, enzymes will only work in the right condition of pH and moisture, pre-incubation is therefore of no use but the enzymes must be carefully mixed with the food.
My cat doesn't like the powdered enzyme supplement. What else can I use?	You can try raw, chopped pancreas, which can be stored frozen for several months.

Akol KG, Washabau RJ, Saunders HM, et al. *Acute pancreatitis in cats with hepatic lipidosis.* J Vet Intern Med 1993; 7: 205-209.

Bauer JE. *Hepatic disease, nutritional therapy, and the metabolic environment.* J Am Vet Med Assoc 1996; 209: 1850-1853.

Beatty JA, Barrs VR, Martin PA, et al. *Spontaneous hepatic rupture in six cats with systemic amyloidosis.* J Small Anim Pract 2002; 43: 355-363.

Biourge V. *Clinical nutrition in liver disease, in* Proceedings. 14th Annu ECVIM-CA Congress 2004; 63-65.

Biourge V. *Nutrition and liver disease.* Semin Vet Med Surg 1997; 12: 34-44.

Biourge V, Groff JM, Fisher C, et al. *Nitrogen balance, plasma free amino acid concentrations and urinary orotic acid excretion during long-term fasting in cats.* J Nutr 1994a; 124: 1094-1103.

Biourge VC, Groff JM, Munn RJ, et al. *Experimental induction of hepatic lipidosis in cats.* Am J Vet Res 1994b; 55: 1291-1302.

Biourge VC, Massat B, Groff JM, et al. *Effect of protein, lipid, or carbohydrate supplementation on hepatic lipid accumulation during rapid weight loss in obese cats.* Am J Vet Res 1994c; 55: 1406-1415.

Biourge VC, Fontaine J. *Exocrine pancreatic insufficiency and adverse reaction to food in dogs: a positive response to a high-fat, soy isolate hydrolysate-based diet.* J Nutr 2004, 134: 2166s-2168s.

Blanchard G, Paragon BM, Milliat F, et al. *Dietary L-carnitine supplementation in obese cats alters carnitine metabolism and decreases ketosis during fasting and induced hepatic lipidosis.* J Nutr 2002; 132: 204-210.

Caney SMA, Gruffydd-Jones TJ. *Feline inflammatory liver disease.* In: Ettinger SJ, Feldman EC, eds. Textbook of Veterinary Internal Medicine Diseases of the Dog and Cat. 6th edition. Philadelphia: WB Saunders Co, 2005; 1448-1453.

Center SA. *Chronic hepatitis, cirrhosis, breed-specific hepatopathies, copper storage hepatopathy, suppurative hepatitis, granulomatous hepatitis, and idiopathic hepatic fibrosis.* In: Strombeck's Small Animal Gastroenterology. 3rd ed. Philadelphia: WB Saunders Co, 1996: 705.

Center SA. *Feline hepatic lipidosis.* Vet Clin Small Anim 2005; 35: 225-269.

Center SA. *Nutritional support of dogs and cats with hepatobiliary disease.* J Nutr 1998; 128: 2733S-2746S.

Center SA. *Pathophysiology of liver disease: Normal and abnormal function.* In: Ettinger SJ, Feldman EC, eds. Textbook of Veterinary Internal Medicine Diseases of the Dog and Cat. 5th edition. Philadelphia: WB Saunders Co, 2000a; 533-632

Center SA, Elston TH, Rowland PH, et al. *Fulminant hepatic failure associated with oral administration of diazepam in 11 cats.* J Am Vet Med Assoc 1996; 209: 618-625.

Center SA, Randolph JF, Warner KL, et al. *The effects of S-adenosylmethionine on clinical pathology and redox potential in the red blood cell, liver, and bile of clinically normal cats.* J Vet Intern Med 2005; 19: 303-314.

Center SA, Warner K, Corbett J, et al. *Proteins invoked by vitamin K absence and clotting times in clinically ill cats.* J Vet Int Med 2000b; 14: 292-297.

Center SA, Warner KL, Erb HN. *Liver glutathione concentrations in dogs and cats with naturally occurring liver disease.* Am J Vet Res 2002; 63: 1187-1197.

d'Anjou MA, Penninck D, Cornejo L, et al. *Ultrasonographic diagnosis of portosystemic shunting in dogs and cats.* Vet Radiol Ultrasound 2004; 45: 424-437.

Day MJ. *Immunohistochemical characterization of the lesions of feline progressive lymphocytic cholangitis/cholangiohepatitis.* J Comp Pathol 1998; 119: 135-147.

De Cock HEV, Forman MA, Farver TB, et al. *Prevalence and histopathologic characteristics of pancreatitis in cats.* Vet Pathol 2007; 44: 39-49.

Delaney SJ. *Management of anorexia in dogs and cats.* Vet Clin North Am Small Anim Pract 2006; 36: 1243-1249.

Feher J, Lengyel G, Blazovics A. *Oxidative stress in the liver and biliary tract diseases.* Scand J Gastroenterol Suppl 1998; 38-46.

Ferreri JA, Hardam E, Kimmel SE, et al. *Clinical differentiation of acute necrotizing from chronic nonsuppurative pancreatitis in cats: 63 cases (1996-2001).* J Am Vet Med Assoc 2003; 223: 469-474.

Forman MA, Marks SL, De Cock HE, et al. *Evaluation of serum feline pancreatic lipase immunoreactivity and helical computed tomography versus conventional testing for the diagnosis of feline pancreatitis.* J Vet Intern Med 2004; 18: 807-815.

Fyfe JC. *Feline intrinsic factor (IF) is pancreatic in origin and mediates ileal cobalamin (CBL) absorption.* J Vet Intern Med 1993; 7: 133.

Fuentealba IC, Aburto EM. *Animal models of copper-associated liver disease.* Comp Hepatol 2003; 2: 5

Gagne JM, Armstrong PJ, Weiss DJ, et al. *Clinical features of inflammatory liver disease in cats: 41 cases (1983-1993).* J Am Vet Med Assoc 1999; 214: 513-516.

Gerhardt A, Steiner JM, Williams DA, et al. *Comparison of the sensitivity of different diagnostic tests for pancreatitis in cats.* J Vet Intern Med 2001; 15: 329-333.

Gupta R, Patel K, Calder PC, et al. *A randomised clinical trial to assess the effect of total enteral and total parenteral nutritional support on metabolic, inflammatory and oxidative markers in patients with predicted severe acute pancreatitis.* Pancreatology 2003; 3: 406-413.

Haney DR, Christiansen JS, Toll JD. *Severe cholestatic liver disease secondary to liver fluke (Platynosomum concinnum) infection in three cats.* J Am Anim Hosp Assoc 2006; 42: 234-237.

Harkin KR, Cowan LA, Andrews GA, et al. *Hepatotoxicity of stanozolol in cats.* J Am Vet Med Assoc 2000; 217: 681-684.

Haynes JS, Wade PR. *Hepatopathy associated with excessive hepatic copper in a Siamese cat.* Vet Pathol 1995; 32: 427 – 429.

Hecht S, Penninck DG, Keating JH. *Imaging findings in pancreatic neoplasia and nodular hyperplasia in 19 cats.* Vet Radiol Ultrasound 2007; 48: 45-50.

Hill RC, Van Winkle TJ: *Acute necrotizing pancreatitis and acute suppurative pancreatitis in the cat. A retrospective study of 40 cases (1976-1989).* J Vet Int Med 1993; 7: 25-33.

Holt DE, Schelling CG, Saunders HM, et al. Correlation of ultrasonographic findings with surgical, portographic, and necropsy findings in dogs and cats with portosystemic shunts: 63 cases (1987-1993). J Am Vet Med Assoc 1995; 207: 1190-1193.

Hooser SB. Hepatotoxins. In: Bonagura JD (ed). Kirk's Current Veterinary Therapy XIII. Philadelphia: WB Saunders Co, 2000; 217-219.

Hunt GB, Kummeling A, Tisdall PL, et al. Outcomes of cellophane banding for congenital portosystemic shunts in 106 dogs and 5 cats. Vet Surg 2004; 33: 25-31.

Ibrahim WH, Bailey N, Sunvold GD, et al. Effects of carnitine and taurine on fatty acid metabolism and lipid accumulation in the liver of cats during weight gain and weight loss. Am J Vet Res 2003; 64: 1265-1277.

Jergens AE, Morrison JA, Miles KG, et al. Percutaneous endoscopic gastrojejunostomy tube placement in healthy dogs and cats. J Vet Intern Med 2007; 21: 18-24.

Johnson CD. Antioxidants in acute pancreatitis. Gut 2007; 56: 1344-1345

Johnston K, Lamport A, Batt RM. An unexpected bacterial flora in the proximal small intestine of normal cats. Vet Rec 1993; 132: 362-363.

Johnston KL, Swift NC, Forster-van Hijfte M, et al. Comparison of the bacterial flora of the duodenum in healthy cats and cats with signs of gastrointestinal tract disease. J Am Vet Med Assoc. 2001 Jan 1; 218:48-51

Kim SW, Rogers QR, Morris JG. Maillard reactions products in purified diets induce taurine depletion in cats which is reversed by antibiotics. J Nutr 1996; 126: 195-201.

Kimmel SA, Washabau RJ, Drobatz KJ. Incidence and prognostic value of low plasma ionized calcium concentration in cats with acute pancreatitis: 46 cases (1996-1998). J Am Vet Med Assoc 2001; 219: 1105-1109

Krahenbuhl S, Reichen J. Carnitine metabolism in patients with chronic liver disease. Hepatology 1997; 25: 148-153.

Kyles AE, Hardie EM, Mehl M, et al. Evaluation of ameroid ring constrictors for the management of single extrahepatic portosystemic shunts in cats: 23 cases (1996 – 2001). J Am Vet Med Assoc 2002; 220: 1341 – 1347.

Laflamme DP. Nutritional management of liver disease. In: Kirk's Current Veterinary Therapy XIII, Bonagura JW (ed). WB Saunders Co, Philadephia, 2000: 277-293.

Langdon P, Cohn LA, Kreeger JM, et al. Acquired portosystemic shunting in two cats. J Am Anim Hosp Assoc 2002; 38: 21-27.

Lasztity N, Hamvas J, Biro L, et al. Effect of enterally administered n-3 polyunsaturated fatty acids in acute pancreatitis - a prospective randomized clinical trial. Clin Nutr 2005; 24: 198-205

Leveille R, Biller DS, Shiroma JT. Sonographic evaluation of the common bile duct in cats. J Vet Int Med 1996; 10: 296-299.

Levy JK, Bunch SE, Komtebedde J. Feline portosystemic vascular shunts. In: Bonagura J, ed. Kirk's Current Veterinary Therapy Small Animal Practice XII. Philadelphia: WB Saunders Co, 1995; 743-749.

Lisciandro SC, Hohenhaus A, Brooks M. Coagulation abnormalities in 22 cats with naturally occurring liver disease. J Am Vet Med Assoc 1998; 12: 71-75.

Lucke VM, Davies JD. Progressive lymphocytic cholangitis in the cat. J Small Anim Pract 1984; 25: 247.

Maddison JE. Newest insights into hepatic encephalopathy. Eur J Comp Gastroent 2000; 5: 17-21.

Makola D, Krenitsky J, Parrish CR. Enteral feeding in acute and chronic pancreatitis. Gastroint Endosc Clin N Am 2007; 17: 747-764

Mansfield CS, Jones BR. Review of feline pancreatitis, part one: the normal feline pancreas, the pathophysiology, classification, prevalence and aetiologies of pancreatitis. J Feline Med Surg 2001a; 3: 117-124.

Mansfield CS, Jones BR. Review of feline pancreatitis, part two: clinical signs, diagnosis and treatment. J Feline Med Surg 2001b; 3: 125-132.

Marchesini G, Fabbri A, Bianchi G, et al. Zinc-supplementation and amino-acid-nitrogen metabolism in patients with advanced cirrhosis. Hepatology 1996; 23: 1084-1092.

Marks SL, Rogers QR, Strombeck DR. Nutritional support in hepatic disease. Part I. Metabolic alterations and nutritional considerations in dogs and cats. Comp Cont Educ Pract Vet (Small Anim) 1994; 971-978.

Marik PE, Zatoga GP. Meta-analysis of parenteral nutrition versus enteral nutrition in patients with acute pancreatitis. BMJ 2004; 328: 1407.

Meertens NM, Bokhove CA, van den Ingh TS. Copper-associated chronic hepatitis and cirrhosis in a European Shorthair cat. Vet Pathol 2005; 42: 97-100.

Michel KE. Nutritional management of liver disease. Vet Clin North Am Small Anim Pract 1995; 25: 485-501.

Newell SM, Selcer BA, Girard E, et al. Correlations between ultrasonographic findings and specific hepatic diseases in cats: 72 cases (1985-1997). J Am Vet Med Assoc 1998; 213: 94-98.

Nicholson BT, Center SA, Randolph JF, et al. Effects of oral ursodesoxycholic acid in healthy cats on clinicopathological parameters, serum bile acids and light microscopic and ultrastructural features of the liver. Res Vet Sci 1996; 61: 258-262.

Perry LA, Williams DA, Pidgeon G, et al. Exocrine pancreatic insufficiency with associated coagulopathy in a cat. J Am Anim Hosp Assoc 1991; 27: 109-114.

Remillard RL, Saker KE. Nutritional management of hepatic conditions. In: Ettinger SJ, Feldman EC, eds. Textbook of Veterinary Internal Medicine Diseases of the Dog and Cat. 6th edition. Philadelphia: WB Saunders Co, 2005; 574-577.

Ruaux CG, Steiner JM, Williams DA. Early biochemical and clinical responses to cobalamin supplementation in cats with signs of gastrointestinal disease and severe hypocobalaminemia. J Vet Intern Med 2005; 19: 155 – 160.

Scherk M, Center SA. Toxic, metabolic, infectious, and neoplastic liver diseases. In: Ettinger SJ, Feldman EC, eds. Textbook of Veterinary Internal Medicine Diseases of the Dog and Cat. 6th edition. Philadelphia: WB Saunders Co, 2005; 1464-1477.

Schulz HU, Niederau C, Klonowski-Stumpe H, et al. Oxidative stress in acute pancreatitis. Hepatogastroenterology 1999; 46: 2736-2750

Schunk CM. Feline portosystemic shunts. Semin Vet Med Surg (Small Anim) 1997; 12: 45-50.

Seaman RL. Exocrine pancreatic neoplasia in the cat: a case series. J Am Anim Hosp Assoc 2004; 40: 238-245

Simpson KW. Feline pancreatitis. Waltham Focus 2005; 15:13-19

Simpson KW, Fyfe J, Cornetta A, et al. Subnormal concentrations of serum cobalamin (Vitamin B$_{12}$) in cats with gastrointestinal disease. J Vet Int Med 2001; 15: 26-32.

Sokol RJ, Twedt DJ, McKim J, et al. Oxidant injury to hepatic mitochondria in patients with Wilson's disease and Bedlington terriers with copper toxicosis. Gastroenterology 1994; 107: 1788-1798

Sokol RJ. Fat-soluble vitamins and their importance in patients with cholestatic liver disease. Pediatr Gastroenterol 1994; 23: 673-705.

Steiner JM. Diagnosis of pancreatitis. Vet Clin North Am Small Anim Pract 2003; 33: 1181-1195.

Steiner JM, Williams DA. Feline exocrine pancreatic disorders. Vet Clin North Am Sm Anim Pract 1999; 29: 551-574.

Steiner JM, Williams DA. Serum feline trypsin-like immunoreactivity in cats with exocrine pancreatic insufficiency. J Vet Intern Med 2000; 14: 627-629.

Steiner JM, Williams DA. Feline exocrine pancreatic disease. In: Ettinger SJ, Feldman EC, eds. Textbook of Veterinary Internal Medicine Diseases of the Dog and Cat. 6th edition. Philadelphia: WB Saunders Co, 2005; 1489-1495.

Steiner JM, Wilson BG, Williams DA. Development and analytical validation of a radioimmunoassay for the measurement of feline pancreatic lipase immunoreactivity in serum. Can J Vet Res 2004; 68: 309-314.

Suzuki A, Mizumoto A, Rerknimitz R, et al. Effect of bacterial or porcine lipase with low fat or high fat diets on nutrient absorption in pancreatic-insufficient dogs. Gastroenterology 1999; 116: 431-437.

Swift NC, Marks SL, MacLachlan J, et al. Evaluation of serum feline trypsin-like immunoreactivity for the diagnosis of pancreatitis in cats. J Am Vet Med Assoc 2000; 217: 37-42.

Tillson DM, Winkler JT. Diagnosis and treatment of portosystemic shunts in the cat. Vet Clin North Am Small Anim Pract 2002; 32: 881-899.

Trainor D, Center SA, Randolph F, et al. Urine sulfated and nonsulfated bile acids as a diagnostic test for liver disease in cats. J Vet Intern Med 2003; 17: 145-153.

Van der Linde-Sipman JS, Niewold TA, Tooten PCJ, et al. Generalized AA-amyloidosis in Siamese and Oriental cats. Vet Immunol Immunopath 1997; 56: 1-10.

Wang KY, Panciera DL, Al-Rukibat RK, et al. Accuracy of ultrasound-guided fine-needle aspiration of the liver and cytologic findings in dogs and cats: 97 cases (1990 – 2000). J Am Vet Med Assoc 2004; 224: 75-78.

Webster CRL. New insights into the cytoprotective action of ursodeoxycholate, in Proceedings. ACVIM Forum 2006; 639-641.

Weiss DJ, Gagne J, Armstrong PJ. Inflammatory liver diseases in cats. Comp Cont Educ 2001; 23: 364-373.

Weiss DJ, Gagne JM, Armstrong PJ. Relationship between inflammatory hepatic disease and inflammatory bowel disease, pancreatitis, and nephritis in cats. J Am Vet Med Assoc 1996; 209: 1114-1116.

Whittemore JC, Campbell VL. Canine and feline pancreatitis. Comp Cont Educ Pract Vet (Small Anim) 2005; 766-776.

Williams DA. Diseases of the exocrine pancreas. BSAVA Manual of canine and feline gastroenterology. 2nd edition, 2005: 222-239.

WSAVA Liver Standardization Group. Morphological classification of biliary disorders of the canine and feline liver. In: Rothuizen J, Bunch SE, Charles JA, eds. WSAVA Standards for Clinical and Histological Diagnosis of Canine and Feline Liver Disease. Philadelphia: WB Saunders Co, 2006.

Zoran DL. The carnivore connection to nutrition in cats. J Am Vet Med Assoc 2002; 221: 1559 – 1567.

Zoran DL. Pancreatitis in cats: diagnosis and management of a challenging disease. J Am Anim Hosp Assoc 2006; 42: 1-9.

Focus on:

Vitamin B₁₂ (cobalamin)

Definition and origins

The anti-anemic qualities of calf liver were first discovered in 1925. They were linked to the existence of an "extrinsic dietary factor", which was only isolated mid-century. Given the name vitamin B_{12} or cobalamin, this substance is mainly found in animal products (fish, meat and offal). Whatever the source, vitamin B_{12} is always synthesized by microorganisms. It is very stable during the heat treatment of food products.

Formula

Vitamin B_{12} is the only vitamin to incorporate a mineral element in its chemical formula, namely cobalt.

The molecule's nucleus is a tetrapyrrole with a central cobalt atom, linked to 4 pyrrolic nitrogen atoms, 1 ribonucleotide and 1 anionic ligand (X). There are several types of cobalamin, depending on the nature of the ligand, including:

X = CN (cyanide): cyanocobalamin

X = CH3 (methyl): methylcobalamin

X = OH (hydroxyl): hydroxocobalamin

X = 5'dAd (5'deoxyadenosyl): adenosylcobalamin

In cats, cobalamin is mainly found in the form of hydroxocobalamin and adenosyl cobalamin.

Biological roles

Cobalamin plays an essential role in the synthesis of nucleic acids (in synergy with folic acid). A deficiency disrupts protein synthesis, especially for fast-regenerating tissues like hematopoietic tissue.

Risk of vitamin B₁₂ deficiency in cats

A fall in the body's cobalamin reserves is seen in cats suffering from pancreatic or hepatic disease.

The depletion of reserves may be explained by chronic dysorexia or intestinal malabsorption reducing the quantity of cobalamin available to the animal. The deficiency may also be secondary to an insufficiency of intrinsic factor essential to the absorption of cobalamin. In cats, this glycoprotein is synthesized only by the pancreas, so pancreatic disease is a risk factor for deficiency. Any imbalance in the intestinal bacterial flora is also likely to reduce the absorption of cobalamin, as intestinal bacteria use vitamin B_{12} and may also form connections to intrinsic factor.

Cobalamin supplementation

Cats are not able to store large quantities of cobalamin in the body and quickly become deficient when their homeostasis is disrupted. Supplementation of vitamin B_{12} is essential in the event of pancreatic or hepatic disease. It is also indicated when an underlying intestinal disease is suspected. Because of the above assimilation problems, oral supplementation is ineffective, so parenteral administration is required.

The plasma concentration of cobalamin should be measured prior to initiating supplementation. It is generally recommended to first administer 250-500 µg/kg (on average 1000 µg / cat) SC. Depending on the cobalamin plasma concentration, this dose may be repeated every two to three weeks until the plasma cobalamin concentation normalizes. The benefit of long-term supplementation should be evaluated on the basis of the underlying disease and the response to treatment.

The potential toxicity of large cobalamin doses administered to cats has not been addressed in any publications.

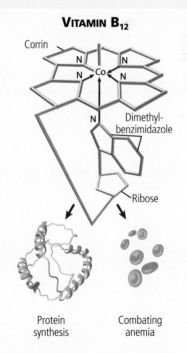

VITAMIN B₁₂

Corrin

Co

Dimethyl-benzimidazole

Ribose

Protein synthesis

Combating anemia

Feline idiopathic hepatic lipidosis

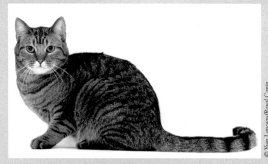

Feline hepatic lipidosis is characterized by the excessive accumulation of hepatic lipids (triglycerides).
When associated with other pathologies (e.g. diabetes mellitus, renal insufficiency, chronic enteritis)
it is qualified as secondary, otherwise it is known as idiopathic hepatic lipdosis (IHL).

Epidemiology

Cats suffering from hepatic lipidosis are generally aged 4-12 years. No particular breed appears to be predisposed, but IHL is most common in neutered cats.

Most cases of IHL are observed after prolonged fasting (4-7 weeks) in cats that were previously obese, although most have already lost at least 30% of their body weight by the time they are taken to the veterinarian. The trigger for anorexia is yet to be identified. Stress factors that should be considered are moving, vacation, arrival of another cat or a baby in the home and poorly palatable food. IHL is said to be more common in cats that live in a group than in those that live alone. IHL "epidemics" are not uncommon in cat colonies in the event of a change of environment or food.

Pathophysiology

Contrary to the process in humans, obesity does not lead to hepatic lipidosis in cats. Some endocrine and/or nutritional imbalances – diabetes mellitus, hyperthyroidism, choline and essential amino acid deficiency, energy overdose during parenteral feeding and a severe diet – do however induce lipidosis in cats. In these situations, lipidosis is generally moderate and does not lead to clinical signs.

The pathophysiological mechanisms responsible for the accumulation of hepatic lipids during prolonged fasting in cats have not yet been fully described (**Figure 1**). This observation constitutes a metabolic particularity in cats, as fasting and hepatic lipidosis are not associated in humans, dogs or rats. In cats, the lipids accumulate from the beginning of the period of fasting (**Figure 2**), but the clinical [anorexia,

---

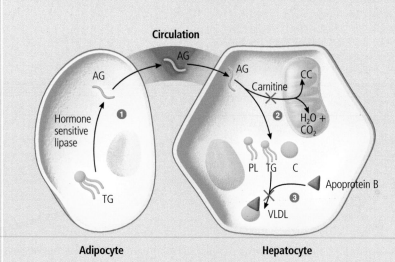

FIGURE 1 - PATHOPHYSIOLOGICAL MECHANISMS INVOLVED IN HEPATIC LIPIDOSIS

FA: fatty acid
C: cholesterol
K: ketones
GH: growth hormone
PL: phospholipids
TG: triglycerides
VLDL: very low density lipoprotein

Metabolic alterations responsible for the accumulation of hepatic lipids might be the result of:
- excessive mobilization of peripheral lipids (1)
- inhibition of fatty acid oxidation (2)
- inhibition of the synthesis and/or transport of lipoproteins (3).

FIGURE 2 - HEPATIC BIOPSIES (AS SEEN WITH AN ELECTRONIC MICROSCOPE)

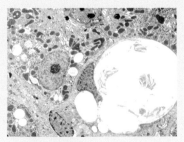
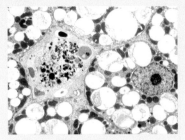
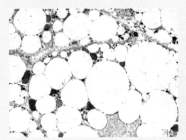

Obese cat. Presence of small vacuoles in the hepatic parenchyma and of a larger vacuole in an endothelial cell.

After 2 weeks of fasting: severe hepatic lipidosis.

After 6 weeks of fasting: very severe hepatic lipidosis. The cell is filled and the nucleus is compressed by the accumulation of intracellular lipid vacuoles.

It is important to note that such histological pictures can be observed in cats who do not present any clinical sign of hepatic lipidosis.

muscular atrophy] and biochemical signs [elevated hepatic enzymes and serum bilirubin (Figure 3)] only appear when the lipidosis becomes very severe.

A preliminary work suggests that cats are not able to efficiently save protein during prolonged fasting. It is therefore possible that the deficiency of one or more indispensable amino acids causes dysfunction in hepatic lipid metabolism, leading to pathological lipidosis.

These observations suggest prudence with respect to a low-calorie diet for cats. Veterinarians must advise owners to make sure their cat actually consumes the recommended food. In case of doubt, the measurement of alkaline phosphatase in the serum can be used as a marker of hepatic lipidosis (Figure 4).

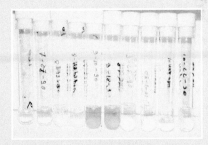

Figure 3 - Hyperbilirubinémie visible. L'évolution de la couleur du sérum a lieu brutalement lors de lipidose hépatique: la transformation se produit environ 3 semaines après le début de la hausse des phosphatases alcalines.

FIGURE 4 - SERUM CONCENTRATIONS OF ALKALINE PHOSPHATASE

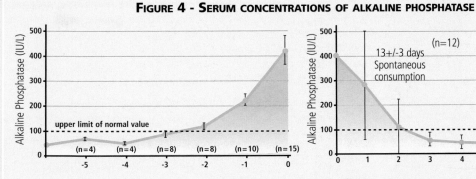
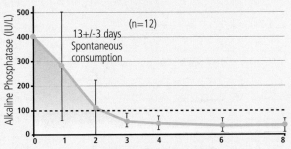

4A - Before the appearance of hyperbilirubinemia (week 0) in anorectic cats. The concentration of alkaline phosphatase is a marker of hepatic lipidosis.

4B - After re-feeding of cats suffering from hepatic lipidosis. The concentration of alkaline phosphatase improves dramatically after 2 weeks and returns to normal within 3 weeks after cats have started to eat again.

ROYAL CANIN

Dietary recommendations

Aggressive nutritional support is the treatment of choice. Our own observations as well as those of other authors show that a highly digestible complete food that respects the following nutritional balances would appear to be appropriate:

- 30-50% calories from protein

- 35-50% calories from fat

- 20-30% calories from carbohydrate

Cats with IHL are glucose-intolerant and preparations rich in rapidly assimilated carbohydrates present a risk of hyperglycemia. In the event of hepatic encephalopathy, limiting the protein content to 20-25% of calories is recommended.

The supplementation of certain nutrients (choline, arginine, citrulline, taurine, thiamine, vitamin C and zinc) has been recommended for the nutritional treatment of IHL. The efficacy of these supplements has not been scientifically demonstrated.

A properly balanced nutritional diet will reduce the bilirubin and the serum hepatic enzymes within 1-2 weeks. They typically return to physiological levels within 4 weeks. Most cats accept food after 2-3 weeks of enteral feeding. The liver regains its normal histological structure within 4-8 weeks.

Feeding practice

The treatment of hepatic lipidosis demands constant attention of the veterinarian. It is not uncommon for the clinical signs to appear to worsen at the start of treatment. It is important to monitor the potassium concentration and reintroduce the cat to food very gradually.

Type of food

Cats with IHL require assisted feeding. A nasoesophageal enteral feeding tube is a cost-effective, rapid and safe way to administer liquid nutrition or wet food homogenized with water. Tube placement requires local anesthesia without expensive equipment. In our experience, it does not prevent cats from eating normally. If the food is not liquid enough, nutritional assistance may be provided via the placement of a gastric or esophageal enteral feeding tube.

It is vital that the cat continues to be fed through vomiting or diarrhea, which are both common during the first week. If the digestive problems are uncontrollable, temporary parenteral feeding may be initiated.

Rationing

During the first day of hospitalization, it is recommended to feed the cat four times at intervals of at least three hours and to limit the serving to 25 mL. Over the following days, increase the serving by multiples of 5 mL until the cat is consuming 60 kcal/kg body weight/day. This will generally be achieved within 5-7 days. Increasing the serving very gradually limits vomiting and diarrhea. After ten days, meal frequency should be reduced to three times per day. If given time to adapt, cats will comfortably tolerate up to 120 ml per serving.

Preventing food aversion

Cats are likely to refuse to eat a food they associate with digestive disorders (nausea, vomiting) that appear during the consumption period. This type of food aversion appears to be a major component in the anorexia associated with hepatic lipidosis.

Recommendations to reduce the risk of food aversion:

- Do not offer multiple types of food to confirm the anorexia

- Use exclusively a feeding tube throughout the period of assisted feeding during the first 10-15 days of treatment

- After 10-15 days of treatment, propose a diet that the cat has not consumed since it has been sick. Don't insist if the cat does not eat immediatly. Repeat the operation after 48 hours until the cat feels like eating spontaneously.

Conclusion

The prognosis of IHL has greatly improved since the recognition of the importance of nutritional support in its treatment. It is nevertheless more reserved when the hepatic lipidosis is complicated by another underlying disease (e.g. chronic gastroenteritis, chronic kidney disease etc.).

FEEDING PROTOCOL DURING THE FIRST WEEK OF TREATMENT

- **Day 1:**
  - 25-50% of MER
  - 20-25 mL/serving, 4 servings/day

- **From day 5-7:**
  - Up to 100% of MER (60-80 kcal/kg)
  - Up to 120 mL/serving, 3-4 servings/day

ROYAL CANIN

References

Barsanti JA, Jones BD, Spano JS, et al. Prolonged anorexia associated with hepatic lipidosis in three cats. Feline Pract 1977; 7: 52-57.

Biourge VC. Feline hepatic lipidosis: characterization of a model. PhD Dissertation. University of California, Davis, 1993.

Biourge VC, Groff JM, Fisher C, et al. Nitrogen balance, plasma free amino-acid concentrations and urinary orotic acid excretion during long term voluntary fasting in cats. J Nutr 1994; 124: 1094-1103.

Biourge VC, Groff JM, Munn R, et al. Experimental induction of feline hepatic lipidosis. Am J Vet Res 1994; 55: 1291-1302.

Biourge VC, Massat B, Groff JM, et al. Effect of protein, lipid, or carbohydrate supplementation on hepatic lipid accumulation during rapid weight loss in obese cats. Am J Vet Res 1994; 55: 1406-1415.

Center SA, Crawford MA, Guida L, et al. A retrospective study of 77 cats with severe hepatic lipidosis: 1975-1990. J Vet Int Med 1993; 7: 349-359.

Center SA, Guida L, Zanelli MJ, et al. Ultrastructural hepatocellular features associated with severe hepatic lipidosis in cats. Am J Vet Res 1993; 5: 724-731.

Jacobs G, Cornelius L, Allen S, et al. Treatment of idiopathic hepatic lipidosis in cats: 11 cases (1986-1987). J Am Vet Med Assoc 1989; 195: 635-638.

Jacobs G, Cornelius L, Keene B, et al. Comparison of plasma, liver, and skeletal muscle carnitine concentrations in cats with idiopathic hepatic lipidosis and in healthy cats. Am J Vet Res 1990; 51: 1349-1351.

National Research Council of the National Academies. Nutrient requirements of dogs and cats; Vitamins: 225-227. The National Academies Press, 2006; Washington DC.

Ruaux CG, Steiner JM, Williams DA. Early biochemical and clinical responses to cobalamin supplementation in cats with signs of gastrointestinal disease and severe hypocobalaminemia. J Vet Intern Med 2005; 19: 155-160.

Ruaux CG, Steiner JM, Williams DA. Metabolism of amino-acids in cats with severe cobalamin deficiency. Am J Vet Res 2001; 62: 1852- 1858.

Simpson KW, Fyfe J, Cornetta A, et al. Subnormal concentrations of serum cobalamin (Vitamin B12) in cats with gastrointestinal disease. J Vet Int Med 2001; 15: 26-32.

Liver/Pancreas

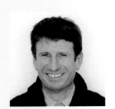

Thomas A. LUTZ
DVM, PhD

Feline diabetes mellitus: nutritional strategies

1 - Prevalence of feline diabetes mellitus 183

2 - Clinical findings 184

3 - Specifics of feline metabolism 184

4 - Classification of diabetes mellitus 185

5 - Introduction to feline diabetes mellitus 186

6 - Physiological aspects of nutrient handling 187

7 - Pathophysiology of feline diabetes mellitus 189

8 - Transient diabetes mellitus 199

9 - Long-term consequences of diabetes mellitus 200

10 - Diagnosis of feline diabetes mellitus 201

11 - Treatment strategies 204

12 - Dietary aspects in the treatment of feline diabetes mellitus 206

13 - Potential problems of high protein, low carbohydrate diets 211

14 - Practical recommendations to feed the diabetic cat 211

Conclusion 212

Frequently asked questions 213

References 214

Royal Canin nutritional information 218

Diabetes

ABBREVIATIONS USED IN THIS CHAPTER		
AST: arginine stimulation test	**GLUT 1, 2 or 4**: glucose transporter type 1, 2, or 4	**NIDDM**: non-insulin-dependent diabetes mellitus
BID: twice daily		
DM: diabetes mellitus	**GST**: glucagon stimulation test	**PPAR** γ: peroxisome proliferator-activated receptor gamma
1DM: type 1 diabetes mellitus	**IAPP**: islet amyloid polypeptide	
2DM: type 2 diabetes mellitus	**IDDM**: insulin-dependent diabetes mellitus	**PUFA**: polyunsaturated fatty acid
DMB: dry matter basis	**IGF-1**: insulin-like growth factor 1	**PUFA n-3**: omega-3 polyunsaturated fatty acid
GIP: glucose-dependent insulinotropic peptide, or gastric inhibitory polypeptide	**IL-1β**: interleukin beta	**TDF**: total dietary fiber
	IVGTT: intravenous glucose tolerance test	**TFA**: trans-fatty acid
GK: glucokinase	**IST**: insulin stimulation test	**TNF-α**: tumor necrosis factor alpha
GLP-1: glucagon-like peptide-1	**NEFA**: non-esterified fatty acid	

Feline diabetes mellitus: nutritional strategies

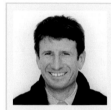

Thomas A. LUTZ
DVM, PhD

Thomas Lutz graduated from the Veterinary School of the Free University in Berlin (FRG) in 1989. He received a first doctoral degree (Dr. med. vet.) at the Institute of Veterinary Physiology from the University of Zurich, in 1991. In 1995, he completed his PhD in feline diabetes mellitus at the University of Queensland (Brisbane, Australia) and in 1999 his Habilitation at the Institute of Veterinary Physiology in Zurich. Since 2004, he is a Professor of Applied Veterinary Physiology in Zurich. His major research areas are the neuroendocrine controls of food intake and feline diabetes mellitus. He has published over 80 scientific articles in peer-reviewed journals.

*D*iabetes mellitus is a common endocrinopathy in cats. Its prevalence has risen over the last 30 years and on average reaches around 1 case per 200 cats. This increase may be directly related to the higher prevalence of obesity in cats. Feline diabetes shares many features of human type 2 diabetes (2DM) in respect to its pathophysiology, underlying risk factors and treatment strategies. General recommendations for feeding diabetic cats has changed over the last few years and now the focus is on diets relatively high in dietary protein and low in carbohydrate. It is clear that not all authors have the same understanding of the composition of high protein or low carbohydrate diets. As a general rule, these terms refer to a protein content (on DMB) of approximately 50% protein or more, and less than 15% carbohydrates. The values will be specified in the chapter when necessary. This high protein, low carbohydrate feeding regimen, combined with rigid and well supervised insulin therapy has resulted in a sharp increase in the remission rate of diabetes mellitus. The present chapter reviews the pathophysiology of feline diabetes and discusses treatment strategies, especially in light of the cats' specific nutrient requirements and the recommended use of high protein, low carbohydrate diets.

Diabetes

1-Prevalence of feline diabetes mellitus

Diabetes mellitus (DM) is a common endocrinopathy in cats. Its prevalence has been reported to be in a range of approximately 1:400 to 1:100 (*Panciera et al, 1990; Rand et al, 1997*). Based on the number of cases presented to veterinary teaching hospitals, a retrospective study showed that the prevalence of feline diabetes increased by a factor of more than 10 over the last 30 years. While in 1970, less than 1 case in 1000 cats was reported, this number increased to more than 12 cases per 1000 cats in 1999 (*Prahl et al, 2003; 2007*). At the same time, however, the fatality rate decreased markedly from over 40% to less than 10% indicating that diabetic cats can be successfully treated. Part of this is certainly due to the better understanding of the pathophysiology of feline diabetes. Important risk factors for the development of the disease are age, gender, neuter status and obesity (**Table 1**).

► Feline diabetes mellitus is associated with obesity

The latter factor is most likely responsible for today's increased prevalence of feline DM because feline obesity is directly associated with insulin resistance (*Scarlett et al, 1994; Hoenig, 2006a; 2007a; see also Pathophysiology of feline diabetes*), and obesity in cats is much more common in today's cat population: at least 20% but more likely 35-40% of cats are considered overweight or obese (*Baral et al, 2003; Lund et al, 2005; Diez & Nguyen, 2006; German, 2006*).

TABLE 1 - RISK FACTORS FOR THE DEVELOPMENT OF DIABETES MELLITUS IN CATS *(Nelson, 2005; Rand & Marshall, 2005; McCann et al, 2007)*	
Age	feline DM occurs more often in old cats
Gender	male cats are affected more often than female cats
Neutering	no independent risk factor, but neutered cats have higher risk to develop obesity
Obesity	increased risk of developing DM in obese cats
Physical activity	feline DM occurs more often in physically inactive cats
Breed	Burmese breed?
Drug treatment	megestrol acetate, glucocorticosteroids
Underlying disease	systemic infection, stomatitis

► Influence of age

Feline DM usually affects middle-aged and older cats with a sharp increase beyond the age of 7 years. Cats below 1 year of age are 50 times less likely to develop diabetes than cats beyond the age of 10 years (*Prahl et al, 2003*).

► Influence of gender and neutering

Male cats seem to be at higher risk of developing diabetes than females. While this situation is similar in humans at least before the average age of menopause, the reason for the gender difference in feline diabetes is unknown at present. The difference seems unlikely to be directly related to the concentration of sexual hormones because most male cats are castrated, and because neutering is not an independent risk factor for the development of diabetes when controlling for body weight (BW) and age (*Prahl et al, 2003*).

► Breed differences

Only a few studies have investigated the possible breed differences in the prevalence of feline diabetes. While a retrospective study in the USA provided no evidence for a higher prevalence in certain breeds of cats with purebred cats actually being at lower risk than mixed breed cats (*Prahl et al, 2003*), some studies performed in Australia reported a higher prevalence among Burmese cats (*Rand et al, 1997*) (**Figure 1**). A similar predisposition was reported from the United Kingdom (UK; *McCann et al, 2007*). The author is unaware of further studies so that it remains unclear

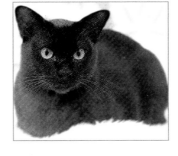

Figure 1 - Burmese Cat.
An Australian study and a study from the UK report that Burmese cats have a genetic predisposition to develop diabetes mellitus (Rand et al, 1997; McCann et al, 2007). However, global breed predispositions are still disputed.

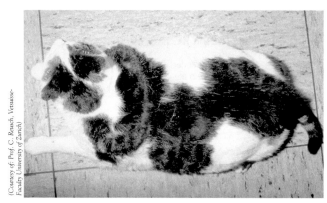

Figure 2 - Obese (10 kg) 11-year old cat with DM.
The risk of diabetes mellitus is increased in obese cats.

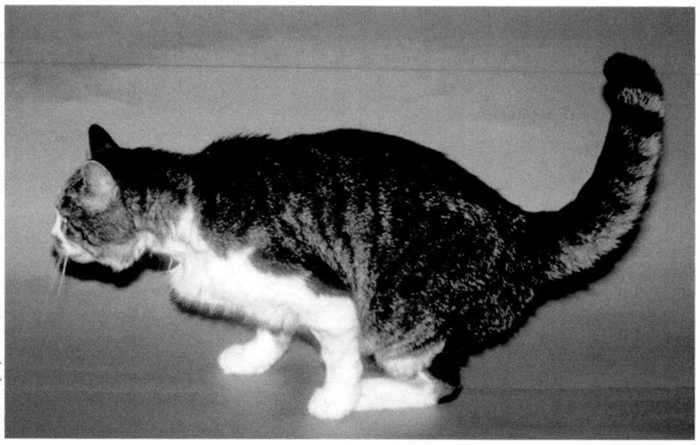

(Courtesy of: Prof. C. Reusch, Vetsuisse-Faculty University of Zurich)

Figure 3 - Neuropathy in a diabetic cat resulting in plantigrade stance. *A plantigrade stance is a typical clinical sign in indicating diabetic neuropathy.*

(Courtesy of: Prof. C. Reusch, Vetsuisse-Faculty University of Zurich).

whether the reported over representation of Burmese cats in Australia and the UK is a global phenomenon.

2 - Clinical findings
(see also: Nelson, 2005)

Most diabetic cats are older than 7 years of age. The classical symptoms are osmotic polyuria which develops subsequent to hyperglycemia, secondary polydipsia and often polyphagia. A large proportion of diabetic cats are overweight at the time of diagnosis (**Figure 2**). Loss of body weight, despite hyperphagia, may occur, but cats are usually still overweight at the time of presentation. Diabetic cats are rarely emaciated when they are first presented to veterinarians.

Due to dehydration, some diabetic cats may be lethargic. Diabetic neuropathy can lead to rear limb weakness and plantigrade gait (**Figure 3**). Rear limb muscle atrophy may be present. Hepatic lipidosis can lead to hepatomegaly. As further complications, diabetic cats may suffer from infection such as stomatitis or cystitis.

3 - Specifics of feline metabolism

▶ Adaptation to a carnivorous diet

The cat is a true carnivore which distinguishes it clearly from the omnivorous dog. The natural diet of wild felids, e.g. mice, contains approximately 70-80% water. On a dry matter basis (on DMB), it contains about 55-60% of protein, 35% of fat, but less than 10% carbohydrate. This is very different from many commonly used commercial dry cat

FIGURE 4A - LACK OF POSTPRANDIAL HYPERGLYCEMIA IN CATS FED A HIGH PROTEIN DIET (54% PROTEIN AND 8% CARBOHYDRATE ON DMB)

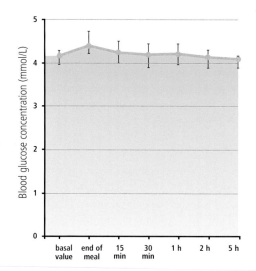

After 24h of fasting, cats were given access to a test meal corresponding to 50% of their normal daily intake. The test meal was offered for 10 minutes during which time all food offered was consumed. The blood glucose concentration in 10 healthy experimental cats just before and after presentation of the test meal is shown.

foods which contain a much higher percentage of carbohydrates, mainly represented by starch from cereals, even if a high digestible dry catfood should not contain more than 40% carbohydrates on DMB. Cats fed a high protein diet (54% on DMB) did not show postprandial hyperglycemia (*Martin & Rand, 1999*) (see also **Figure 4 A & B**), unless relatively high amounts of simple sugars were added **(Figure 4 B)**. This may be one of several reasons why diets high in protein, i.e. near-natural diets, have beneficial effects in controlling nutrient metabolism in diabetic cats (see below).

Cats have a generally high demand for essential amino acids. Arginine and taurine are essential in cats. It has been argued that taurine deficiency may be a causal factor contributing to DM. However the potential usefulness of taurine to prevent or reduce diabetic retinopathy or neuropathy (reviewed in *Franconi et al, 2006*) should not be taken as evidence for a causal relationship. Currently no experimental evidence is available that would suggest such a link in cats.

▶ Intensive gluconeogenesis

In cats, gluconeogenesis from amino acids is not downregulated even if protein intake is deficient (*Rogers et al, 1977*).

The activity of gluconeogenic enzymes is much higher in cats than in dogs (*Washizu et al, 1998; Washizu et al, 1999; Takeguchi et al, 2005*). On the other hand, cats seem to be deficient in hepatic glucokinase (GK) function due to low hepatic GK expression or enzymatic activity (*Washizu et al, 1999; Schermerhorn, 2005; Tanaka et al, 2005; but see section on pancreatic glucose sensing in cats via GK*). However, regulation of GK activity in cats seems to differ from other species because cats have a very low activity in GK regulating protein (*Schermerhorn, 2005*) which in other species would be associated with high GK activity. The activity of other glycolytic key enzymes, including hexokinase which can perhaps partly compensate for low GK activity, is higher in cats than in dogs (*Washizu et al, 1999*).

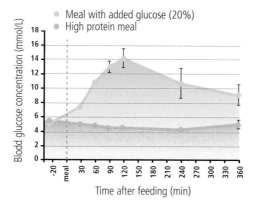

FIGURE 4B - INFLUENCE OF THE DIET ON POSTPRANDIAL HYPERGLYCEMIA IN 12 CATS

● Meal with added glucose (20%)
● High protein meal

Postprandial hyperglycemia does not occur when cats are fed a high protein diet (54% protein and 8% carbohydrate on DMB), unless high amounts of glucose are added (20% per weight).

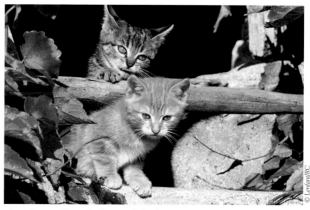

As a direct effect of a low carbohydrate intake under natural feeding conditions, cats have developed a high capacity for intensive gluconeogenesis from glucogenic amino acids.

4 - Classification of diabetes mellitus

Different terminology has been used to describe the different forms of diabetes mellitus in humans and other species. The following terminology, based on the underlying pathophysiology, will be used throughout this chapter. Primary diabetes mellitus can be subdivided into type 1 diabetes mellitus (1DM) and type 2 diabetes (2DM) **(Table 2)**.

In humans, these were formerly also named juvenile and adult-onset diabetes, respectively. However, due to the massive increase in childhood obesity, up to 50% of diabetic children now suffer from 2DM compared to only 5-10% as observed previously. Therefore, the terms of juvenile or adult-onset diabetes should no longer be used.

Insulin-dependent (IDDM) and non-insulin-dependent diabetes mellitus (NIDDM) are purely descriptive terms which define the necessity of a diabetic human or animal to be treated with insulin to achieve metabolic control. The underlying pathophysiology is not reflected in these terms and will therefore not be used here.

The most common type of feline DM is pathophysiologically similar to 2DM in humans (for review, see *Henson & O'Brien, 2006*) and will be described in the following paragraph. Even though

TABLE 2 - CLASSIFICATION OF FELINE DIABETES MELLITUS

Type of DM			Occurrence in cats	Major defects
Primary DM	Type 1 DM (1DM)		rare	autoimmune mediated destruction of pancreatic beta-cells
	Type 2 DM (2DM)		at least 90% of cases	disturbed beta-cell function insulin resistance pancreatic islet amyloid
Other causes of DM (formerly called secondary DM)	Antagonistic disease	Infection	approx. 10% of cases	insulin resistance
		Pancreatitis, pancreatic tumor		destruction of functional beta-cells
		Acromegaly		insulin antagonistic effect of GH
	Steroid-induced			e.g. cats treated with progesterone derivatives (megestrol acetate)

DM = diabetes mellitus GH = growth hormone

histological changes in pancreatic islets suggestive of a 1DM like syndrome have been described in cats (*Nakayama et al, 1990*), this seems to be an uncommon finding. Further, cats do not develop autoantibodies against beta-cell antigens or insulin (*Hoenig et al, 2000*), arguing against an autoimmune-induced form of diabetes typical for 1DM. Finally, it is now recognized that the pathophysiology of 2DM also involves inflammatory, immune-mediated processes (*Donath et al, 2005*). Therefore, the presence of inflammatory processes does not exclude a 2DM like pathophysiology.

5 - Introduction to feline diabetes mellitus

▶ Major defects in feline diabetes mellitus

Feline diabetes and human 2DM are pathophysiologically comparable endocrinopathies. When necessary for the understanding of underlying disturbances, reference to data from experimental models, mostly from rodents, will be made in this chapter.

The major defects in diabetic cats and 2DM humans are:
- insulin resistance resulting in disturbed utilization of nutrients in insulin-sensitive tissues.
- disturbed pancreatic beta-cell function, resulting in the abnormal release and lack of insulin and amylin.
- deposition of pancreatic islet amyloid resulting from precipitation of amylin (islet amyloid polypeptide) **(Figure 5).**

Further defects will also be discussed in this paragraph. It is still debated whether the primary defect in 2DM or feline diabetes is disturbed beta-cell function or impaired insulin action. However, at the time of diagnosis both defects are usually present and contribute to the deterioration of the metabolic situation. Due to glucotoxicity, both defects also contribute to the self-perpetuation of the disease that usually can be observed.

▶ Genetics and feline diabetes mellitus

In human 2DM, genetics determining the predisposition of individuals to the development of 2DM are an area of intensive research. Several mutations and gene polymorphisms have been identified which are linked to an increased risk to develop 2DM in certain diabetic patients (for review, see e.g. *Barroso, 2005; Malecki, 2005*). However, it is clear that the massive increase in the occurrence of human 2DM is not the result of a major change in the genetic background but rather the result of life style changes such as abundance of food and lack of physical activity that make us more vulnerable to the development of obesity and subsequently 2DM. Hence, a previously beneficial genetic background may have deleterious effects in today's life.

FIGURE 5 - MAJOR PHYSIOLOGICAL DISTURBANCES IN FELINE DIABETES MELLITUS

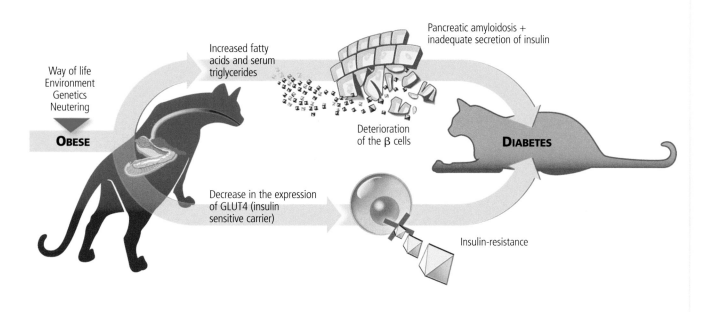

Way of life
Environment
Genetics
Neutering

OBESE

Increased fatty acids and serum triglycerides

Pancreatic amyloidosis + inadequate secretion of insulin

Deterioration of the β cells

DIABETES

Decrease in the expression of GLUT4 (insulin sensitive carrier)

Insulin-resistance

Studies on a possible role of genetic factors in the development of feline diabetes are far less advanced than in humans. Some cats may have an underlying predisposition for glucose intolerance because it was found that baseline insulin levels were higher while first phase insulin response and insulin sensitivity were lower in cats that developed a more severe reduction in insulin sensitivity when gaining body weight *(Appleton et al, 2001b)*. Similar findings were reported by *Wilkins et al (2004)*. Further, at least some studies suggest a breed disposition for the development of feline DM with Burmese cats being at higher risk *(Rand et al, 1997)*. Despite these indications for a possible role of genetic factors, nothing is known about the mode of inheritance and about the nature of the genes that could possibly be affected.

6 - Physiological aspects of nutrient handling

Before discussing details of the pathophysiology of feline diabetes, a few aspects of the physiological role of the key hormonal players will be briefly summarized. In healthy animals, pancreatic insulin secretion is controlled mainly by nutrients **(Figures 6 & 7)**. Insulin action in target tissues is mediated by the insulin receptor. Binding of insulin to its receptor activates the receptor intrinsic tyrosine kinase which then triggers rapid effects (e.g., translocation of the insulin-sensitive glucose transporter GLUT4 and modification of the activity of metabolic enzymes) and delayed effects relying on influences on gene transcription. The latter are mediated by the transcription factor peroxisome proliferator-activated receptor γ (PPARγ). This transcription factor is targeted by the antidiabetic drugs thiazolidinediones which increase insulin sensitivity.

FIGURE 6 - REGULATION OF INSULIN SECRETION BY GLUCOSE IN PANCREATIC BETA-CELLS

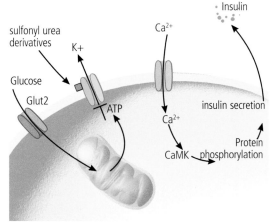

sulfonyl urea derivatives

$K+$

Ca^{2+}

Insulin

Glucose

Glut2

ATP

Ca^{2+}

CaMK

insulin secretion

Protein phosphorylation

Glucose is taken up by the beta-cells via the GLUT2 glucose transporter and subjected to metabolism via glycolysis and the Krebs cycle in mitochondria. Adenosine triphosphate (ATP) leads to closure of ATP-sensitive K+ channels which are also the target structures for sulfonylurea drugs. The resulting depolarization opens voltage-sensitive Ca²⁺ channels, Ca²⁺ influx leads to activation of Ca²⁺ dependent kinases (CaMK) and finally secretion of insulin.

FIGURE 7 - REGULATION OF INSULIN SECRETION BY AMINO ACIDS AND FATTY ACIDS IN PANCREATIC BETA-CELLS

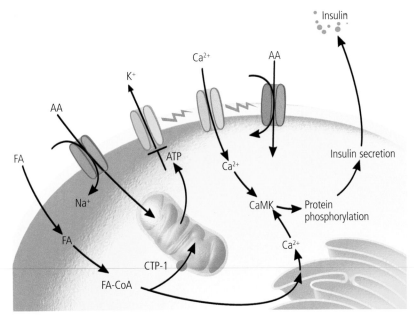

Metabolism of amino acids (AA) and fatty acids (FA) results in the formation of ATP, similar to glucose metabolism (see Figure 6). Alternatively, some amino acids, e.g. arginine, cause direct depolarization (electrogenic transport) of the beta-cell membrane and subsequent Ca²⁺ influx. Activated fatty acids (FA-CoA) can also release Ca²⁺ from intracellular Ca²⁺ stores.
CPT-1: carnitine palmitoyl transferase-1

▶ Pancreatic glucose sensing in cats

Cats given intravenous or peroral glucose loads exhibit a strong increase in insulin secretion. Similarly, intravenous administration of amino acids, such as arginine, increases insulin secretion in cats. Under natural feeding conditions, nutrient induced insulin release seems to be very efficient because postprandial hyperglycemia is absent in cats fed a high protein diet (**Figure 4**). However, the relative contribution of amino acids versus glucose in respect to the meal induced increase in circulating insulin levels is less clear. In recent years, the nutrient sensing machinery in the feline pancreas has been partly elucidated (*Schermerhorn, 2006*). Despite the low activity of hepatic glucokinase (GK), pancreatic GK is present in cats and its activity seems to be comparable to other species. GK is one of the main components of the glucose sensing mechanism (*Schuit et al, 2001*). Other essential components such as subunits of ATP-sensitive K+ channels (**Figures 6 & 7**), Kir6.2 and SUR1, have also been characterized in cats (*Schermerhorn, 2006*).

▶ Potentiation of nutrient-stimulated insulin secretion by incretins

Nutrient-stimulated insulin secretion is potentiated by incretin hormones, the most important being glucagon-like peptide-1 (GLP-1) and glucose-dependent insulinotropic polypeptide (GIP; formerly known as gastric inhibitory polypeptide). Incretins are defined as hormones that are released in response to nutrients and that potentiate nutrient-induced pancreatic insulin secretion. Due to incretin action, a given glucose load triggers a more pronounced insulin response when administered orally than parenterally (for review: *Drucker, 2001*).

In humans and laboratory rodents, GLP-1 is secreted in response to meal ingestion with blood levels rising postprandially. Part of GLP-1 secretion is due to a direct effect of luminal glucose on the ileal L-cells through a glucose sensing mechanism. It is believed, however, that nutrients also indirectly trigger the release of ileal GLP-1 because plasma GLP-1 levels rise within minutes after meal onset, i.e. long before any ingested nutrient might reach the ileum (*Drucker, 2001*). GLP-1's potent insulinotropic effect is glucose-dependent and disappears at plasma glucose levels below approximately 4.5 mmol/l (80 mg/dL). Therefore, GLP-1 usually does not induce hypoglycemia. GLP-1 acts via a potentiation of glucose-induced insulin release, most likely by an interaction at the ATP-dependent K+-channel (see above; **Figure 6**), but also through effects directly involving the secretion of insulin granula.

GLP-1 also seems to stimulate insulin biosynthesis and the synthesis of the glucose sensing machinery, mainly the GLUT2 glucose transporter and glucokinase. Finally, GLP-1 also exerts trophic effects on beta-cells and its precursors, thereby stimulating beta-cell differentiation and proliferation. This is accompanied by an inhibition of beta-cell apoptosis which seems to play a major role in the development of human 2DM (*Donath et al, 2005*) and most likely feline DM.

Similar to amylin, GLP-1 has been shown to diminish glucagon release. This effect is glucose-dependent in that GLP-1 inhibits glucagon release at euglycemic or hyperglycemic levels but not at hypoglycemic levels when glucagon's effect to defeat hypoglycemia is necessary and important.

► Pancreatic amylin

Pancreatic beta-cells are also the major source for amylin which is co-synthesized and co-secreted with insulin in response to appropriate stimuli (*Lutz & Rand, 1996*). The lack of amylin and its metabolic effects may play a role in the development of human 2DM and feline DM. These effects are unrelated to the propensity of human and feline amylin to form amyloid deposits which is another important contributing factor to feline DM (see below; *O'Brien, 2002*). At least three hormonal effects of amylin are of physiological relevance and contribute to the regulation of nutrient metabolism:
- inhibition of food intake (*Lutz, 2005*)
- modulation of pancreatic glucagon release by reducing excessive postprandial hyperglycemia (*Edelman & Weyer, 2002*)
- regulation of gastric emptying (*Edelman & Weyer, 2002*).

It should be mentioned that none of these effects has so far been confirmed in cats but their physiological relevance has clearly been shown in both humans and rodents. However, a preliminary study in healthy cats has shown that amylin may reduce circulating glucagon levels in cats (*Furrer et al, 2005*) (see also below and **Figure 16**). In humans, the amylin analogue pramlintide (Symlin[R]) is now an approved adjunct treatment to insulin for diabetic patients for its effects to reduce glucagon secretion and to inhibit gastric emptying.

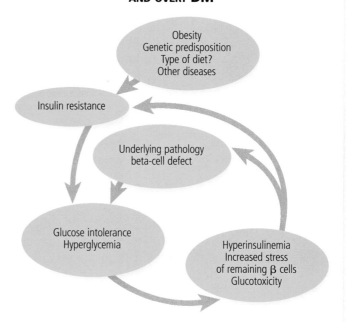

FIGURE 8 - THE VICIOUS CIRCLE OF INSULIN RESISTANCE, DEFECT IN BETA-CELL FUNCTION AND GLUCOTOXICITY, THAT EVENTUALLY LEADS TO BETA-CELL EXHAUSTION AND OVERT DM

Insulin resistance, which can be caused by obesity or genetic predisposition, and possibly beta-cell defects, that cause reduced insulin secretory capacity, lead to glucose intolerance and subsequently hyperglycemia. This causes an increased secretory demand on the remaining beta-cells. Further, glucotoxicity progressively disturbs beta-cell function and promotes insulin resistance. Eventually, the pancreatic beta-cells will fail to produce sufficient amounts of insulin leading to overt DM.

7 - Pathophysiology of feline diabetes mellitus

► Insulin resistance in feline diabetes mellitus

One of the two major metabolic hallmarks of human 2DM and feline DM, next to disturbed pancreatic beta-cell function, is insulin resistance. Insulin resistance, or lower than normal insulin sensitivity, is characterized by a reduced response of insulin target tissues to a given amount of insulin. This can be assessed via insulin-sensitive glucose uptake which is markedly reduced in insulin resistant individuals. While oversecretion of insulin may compensate at least partly for insulin resistance, measurable glucose intolerance or overt hyperglycemia will develop once hyperinsulinemia cannot be sustained, or when maintained stress on beta-cells leads to their exhaustion (**Figure 8**).

> Tests to assess insulin sensitivity

The classical clinical tests to assess insulin sensitivity and secretion are the intravenous glucose tolerance test (IVGTT; *O'Brien et al, 1985; Appleton et al, 2001a,b*) or the insulin sensitivity test (IST; *Feldhahn et al, 1999; Appleton et al, 2001a,b*). In the IVGTT, the increase in blood glucose and insulin concentrations are measured following an intravenous glucose bolus. Reported upper limits of the normal range for glucose half-life in plasma (glucose T1/2) in healthy cats are approximately 75-80 min (*Lutz and Rand, 1996; Appleton et al, 2001a,b*). In the IST, the glucose-lowering effect of insulin is assessed directly (*Appleton et al, 2001a,b*).

Glucose intolerant "pre-diabetic" and diabetic cats typically present with higher glucose concentrations in IVGTTs and with glucose T1/2 that is prolonged. Fasting insulin levels seem to be more variable because they have been reported to be elevated in some studies (*e.g., Nelson et al, 1990*) but not in others (*e.g., Lutz & Rand, 1996*).

> Mechanisms for insulin resistance

Impaired glucose tolerance in diabetic cats is the result of a reduced insulin response (*O'Brien et al, 1985*) and reduced insulin sensitivity. Insulin sensitivity in diabetic cats is approximately 6 times lower than in healthy cats (*Feldhahn et al, 1999*). The exact underlying mechanisms for insulin resistance in human 2DM and in feline DM are still unknown (*Reaven, 2005; Reusch et al, 2006b*). Similar to humans, the major cause of insulin resistance in cats is obesity and physical inactivity. Insulin sensitivity in obese cats is markedly reduced compared to lean control animals (see below).

> Factors contributing to insulin resistance

Genetic causes of receptor or post-receptor defects have not been analyzed in detail in cats, but some molecular tools have become available lately that will allow us to study some of the underlying mechanisms of peripheral insulin resistance in more detail. Most attention has been drawn to glucose transporters in insulin-sensitive tissues and to metabolically active cytokines released from adipose tissue (*e.g., Brennan et al, 2004; Hoenig et al, 2007a; Zini et al, 2006*).

Whether there is a systemic **difference in insulin sensitivity between male and female cats** is less clear. On the one hand, it has been reported that male cats have lower insulin sensitivity and higher baseline insulin concentrations than female cats (*Appleton et al, 2001a; Rand & Marshall, 2005*). The latter study was performed in lean animals which were fed a diet relatively high in carbohydrate. However, all animals, males and females, were castrated at the time of study. Therefore, it is unlikely that direct effects of sexual hormones can explain the difference in insulin sensitivity. Either early effects of sexual hormones, acting before the time of castration, or indirect effects of sexual hormones may account for these differences.

On the other hand, **obesity** is well recognized as the main risk factor to induce insulin resistance, and relative body weight (BW) gain after castration appears to occur more rapidly in females than in males (*Martin & Siliart, 2005*). This somehow contrasts to a study by Hoenig et al (*2007b*) who reported that insulin leads to increased glucose oxidation in obese castrated males while castrated females maintain greater fat oxidation in response to insulin. This metabolic gender difference was therefore supposed to favor more rapid fat accumulation in males than females, which may explain the greater risk of DM in neutered males. However, the same authors also reported that gender was not an independent risk factor in a study comparing glucose kinetics parameters between lean and obese cats (*Hoenig et al, 2007a,b*).

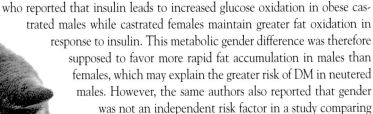

More research is needed to investigate the possible gender differences in insulin sensitivity and the development of feline DM.

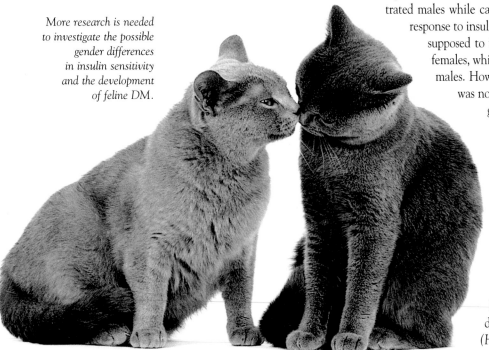

Other causes of insulin resistance include insulin antagonistic hormones, e.g. **glucocorticosteroids and progestins**, which directly counteract insulin action. Further, at least in other species, glucocorticosteroids increase food intake and may therefore contribute to the development of obesity. Presumably, they have similar effects in cats. Hyperthyroidism and growth hormone excess (acromegaly) have also been shown to reduce glucose tolerance, possibly due to the induction of peripheral insulin resistance (*Hoenig & Ferguson, 1989; Feldman & Nelson, 2004*).

FIGURE 9 - PLASMA AMYLIN AND PLASMA INSULIN CONCENTRATIONS IN CATS WITH NORMAL AND DISTURBED GLUCOSE TOLERANCE

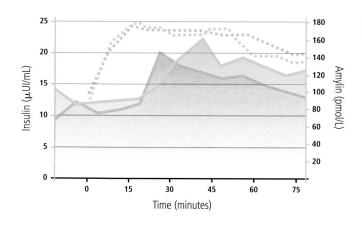

Glucose tolerant
Glucose intolerant

Glucose (1 g/kg BW) was infused intravenously and the plasma concentrations of amylin and insulin were determined by radioimmunoassay. Despite unchanged baseline amylin and insulin concentrations, the overall beta-cell secretory capacity is clearly reduced in cats with disturbed glucose tolerance. Glucose tolerant cats had glucose T1/2 below 80 min. Glucose intolerant cats had glucose T1/2 above 80 min. (See also **Figure 22**).

► Disturbed pancreatic beta-cell function

The second major hallmark of feline diabetes is disturbed beta-cell function. Typical defects are a markedly reduced or missing first phase insulin secretion and a delayed onset of second phase insulin release which mainly relies on insulin synthesis. Even though the baseline insulin concentration may be unchanged, the overall insulin secretory capacity is clearly reduced in diabetic cats **(Figure 9)**. In most cases, the underlying defect of disturbed beta-cell function at the molecular level is completely unknown.

Because insulin and amylin are usually cosecreted, similar defects also refer to amylin secretion **(Figure 9)**. However, early phases of feline DM seem to be associated with relative hyperamylinemia *(Lutz & Rand, 1996)*. It is currently unknown whether initial hypersecretion of amylin contributes to accelerated deposition of pancreatic islet amyloid (see below) or whether it may rather be regarded as an adaptive response to help control blood glucose due to amylin's metabolic effects such as inhibition of postprandial glucagon secretion (see below).

Once established, deficient insulin secretion leads to overt hyperglycemia. Sustained hyperglycemia then causes progressive disruption of normal beta-cell function. This phenomenon is called glucotoxicity *(Prentki et al, 2002)* and will be discussed below. Further complication results from inflammatory events which are now considered an important feature in the pathophysiological sequence leading to beta-cell insufficiency in 2DM like syndromes *(Donath et al, 2005; see below)*.

► Obesity and the development of diabetes mellitus

The higher prevalence of feline DM in recent years is most likely caused by the rise in obesity in our cat population. Obesity considerably increases the risk to become diabetic about 4 times compared to lean cats, and at least 60% of obese cats seem to become diabetic over time *(Hoenig, 2006a,b)*. Further, and similar to humans, the degree of overweight seems to be directly linked to the increased risk of developing DM. In studies by Scarlett and coworkers

FIGURE 10 - BODY CONDITION SCORING IN CATS

Scoring	Characteristics
Emaciated: 1 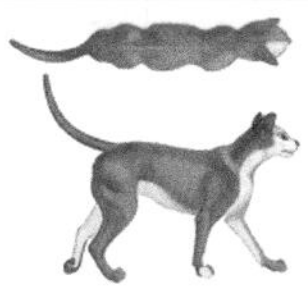	- Ribs, spine, pelvic bones easily visible (short hair) - Obvious loss of muscle mass - No palpable fat on rib cage
Thin: 2 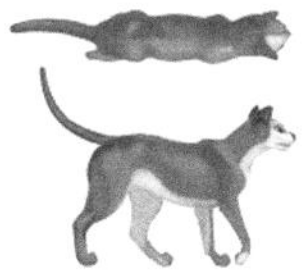	- Ribs, spine, pelvic bones visible - Obvious abdominal tuck (waist) - Minimal abdominal fat
Ideal: 3 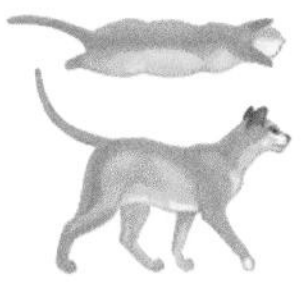	- Ribs, spine not visible, but easily palpable - Obvious abdominal tuck (waist) - Few abdominal fat
Overweight: 4 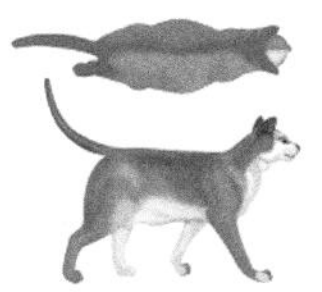	- Ribs, spine not easily palpated - Abdominal tuck (waist) absent - Obvious abdominal distention
Obese: 5 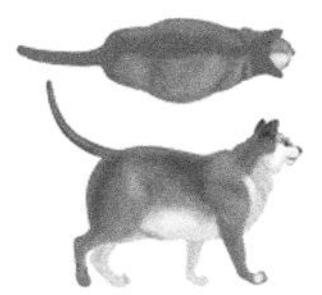	- Massive thoracic, spinal and abdominal fat deposits - Massive abdominal distention

FIGURE 11 - ASSOCIATION BETWEEN GLUCOSE TOLERANCE (ASSESSED BY GLUCOSE HALF-LIFE IN AN IVGTT) AND BODY WEIGHT IN CLINICALLY HEALTHY CATS

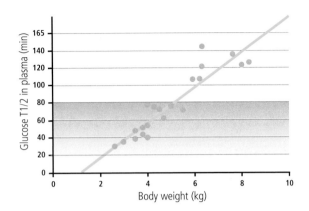

The upper limit of normal was a glucose T1/2 of less than 80 min. Glucose T1/2 was significantly higher in overweight compared to normal weight cats (Lutz & Rand, 1995).

(Scarlett et al, 1994; Scarlett & Donoghue, 1998), overweight cats were 2.2 times as likely, and obese cats were 6 times as likely to be diabetic than optimal weight cats. Different scoring systems have been described but the most common scoring systems used are the 5-point system **(Figure 10)** (where a BCS of 3 is considered ideal) or the 9-point system (where a BCS of 5 is considered ideal); (see Obesity chapter).Therefore, any increase in body weight above normal should be avoided to reduce the risk of cats to develop DM *(Scarlett & Donoghue, 1998)*.

Once obesity is established, the heat production and hence the energy requirement, is reduced in obese cats when corrected for metabolic BW *(Hoenig et al, 2006c; 2007a,b)*. This will help to perpetuate obesity unless food intake is rigorously adjusted. In another study *(Nguyen et al, 2004a,b)*, it was reported that total energy expenditure is unchanged in neutered or intact cats of different BW if values are corrected for metabolic BW or for lean body mass. However, *Nguyen et al* (2004a,b) used a different technique to determine total energy expenditure than *Hoenig et al* (2007b) which may explain the different outcome.

> Obesity and insulin resistance

A number of studies have shown that obese cats face a high risk of developing DM because they have a higher baseline insulin concentration, show an abnormal insulin secretion pattern in IVGTT and euglycemic hyperinsulinemic clamp studies, and are insulin resistant *(Biourge et al, 1997; Scarlett & Donoghue, 1998; Appleton et al, 2001b; Hoenig et al, 2002; 2007b)*. Depending on the experimental technique and the degree of obesity, insulin sensitivity was reported to be reduced by 50 to over 80%. Figure 11 shows one example of how glucose tolerance in cats is affected by body weight (see also **Figure 13**). A cat was considered having abnormal glucose tolerance when glucose half-life was above 80 min in an IVGTT *(Lutz & Rand, 1995)*.

Insulin resistance seems to be associated with a decreased expression in the insulin-sensitive glucose transporter GLUT4, while the expression of GLUT1, which mediates insulin-independent glucose transport, is unaltered *(Brennan et al, 2004)*. This effect occurs early in the development of obesity, before overt glucose intolerance is observed. Interestingly, at basal insulin levels glucose utilization seems to be normal in obese cats. However, in a stimulated state (e.g. by IVGTT), not only insulin sensitivity but also glucose effectiveness, that is, the ability of glucose to promote its own utilization at baseline insulin levels, was reduced by approximately 50% *(Appleton et al, 2001b; Hoenig et al, 2006c; 2007a,b)*.

> Obesity and lipid metabolism

Obese cats have higher baseline concentrations of non-esterified fatty acids (NEFA) than lean cats. This may reflect in part a general change from glucose to fat metabolism in skeletal muscle of obese cats. Lower activity of lipoprotein lipase in body fat combined with higher activity of lipoprotein lipase and of hormone-sensitive lipase in the muscle in obese cats may favor the redistribution of fatty acids from adipose tissue to skeletal muscle *(Hoenig et al, 2006b; 2007b)*. The lipid accumulation in skeletal muscle seen in obese cats could then result in a lower insulin sensitivity because changes in lipid metabolism lead to altered insulin signaling and affect GLUT4 expression *(Wilkins et al, 2004; Brennan et al, 2004)*. In obese cats, both intramyocellular and extramyocellular lipids increase. Whether and how elevated intramyocellular lipids affect GLUT4 expression, and hence insulin sensitivity directly remains to be study. All in all, general obesity clearly favors the development of insulin resistance in muscle *(Wilkins et al, 2004)*.

The link between obesity and the changes in metabolic handling of nutrients in adipose and skeletal muscle tissue may be represented by differential expression of tumor necrosis factor-alpha (TNFα). TNFα reduces lipoprotein lipase, and a study has shown that TNFα is upregulated in adipocytes, but downregulated in skeletal muscle of obese cats (*Hoenig et al, 2006b*).

TNFα is one of the numerous hormones and cytokines that are released by adipose tissue and that are now considered of pivotal importance for regulating nutrient handling (for review, see *Lazar, 2005*). All endocrine factors released from adipose tissue are collectively called adipokines. TNFα in particular is not only produced by adipocytes, but also by macrophages. In fact, obesity is considered a low grade inflammatory disease of adipose tissue. Many cytokines released from adipose tissue induce peripheral insulin resistance. For example, TNFα, which is among the best investigated, interferes with insulin signalling and causes insulin resistance.

Adiponectin is the only adipokine known which is inversely related to the amount of body adiposity (for review, see *Ahima, 2005*). Adiponectin improves insulin sensitivity by increasing fatty acid oxidation, reducing hepatic gluconeogenesis, and by inhibiting inflammatory responses. Because its concentration is reduced in obesity, it combines with increased release of TNFα to promote insulin resistance. However, it has to be pointed out that none of these effects have been investigated in detail in cats (see also **Figure 12**). It was also claimed that elevated levels of insulin-like growth factor-1 (IGF-1) may constitute the link between obesity and insulin resistance (*Leray et al, 2006*). However, this has never been shown in cats and the data in other species are also conflicting. *Reusch et al* (2006a) have shown that diabetic cats have lower IGF-1 levels which increase in response to insulin treatment.

Despite many similarities between human 2DM and feline DM, it should be highlighted that there may also be some distinct differences. One of them being that in cats, insulin suppresses the serum concentration of NEFA's more in obese than in lean cats. This appears to be due to an increased sensitivity to insulin-induced fatty acid uptake (*Hoenig et al, 2003*). Further, obese cats seem to accumulate similar amounts of subcutaneous and visceral fat. This may be of importance because in humans, visceral fat in particular has been associated with the metabolic derangements of obesity.

> Reversibility of insulin resistance

Regarding the possible treatment outcome for diabetic cats, it is important to note that insulin resistance induced by obesity in cats is reversible after the correction of body weight (**Figure 13**) (*Biourge et al, 1997*). Hence, if diabetic cats are obese, lowering their body weight to normal should always be part of the therapy. In the course of the above mentioned study (*Biourge et al, 1997*), cats were also exposed to a poorly palatable diet which resulted in a voluntary decrease in food intake. The ensuing rapid body weight loss led to a deterioration of glucose tolerance and severely depressed insulin secretion. This was, however, temporary. Presumably, insulin resistance was caused by an adaptation to nutrient deprivation and a shift from carbohydrate to fat catabolism. This may result in elevated levels of triglycerides and free fatty acids. Hence, these are increased in obesity, but also during massive caloric restriction and must be considered a normal metabolic adaptation (see also *Banks et al, 2006*).

FIGURE 12 - INSULIN RESISTANCE

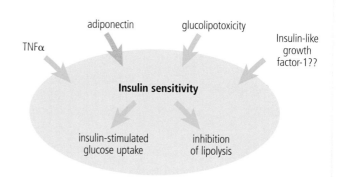

Tumor necrosis factor-alpha and glucolipotoxicity reduce insulin sensitivity in insulin target tissues (Rossetti et al, 1990; Hoenig et al, 2006), resulting in reduced insulin-stimulated glucose uptake and decreased inhibition of lipolysis. Adiponectin increases insulin sensitivity (Ahima, 2005). Insulin-like growth factor-1 has been hypothesized to reduce insulin sensitivity, but data are conflicting (Leray et al, 2006; Reusch et al, 2006).

FIGURE 13 - THE EFFECT OF BODY WEIGHT GAIN AND RECOVERY TO NORMAL BODY WEIGHT ON PLASMA INSULIN LEVELS
(Biourge et al, 1997)

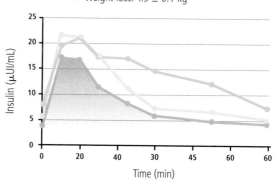

- Baseline: 4.7 ± 0.1 kg
- Weight gain: 6.0 ± 0.2 kg
- Weight loss: 4.9 ± 0.1 kg

Cats were tested with an IVGTT. 0.5 g/kg glucose was injected at t=0 min

Even though the phenomenon of increased body weight in neutered cats has been known for a long time, more in-depth studies on underlying causes have only recently been performed. The increase in body weight, and hence the decrease in insulin sensitivity, in cats after neutering appears to result from both an increase in food intake and a decrease in energy requirement *(Root et al, 1996; Biourge et al, 1997; Fettman et al, 1997; Harper et al, 2001; Hoenig & Ferguson, 2002; Kanchuk et al, 2002; Kanchuk et al, 2003)*. The latter effect, however, has been disputed because it was not consistently observed in male cats *(Kanchuk et al, 2003)*. The different outcome of studies may be due to procedural differences. *Kanchuk et al* (2003), determined energy expenditure as expressed per lean body mass. This was done on the understanding that BW gain in overfed cats results mainly from an increase in adipose tissue mass which is metabolically relative inactive *(Kanchuk et al, 2003; see also Martin et al, 2001)*. In any case, neutered cats have a much higher risk of becoming obese.

▶ General concepts of glucotoxicity, lipotoxicity, and glucolipotoxicity

Glucose sensing in the feline pancreas seems to be similar to other species. Via the pathways outlined in **Figure 6 & 7**, glucose and free fatty acids (or NEFA) normally increase insulin secretion. Glucose also promotes normal expansion of beta-cell mass, and the two mechanisms, glucose stimulation and uptake via GLUT2, and glucose-induced cell proliferation seem to be directly linked through distinct intracellular signaling pathways (reviewed in *Prentki & Nolan, 2006*). The effect of glucose on beta-cell proliferation is further stimulated by incretins such as GLP-1 and free fatty acids. Hence, GLP-1 protects beta-cells from apoptosis and promotes beta-cell growth.

As reviewed by *Prentki et al* (2002), glucose concentrations below 10 mmol/L (180 mg/dL) normally are not toxic to the pancreatic beta-cells. This refers to physiological postprandial hyperglycemia which triggers beta-cell proliferation *(Donath et al, 2005)*. Similarly, physiologically elevated fatty acid concentrations alone are not toxic, at least when malonyl-CoA, which is a side product of glucose metabolism in beta-cells and which inhibits uptake of fatty acids in mitochondria for subsequent beta-oxidation, is low. Fatty acids increase insulin secretion via increases in Ca^{2+} and diacylglycerol **(Figure 7)**. Problems only arise when hyperglycemia and elevated fatty acids occur simultaneously and for prolonged periods. While insulin secretion initially is increased via glucose and long chain fatty acid-CoA **(Figures 6 & 7)**, a marked elevation of glucose, and activated fatty acids and further lipid signalling molecules reduce insulin secretion and promote apoptosis. These effects are called glucotoxicity and lipotoxicity, respectively. Because lipotoxicity is most apparent under prevailing hyperglycemia, the term glucolipotoxicity has been coined *(Prentki & Nolan, 2006)*.

It has to be made clear that only few aspects of gluco- and lipotoxicity have been studied in cats so far. Nonetheless, the author believes that due to the many similarities between rodent models of 2DM and especially human 2DM and feline DM *(Henson & O'Brien, 2006)*, many aspects discussed in the following section are probably also valid for cats (see below).

The reduction in beta-cell mass caused by chronic hyperglycemia and glucotoxicity results from an imbalance between beta-cell neogenesis and proliferation, and beta-cell apoptosis *(Donath et al, 2005)*. During chronic hyperglycemia and hyperlipidemia, glucose, saturated fatty acids and triglycerides accumulate in beta-cells, triggering the release of cytokines. All these factors reduce insulin secretion and favor beta-cell apoptosis. At the cellular level, glucotoxicity is associated with mitochondrial dysfunction which, due to enhanced oxidative glucose metabolism, may be linked to increased oxidative stress in pancreatic beta-cells *(Prentki & Nolan, 2006)*. Reactive oxygen species can be "detoxified", but this happens at the expense of ATP and hence lower insulin secretion **(Figures 6 & 7)**.

Dysfunctional lipid metabolism, triglyceride and free fatty acid cycling also contribute to beta-cell failure. This results in the accumulation of long chain fatty acid-CoA which directly influences the ATP-sensitive K channel that is involved in glucose-stimulated insulin release. Further, elevated intracellular malonyl-CoA levels reduce the uptake of fatty acids into mitochondria and thereby shift fat metabolism from fatty acid oxidation to fatty acid esterification and lipid accumulation. This results in a lower production of intracellular ATP which is important for stimulus-secretion coupling *(Prentki & Nolan, 2006)*.

In recent years, evidence has also accumulated that glucotoxic and lipotoxic events are directly linked to islet inflammation. Among other factors, interleukin 1-beta (IL-1beta) has been identified as one of the key molecules *(Donath et al, 2005)*. Even though IL-1beta upregulation has now been reported in several animal models of 2DM, further studies are clearly required to investigate the link between hyperglycemia and inflammation *(Prentki & Nolan, 2006)*. The author is not aware of any such studies having been performed in cats to date.

► Gluco- and lipotoxicity in cats

In their paper entitled *Experimental diabetes produced by the administration of glucose*, Dohan and Lukens (1948) described the effect of sustained hyperglycemia on the islets of Langerhans. They report that cats developed degranulation of beta-cells followed by degeneration of islets. Many cats developed overt diabetes mellitus, at that time characterized by massive glucosuria.

> Glucotoxicity

Glucotoxicity clearly contributes to beta-cell failure in cats but it is reversible if hyperglycemia resolves. However if maintained, permanent loss of beta-cells may ensue. In healthy cats, sustained hyperglycemia of about 30 mmol/L (540 mg/dL) induced by chronic glucose infusion almost completely shut down insulin secretion three to seven days after the start of infusion. Pancreatic histology revealed massive changes in beta-cell morphology. Pancreatic beta-cells showed vacuolation, glycogen deposition, loss of insulin staining and pyknosis. However, even profound histological changes appeared to be reversible upon early resolution of hyperglycemia *(Rand & Marshall, 2005)*. The author's unpublished studies also clearly show that hyperglycemia of about 25 mmol/L (450 mg/dL) for only 10 days is sufficient to cause a massive decrease in the insulin secretory capacity of pancreatic beta-cells in healthy cats.

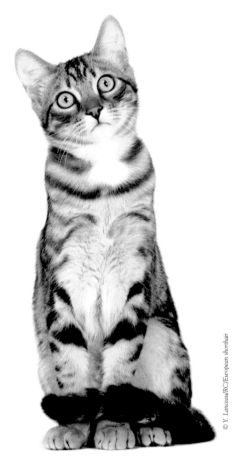

Interestingly, the first report on glucotoxicity in cats by was published in 1948.

> Lipotoxicity

Lipotoxicity has not been investigated in detail in cats. However, *Hoenig (2002)* hypothesized that lipotoxicity might also play a pathogenic role in the diabetic cat. As first described in the glucose fatty acid cycle (Randle cycle; *Randle, 1998*), glucose inhibits fatty acid oxidation, and vice versa **(Figure 14)**. Because NEFA concentrations are elevated in obese cats and because obese cats are most prone to developing diabetes mellitus, it is plausible to suggest that NEFA reduces glucose metabolism in beta-cells. However glucose metabolism is a necessary component in glucose-stimulated insulin release. Hence, glucose-stimulated insulin release would be decreased. A study by the same group has shown that saturated fatty acids in particular seem to be detrimental to glucose control in cats while polyunsaturated fatty acids (3-PUFA) may have beneficial effects *(Wilkins et al, 2004)*.

Similar cellular mechanisms as just described for the pancreatic beta-cell also seem to play a role in glucolipotoxicity in insulin target tissues. This has been investigated

FIGURE 14 - SIMPLIFIED CONCEPT OF THE GLUCOSE FATTY ACID CYCLE
(Randle cycle; Randle, 1998).

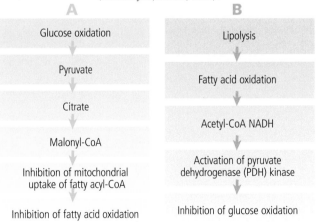

A

Glucose oxidation → Pyruvate → Citrate → Malonyl-CoA → Inhibition of mitochondrial uptake of fatty acyl-CoA → Inhibition of fatty acid oxidation

B

Lipolysis → Fatty acid oxidation → Acetyl-CoA NADH → Activation of pyruvate dehydrogenase (PDH) kinase → Inhibition of glucose oxidation

Glucose supply promotes glucose oxidation, glucose and lipid storage and inhibits fatty acid oxidation (A). Fatty acid oxidation impairs glucose oxidation (B) and may promote glucose storage in the form of glycogen if glycogen reserves are depleted.

in less detail but as mentioned earlier, intramyocellular lipid accumulation in skeletal muscle cells reduces their insulin sensitivity (*Wilkins et al, 2004*; see also *Hoenig, 2002*). Hence, elevated glucose levels and perturbed lipid metabolism in diabetic cats not only lead to beta-cell failure but may also reduce insulin sensitivity in insulin-target tissues.

All in all, gluco- and lipotoxicity seem to be phenomena which contribute to the progressive deterioration of metabolic control in diabetic cats, both via an effect on pancreatic beta-cells and via an effect on insulin-sensitive target tissue. This clearly underlines the pivotal importance of glucose lowering strategies to curtail this progressive deterioration. Hence, early reversal of hyperglycemia, preferentially by aggressive insulin treatment, reverses glucolipotoxicity, and this will help to achieve diabetic remission in a large number of diabetic cats (see also paragraph on transient diabetes; *Nelson et al, 1999*).

▶ Amylin as a circulating hormone in the development of feline diabetes mellitus

As discussed, amylin is a normal secretory product of pancreatic beta-cells in all species. Amylin is co-synthesized and co-secreted in parallel with insulin in response to appropriate stimuli (*Lutz & Rand, 1996*). Hence, changes in plasma insulin levels are usually associated with corresponding changes in plasma amylin levels. In human 2DM and in feline DM, the hormonal situation changes over the course of the disease. Early phases of feline 2DM or mild forms of the disease are often characterized by (compensatory) hyperinsulinemia and absolute or relative hyperamylinemia (*O'Brien et al, 1991; Lutz & Rand, 1996*). Early hyperamylinemia may favor the deposition of feline amylin as pancreatic amyloid (see below). Progressive beta-cell failure in more severe forms and late stages of feline DM, however, leads to overt hypoinsulinemia and hypoamylinemia (*Johnson et al, 1989; Ludvik et al, 1991*). Most clinical cases of feline DM are probably presented to veterinarians at that stage.

The regulation of nutrient metabolism by amylin involves modulation of pancreatic glucagon release, the regulation of gastric emptying (for review: *Edelman & Weyer, 2002*), and an inhibition of food intake (*Lutz, 2005*). Hence, the lack of amylin in DM results in oversecretion of glucagon, accelerated gastric emptying and overeating. At least in humans and rodents, amylin has been shown to decrease excessive postprandial hyperglucagonemia observed in DM (*Fineman et al, 2002*) and to normalize gastric emptying. Hyperglucagonemia is also present in diabetic cats (**Figure 15**; *Tschuor et al, 2006*), but it is unknown at present whether this is due to the lack of amylin in these animals. However, preliminary studies in healthy cats show a trend for an effect of amylin to reduce glucagon output (**Figure 16**; *Furrer et al, 2005*). Similar studies in diabetic cats have not been performed yet. Further, it has not been investigated in detail whether, similar to humans or rodents, gastric emptying in diabetic cats is accelerated. Hence, it is unknown if presuming that such defect were present, this would be due to amylin deficiency.

In summary, there is reason to believe that the lack of amylin in diabetic cats contributes to metabolic dysregulation. The most prominent effect in this regard is the lack of amylin's suppression

FIGURE 15 - BASELINE HYPERGLUCAGONEMIA IN DIABETIC CATS AFTER 12H OF FASTING

(Tschuor et al, 2006)

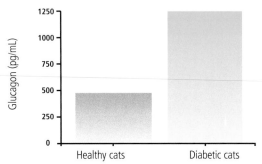

Median values of 7 healthy and 10 diabetic cats are shown.

FIGURE 16 - AMYLIN SLIGHTLY REDUCES MEASURED GLUCAGON BLOOD LEVELS IN AN ARGININE STIMULATION TEST (AST; FIGURE 16A) AND A MEAL RESPONSE TEST (MRT; FIGURE 16B)

(Furrer et al, 2005)

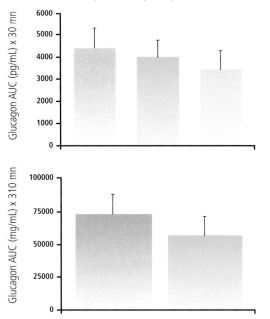

AUC = area under the curve, n = 6.
The effects approached significance.

of prandial glucagon secretion. Amylin replacement is now a common form of therapy in human DM but is so far unknown in the treatment of diabetic cats.

► Pancreatic glucagon as a circulating hormone in the development of feline diabetes mellitus

Pancreatic glucagon as a pathogenic factor in the development of DM has been neglected for many years due to the overwhelming importance that was given to insulin deficiency as the critical factor. Notwithstanding, deficient suppression of glucagon secretion, especially in the immediate postprandial period, seems to be a major contributor to postprandial hyperglycemia **(Figure 15)** *(O'Brien et al, 1985; Furrer et al, 2005; Tschuor et al, 2006)*. Diabetic hyperglucagonemia seems to be directly linked to amylin deficiency and hence disinhibition of glucagon release. This may also be true for the cat **(Figure 16)** *(Furrer et al, 2005)*. To what extent reduced insulin suppression of glucagon release also contributes to the phenomenon in cats, remains to be determined.

► Pancreatic amyloidosis

The most common and consistent morphological feature is islet amyloidosis **(Figure 17)** *(Yano et al, 1981; O'Brien et al, 1985; Johnson et al, 1986; Johnson et al, 1989; Lutz et al, 1994; Lutz & Rand, 1997)*. Amyloid deposition is found in a large proportion of overtly diabetic cats and cats with impaired glucose tolerance, a state also referred to as pre-diabetic *(Johnson et al, 1986; Westermark et al, 1987; Lutz & Rand, 1995)*. Islet amyloidosis is thought to play an important role in the pathogenesis of 2DM and feline DM because it contributes to progressive beta-cell loss which is typically observed over the course of the disease *(Höppener et al, 2002)*.

Pancreatic amyloid deposits consist mainly of amylin, hence amylin's other name islet amyloid polypeptide, or IAPP *(Westermark et al, 1987)*. Pancreatic amylin has the propensity to precipitate as amyloid deposits only in a small number of species such as humans, non-human primates and cats *(Johnson et al, 1989; Westermark et al, 1987)*, and only these species naturally develop a 2DM like syndrome. A necessary precondition is a certain amino acid sequence in the middle part of the amylin molecule in humans and cats (but not rats) that is unrelated to amylin's hormonal action, but predisposes amylin to form insoluble fibrillar aggregates. A second prerequisite appears to be hypersecretion of amylin leading to high local amylin concentrations in pancreatic islets *(Cooper, 1994)*. Especially during early islet amyloid formation, soluble amylin fibril oligomers contribute to beta-cell toxicity and subsequent beta-cell loss *(Höppener et al, 2002; Butler et al, 2003; Konarkowska et al, 2006; Matveyenko & Butler, 2006)*. A third and only poorly defined factor in the development of islet amyloidosis seems to be some malfunction of pancreatic beta-cells leading to aberrant processing of amylin *(Ma et al, 1998)*.

As mentioned, early phases of feline DM are characterized by hyperamylinemia *(O'Brien et al, 1991; Lutz & Rand, 1996)*. This may favor the deposition of feline amylin as pancreatic amyloid. Progressive beta-cell failure in late stages of feline DM leads to low circulating amylin levels *(Johnson et al, 1989; Ludvik et al, 1991; Cooper 1994)*.

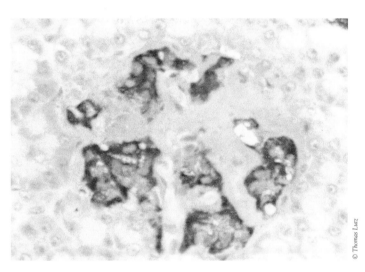

© Thomas Lutz

Figure 17A - Pancreatic islet of a cat with massive deposition of islet amyloid *which consists mainly of precipitates of the beta-cell hormone amylin.*

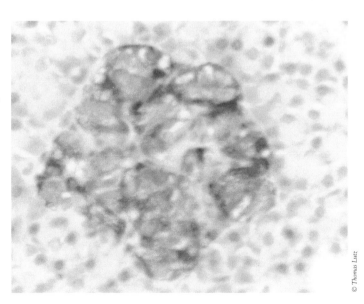

© Thomas Lutz

Figure 17 B - The pancreatic islet of a healthy control cat *is shown for comparison. Immunohistochemical stain for amylin. Intact beta-cells stain in red, islet amyloid stains in pink.*

FIGURE 18 - FREQUENCY OF ISLET AMYLOID DEPOSITION IN 84 CLINICALLY HEALTHY CATS

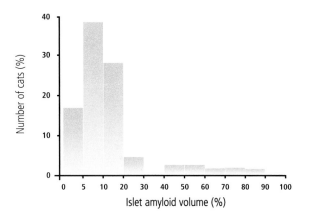

Some cats have large amyloid deposits without developing clinical signs of DM (Lutz et al, 1994). Volume percent of islet amyloid is referred to the total islet volume (=100%).

FIGURE 19 - ISLET AMYLOID DEPOSITION INCREASES WITH AGE

(Lutz et al, 1994)

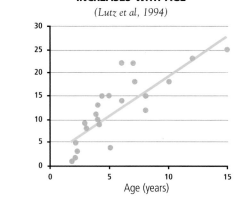

Young clinically healthy cats have no or only minor detectable deposition of pancreatic amyloid.

► Quantitative aspects of islet amyloid in cats

Being the most prominent histological finding in diabetic cats, it was very interesting to note that islet amyloid deposition also occurs in non-diabetic, healthy cats. Some of these cats appeared to develop relatively large amounts of islet amyloid without obvious clinical signs (**Figure 18**) (*Lutz et al, 1994*). The prevalence of pancreatic amyloid increased with age (**Figure 19**), hence a finding similar to the general observation of an increased prevalence of feline diabetes in older animals. Most important, however, diabetic cats had markedly larger deposits of pancreatic amyloid than healthy cats, and the extent of amyloid deposition seemed to be directly related to the severity of clinical signs in feline DM (*O'Brien et al, 1985; Johnson et al, 1989; Lutz et al, 1994*). This is also reflected in the association between the amount of pancreatic islet amyloid and the occurrence of glucose intolerance as assessed via glucose half-life in plasma in an IVGTT (**Figure 20**).

Unfortunately, even though pancreatic islet amyloid is an important factor in the pathophysiology of feline DM, it cannot be assessed under *in vivo* conditions. Therefore, it is currently not a helpful prognostic marker for the development of the disease.

Studies in transgenic rodents have clearly pointed to an important role of amylin-derived amyloid in the development and progression of 2DM. Small molecular weight, soluble amylin oligomers in species with an amyloidogenic amino acid sequence, are causative for beta-cell apoptosis (for review: see *Muff et al, 2004*). Nonetheless, the primary events leading to the formation of these cytotoxic oligomers in 2DM remain to be resolved.

► The link between hyperglycemia and the formation of islet amyloid

Now that the major pathogenetic factors (gluco-lipotoxicity and amylin-derived islet amyloid) contributing to progressive beta-cell failure in diabetic cats have been reviewed, it should be noted that it is as yet completely unknown whether and how there may be a link between these factors. However, it seems possible that changes in the intracellular milieu induced by elevated glucose or fatty acid levels (intracellular stress) may create conditions that promote the formation and precipitation of islet amyloid fibrils. The most toxic form to beta-cells are small molecular oligomers of amylin fibrils which are most likely formed early in the disease process. Hence, any therapy aimed at reducing blood glucose levels, and subsequently at reducing the secretory stress on pancreatic beta-cells, as early as possible in the disease process may favor diabetic remission as seen in transient DM (see below).

► Reduced insulin sensitivity in diseased cats

Similar to humans, glucose homeostasis seems to be frequently impaired in cats suffering from various diseases including severe inflammation, malignant neoplasia, sepsis, viral infection, end-stage renal disease, and chronic heart failure. As an underlying cause, a combination of augmented synthesis of pro-inflammatory cytokines and the presence of insulin counter-regulatory hormones has been hypothesized. This has been substantiated in cats with congestive heart failure which have elevated levels of TNFα (*Meurs et al, 2002*).

Further, stomatitis, pulmonary lesions (*Mexas et al, 2006*), and urinary tract infections (*Jin & Lin, 2005*) seem to be more frequent in diabetic cats. Seriously ill cats may show profound stress-induced hyperglycemia. They do not always suffer from concomitant hyperinsulinemia which would be indicative of insulin resistance (*Chan et al, 2006*).

The exact mechanisms linking disturbed glucose homeostasis and various illnesses in cats are still largely unknown. Various cytokines are most likely involved. A recent preliminary study has shown that a 10-day infusion of lipopolysaccharide, which is a cell wall component of Gram negative bacteria and which causes the release of various cytokines, leads to impaired glucose tolerance (*unpublished*). It could also be speculated that these disorders are associated with reduced levels of the adipocyte hormone adiponectin which appears to be an important factor in regulating insulin sensitivity in insulin target tissues (*Hoenig et al, 2007a*). Apart from effects of cytokines on insulin-sensitive tissues, various cytokines directly reduce pancreatic endocrine secretion.

Finally, it should also be recognized that one is faced with a typical chicken and the egg conundrum. On one hand, hyperglycemia in DM reduces the body defense against infection, for example, in the urogenital tract (*e.g., Lederer et al, 2003; Bailiff et al, 2006*). On the other hand, infection and inflammatory disorders, perhaps through TNFα, are associated with insulin resistance which may ultimately lead to DM **(Figure 21)**.

8 - Transient diabetes

Transient DM occurs relatively frequently in diabetic cats. Historically, approximately 20% of diabetic cats were reported to fall into this category (*Nelson et al, 1999; Nelson, 2005*). However, the proportion of transiently diabetic cats seems to have increased recently (see below). Transiently diabetic cats go into spontaneous remission, that is, clinical symptoms such as polyuria and polydipsia resolve, blood glucose levels normalize and glucosuria disappears. This usually happens within one to four months after the initation of therapy (*Nelson et al, 1999*). At that time, specific antidiabetic glucose-lowering therapy can be discontinued. Once DM resolves, the glucose induced insulin secretion is normalized. Nevertheless, beta-cell density is still decreased and islet pathology is present. Therefore, most of these cases correspond to a subclinical phase of DM (*Nelson et al, 1999*).

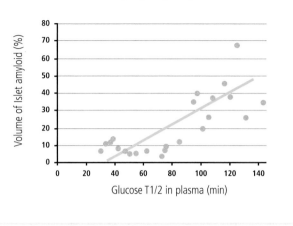

FIGURE 20 - THE AMOUNT OF PANCREATIC ISLET AMYLOID IS POSITIVELY CORRELATED TO GLUCOSE T1/2 AS DETERMINED IN AN IVGTT

(*Lutz et al, 1994*)

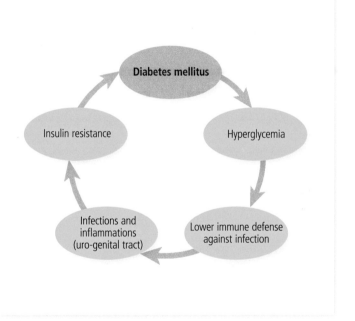

FIGURE 21 - SELF-PERPETUATION OF DIABETES MELLITUS

▶ Conditions for diabetic remission

The conditions that need to be fulfilled for diabetic remission to occur are not yet completely clear. Obviously, an adequate number of functional beta-cells still needs to be present (*Nelson et al, 1999*). One important factor seems to be the early resolution of hyperglycemia and hence the disappearance, or at least reduction, of glucotoxicity. Intensive glucose-lowering therapy, perhaps supported by an appropriate diet (see below), can terminate the vicious circle of chronic hyperglycemia leading to an impairment of pancreatic beta-cell function and decreased insulin sensitivity. Because glucotoxicity is initially reversible, it seems plausible that the earlier glucose-lowering therapy is initiated in diabetic cats, the higher the likelihood for diabetic cats to go into remission. However, hard scientific data to support this idea are lacking.

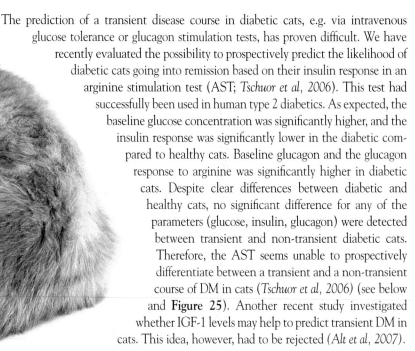

► Differences between transient and non-transient diabetic cats?

The prediction of a transient disease course in diabetic cats, e.g. via intravenous glucose tolerance or glucagon stimulation tests, has proven difficult. We have recently evaluated the possibility to prospectively predict the likelihood of diabetic cats going into remission based on their insulin response in an arginine stimulation test (AST; *Tschuor et al, 2006*). This test had successfully been used in human type 2 diabetics. As expected, the baseline glucose concentration was significantly higher, and the insulin response was significantly lower in the diabetic compared to healthy cats. Baseline glucagon and the glucagon response to arginine was significantly higher in diabetic cats. Despite clear differences between diabetic and healthy cats, no significant difference for any of the parameters (glucose, insulin, glucagon) were detected between transient and non-transient diabetic cats. Therefore, the AST seems unable to prospectively differentiate between a transient and a non-transient course of DM in cats (*Tschuor et al, 2006*) (see below and **Figure 25**). Another recent study investigated whether IGF-1 levels may help to predict transient DM in cats. This idea, however, had to be rejected (*Alt et al, 2007*).

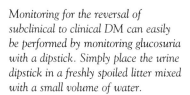

Monitoring for the reversal of subclinical to clinical DM can easily be performed by monitoring glucosuria with a dipstick. Simply place the urine dipstick in a freshly spoiled litter mixed with a small volume of water.

In diabetic cats that go into remission, recurrence of clinically overt DM is always possible. Islet pathology is usually present in transiently diabetic cats. Therefore, the susceptibility to revert to overt DM is probably higher than in previously healthy cats. This may be caused by additional stressors such as insulin-antagonistic drugs (e.g. glucocorticoids, megestrol acetate) or obesity. It is usually impossible to predict if or when clinical signs will recur, underlying the necessity to monitor cats in diabetic remission carefully for recurrence. In some cases, cats have been reported to revert from subclinical to clinical DM more than 3 years after the first resolution of symptoms (*Nelson et al, 1999*).

► Evolution of the remission rate of diabetic cats

The proportion of transiently diabetic cats seemed to have increased over the last years, reaching 70% in some studies. This may be related to the recent recommendation to feed diabetic cats a diet relatively high in protein and low in carbohydrate, respectively. Whether the improvement of the metabolic situation depends on the high protein content (49-57% DMB in studies by *Frank et al, 2001; Mazzaferro et al, 2003*), the low carbohydrate (18% in the study by *Bennett et al, 2006*), or both, may require further investigation (see also below). We have also confirmed that the remission rate of diabetic cats is higher than previously reported when the cats were fed a high-protein diet (approx. 54% protein, 8% carbohydrate DMB; *Tschuor et al, 2006*). In our study, approximately 50% of insulin-treated cats went into remission within 4 weeks of intensive therapy. Interestingly, remission occurred before considerable weight loss was observed.

9 - Long-term consequences of diabetic hyperglycemia

Chronic hyperglycemia has deleterious effects on insulin-producing pancreatic beta-cells and on insulin target tissues (glucotoxicity; see above). But long-term hyperglycemia also seems to be the major factor contributing to other complications frequently seen in diabetic cats. These are diabetic neuropathy, nephropathy and retinopathy. The two main underlying mechanisms are glycation of proteins and osmotic damage due to the accumulation of sugar alcohols.

► Glycation of proteins and accumulation of sugar alcohols

An early pathologic change of DM is increased unspecific, non-enzymatic glycosylation (or glycation) of proteins, which cause abnormal aggregation of collagen fibrils and the production of superoxide radicals. This results in damage to the connective tissue and basal membranes. Further, osmotic cell damage seems to occur due to the accumulation of the sugar alcohol sorbitol which is not freely permeable to the cell membrane. Sorbitol is generated from glucose through aldose reductase activity. While only small amounts of sorbitol are generated under normal conditions, hyperglycemia can lead to the accumulation of considerable amounts of sorbitol by an "overflow" mechanism when normal glucose utilization via hexokinase is saturated.

► Diabetic neuropathy, retinopathy and cataract

The exact prevalence of diabetic neuropathy, nephropathy and retinopathy in cats is unknown. Diabetic neuropathy leads to hindlimb weakness and a typical plantigrade stance **(Figure 3)**. The pathology seems to share many similarities with human diabetic neuropathy *(Mizisin et al, 2007)*.

Interestingly, if intensive glucose-lowering therapy is initiated rapidly after diagnosis, at least some of these changes seem to be reversible and gait normalizes. Even though diabetic nephropathy and retinopathy also occur in cats, diabetic retinopathy is only rarely observed in clinical practice. Experimentally induced hyperglycemia has been shown to lead to retinal changes only after several years of duration, and these changes could only be detected using specific diagnostic techniques *(personal communication; Dr. M. Richter, Division of Ophthalmology, Vetsuisse Faculty, University of Zurich)*.

Similarly, and in contrast to dogs, diabetic cataracts are also very rare in diabetic cats **(Figure 22)**. It has been suggested that the generation of sorbitol in older diabetic cats was much lower than in dogs and young cats because of the lower aldose reductase activity in old cats *(Richter et al, 2002)*. Excess sorbitol is responsible for the damage to the lens. Even though DM is very infrequent in young cats, young diabetic cats often present typical lens opacity as in diabetic dogs, probably because of their high aldose reductase activity *(Richter et al, 2002)*. A recent study challenged the view of a generally low occurrence of diabetic cataracts in cats *(Williams & Heath, 2006)*. This study showed that lens opacities occur much more frequently than previously suggested. In addition, these opacities occurred at a much younger age in diabetic than in non-diabetic cats.

10 - Diagnosis of feline diabetes mellitus

Diagnosis of feline DM should always include an assessment of the key clinical features that typically occur in uncomplicated forms of diabetes, i.e. polyuria, polydipsia, polyphagia, loss of body weight. Obviously, the presence of one or all features, although indicative, is not sufficient for establishing the diagnosis. Therefore, laboratory parameters need to be assessed.

Figure 22 - Cataract in a diabetic cat.

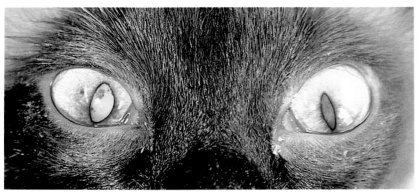

(by courtesy: Prof. B. Spiess, Vetsuisse-Faculty University of Zurich)

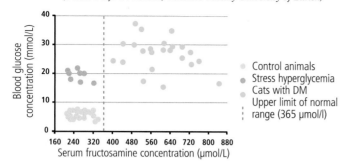

FIGURE 23 - SERUM FRUCTOSAMINE CONCENTRATIONS IN NORMOGLYCEMIC AND HYPERGLYCEMIC CATS WITH STRESS-INDUCED OR CHRONIC DIABETIC HYPERGLYCEMIA

(From: Prof. C. Reusch, Vetsuisse-Faculty University of Zurich)

► Fasting hyperglycemia

Fasting hyperglycemia is one of the key symptoms in diabetic cats, but fasting hyperglycemia alone is not reliable due to the phenomenon of stress hyperglycemia **(Figure 23)**. Cats are much more prone to stress-induced hyperglycemia than dogs. Blood glucose levels in stressed cats often exceed 20 mmol/L (360 mg/dL) *(Laluha et al, 2004)*. Therefore, stress-induced hyperglycemia has to be excluded before initiating insulin therapy (see below). Similar to fasting blood glucose, glucosuria may be misleading. While glucosuria is present in diabetic cats and is normally absent in healthy cats, stress-induced hyperglycemia can occur to such an extent that spill over of glucose into the urine is not uncommon.

► Plasma insulin

Diabetic cats are not able to secrete enough insulin to maintain blood glucose levels in the normal range. This deficiency, however, might be referred to as relative, i.e. the plasma insulin level may seem normal but for the level of glycemia, these cats are hypoinsulinemic. Having said this, it is clear that the determination of fasting insulin levels is usually not helpful, unless there is massive absolute hypoinsulinemia. Further, insulin levels are not measured routinely due to the high cost involved, and the limited availability of species specific insulin assays.

It was proposed that proinsulin, or the insulin: proinsulin ratio, respectively, may be a helpful tool to diagnose DM in cats. In humans, elevated fasting levels of proinsulin seem to be indicative of beta-cell damage and proinsulin may serve as an early marker for beta-cell dysfunction. The amino acid sequence of feline proinsulin has been published. Therefore it is possible that assays may become available to assist in the early diagnosis of feline DM *(Hoenig et al, 2006a)*. Interestingly, pro-insulin secretion appears to be elevated in obese cats.

TABLE 3 - COMPARISON OF FRUCTOSAMINE AND GLYCATED HEMOGLOBIN FOR THE ASSESSMENT OF SUSTAINED HYPERGLYCEMIA

	Fructosamine	Glycated hemoglobin
Common characteristics	- Derive from irreversible, non-enzymatic and unspecific binding of glucose to amino acid residues. - Directly proportional to the average blood glucose concentration over time. - Depend on the average turnover rate of the respective protein which is shorter for serum proteins than for hemoglobin.	
Respective characteristics	- Fructosamine refers to the sum of glycated serum proteins which can be measured by colorimetric assays. - A marker for the average glycemia over the last 10-14 days. - Affected by changes in serum protein levels.	- Glycated hemoglobin is a glycosylation product of hemoglobin and glucose. It is measured by chromatography. - Indicative for the average blood glucose level over the previous 4-8 weeks. - Affected by the hemoglobin concentration.

► Fructosamine and glycated hemoglobin

As mentioned, neither fasting blood or urine glucose levels are reliable markers for feline DM. As such, fructosamine and glycated (glycosylated) hemoglobin are now two frequently used markers for the long-term assessment of glycemia in the diagnosis and the monitoring of feline DM **(Tables 3 & 4)**. Both products derive from irreversible, non-enzymatic and unspecific binding of glucose to amino acid residues.

- **Fructosamine** refers to the sum of glycated serum proteins which can be measured by colorimetric assays.
- **Glycated hemoglobin**, especially the fraction of glycated hemoglobin A1c (HbA1c), is a glycosylation product of hemoglobin and glucose. It is measured by chromatography. Glycated hemoglobin is only rarely used as a diagnostic marker in cats.

The level of fructosamine and glycated hemoglobin is directly proportional to the average blood glucose concentration over time. Both also depend on the average turnover rate of the respective protein which is shorter for serum proteins than for hemoglobin. Therefore, the serum fructosamine concentration is a marker for the average glycemia over the last 10-14 days while the concentration of glycated hemoglobin is indicative for the average blood glucose level over the previous four to eight weeks. The levels of fructosamine and glycated hemoglobin are also affected by changes in serum protein levels and the hemoglobin concentration, respectively. These have to be taken into account when interpreting laboratory data (*Nelson, 2005*).

Fructosamine is used more frequently in clinical practice because it can be easily and rapidly measured. Since the original report about fructosamine as an indicator of blood glucose levels in diabetic cats (*Kaneko et al, 1992*), numerous subsequent publications supported the usefulness of fructosamine as an easy-to-use and reliable marker for the assessment of chronic hyperglycemia (e.g., *Reusch et al, 1993; Lutz et al, 1995; Crenshaw et al, 1996; Thoresen & Bredal, 1996; Plier et al, 1998; Elliott et al, 1999; Reusch & Haberer, 2001*). Normal values show some variation between different laboratories but are all in the same order of magnitude **(Table 4)**. Compared to blood glucose levels, one of the major advantages of the assessment of serum fructosamine is that its level is unaffected by short-term, stress induced hyperglycemia which can clearly be distinguished from diabetic hyperglycemia **(Figure 23)**.

▶ Other tests

Even though not routinely performed in clinical practice, more elaborate tests are available to assess glucose metabolism in cats. Most commonly used are:
- the intravenous glucose tolerance test (IVGTT) (*O'Brien et al, 1985; Link & Rand, 1998; Appleton et al, 2001a,b*)
- the arginine stimulation test (AST) (*Kitamura et al, 1999*)
- the glucagon stimulation test (GST)

Less common are insulin sensitivity tests (IST) (*Feldhahn et al, 1999; Appleton et al, 2001a,b*), while the euglycemic hyperinsulinemic clamp (*Petrus et al, 1998*) and the hyperglycemic glucose clamp (*Slingerland et al, 2007*) are only used for research purposes. In the euglycemic hyperinsulinemic clamp, a constant dose of insulin is infused and glucose metabolism parameters are derived from the amount of glucose that has to be infused to maintain blood glucose levels in the normal range. In the hyperglycemic glucose clamp, the blood glucose concentration is clamped to a fixed value and glucose metabolism parameters are derived from glucose and insulin levels throughout the clamp period.

With the IVGTT, glucose tolerance is assessed by calculating glucose half-life in plasma (glucose T1/2; upper limit of normal: approximately 75-80 min) (*Lutz & Rand, 1996; Appleton et al, 2001a*). Insulin sensitivity and the insulin secretory pattern, indicative of beta-cell function, can also be estimated **(Figures 9 & 24)**. Even though IVGTT are mostly used under standardized conditions, a study suggested that uniform and reliable reference values for the IVGTT cannot be established (*Hoenig et al, 2002*). Environmental factors like diet, housing, husbandry, and laboratory equipment, substantially influence the results. Therefore, the pattern of response to IV glucose injection should be evaluated rather than absolute concentrations of glucose or insulin (*Hoenig et al, 2002*). In the same study, it was proposed that glucose should be injected at a dose of at least 0.8 g/kg (a dose of 1 g/kg is used routinely) because lower doses which have been used in some studies (e.g., *Nelson et al, 1990*) may not enable the full assessment of the insulin response in cats of different body weight and body condition.

The AST, which triggers the release of both insulin and glucagon, has been used less often in diagnosing feline DM. Differentiation between healthy and diabetic cats is easily possible using this test, but permanently diabetic cats cannot be distinguished from cats going into diabetic remission (transient diabetes; **Figure 25**; *Tschuor et al, 2006*).

TABLE 4 - INTERPRETATION OF SERUM FRUCTOSAMINE AND GLYCATED HEMOGLOBIN LEVELS IN DIABETIC CATS
(adapted from Nelson, 2005)

Monitoring of diabetic cats	Fructosamine (µmol/L)	Glycated hemoglobin (%)
normal values	190-365 µmol/L (mean 240)	0.9 - 2.5% (mean 1.7)
excellent glycemic control	350 - 400	1.0 - 2.0
good control	400 - 450	2.0 - 2.5
fair control	450 - 500	2.5 - 3.0
poor control	> 500	> 3.0
sustained hypoglycemia	< 300	< 1.0

Normal values differ slightly between different laboratories.

FIGURE 24 - GLUCOSE TOLERANCE TEST

Glucose concentration

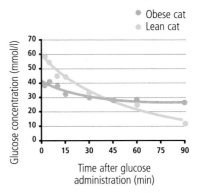

Insulin concentration

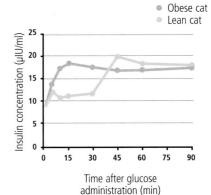

Glucose tolerance test in a lean cat (BW 3.5 kg) with normal glucose tolerance (glucose T1/2 37 min) and an obese cat (BW 6.5 kg) with abnormal glucose tolerance (glucose T1/2 125 min). Glucose (1 g/kg BW) was injected at t=0 min.

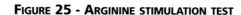

FIGURE 25 - ARGININE STIMULATION TEST

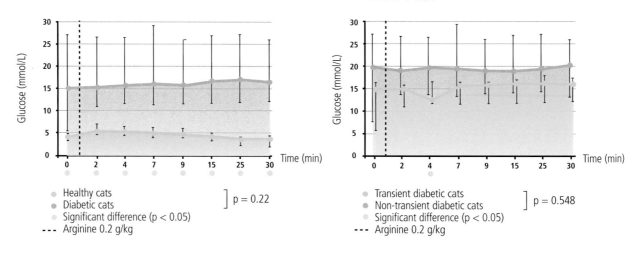

In an arginine stimulation test (arginine injection at t=0 min; 0.2 g/kg BW), blood glucose concentration in healthy cats is significantly lower than in diabetic cats.

However, this test can not differentiate between permanently and transiently diabetic cats (Tschuor et al, 2006).

11 - Treatment strategies

► Key issues in treating diabetic cats

Treatment beyond the disappearance of clinical signs (polyuria, polydipsia), which has traditionally been considered sufficient for treating diabetic cats, offers additional benefits. The benefits are linked to the possibility of spontaneous remission of feline DM, i.e. the transition into a subclinical form of DM. Remission of DM is thought to be mainly due to the disappearance of glucotoxicity once hyperglycemia is controlled. The key issues in treating diabetic cats must focus on lowering the blood glucose level into a range of 5-15 mmol/L (90-270 mg/dl).

Another key issue is that glucose lowering therapy should be initiated as soon as possible after the diagnosis of DM has been established. Early initiation of therapy is warranted because glucotoxic changes in pancreatic islets are at first reversible, but with time will become irreversible (*Prentki & Nolan, 2006*). Although it has not been unequivocally demonstrated, it is the author's clinical impression that early intervention leads to a higher percentage of diabetic cats that go into remission.

Overall, the recommendation is to treat early and intensively. Today, this is typically coupled with dietary intervention, especially the use of high-protein (> 50% protein DMB), low-carbohydrate (< 15% DMB) diets (see below).

► Insulin as a glucose lowering drug

Insulin therapy is by far the most effective means to achieve good glycemic control in diabetic cats. Feline insulin is not available for therapy, but insulin of animal origin (bovine or porcine), human recombinant insulin and a synthetic analogue of human insulin have been used for the treatment of diabetic cats (*Goossens et al, 1998; Marshall & Rand, 2002; Weaver et al, 2006*). The different types of insulin that are currently used are summarized in **Table 5**.

The exact treatment schedules for diabetic cats can be found in textbooks of veterinary internal medicine, e.g. *Nelson* (2005). Except for the treatment of an acute diabetic crisis (e.g. acute diabetic ketoacidosis), when regular crystalline insulin may be administered intramuscularly or intravenously, insulin is normally injected subcutaneously. Most diabetic cats will need insulin injections BID because of the short duration of action of insulin preparations in that species compared to humans.

TABLE 5 - TYPES OF INSULIN COMMONLY USED FOR THE TREATMENT OF DIABETIC CATS

Type of insulin	Route of administration	Onset of effect	Maximum effect	Duration of effect
Regular crystalline	IV IM SC	immediate 10 - 30 min 10 - 30 min	0.5 - 2 h 1 - 4 h 1 - 5 h	1 - 4 h 3 - 8 h 4 - 10 h
NPH (neutral protamine Hagedorn)	SC	0.5 - 2 h	2 - 8 h	4 - 12 h
Lente	SC	0.5 - 2 h	2 - 10 h	6 - 18 h
Ultralente	SC	0.5 - 8 h	4 - 16 h	6 - 24 h
PZI (protamine zinc insulin)	SC	0.5 - 4 h	4 - 14 h	6 - 20 h
commonly used insulin preparations				
Caninsulin® (intermediate insulin; porcine)	SC	1 - 2 h	4 - 6 h	8 - 12 h
Lantus® (long acting; human insulin analogue, glargine)	SC		16 h	24 h

The use of these agents in cats can be restricted according to the licence applicable in each country.

The only registered insulin preparation for dogs and cats in some countries is lente porcine insulin consisting of 30% amorphous and 70% crystalline Zn-insulin (e.g., Caninsulin[R]). Insulin therapy typically is initiated with BID injections of this intermediate-type insulin. Dosing in cats typically starts at 1-2 U/cat. Recommendations for dose adjustments vary with the type of insulin used. This usually requires serial blood curves which can be either produced at home (home monitoring) or under clinical settings.

A new preparation of human synthetic insulin is now also used in diabetic cats *(Marshall & Rand, 2002; Marshall & Rand, 2004; Weaver et al, 2006; Rand, 2006)*. Glargine insulin is an insulin analogue which is released slowly from subcutaneous depots. It is used in humans to provide a constant, peakless baseline insulin supply. In humans, glargine is often combined with meal associated injections of short acting insulins.

In cats, glargine is thought to result in better glycemic control over an entire 24h-period. In the study by *Weaver et al (2006)*, glargine was shown to provide good glycemic control in cats even if only administered SID. Obviously, this would constitute an important advantage for cat owners, but most cats will require BID injections.

▶ Other forms of therapy

Because feline DM is a type of DM corresponding to human type 2 DM, forms of therapy other than insulin have been tested. It should however be clearly stated that by far the best outcome of diabetic therapy is obtained with insulin, complemented by an appropriate diet (see below).

The use of sulfonylurea derivates, which stimulate pancreatic beta-cell secretion **(Figure 6)** and may improve peripheral insulin sensitivity, is probably the most advanced non-insulin form of therapy. The sulfonylurea of choice is glipizide *(Nelson et al, 1993; Feldman et al, 1997)*. Considering the outcome of various studies, it seems safe to state that at best only 25% of diabetic cats will respond to glipizide treatment. Secondary failures to treat diabetics with sulfonylureas are not uncommon because sulfonylureas not only stimulate insulin but also amylin secretion *(Hoenig et al, 2002)*. The high local amylin concentrations and progressive deposition of pancreatic islet amyloid may be a long-term detrimental sequelae of treatment with these drugs *(Hoenig et al, 2002)*.

Another class of orally available antidiabetic drugs are the thiazolidinediones (glitazones) which are ligands of PPARγ. Glitazones therefore increase insulin sensitivity of insulin target tissues. Darglitazone, one member of this group of compounds, increased insulin sensitivity in obese cats

(*Hoenig et al, 2003*). The usefulness of these drugs in the routine treatment of feline DM, however, remains largely unknown.

Metformin improves insulin sensitivity mainly via inhibition of hepatic gluconeogenesis and glycogenolysis. Even though metformin can have beneficial metabolic effects in diabetic cats, its use for routine treatment was largely questioned: only few of the treated cats improved after treatment. Metformin does not seem to offer any advantage over conventional treatment (*Nelson et al, 2004*).

Postprandial hyperglycemia is one key feature of DM. Therefore, slowing down postprandial intestinal glucose absorption appears as a viable alternative in diabetic therapy. The competitive inhibitor of pancreatic amylase and glucosidases in the intestinal brush border membrane, acarbose, has been proposed for this purpose (*Nelson, 2005*). Even though acarbose may slow gastrointestinal glucose absorption, the recommendation of feeding diabetic cats with a high protein diet seems to largely outweigh the benefit of using acarbose.

▶ Future therapeutic options

The metabolic effects of amylin and GLP-1 have been described previously in this chapter. Beneficial effects of both amylin and GLP-1 are an inhibition of gastric emptying and of postprandial glucagon release (for amylin, see **Figure 16**). Not all of these effects have been investigated in cats so far. The amylin analogue pramlintide (Symlin[R]), which is combined with insulin, and the GLP-1 agonist exendin-4 (Byetta[R]) are now in clinical use for the treatment of human diabetics. Neither drug has been tested in diabetic cats so far and whether these treatments would constitute considerable advantages over current treatment options with insulin is not clear.

Chemical compounds that activate glucokinase have been considered interesting targets for diabetic therapy (*Schermerhorn, 2006*). Clinical usefulness of these drugs is unlikely in the foreseeable future.

12 - Dietary aspects in the treatment of feline diabetes mellitus

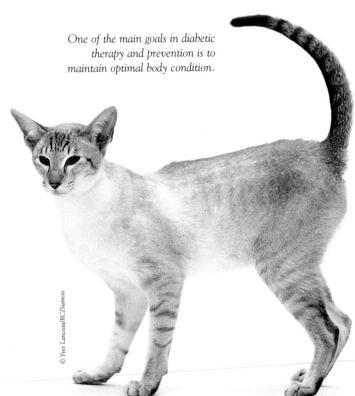

One of the main goals in diabetic therapy and prevention is to maintain optimal body condition.

© Yves Lanceau/RC/Siamois

The optimal diet for feeding the diabetic cat may not yet be known. However, the concept of the most beneficial diet in feline diabetes has seen some major changes over the last few years. Certainly the major step to better glycemic control was the introduction and recommendation of diets high ($\geq$ 45 % of calories) in protein and low ($\leq$ 20 % of calories) in carbohydrate.

Retrospectively, it seems obvious to feed cats a high protein diet which closely resembles their natural diet. Nonetheless, recognition that this may be particularly useful for the diabetic cat has revolutionized diabetic therapy. The traditional high ($\geq$ 30 % of calories) carbohydrate (mainly starch), high ($\geq$ 50 g total dietary fiber (TDF)/ 1000 kcal) fiber diet, which probably was adopted indiscriminately from the recommended diet in diabetic dogs or humans, is no longer recommended for cats. This mainly refers to the carbohydrate content of diets.

▶ General goals for feeding the diabetic cat

(*see also: Biourge, 2005*)

Because feline DM is a lifestyle disease similar to human type 2 DM, one of the main goals in diabetic therapy and prevention is to maintain optimal body condition. As will be discussed below, high protein diets are of particular benefit in feeding diabetic cats. However, the use of these specific diets is most effective when combined with aggressive glucose lowering therapy. For this, insulin therapy is the most useful. This will help to control for glucotoxicity (see above). The best results have been obtained with twice daily insulin injections. Without insulin therapy (or other glucose lowering therapies), it is extremely unlikely that one will be able to successfully treat diabetic cats, at least in the initial phase of treatment. With the combination of insulin and diet, however, there is a good chance for diabetic remission which may allow discontinuation of insulin administration. To achieve good metabolic control and to avoid the risk of insulin-induced hypoglycemia, consistency in timing and in the diet's caloric content is also important.

The three main goals in the nutritional management of diabetic cats are:
1. to control excess body weight.
2. to reduce postprandial hyperglycemia.
3. to stimulate endogenous insulin secretion.

► Prevent or correct obesity

Obesity is directly linked with insulin resistance which predisposes cats to develop overt diabetes mellitus *(Scarlett et al, 1994; Scarlett & Donoghue, 1998)*. Prevention of obesity must therefore be one of the main goals when feeding cats.

Veterinarians should clearly council cat owners to restrict feeding immediately after neutering. Diets with low energy density, i.e. with a restricted amount of fat should be used. Dry diets that are high in fat ($\geq$ 40 % of calories), especially if fed free choice in neutered cats, have been linked to weight gain and the development of obesity in numerous studies (e.g., *Scarlett et al, 1994; Scarlett & Donoghue, 1998*). To the contrary, feeding a moderate fat (25% of calories), moderate carbohydrate diet (35% of calories) reduced weight gain following neutering compared to a high fat (> 40 % of calories) dry diet *(Nguyen et al, 2004b)*.

Weight loss is encouraged if the cat is fed a high protein diet (45% protein; 25% carbohydrates on DM) rather than a diet richer in carbohydrates (28% protein, 38% carbohydrates) *(Hoenig et al, 2007a)*. Restricting caloric intake to the actual needs is important, even if cats are fed diets that closely resemble their natural diet because, at least in the short term, high protein diets do not lead to a significant amount of weight loss if fed ad libitum. However, during restricted feeding, when cats loose body weight, high protein diets may have an additional beneficial effect of favoring the loss of body fat over lean body mass *(Mazzaferro et al, 2003; Hoenig et al, 2007a)*.

A moderate increase in dietary fiber (25-30 g/1000 kcal) might be of interest to moderate the energy density of the diet and to reduce the concentration of fat and carbohydrates. The amount of food offered has to be adjusted to the body composition *(Nguyen et al, 2004a,b)*. On average, this translates into a daily energy requirement of approximately 45-55 kcal/kg of body weight. Because most of our pet cats are neutered and have a sedentary lifestyle, feeding highly palatable, energy rich diets should be reduced. It should be made clear to the owner that any increase in body weight above normal increases the risk of cats to develop DM and should therefore be avoided *(Scarlett & Donoghue, 1998)*. Once established, obesity is the major risk factor for the development of feline DM because of decreased insulin sensitivity *(Biourge et al, 1997; Appleton et al, 2001b)*. Obese cats with insulin resistance have a disturbed insulin secretory pattern even before glucose tolerance is affected *(Hoenig, 2002)*.

► Minimize postprandial glucose excursions

Apart from body weight alone, however, there may also be an additional influence of diet. High carbohydrate (50% of calories) intake will promote postprandial glycemia, especially if the carbohydrate source has a high glycemic index **(Figure 26)**. Hyperglycemia will stimulate pancreatic beta-cells to secrete more insulin. This stress might become overwhelming on the pancreas of overweight cats in which insulin resistance is present. However, there are no studies to date to show that high carbohydrate diets are directly linked to the development of insulin resistance or overt DM.

> **PRINCIPLES IN THE FORMULATION OF DIETS FOR DIABETIC CATS**
> The ideal diet for the diabetic cat should be:
> - moderate in energy (< 4,000 kcal/kg DMB)
> - moderate in fat (< 30% of the calories)
> - rich in protein (>45% of the calories)

FIGURE 26 - WHAT IS THE GLYCEMIC INDEX?

Measuring method in man:
- *amount of food, equivalent to 50 g carbohydrate
  eaten within 13 minutes*
- *blood glucose levels are measured in the next 2 to 3 hours:
  measurement of the Area Under the Curve (AUC)*
- *trial replicated with 8-10 individuals*
- *Glycemic Index (GI) = ratio of curve integrals compared
  to a control (glucose = 100%)*
- *classification:*
    < 55 : low GI
    between 55 and 70: medium GI
    > 70 : high GI

*In man, GI does not necessarily represent a practical guide for evaluating
foods because data can be in conflict depending on the composition
of the meal, the processing method, cooking, etc. Answers can also vary
amongst individuals. In animals, results are more reliable because the diet
can be better controlled.*

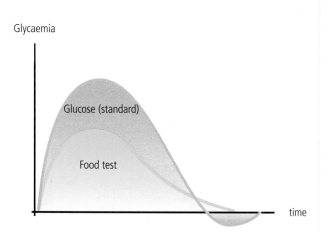

Diabetic cats fed a high protein diet (protein 57%; carbohydrate 8% DMB) achieve better metabolic control than cats fed a high carbohydrate diet (protein 40%, carbohydrate 24%; *Frank et al, 2001*). The use of high protein diets also helps to reduce postprandial hyperglycemia **(Figure 4)** (63% protein DMB, 8% carbohydrate in the study by *Kettelhut et al, 1980*; 54% and 8% in the study by *Tschuor et al, 2006*).

Not only the high protein and low carbohydrate content are of importance, but also the source of carbohydrate. Carbohydrates in diets for diabetic cats were recommended to be complex with a low glycemic index (i.e. barley, corn). Rice, which has a higher glycemic index than corn, resulted in a more pronounced increase of postprandial glucose and insulin levels (*Rand et al, 2004*).

It is unknown at present if this aspect is still relevant considering the low amount of carbohydrates in today's typical diabetic diets. The glycemic index in high carbohydrate diets for diabetic cats would have played a more considerable role than in diets following today's recommendations. Neither the specific role of the glycemic index in low carbohydrate diets nor the effect of mixed carbohydrate sources have so far been investigated.

▶ Stimulate endogenous insulin secretion

The third goal can also be achieved by high protein diets because the response of pancreatic beta-cells to amino acids in diabetic cats is usually maintained for longer periods than their response to glucose (*Kitamura et al, 1999*). Arginine has a strong effect on pancreatic insulin secretion.

▶ Use of high protein diets in the treatment of feline diabetes mellitus

Introduction of high protein diets to feed diabetic cats has been a major step forward in improving therapy in feline DM. Several studies have shown that high protein diets improve the metabolic situation in diabetic and obese cats.

- *Hoenig* (2006a,b) reported that insulin sensitivity of fat metabolism was not normalized in obese cats after body weight loss when the cats were fed a high carbohydrate diet but a high protein diet (45% DMB) improves insulin sensitivity in obese cats. Diabetic cats were not tested in this study.

- The use of a high protein (57% DMB and 50% of calories) low carbohydrate (8% DMB and 13% of calories), canned diet *(Frank et al, 2001)* showed a clear beneficial effect over a higher carbohydrate (24% DMB and 23% of calories), high fiber (56 g TDF/1000 kcal) diet. In diabetic cats fed the high protein diet, the insulin dose could be reduced by up to 50%, and completely withdrawn in 3 of 9 cats *(Frank et al, 2001; Bennett et al, 2006)*.

- In our own experience *(Tschuor et al, 2006)*, the use of a high protein (54% DMB) low carbohydrate (8%), canned diet led to a much higher rate of diabetic remission (50-70%) than previously observed. Interestingly, this occurred even before any marked body weight loss was apparent. Therefore, even though high protein diets have been reported to make weight loss easier in cats *(Szabo et al, 2000; Michel et al, 2005)*, this does not seem to be required for the beneficial effects observed in diabetic individuals.

► Use of high protein diets in the prevention of feline diabetes mellitus

It has been hypothesized that feline pancreatic beta-cells may not be well adapted to high dietary carbohydrate loads and that high carbohydrate diets may be detrimental in cats. Nonetheless, the long-term consequences of overfeeding healthy cats with carbohydrates in respect to their contribution to the development of feline diabetes is currently unknown. One report mentions that insulin sensitivity is decreased and that hyperinsulinemia prevails in cats fed a high carbohydrate diet compared to cats fed a high protein diet *(Hoenig, 2002)*. On the other hand, another study did not reveal any effect of a high protein (approx. 57% DMB protein 22% DMB carbohydrate) versus a medium protein (32% DMB protein, 49% DMB carbohydrate) diet on insulin concentration and insulin sensitivity during an IVGTT or an arginine stimulation test in normal weight cats *(Leray et al, 2006)*. More detailed experiments on a possible direct influence of high protein versus high carbohydrate diets to the development of insulin resistance, beta-cell failure and eventually DM in cats are clearly warranted.

The underlying mechanisms that could explain the positive effects of high protein, low carbohydrate diets are not clear. It has been suggested that the positive effect of these diets may be linked to a decrease in IGF-1 levels *(Leray et al, 2006; but see Alt et al, 2007 reporting low IGF-1 levels in diabetic cats that normalize upon insulin treatment)*. Interestingly, in the study by Leray and colleagues no effect of a high protein (50% protein calories) dry diet on insulin sensitivity was observed in normal weight cats *(Leray et al, 2006)*. This was different from findings in other species. Therefore, it is unknown whether feeding cats with high protein diets is an effective means to prevent the development of diabetes mellitus. Clearly, this question remains unanswered at present.

► Dietary carbohydrate and fiber content in the diet of the diabetic cat

The traditional diet for the diabetic cat contained relatively high ($\geq$ 30 % of calories) amounts of carbohydrate and of dietary fiber ($\geq$50 g TDF/1000 kcal). Dietary fiber is considered beneficial because it slows gastric emptying, gastrointestinal glucose absorption, increases insulin sensitivity and improves the control of nutrient metabolism by releasing gut hormones *(Nelson et al, 2000)*. Viscous soluble fibers were considered of most value because they slow the transport of glucose to the surface of the gastrointestinal mucosa *(Nelson, 2005)*.

A study compared the outcome on the diabetic management of two canned diets with a protein content of approximately 40% of energy, one containing low amounts of carbohydrate (12% of energy) and dietary fiber (0.1g/100kcal), and one containing moderate amounts of carbohydrate (26% of energy) and high amounts of fiber (approximately 5 g/100 kcal) *(Bennett et al, 2006)*. The rate of diabetic remission was higher in the former diet (> 60% versus approx. 40%). Hence, a low content of carbohydrate clearly seems to be beneficial, and seems to outweigh the relatively low fiber content in this diet.

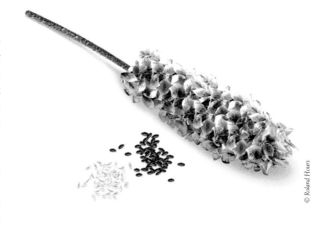

© Roland Hours

Psyllium seeds have been traditionally used in weight loss diets. Mucilage is able to absorb a great deal of water in the stomach, forming a voluminous gel. This slows down gastric emptying.

TRANS- AND CIS-CONFIGURATION OF FATTY ACIDS

Configuration *cis*

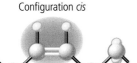

Configuration *trans*

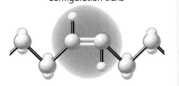

In the trans-configuration, the hydrogen atoms are on the opposite sides of the double bond.

A study by *Nelson et al* (2000) compared two diets with similar amounts of protein (44% of dry matter), one containing a high amount (13% DMB), and one containing a low amount of fiber (2% DMB). The high fiber diet was beneficial. However, it also contained markedly less carbohydrate (27 versus 38% DMB) and slightly more protein. All factors combined might therefore have been responsible for the beneficial effect.

Overall, there is good evidence that the optimal diet for a diabetic cat should have a high protein and low carbohydrate content. Under these conditions, a high fiber content may be of slightly less importance than previously thought. However, by slowing gastrointestinal transit, dietary fiber still has its place in diets for diabetic cats. Further, a high fiber content leads to overall caloric dilution of the diet which clearly may help to control body weight in cats.

▶ The role of specific fatty acids

The role of different types of fatty acids in obese cats has also been evaluated. One diet was enriched in omega-3 polyunsaturated fatty acids (n-3 PUFA; total fat content 20.1% on DMB; 9.6% of fat consisting of n-3 PUFA), the control diet contained reduced amounts of n-3 PUFA (total fat content 19.8%; 1.5% of n-3 PUFA). The diet high in n-3 PUFA was shown to improve the long-term control of glycemia and lower plasma insulin levels *(Wilkins et al, 2004)*. In contrast, saturated fatty acids were considered to have detrimental effects on glucose control. The proposed underlying mechanism of omega 3-PUFA's role in metabolism may include an activation or increased expression of PPAR-gamma, and thus an increase in insulin sensitivity.

▶ Trace elements and antioxidants

The trace element **chromium** has been considered an essential cofactor for insulin action. The exact mechanism of chromium action to increase insulin sensitivity is unknown. However, the data are conflicting and far from conclusive. At present, there is no clear evidence to recommend the use of chromium. To the author's knowledge, the effect of chromium in diabetic cats has not been tested. Compared to other treatment options, chromium's beneficial effect appears negligible.

Vanadium, another trace element, seems to have comparable effects to chromium yet may act through different mechanisms. Only preliminary results are available which suggest that vanadium may have some beneficial effects in diabetic cats. The recommended dose was 0.2 mg/kg per day, administered via food or water *(Nelson, 2005)*.

Glucotoxicity induced by chronic hyperglycemia contributes to progressive beta-cell damage and insulin resistance. In part, this is due to increased intracellular oxidative stress. Whether widespread use of antioxidants may help to reduce these effects, has, to the authors' knowledge, not been investigated in well-controlled studies in cats. However, these compounds are considered safe based on the current scientific data. One may therefore consider fortifying diets with antioxidants.

TRANS-FATTY ACIDS

Patricia A. Schenck, DVM, PhD

Trans-fatty acids (TFA) are a specific type of unsaturated fat. Naturally occurring unsaturated fatty acids are mostly in the cis-configuration. In TFA, the spatial configuration is different because the hydrogen atoms are on the opposite sides of the double bond. TFA are found naturally in ruminant meats and dairy products. They are created by microbial transformation of cis-unsaturated fatty acids in the forestomachs. High levels of TFA, however, are also created during industrial hydrogenation or deodorization mainly of plant oils. The concentration of TFA in ruminant fats is approximately 5 to 8 g/100g fat, whereas the TFA of partially hydrogenated vegetable oils averages 45g TFA/100g oil.

TFA and human nutrition
Recently, public interest has focused on the potential health risks associated with TFA intake in humans. Dietary TFA have been suggested to increase insulin resistance in humans, increasing the risk for the development of type 2 diabetes mellitus. Therefore, the replacement of TFA with polyunsaturated fat was postulated to markedly reduce the risk for the development of diabetes. Because of these potential health risks, some government agencies require the clear labeling of TFA contents in human foods, and some countries such as Denmark restrict the sale of processed oils containing high levels of TFA (e.g., more than 2% TFA in Denmark). In the United States, TFA have to be itemized separately in the Nutrition Facts label of food products.

Not all TFA are equal
It is very important to stress that not all TFA are equal. The negative effects of some TFA that are mainly created during industrial processing of vegetable fat have to be clearly separated from effects of other TFA that are created by microbial fermentation in the ruminants' forestomachs. At least some of the latter TFA, e.g. the C-18 trans-vaccen acid, may rather have beneficial health effects. Trans-vaccen acid can be metabolized to conjugated linoleic acid which has been shown to have antidiabetic effects and anti-cancerogenic effects in animal experiments.

TFA in cat and dog food
Currently, there is no reason to believe that pet food containing TFA derived from ruminant sources has any deleterious effects on animal health. To my knowledge, no studies evaluating the effects of TFA in pets have been reported at this time nor have the different effects of TFA derived from ruminant sources versus industrially processed vegetable oils been looked at in cats or dogs.

13 - High protein diet and renal function

The question about the long-term effect of high protein diets on renal function has been raised. However, it should be stressed that there is no indication that the long term feeding of diets high in protein causes a deterioration of kidney function in normal cats or in cats with early kidney disease (*Finco et al, 1998*). Obviously, high protein diets are contraindicated for cats with uremia, and nephropathy is a relatively common finding in diabetic cats (*Nelson, 2005*). To the author's knowledge, however, no study has investigated this question in detail.

In cases where impaired renal function and azotemia occur concurrently in diabetic cats, the use of diets with reduced amounts of protein may be warranted to minimize the risk of a uremic crisis. In these cases, one may envisage the combination of such a diet with drugs like acarbose, which limits gastrointestinal carbohydrate absorption. However, hard data to support this idea are lacking.

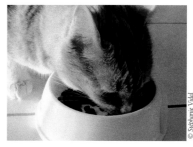

In our experience, most cats readily accept the currently available diets that are high in protein and low in carbohydrate. Cats like these diets, and many cats are rather polyphagic in the initial stages of treatment.

Despite a clear improvement in the management of diabetic cats since the introduction of diets high in protein and low in carbohydrate, many questions remain to be answered.
- Is protein or carbohydrate the key factor, i.e. is it the high protein or the low carbohydrate content that is most important?
- Do some particular amino acids such as arginine, have beneficial effects? Hence, would different sources of protein play a role (*Leray et al, 2006*)?
- What are the long term consequences of feeding these diets for the risk of diabetic ketosis or diabetic nephropathy? At present, there is no indication that the long term feeding of diets high in protein leads to a deterioration of kidney function in normal cats or in cats with early kidney disease (*Finco et al, 1998*).
- What are the long term consequences of feeding high protein diets on body weight and body composition?

14 - Practical recommendations to feed the diabetic cat

▶ Format of the food

Today, special diets for diabetic cats are available both as canned or dry food. Extrusion technology has been improved to such a degree where dry diets with high protein and low carbohydrate content have become available. Clearly, there is no indication whether a canned versus a dry diet offers a major advantage as long as the composition of the diet with a high protein and low carbohydrate content is controlled.

▶ Method of feeding

Most diabetic cats can best be fed twice a day, with insulin being injected just before or after meals. Obviously, this feeding regimen does not correspond to the natural feeding rhythm in cats which, when fed ad libitum, may consume up to 15 small meals throughout the day. Nevertheless, especially with the use of high protein diets, postprandial glucose levels increase only slightly compared to high carbohydrate diets (*Kettelhut et al, 1980; Kienzle, 1994; Martin & Rand, 1999*). Therefore, the timing of insulin injection relative to offering food, may seem less important. This was confirmed in an unpublished study indicating that the timing of insulin injection, which was supposed to be optimized for insulin action to occur (45 minutes before meal versus at the onset of the meal), had little effect on metabolic control (*Alt, 2006*). Hence, the composition of the diet is much more important than the timing of meals. It needs to be stressed, however, that food must be available once insulin action occurs to prevent life-threatening hypoglycemia.

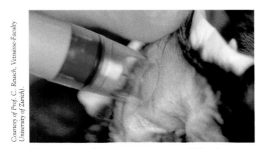

Courtesy of Prof. C. Reusch, Vetsuisse-Faculty University of Zurich).

Figure 27 - Home monitoring of blood glucose concentration in cats.

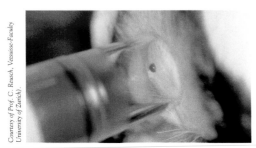

Courtesy of Prof. C. Reusch, Vetsuisse-Faculty University of Zurich).

Capillary blood obtained from the cat's ear.

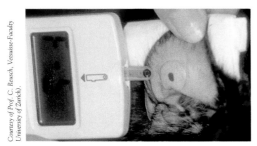

Courtesy of Prof. C. Reusch, Vetsuisse-Faculty University of Zurich).

Glucose is easily checked with portable glucometers.

► Medical checks

Caution must be taken to avoid hypoglycemia when insulin-treated diabetic cats are shifted to a high protein, low carbohydrate diet.

This point also stresses that throughout therapy, diabetic cats should be regularly monitored. This can be achieved by home monitoring for the blood glucose level with portable glucometers (**Figure 27**) *(Reusch et al, 2006b)* coupled with regular laboratory determination of serum fructosamine concentrations. Owners should also be aware of the possible clinical signs associated with hypo- or hyperglycemia. Throughout therapy, but also when insulin therapy is no longer necessary (transient diabetes mellitus), owners can easily check their cats for the recurrence of glucosuria using glucose sticks in fresh cat litter that is mixed with a small volume of water. This will provide at least some information to consider adjustment in the insulin regimen.

Remission of diabetes mellitus is possible in many cats if the blood glucose concentration can be controlled with insulin therapy combined with a high protein diet. Therefore, many cats may not need lifelong insulin therapy. Insulin is discontinued with acquisition of glycemic control. It is recommended to maintain the high protein diet during remission. In addition, the cat should be regularly reevaluated to monitor for recurrence of clinical signs of diabetes mellitus. If or when the diabetes returns, specific treatment must be immediately reinstated.

Conclusion

Feline DM is a frequent metabolic disorder and its prevalence has increased over the last 30 years. This is most likely linked to the obesity problem in our pet population, especially in cats. However, at the same time treatment has become much more successful and the fatality rate in diabetes mellitus decreased tremendously over the last 10-20 years. Considering the major underlying pathophysiological disorder, i.e. the lack of insulin and insulin action, most diabetic cats have traditionally been treated with insulin. Insulin is still the treatment of choice because it is best suited to control metabolism and to help reduce glucolipotoxicity. This may result in complete resolution of clinical signs. Over the last few years, it has become very clear that insulin therapy should be supported by switching the diet of diabetic cats to a high protein (> 50%) low carbohydrate (<15%) diet. The remission rate has increased markedly since the introduction of these diets in the treatment regimen. Overall, feline DM clearly is a disease that can and should be treated.

Frequently asked questions about dietetic treatment of feline diabetes mellitus

Q	A
What is the most effective way to treat diabetic cats?	Experience over the last few years clearly favors intensive insulin therapy (mostly BID), combined with feeding a high protein diet, low carbohydrate diet.
Do diabetic cats have postprandial hyperglycemia?	This seems to depend largely on the composition of the diet. Cats fed high protein diets that are now recommended for diabetic cats show no or only a slight postprandial increase in glycemia. The higher the carbohydrate content of a diet, the stronger the postprandial hyperglycemia will be.
What is the effect of different diets on average blood glucose levels?	In general, it is much easier to maintain near-normal glycemia in insulin-treated, diabetic cats when they are fed a high-protein, low-carbohydrate diet. Postprandial hyperglycemia is almost absent, and the average blood glucose level is reduced.
How long before or after insulin injection should a diabetic cat be fed?	If meal-fed, diabetic cats can be injected just after feeding but no clear recommendation can be given. A study compared feeding immediately after injection or 45 min after injection. No major differences on metabolic control were observed.
What feeding paradigm is best for diabetic cats?	If maintenance of body weight is not a problem, it appears possible to feed diabetic cats ad libitum. If obesity is of concern, restricted feeding requires that food is not available ad libitum. In this situation, two meals per day, just followed by insulin injection, may be most appropriate.
What do you do if a diabetic cat does not eat after the insulin injection?	In an emergency situation, when a diabetic cat has received its full dose of insulin and does not eat, the cat should be offered rapidly absorbable carbohydrates, e.g. honey, to prevent life-threatening hypoglycemia. If a diabetic cat suddenly refuses to eat the diet, another formulation should be tested, preferably also with a high protein content. Such an emergency situation can be prevented if insulin is injected only after the cat has eaten the meal. Obviously, this may be difficult for some owners for practical or time reasons.
Can the diet for a diabetic cat be varied from day to day?	Ideally, diabetic cats should be fed with high protein diets throughout the remainder of their lives, even if diabetic remission occurs. Anecdotal reports indicate that hyperglycemia will reappear within a few days when switching a cat in diabetic remission to a high carbohydrate diet. Therefore, given the metabolic situation in cats and the specific benefit of high protein, low carbohydrate diets in diabetic cats, it appears safe to recommend the long term use of these diets, even after resolution of clinical signs.
Does physical activity play a role in therapy?	It may be very difficult to control physical activity in cats. However, it is recommended to keep physical activity at a relatively constant level so that energy intake and energy expenditure are well matched to the treatment regime with insulin and diet.
Should the diet for diabetic cats contain high levels of dietary fibers?	Traditionally, high fiber diets were recommended for diabetic cats. However, the high fiber content does not seem to be the most important factor. High protein low carbohydrate diets seem to be very effective. It is currently not completely clear if high protein high fiber diets would offer an additional benefit. In any case, however, the lower caloric density in high fiber diets will render the control of body weight easier.
What should be done to achieve ideal body weight in diabetic cats?	Most diabetic cats are obese. Therefore, treatment should also aim at reducing body weight to normal levels. A decrease of 1.5% of body weight per week appears to be safe (see Obesity chapter). When fed high protein diets, cats loose mainly body fat and maintain lean body mass.
Can diabetes mellitus be prevented?	The risk for becoming diabetic increases dramatically in overweight cats. Therefore, preventing obesity seems to be the most important factor to lower the risk of developing the disease. This is true in particular for neutered cats, because neutered cats eat more and need less energy. Neutered cats are three to four times more likely to become obese, and obese cats are four times more likely to become diabetic.

References

Ahima RS. *Central actions of adipocyte hormones.* Trends Endocrinol Metab 2005; 16: 307-313.

Alt N. *The effect of feeding time on the quality of metabolic control, day-to-day variability of blood glucose curves and evaluation of IGF-1 levels in cats with diabetes mellitus.* Dissertation, University of Zurich, 2006.

Alt N, Kley S, Tschuor F, et al *Evaluation of IGF-1 levels in cats with transient and permanent diabetes mellitus.* Res Vet Sci 2007; doi: 10.1016/j. rvsc.2007.01.014.

Appleton DJ, Rand JS, Sunvold GD. *Plasma leptin concentrations in cats: reference range, effect of weight gain and relationship with adiposity as measured by dual energy X-ray absorptiometry.* J Fel Med Surg 2000; 2: 191-199.

Appleton DJ, Rand JS, Priest J, et al. *Determination of reference values for glucose tolerance, insulin tolerance, and insulin sensitivity tests in clinically normal cats.* Am J Vet Res 2001a; 62: 630-636.

Appleton DJ, Rand JS, Sunvold GD. *Insulin sensitivity decreases with obesity, and lean cats with low insulin sensitivity are at greatest risk of glucose intolerance with weight gain.* J Fel Med Surg 2001b; 3: 211-228.

Bailiff NL, Nelson RW, Feldman EC, et al. *Frequency and risk factors for urinary tract infection in cats with diabetes mellitus.* J Vet Intern Med 2006; 20: 850-855.

Banks WA, Farr SA, Morley JE. *The effects of high fat diets on the blood-brain barrier transport of leptin: failure or adaptation?* Physiol Behav 2006; 88: 244-248.

Baral RM, Rand JS, Catt MJ. *Prevalence of feline diabetes mellitus in a feline private practice.* J Vet Intern Med 2003; 17: 433.

Barroso I. *Genetics of type 2 diabetes.* Diabet Med 2005; 22: 517-535.

Bennett N, Greco DS, Peterson ME, et al. *Comparison of low carbohydrate-low fiber diet and a moderate carbohydrate-high fiber diet in the management of feline diabetes mellitus.* J Fel Med Surg 2006; 8: 73-84.

Biourge V, Nelson RW, Feldman EC, et al. *Effect of weight gain and subsequent weight loss on glucose tolerance and insulin response in healthy cats.* J Vet Intern Med 1997; 11: 86-91.

Biourge VC. *Feline diabetes mellitus: nutritional management.* Waltham Focus 2005; 15: 36-40.

Brennan CL, Hoenig M, Ferguson DC. *GLUT4 but not GLUT1 expression decreases early in the development of feline obesity.* Domest Anim Endocrinol 2004; 26: 291-301.

Butler AE, Janson J, Soeller WC, et al. *Increased beta-cell apoptosis prevents adaptive increase in beta-cell mass in mouse model of type 2 diabetes: evidence for role of islet amyloid formation rather than direct action of amyloid.* Diabetes 2003; 52: 2304-14.

Chan DL, Freeman LM, Rozanski EA, et al. *Alterations in carbohydrate metabolism in critically ill cats.* J Vet Emerg Crit Care 2006; 16: S7-S13.

Cooper GJS. *Amylin compared with calcitonin-gene related peptide: structure, biology and relevance to metabolic disease.* Endocr Rev 1994; 15: 163-201.

Crenshaw KL, Peterson ME, Heeb LA, et al. *Serum fructosamine concentration as an index of glycemia in cats with diabetes mellitus and stress hyperglycemia.* J Vet Intern Med 1996; 10: 360-364.

Diez M, Nguyen P. *The epidemiology of canine and feline obesity.* Waltham Focus 2006; 16: 2-8.

Dohan FC, Lukens FDW. *Experimental diabetes produced by the administration of glucose.* Endocrinol 1948; 42: 244-262.

Donath MY, Ehses JA, Maedler K, et al. *Mechanisms of beta-cell death in type 2 diabetes.* Diabetes 2005; 54 suppl. 2: S108-S113.

Drucker DJ. *Minireview: the glucagon-like peptides.* Endocrinol 2001; 142: 521-527.

Edelman SV, Weyer C. *Unresolved challenges with insulin therapy in type 1 and type 2 diabetes: potential benefit of replacing amylin, a second beta-cell hormone.* Diab Technol Therapeut 2002; 4: 175-189.

Elliott DA, Nelson RW, Reusch CE, et al. *Comparison of serum fructosamine and blood glycosylated hemoglobin concentrations for assessment of glycemic control in cats with diabetes mellitus.* J Am Vet Med Assoc 1999; 214: 1794-1798.

Feldhahn JR, Rand JS, Martin G. *Insulin sensitivity in normal and diabetic cats.* J Fel Med Surg 1999; 1: 107-115.

Feldman EC, Nelson RW, Feldman MS. *Intensive 50-week evaluation of glipizide administration in 50 cats with previously untreated diabetes mellitus.* J Am Vet Med Assoc 1997; 210: 772-777.

Feldman EC, Nelson RW. *Feline diabetes mellitus.* In: Feldman EC, Nelson RW, eds. Canine and Feline Endocrinology and Reproduction. 3rd ed. St. Louis: Saunders, 2004; 539-579.

Fettman MJ, Stanton CA, Banks LL, et al. *Effects of neutering on bodyweight, metabolic rate and glucose tolerance of domestic cats.* Res Vet Sci 1997; 62: 131-136.

Finco DR, Brown SA, Brown CA, et al. *Protein and calorie effects on progression of induced chronic renal failure in cats.* Am J Vet Res 1998; 59: 575-82.

Fineman M, Weyer C, Maggs DG, et al. *The human amylin analog, pramlintide, reduces postprandial hyperglucagonemia in patients with type 2 diabetes mellitus.* Horm Metab Res 2002; 34: 504-508.

Franconi F, Loizzo A, Ghirlanda G, et al. *Taurine supplementation and diabetes mellitus.* Curr Opin Clin Nutr Metab Care 2006; 9: 32-36.

Frank G, Anderson W, Pazak H, et al. *Use of high-protein diet in the management of feline diabetes mellitus.* Vet Therapeut 2001; 2: 238-245.

Furrer D, Tschuor F, Reusch C, et al. *Effect of amylin on plasma concentrations of glucose, insulin and glucagon in an arginine stimulation and meal response test in cats,* in: Proceedings ECVIM Forum 2005.

German AJ. *The growing problem of obesity in dogs and cats.* J Nutr 2006; 136: 1940S-1946S.

Goossens MMC, Nelson RW, Feldman EC, et al. *Response to insulin treatment and survival in 104 cats with diabetes mellitus (1985-1995).* J Vet Intern Med 1998; 12: 1-6.

Harper EJ, Stack DM, Watson TDG, et al. *Effects of feeding regimens on bodyweight, composition and condition score in cats following ovariohysterectomy.* J Small Anim Pract 2001; 42: 433-438.

Henson MS, O'Brien TD. *Feline models of type 2 diabetes mellitus.* ILAR J 2006; 47: 234-242.

Hoenig M. *Comparative aspects of diabetes mellitus in dogs and cats.* Mol Cell Endocrinol 2002; 197: 221-229.

Hoenig M. The cat as a model for human nutrition and disease. Curr Opin Nutr Metab Care 2006a; 9: 584-588.

Hoenig M. Unique aspects of metabolism in obese cats, in Proceedings. 24th ACVIM Forum 2006b; 432.

Hoenig M, Alexander S, Holson J, et al. Influence of glucose dosage on interpretation of intravenous glucose tolerance tests in lean and obese cats. J Vet Intern Med 2002; 16: 529-532.

Hoenig M, Caffall ZF, McGraw RA, et al. Cloning, expression and purification of feline proinsulin. Domest Anim Endocrinol 2006a; 30: 28-37.

Hoenig M, Ferguson DC. Effect of darglitazone on glucose clearance and lipid metabolism in obese cats. Am J Vet Res 2003; 64: 1409-1413.

Hoenig M, Ferguson DC. Effects of neutering on hormonal concentrations and energy requirements in male and female cats. Am J Vet Res 2002; 63: 634-639.

Hoenig M, Ferguson DC. Impairment of glucose tolerance in hyperthyroid cats. J Endocrinol 1989; 121: 249-251.

Hoenig M, Hall G, Ferguson D, et al. A feline model of experimentally induced islet amyloidosis. Am J Pathol 2000; 157: 2143-2150.

Hoenig M, McGoldrick JB, deBeer M, et al. Activity and tissue-specific expression of lipases and tumor-necrosis factor alpha in lean and obese cats. Domest Anim Endocrinol 2006b; 30: 333-344.

Hoenig M, Thomaseth K, Brandao J, et al. Assessment and mathematical modeling of glucose turnover and insulin sensitivity in lean and obese cats. Domest Anim Endocrinol 2006c; 31: 373-389.

Hoenig M, Thomaseth K, Waldron M, et al. Fatty acid turnover, substrate oxidation, and heat production in lean and obese cats during the euglycemic hyperinsulinemic clamp. Domest Anim Endocrinol 2007b; 32: 39-338.

Hoenig M, Thomaseth K, Waldron M, et al. Insulin sensitivity, fat distribution and adipocytokine response to different diets in lean, and obese cats before and after weight loss. Am J Physiol Regul Integr Comp Physiol 2007a; 292: R227-R234.

Höppener JWM, Nieuwenhuis MG, Vroom TM, et al. Role of islet amyloid in type 2 diabetes mellitus: consequence or cause? Mol Cell Endocrinol 2002; 197: 205-212.

Jin Y, Lin D. Fungal urinary tract infections in the dog and cat: a retrospective study (2001-2004). J Am Anim Hosp Assoc 2005; 41: 373-381.

Johnson KH, Hayden DW, O'Brien TD, et al. Spontaneous diabetes mellitus - islet amyloid complex in adult cats. Am J Pathol 1986; 125: 416-419.

Johnson KH, O'Brien TD, Betsholtz C, et al. Islet amyloid, islet-amyloid polypeptide and diabetes mellitus. New Engl J Med 1989; 321, 513-518.

Kanchuk ML, Backus RC, Calvert CC, et al. Neutering induces changes in food intake, body weight, plasma insulin and leptin concentrations in normal and lipoprotein lipase-deficient male cats. J Nutr 2002; 132: 1730S-1732S.

Kanchuk ML, Backus RC, Calvert CC, et al. Weight gain in gonadectomized normal and lipoprotein lipase-deficient male domestic cats results from increased food intake and not decreased energy expenditure. J Nutr 2003; 133: 1866-1874.

Kaneko JJ, Kawamoto M, Heusner AA, et al. Evaluation of serum fructosamine concentration as an index of blood glucose control in cats with diabetes mellitus. Am J Vet Res 1992; 53: 1797-1801.

Kettelhut IC, Foss MC, Migliorini RH. Glucose homeostasis in a carnivorous animal (cat) and in rats fed a high-protein diet. Am J Physiol 1980; 239: R437-R444.

Kienzle E. Blood sugar levels and renal sugar excretion after the intake of high carbohydrate diets in cats. J Nutr 1994; 124: 2563S-2567S.

Kitamura T, Yasuda J, Hashimoto A. Acute insulin response to intravenous arginine in nonobese healthy cats. J Vet Intern Med 1999; 13: 549-556.

Konarkowska B, Aitken J, Kistler J, et al. The aggregation potential of human amylin determines its cytotoxicity towards islet beta-cells. FEBS J 2006; 273: 3614-3624.

Laluha P, Gerber B, Laluhova D, et al. Stress hyperglycemia in sick cats: a retrospective study over 4 years. Schweiz Arch Tierheilk 2004; 146: 375-383.

Lazar MA. How obesity causes diabetes: not a tall tale. Science 2005; 307: 373-375.

Lederer R, Rand JS, Hughes IP, et al. Chronic or recurring medical problems, dental disease, repeated corticosteroid treatment, and lower physical activity are associated with diabetes in burmese cats. J Vet Intern Med 2003; 17: 433.

Leray V, Siliart B, Dumon H, et al. Protein intake does not affect insulin sensitivity in normal weight cats. J Nutr 2006; 136:2028S-2030S.

Link KRJ, Rand JS. Reference values for glucose tolerance and glucose tolerance status in cats. J Am Vet Med Assoc 1998; 213: 492-496.

Ludvik B, Lell B, Hartter E, et al. Decrease of stimulated amylin release precedes impairment of insulin secretion in type II diabetes. Diabetes 1991; 40: 1615-1619.

Lund EM, Armstrong PJ, Kirk CA, et al. Prevalence and risk factors for obesity in adult cats from private US veterinary practices. Intern J Appl Res Vet Med 2005; 3: 88-96

Lutz TA, Ainscow J, Rand JS. Frequency of pancreatic amyloid deposition in cats from south-eastern Queensland. Aus Vet J 1994; 71: 254-256.

Lutz TA, Rand JS. Pathogenesis of feline diabetes mellitus. Vet Clin North Am Small Anim Pract 1995; 25: 527-552.

Lutz TA, Rand JS, Ryan E. Fructosamine concentrations in hyperglycemic cats. Can Vet J 1995; 36: 155-159.

Lutz TA, Rand JS. Plasma amylin and insulin concentrations in normoglycemic and hyperglycemic cats. Can Vet J 1996; 37: 27-34.

Lutz TA, Rand JS. Detection of amyloid deposition in various regions of the feline pancreas by different staining techniques. J Comp Pathol 1997; 116: 157-170.

Lutz TA. The pancreatic hormone amylin as a centrally acting satiating hormone. Curr Drug Targets 2005; 6: 181-189.

Ma Z, Westermark GT, Johnson KH, et al. Quantitative immunohistochemical analysis of islet amyloid polypeptide (IAPP) in normal, impaired glucose tolerant, and diabetic cats. Amyloid 1998; 5: 255-261.

Malecki MT. Genetics of type 2 diabetes mellitus. Diabetes Res Clin Pract 2005; 68 suppl. 1: S10-S21.

Marshall RD, Rand JS. Comparison of the pharmacokinetics and pharmacodynamics of once versus twice daily administration of insulin glargine in normal cats. J Vet Intern Med 2002; 16: 373.

Marshall RD, Rand JS. Insulin glargine and a high protein-low carbohydrate diet are associated with high remission rates in newly diagnosed diabetic cats. J Vet Intern Med 2004; 18: 401.

Martin GJW, Rand JS. Food intake and blood glucose in normal and diabetic cats fed ad libitum. J Fel Med Surg 1999; 1: 241-251.

Martin L, Siliart B, Dumon H, et al. Leptin, body fat content and energy expenditure in intact and gonadectomized adult cats: a preliminary study. J Anim Physiol Anim Nutr 2001; 85; 195-199.

Martin L, Siliart B. Hormonal consequences of neutering in cats. Waltham Focus 2005; 15: 32-35.

Matveyenko AV, Butler PC. Beta-cell deficit due to increased apoptosis in the human islet amyloid polypeptide transgenic (HIP) rat recapitulates the metabolic defects present in type 2 diabetes. Diabetes 2006; 55: 2106-2114.

Matveyenko AV, Butler PC. Islet amyloid polypeptide (IAPP) transgenic rodents as models for type 2 diabetes. ILAR J 2006; 47: 225-233.

Mazzaferro EM, Greco DS, Turner AS, et al. Treatment of feline diabetes mellitus using an alpha-glucosidase inhibitor and a low-carbohydrate diet. J Fel Med Surg 2003; 5: 183-189.

McCann TM, Simpson KE, Sham DJ, et al. Feline diabetes mellitus in the UK: the prevalence within an insured cat population and a questionnaire-based putative risk factor analysis. J Fel Med Surg 2007; 9: 289-299.

Meurs KM, Fox PR, Miller MW, et al. Plasma concentrations of tumor necrosis factor-alpha in cats with congestive heart failure. Am J Vet Res 2002; 63: 640-642.

Mexas AM, Hess RS, Hawkins EC, et al. Pulmonary lesions in cats with diabetes mellitus. J Vet Intern Med 2006; 20: 47-51.

Michel KE, Bader A, Shofer FS, et al. Impact of time-limited feeding and dietary carbohydrate content on weight loss in group-housed cats. J. Fel Med Surg 2005; 7: 349-355.

Mizisin AP, Nelson RW, Sturges BK, et al Comparable myelinated nerve pathology in feline and human diabetes mellitus. Acta Neuropathol 2007; 113: 431-442.

Muff R, Born W, Lutz TA, et al. Biological importance of the peptides of the calcitonin family as revealed by disruption and transfer of corresponding genes. Peptides 2004; 25: 2027-2038.

Nakayama H, Uchida K, Ono K, et al. Pathological observation of six cases of feline diabetes mellitus. Jpn J Vet Sci 1990; 52: 819-825.

Nelson RW, Himsel CA, Feldman EC, et al. Glucose tolerance and insulin response in normal-weight and obese cats. Am J Vet Res 1990; 51: 1357-1362.

Nelson RW, Feldman EC, Ford SL, et al. Effect of an orally administered sulfonylurea, glipizide, for treatment of diabetes mellitus in cats. J Am Vet Med Assoc 1993; 203: 821-827.

Nelson RW, Griffey SM, Feldman EC, et al. Transient clinical diabetes mellitus in cats: 10 cases (1989-1991). J Vet Intern Med 1999; 13: 28-35.

Nelson RW, Scott-Moncrieff JC, Feldman EC, et al. Effect of dietary insoluble fiber on control of glycemia in cats with naturally acquired diabetes mellitus. J Am Vet Med Assoc 2000; 216: 1082-1088.

Nelson RW, Spann D, Elliott DA, et al. Evaluation of the oral antihyperglycemic drug metformin in normal and diabetic cats. J Vet Intern Med 2004; 18: 18-24.

Nelson RW. Diabetes mellitus. In: Ettinger SJ, Feldman EC, eds. Textbook of Veterinary Internal Medicine. 6th ed. St. Louis: Elsevier Saunders, 2005; 1563-1591.

Nguyen P, Leray V, Dumon H, et al. High protein intake affects lean body mass but not energy expenditure in nonobese neutered cats. J Nutr 2004a; 134 suppl.: 2084S-2086S.

Nguyen P, Dumon HJ, Siliart BS, et al. Effects of dietary fat and energy on body weight and composition after gonadectomy in cats. Am J Vet Res 2004b; 65: 1708-1713.

O'Brien TD, Hayden DW, Johnson KH, et al. High dose intravenous glucose tolerance test and serum insulin and glucagon levels in diabetic and non-diabetic cats: relationships to insular amyloidosis. Vet Pathol 1985; 22: 250-261.

O'Brien TD, Westermark P, Johnson KH. Islet amyloid polypeptide and insulin secretion from isolated perfused pancreas of fed, fasted, glucose-treated and dexamethasone treated rats. Diabetes 1991; 40: 1701-1706.

O'Brien TD. Pathogenesis of feline diabetes mellitus. Mol Cell Endocrinol 2002; 197: 213-219.

Panciera DL, Thomas CB, Eicker SW, et al. Epizootiologic patterns of diabetes mellitus in cats: 333 cases (1980-1986). J Am Vet Med Assoc 1990; 197: 1504-1508.

Petrus DJ, Jackson MW, Kemnitz JW, et al. Assessing insulin sensitivity in the cat: evaluation of the hyperinsulinemic euglycemic clamp and the minimal model analysis. Res Vet Sci 1998; 65: 179-181.

Plier ML, Grindem CB, MacWilliams PS, et al. Serum fructosamine concentration in nondiabetic and diabetic cats. Vet Clin Pathol 1998; 27: 34-39.

Prahl A, Glickman L, Guptill L, et al. Time trends and risk factors for diabetes mellitus in cats. J Vet Intern Med 2003; 17: 434.

Prahl A, Guptill L, Glickman NW, et al. Time trends and risk factors for diabetes mellitus in cats presented to veterinary teaching hospitals. J Fel Med Surg 2007, doi:10.1016/j. jfms.2007.02.004.

Prentki M, Joly E, El-Assad W, et al. Malonly-CoA signaling, lipid partitioning, and glucolipotoxicity. Diabetes 2002; 51 suppl. 3: S405-S413.

Prentki M, Nolan CJ. Islet beta cell failure in type 2 diabetes. J Clin Invest 2006; 116: 1802-1812.

Rand JS, Bobbermien LM, Hendrikz JK, et al. Over representation of Burmese cats with diabetes mellitus. Aust Vet J. 1997; 75: 402-405.

Rand JS, Fleeman LM, Farrow HA, et al. Canine and feline diabetes mellitus: nature or nurture? J Nutr 2004; 134 suppl.: 2072S-2080S.

Rand JS, Marshall RD. Diabetes mellitus in cats. Vet Clin North Am Small Anim Pract 2005; 35: 211-224.

Rand J. Editorial: Glargine, a new long-acting insulin analog for diabetic cats. J Vet Intern Med 2006; 20: 219-220.

Randle PJ. Regulatory interactions between lipids and glucides: the glucose fatty acid cycle after 35 years. Diabetes Metab Rev 1998; 14: 263-283.

Reaven GM. The insulin resistance syndrome: definition and dietary approaches to treatment. An Rev Nutr 2005; 25: 391-406.

**Patricia A.
SCHENCK**
DMV, PhD

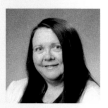

Diagnostic approach to the hyperlipidemic cat and dietary treatment

1 - Lipid metabolism 225

2 - Diagnostic approach to the hyperlipidemic patient 229

3 - Causes of hyperlipidemia 231

4 - Primary hyperlipidemia 233

5 - Effects of persistent hyperlipidemia 235

6 - Treatment of hyperlipidemia 236

Conclusion 238

Frequently asked questions 239

References 240

Royal Canin nutritional information 244

ABBREVIATIONS USED IN THIS CHAPTER

ACAT: acyl-coenzyme A cholesterol acyltrans-
ferase
ALT: alanine aminotransferase
AST: aspartate aminotransferase
CETP: cholesteryl ester transfer protein
DHA: docosahexaenoic acid

EPA: eicosapentaenoic acid
HDL: high density lipoproteins
HMGCoA reductase: 3-hydroxy-3-methylglu-
taryl coenzyme A reductase
IDL: intermediate density lipoproteins
LCAT: lecithin cholesterol acyltransferase

LDH: lactate deshydrogenase
LDL: low density lipoproteins
LPL: lipoprotein lipase
ME: metabolizable energy
VLDL: very low density lipoproteins

Diagnostic approach to the hyperlipidemic cat and dietary treatment

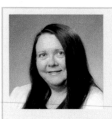

Patricia A. SCHENCK
DVM, PhD

Dr. Schenck received her Masters degree in Animal Science and her DVM degree from the University of Illinois in Champaign-Urbana. After owning her own small animal practice, she returned to the University of Florida where she completed her PhD in lipid biochemistry. After completing a post-doc at the USDA in Peoria Illinois, she joined the Ohio State University, where she became interested in research in calcium regulation. After working in the pet food industry for a number of years, she joined the Endocrinology section in the Diagnostic Center for Population and Animal Health at Michigan State University in 2001. Her current research interests include developing new tests for increasing diagnostic utility in calcium and lipid disorders, hyperlipidemias in the dog, idiopathic hypercalcemia in the cat, and the relationships between lipids and parathyroid hormone.

Hyperlipidemia or hyperlipemia *refers to an abnormally high lipid concentration in serum or plasma. Normally hyperlipidemia occurs after ingesting a meal, especially a meal high in fat, but fasting hyperlipidemia is indicative of abnormal lipid metabolism. (The term lipemia, the presence of lipids in serum or plasma, is often incorrectly used to describe an abnormal excess concentration of circulating lipids).*

Hyperlipidemia *and* hyperlipoproteinemia *are often used interchangeably, but hyperlipoproteinemia more correctly refers to an excess of circulating lipoproteins.*

Hypercholesterolemia *and* hypertriglyceridemia *refer respectively to an abnormally high concentration of circulating cholesterol or triglyceride. They both may occur alone or in combination with hyperlipoproteinemia.*

1 - Lipid metabolism

Perturbations in any aspect of lipid metabolism may result in abnormal hyperlipidemia. Abnormalities may occur in:
- lipid absorption, synthesis, esterification
- lipoprotein synthesis, receptor-mediated uptake
- bile formation and circulation or reverse cholesterol transport.

► Lipid absorption

Cholesterol and triglycerides are absorbed in the small intestine. Cholesterol may be ingested in the diet (exogenous), or is derived from biliary secretion and desquamation of intestinal epithelial cells (endogenous) which may account for up to 50% of the total cholesterol present in the small intestinal lumen (*Holt, 1972*).

Absorption requires bile acids and micelle formation. Salts of bile acids are secreted by the liver and enter the small intestine via the bile, and most secreted salts exist as conjugates with taurine in cats. When the concentration of bile salts reaches a high enough level, bile salts form aggregates or micelles (*Feldman et al, 1983*), and allow approximately 30 to 60% of available cholesterol to be absorbed. Within the lumen of the intestine, cholesteryl esters from micelles are hydrolysed by pancreatic cholesterol esterase. Free cholesterol passively diffuses across the intestinal mucosal cell wall (*Westergaard & Dietschy, 1976*). Within the intestinal cell, free cholesterol is re-esterified with fatty acids, and is mediated by the enzyme acyl CoA: cholesterylacyltransferase (ACAT). A combination of free cholesterol and cholesteryl esters are then secreted into chylomicron particles.

Within the intestinal lumen, triglycerides are hydrolysed by pancreatic lipase to monoglycerides, diglycerides, and free fatty acids **(Figure 1)**. In combination with cholesterol, phospholipid, and bile salts, these monoglycerides, diglycerides, and free fatty acids form mixed micelles. These micelles release monoglycerides, diglycerides, and free fatty acids at the intestinal cell wall where they are absorbed. Within the intestinal cell, monoglycerides and diglycerides are re-esterified to form triglycerides. Triglycerides along with cholesteryl esters, free cholesterol, phospholipid, and proteins will be incorporated into chylomicron particles for release into the circulation via the lymphatic system by way of the thoracic duct.

► Cholesterol synthesis

Endogenous cholesterol synthesis contributes to the total body cholesterol concentration. Cholesterol can be synthesized by almost all cells, with the highest rate of synthesis in the liver and intestine (*Turley & Dietschy, 1981*). In humans, approximately 1 g cholesterol per day is synthesized within the body from acetyl CoA, and the enzyme 3-hydroxy-3-methylglutaryl coenzyme A reductase (HMGCoA reductase) is the rate-limiting enzyme in cholesterol synthesis (*Alberts, 1988*).

► Lipoprotein production

Lipoproteins are the main carriers of cholesterol in the blood and are important in the delivery of cholesterol to all tissues. Circulating lipoproteins are classified by their size, density, and electrophoretic behavior (*Mahley & Weisgraber, 1974*). Lipoproteins in humans have been well characterized (*Alaupovic et al, 1968; Assmann, 1982; Shepherd & Packard, 1989*), but direct correlations cannot be made to the feline due to many differences in lipoprotein characteristics (*Mahley et al, 1974; Mahley & Weisgraber, 1974*).

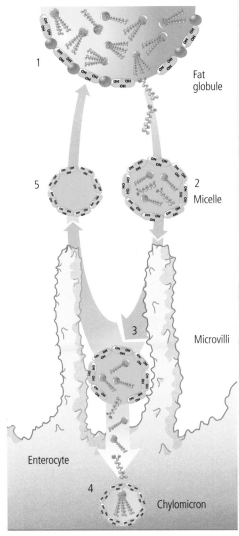

FIGURE 1 - DIGESTION AND ABSORPTION OF LIPIDS
(*From Gogny, 1994*)

1- Fat globules: lipases act on the surface of the emulsion

2- Micelle: transport form for fatty acids

3- Fat release to the enterocytes

4- Triglycerides resynthesis and incorporation in chylomicrons

5- Absorption of biliary salts in the ileum

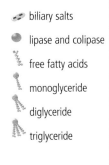
biliary salts
lipase and colipase
free fatty acids
monoglyceride
diglyceride
triglyceride

Lipoproteins are micellar particles with a hydrophobic core containing triglycerides and cholesteryl esters, and an amphipathic outer surface containing phospholipid, unesterified cholesterol, and proteins (*Assmann, 1982*). Proteins within a lipoprotein tend to be specific for that lipoprotein class. Lipoprotein particles are not static, but are in a dynamic state of equilibrium, with transfer of components occurring between lipoproteins.

Five major classes of lipoproteins have been characterized, including:

- chylomicrons
- very low density lipoproteins (VLDL)
- intermediate density lipoproteins (IDL)
- low density lipoproteins (LDL)
- and high density lipoproteins (HDL).

Some mammals (humans and most monkeys) have a predominance of LDL and are classified as "LDL mammals" (*Chapman, 1986*). LDL mammals are more sensitive to elevations in LDL cholesterol and the development of atherosclerosis. Cats and most other mammals are considered "HDL mammals" due to the predominance of circulating HDL. HDL mammals are less sensitive to elevated LDL cholesterol concentrations, and are more resistant to the development of atherosclerosis (**Table 1**).

► Chylomicrons

Chylomicrons are the largest of the lipoproteins with the lowest density (**Table 2**). Chylomicrons have a high triglyceride content, low protein content and remain at the origin on lipoprotein electrophoresis (*Bauer, 1996*). Chylomicrons contain different types of apoproteins. In the peripheral circulation, chylomicrons contribute apoprotein A to HDL in exchange for apoprotein C and E (**Figure 2**), increasing their protein content (*Capurso, 1987*). A chylomicron remnant is formed.

Lipoprotein lipase (LPL) activated by apoprotein C-II of chylomicrons hydrolyzes the triglyceride present in chylomicrons, creating a phos-

TABLE 1 - PREDOMINANCE OF CERTAIN LIPOPROTEINS BY SPECIES	
"LDL mammals"	**"HDL mammals"**
Humans and most Monkeys	Dogs
Rabbits	Cats
Hamsters	Horses
Guinea pigs	Ruminants
Pigs	Rats
Camels	Mice
Rhinoceros	Most other mammals

LDL: Low Density Lipoproteins
HDL: High Density Lipoproteins

TABLE 2 - FELINE LIPOPROTEIN CHARACTERISTICS								
			APPROXIMATE COMPOSITION (%)					
Lipoproteins	Hydrated density g/mL	Electrophoretic mobility	Triglycerides	Cholesteryl ester	Free cholesterol	Proteins	Phospholipids	Major apoproteins
Chylomicrons	0.960	Origin	**90**	2	1	2	6	B_{48}
VLDL	< 1.006	β (pre-β)	**60**	13	7	5	15	B_{100}, E, C
LDL	1.030 – 1.043	β	10	**38**	8	22	22	B_{100}
HDL	-	-	4	16	6	50	25	-
- HDL2	1.063 – 1.100	α1	-	-	-	-	-	E, A-1, C
- HDL3	1.100 – 1.210	α1	-	-	-	-	-	A, C

FIGURE 2 - CHYLOMICRON METABOLISM

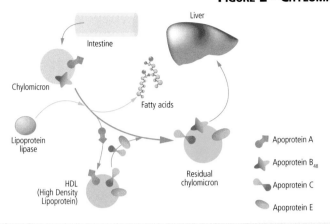

Chylomicron particles containing a high concentration of triglyceride are released from the intestinal mucosal cell into the lymphatics and to the circulation. Lipoprotein lipase hydrolysis of triglycerides within chylomicrons releases fatty acids and decreases the triglyceride content of chylomicrons, creating a chylomicron remnant. In addition, there is an exchange of apoproteins between HDL and chylomicrons. Chylomicrons contribute apoprotein A to HDL in exchange for apoproteins C and E. The chylomicron remnant formed is recognized by an apoprotein E receptor on hepatocytes and is removed from the circulation. A deficiency of lipoprotein lipase activity can result in decreased metabolism of chylomicrons to chylomicron remnants and thus a prolonged appearance of chylomicrons in the circulation.

FIGURE 3 - CHYLOMICRON, VLDL, LDL, AND LIVER CHOLESTEROL METABOLISM

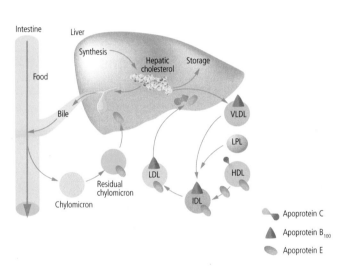

Chylomicron particles containing lipids are released from the intestine into the circulation. Cholesterol-rich chylomicron remnants form and are recognized by the apoprotein E receptor on hepatocytes. Once in the hepatocyte, cholesterol can be stored as cholesteryl ester (via the action of ACAT), can be excreted into bile as cholesterol or bile acids, or secreted into VLDL particles. Synthesis of cholesterol in the hepatocyte (via HMGCoA reductase) contributes to the available cholesterol pool. Lipoprotein lipase hydrolysis of triglyceride within secreted VLDL and exchange of apoproteins create a triglyceride-depleted IDL which forms the triglyceride-poor, cholesterol-enriched LDL particle. The LDL receptor recognizes apoproteins B and E and mediates uptake and removal of LDL from the circulation. A deficiency of lipoprotein lipase activity can result in decreased metabolism of VLDL to LDL and thus a prolonged appearance of VLDL in the circulation.

pholipid-rich particle. Lipoprotein lipase is associated with endothelial cell surfaces, interacting with membrane associated heparan sulfate (*Nilsson-Ehle et al, 1980*). Chylomicron remnant formation is necessary for hepatic clearance of chylomicrons (*Cooper, 1977*). Once chylomicron remnants are formed, they are rapidly removed from the circulation by the apoprotein E receptor in liver cells (*Mahley et al, 1989*).

► Very low density lipoproteins (VLDL)

VLDL are synthesized by hepatocytes **(Figure 3)**, and are a major transporter of triglyceride (*Mills & Taylaur, 1971*). VLDL are smaller and heavier than chylomicrons, have a density of < 1.006 g/mL, and contain apoproteins B100, E, and C. VLDL binds to LPL, and LPL hydrolyzes the triglyceride present in VLDL. This process may create VLDL remnants which can be removed by the liver via receptor or non-receptor-mediated uptake (*Havel, 1984*). Feline VLDL exhibits pre-β migration on lipoprotein electrophoresis, which is similar to human VLDL.

► Low density lipoproteins (LDL)

HDL transfers apoprotein E to VLDL, creating an IDL particle. With further loss of triglyceride, phospholipid, and apoprotein, LDL is formed. Removal of LDL from the circulation is via the LDL receptor which binds both apoprotein B and apoprotein E (*Goldstein & Brown, 1984*). Feline

LDL exhibits β migration on lipoprotein electrophoresis, have a density of 1.030 - 1.043 g/mL, and contain apoprotein B100.

► High density lipoproteins (HDL)

HDL are the smallest and heaviest of the lipoproteins, with the greatest quantity of protein and least quantity of triglyceride of any of the lipoproteins. Cats have approximately 5 times more HDL than LDL unlike humans, but similar to the canine. Feline HDL is divided into 2 subclasses based on composition and density:

- HDL2 has a density of 1.063 – 1.100 g/mL, and contains apoproteins E, A-1, and C.
- HDL3 is smaller than HDL2 with a density of 1.100 – 1.210 g/mL, and contains apoproteins A and C.

Both HDL2 and HDL3 exhibit α1-migration on lipoprotein electrophoresis (*Demacker et al, 1987*).

Nascent HDL is secreted by the liver **(Figure 4)**, and contains very little free cholesterol and cholesteryl ester. Free cholesterol is transferred from peripheral cells to nascent HDL, and these cholesterol-rich particles serve as substrate for lecithin cholesterol acyltransferase (LCAT), converting free cholesterol to cholesteryl esters. With the increased concentration of cholesteryl esters, the core of HDL enlarges and becomes more spherical. Hepatic lipase may also play a role in the interconversion of HDL subfractions (*Groot et al, 1981*). The conversion of free cholesterol to cholesteryl esters and its subsequent transfer to other lipoproteins allows additional free cholesterol to transfer from the surface of cells and other lipoproteins to HDL (*Kostner et al, 1987*). Thus LCAT plays a key role in the transfer of free cholesterol from peripheral tissues to the liver (*Albers et al, 1986*).

In humans, cholesteryl ester transfer protein (CETP) is responsible for cholesteryl ester and triglyceride exchange between HDL and LDL or VLDL. Cholesteryl ester derived from free cholesterol in peripheral cells is transferred to LDL, which can then return to the liver via receptor-mediated uptake (reverse cholesterol transport) (*Noel et al, 1984*). This mechanism for returning peripheral cholesterol to the liver has been termed reverse cholesterol transport. Cats however have low levels of CETP (*Guyard-Dangremont et al, 1998*), and thus there is little transfer of cholesteryl ester to LDL. Without cholesteryl ester transfer, HDL remains enriched with cholesteryl esters, and is designated HDL1, or HDLc. In the cat, reverse cholesterol transport is completed via HDL uptake by the liver. The cat is a "HDL mammal" since most of the circulating cholesterol is carried by HDL and cannot be transferred to LDL as in humans (a "LDL mammal").

FIGURE 4 - REVERSE CHOLESTEROL TRANSPORT

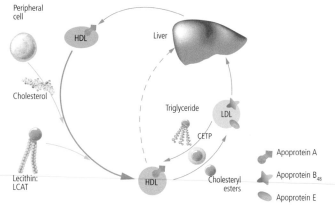

Discoidal HDL (nascent HDL) is secreted by the liver and obtains unesterified cholesterol from peripheral cells. LCAT in the circulation esterifies this cholesterol, resulting in a more spherical cholesteryl ester-rich particle. If cholesteryl ester transfer protein (CETP) is present, cholesteryl ester is transferred from HDL to LDL, with exchange of triglyceride from LDL to HDL. LDL carrying cholesteryl ester derived from peripheral cells returns to the liver completing reverse cholesterol transport. In dogs with little CETP, other mechanisms exist to return cholesterol to the liver via HDL directly.

2 - Diagnostic approach to the hyperlipidemic patient

When a patient exhibits serum hyperlipidemia after a 10 to 12 hour fast **(Figure 5)**, investigation into the cause is warranted **(Figure 6)**. The presumption that the cat was fasted should be verified, to ensure that all access to food has been withheld. Once fasting hyperlipidemia has been confirmed, the causes of hyperlipidemia secondary to other disorders should be ruled out. If no secondary disorder resulting in hyperlipidemia is evident, then a primary hyperlipidemia should be considered.

► Serum turbidity

Visual evaluation of the degree of serum turbidity can provide an estimation of serum triglyceride concentration:
- normal, clear serum: typical triglyceride concentration < 200 mg/dL (2.3 mmol/L)
- hazy serum: triglyceride concentration around 300 mg/dL (3.4 mmol/L)
- opacity of the serum: triglyceride concentration approaches 600 mg/dL (6.8 mmol/L)
- serum with the appearance of skim milk: triglyceride concentration is usually around 1000 mg/dL (11.3 mmol/L)
- serum with the appearance of whole milk: triglyceride concentration as high as 2500 (28.2 mmol/L) to 4000 mg/dL (45.2 mmol/L)

► Refrigeration test

To ascertain the lipoprotein classes that may be present in excess, a simple refrigeration test can be performed **(Figure 7)**. The serum sample is refrigerated and left undisturbed overnight. Chylomicrons, being the least dense lipoprotein, will "float" forming a "cream layer" on the top of the serum sample *(Rogers, 1977)*. If the serum below the chylomicron layer is clear, then only

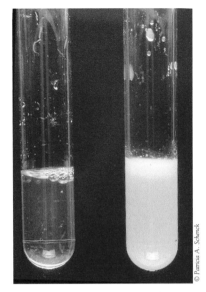

Figure 5 - The appearance of normal and hyperlipidemic serum. Normal serum should be clear, with no evidence of turbidity (left tube). Fasting serum that is turbid indicates the presence of excess lipid in the serum (right tube).

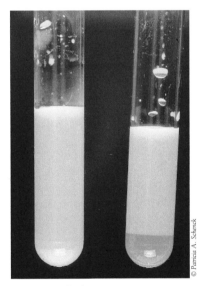

Figure 7 - Refrigeration test of hyperlipidemic serum. On the left, a fasting serum sample shows hyperlipidemia. After the refrigeration test, there is the appearance of a lactescent layer ("cream layer") floating on top of the serum. This layer is due to increased chylomicron particles present in the serum sample. Note that the serum below the top lactescent layer is also turbid, indicating the presence of other lipoproteins in excess (in addition to the excess chylomicron particles).

FIGURE 6 - ALGORITHM TO DETERMINE THE CAUSE OF HYPERLIPIDEMIA

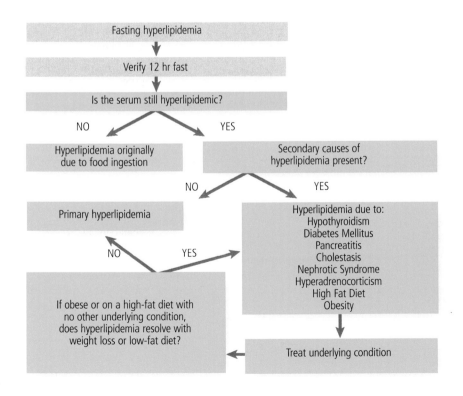

FIGURE 8 - DENSITOMETRIC TRACING OF A LIPOPROTEIN ELECTROPHORETOGRAM FROM A NORMAL CAT.

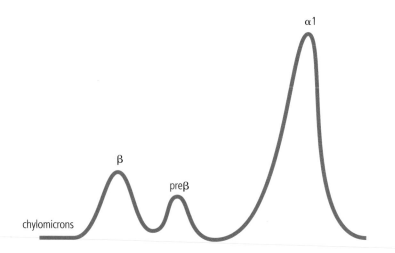

The peaks from left to right represent the relative concentrations of β-migrating lipoproteins (LDL), preβ-migrating lipoproteins (VLDL), and α1-migrating lipoproteins (HDL2/HDL3). Note the predominance of α1-migrating lipoproteins in the normal cat (a HDL mammal). A small percentage of chylomicrons may be present in normal cats; chylomicrons will exhibit a small peak at the origin if present.

chylomicrons are present in excess, and either a non-fasted sample, or primary hyperchylomicronemia should be suspected. If the serum below the chylomicron layer is turbid, then other lipoproteins are present in excess in addition to the hyperchylomicronemia. If a "cream layer" does not form after refrigeration, then chylomicrons are not present, and the visible hyperlipidemia is due to an excess of other lipoproteins.

► Lipoprotein electrophoresis

Lipoprotein electrophoresis can be used to characterize lipoproteins in serum. With electrophoresis, lipoproteins separate based on their charge and mobility on agarose gel. The agarose gel is then stained and scanned using a densitometer to semi-quantify classes of lipoproteins **(Figure 8)**. Lipoprotein electrophoresis should be performed on fresh, not-previously-frozen serum, and the scan interpreted by someone knowledgeable of feline lipoprotein characteristics (i.e. not a human laboratory), since differences exist between humans and cats in electrophoretic pattern. Lipoprotein electrophoresis is not quantitative, but is useful to identify an excess in a particular lipoprotein class.

► Ultracentrifugation

Ultracentrifugation can be utilized to separate lipoproteins based on density. Ultracentrifugation is time-consuming, requires expensive equipment, and considerable skill to produce reliable results. Thus ultracentrifugation is rarely available except in the research setting.

► Serum interferences

Excess of other analytes present in serum may interfere with the measurement of lipids:
- hyperbilirubinemia may cause a false lowering of cholesterol measurement
- if cholesterol is present at a concentration of greater than 700 mg/dL, the measured triglyceride concentration may be falsely lowered (*Shephard & Whiting, 1990*)
- hypertriglyceridemia may result in a falsely lower cholesterol concentration (*Cobbaert & Tricarico, 1993*)
- pentobarbital may falsely increase triglyceride measurement (*Hata et al, 1978*), but phenobarbitone has no effect on cholesterol concentration (*Foster et al, 2000*).

Depending on the methodology utilized for analysis, hyperlipidemia may interfere with a number of assays. Hyperlipidemia may result in an approximately 2% increase in sodium, urea, glucose, chloride, and total protein measurement (*Miyada et al, 1982*). Total calcium measurement may be slightly elevated (*Darras et al, 1992*), and cortisol may be slightly elevated, but not clinically significant (*Lucena et al, 1998*). Bilirubin concentration may be falsely increased (*Ng et al, 2001*), and immunoglobulin A, immunoglobulin M, haptoglobin and α1-antitrypsin concentration may also be falsely increased (*Bossuyt & Blanckaert, 1999*). Concentration of LDH is decreased and AST and ALT concentrations are increased (*Miyada et al, 1982*). Hypertriglyceridemia may interfere with WBC, RBC, hemoglobin and platelet measurements (*Peng et al, 2001*), and causes a false increase in haptoglobin concentration (*Weidmeyer & Solter, 1996*). Glycated hemoglobin measurement may be falsely decreased (*Garrib et al, 2003*), and free thyroxine measured by ELISA may be increased (*Lucena et al, 1998*). However, triglyceride concentration up to 10mg/dL will not interfere with phenobarbital measurement (*Baer & Paulson, 1987*).

3 - Causes of hyperlipidemia

Hyperlipidemia may be the result of lipid abnormalities secondary to other conditions, or may be a primary disorder of lipid metabolism (**Table 3**). In the cat, recognized primary disorders include inherited hyperchylomicronemia, and idiopathic hypercholesterolemia. Conditions that can result in secondary hyperlipidemia include hypothyroidism, pancreatitis, diabetes mellitus, nephrotic syndrome, hyperadrenocorticism, cholestasis, obesity or the feeding of very high fat diets.

▶ Hypothyroidism

Naturally occurring hypothyroidism is rare in cats, and may be congenital or acquired. Iatrogenically-induced hypothyroidism is more common in the cat, arising from treatment for hyperthyroidism. Increases in both serum cholesterol and triglyceride concentrations have been associated with canine hypothyroidism (*Boretti et al, 2003; Rogers et al, 1975*), and cholesterol elevations are usually moderate (*Jaggy et al, 1994*). Both serum cholesterol and triglyceride concentrations return to normal with adequate thyroid replacement therapy (*Rogers et al, 1975*). Changes in lipoproteins have not been evaluated in hypothyroid cats.

In humans with hypothyroidism, mRNA for LDL receptors is decreased resulting in decreased cholesterol and chylomicron clearance (*Kovanen, 1987*). Lipoprotein lipase activity may be altered (*Hansson et al, 1983; Pykalisto et al, 1976*), and there is decreased excretion of cholesterol into bile (*Gebhard & Prigge, 1992*). Cholesterol synthesis is also decreased, but the decrease in clearance is greater than the decrease in synthesis, leading to a net increase in cholesterol concentration (*Field et al, 1986*).

Naturally occurring atherosclerosis has been noted in dogs with hypothyroidism (*Manning, 1979*), but has not been observed in the cat.

▶ Pancreatitis

In humans, there is evidence that pancreatitis is associated with decreased LPL activity (*Hazzard et al, 1984*). This decreased activity of LPL may result in increased triglyceride concentrations with slower clearance of chylomicrons. Two dogs with pancreatitis also exhibited a moderate decrease in LPL activity, which returned to normal with treatment and resolution of the pancreatitis (*Schenck, unpublished observations*).

In cats, pancreatitis usually results in hyperlipidemia with elevations in serum cholesterol (*Hill & Van Winkle, 1993*) and possibly triglyceride concentrations. Pancreatitis can be a cause of hyperlipidemia, or a sequel to hyperlipidemia. Little is known regarding lipoprotein abnormalities in the cat with pancreatitis.

▶ Diabetes mellitus

In diabetes mellitus, elevations of both serum triglyceride and cholesterol concentrations are typically observed (*Rogers et al, 1975*). Lipoproteins have not been characterized in the diabetic cat, but abnormalities have been well characterized in humans.

In humans with diabetes mellitus, LPL activity is decreased, with an increase in free fatty acids (*Steiner et al, 1975*) and hepatic lipase activity (*Muller et al, 1985*). Urinary mevalonate concentration is elevated approximately six-fold, indicating an increase in whole-body cholesterol synthesis, and HMGCoA reductase activity is increased in both the liver and intestine (*Feingold et al, 1994; Kwong et al, 1991*). There is impaired removal of VLDL from the circulation (*Wilson et al, 1986*), and a decrease in the number and affinity of LDL receptors (*Takeuchi, 1991*). Prolonged retention of lipoprotein rem-

TABLE 3 - CAUSES OF HYPERLIPIDEMIA IN THE CAT
Postprandial
Primary
Inherited hyperchylomicronemia
Idiopathic hypercholesterolemia
Secondary
Hypothyroidism
Pancreatitis
Diabetes Mellitus
Nephrotic Syndrome
Hyperadrenocorticism
Cholestasis
Obesity
"High fat" diets

Since cats and humans both typically exhibit Type 2 diabetes mellitus characterized by insulin resistance, it is likely that there are lipoprotein similarities.

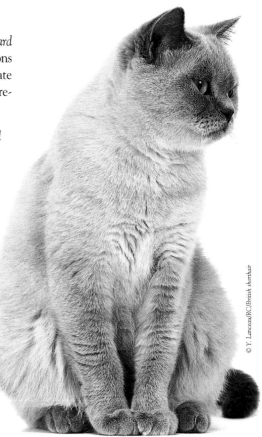

© Y. Lanceau/RC/British shorthair

231

nants may contribute to an increased delivery of cholesterol to extrahepatic tissues, and the increased concentration of HDL1 reflects a disturbance in cholesterol transport from peripheral cells back to the liver *(Wilson et al, 1986)*.

Naturally occurring atherosclerosis has been observed at necropsy in a dog with diabetes mellitus *(Sottiaux, 1999)*, but this has not yet been noted in the diabetic cat.

► Nephrotic syndrome

Lipoprotein abnormalities have not been characterized in cats with nephrotic syndrome. Cats with nephrotic syndrome may exhibit mild elevations in serum cholesterol and triglyceride.

Lipoprotein abnormalities in nephrotic syndrome and chronic renal disease have been well characterized in humans, and the progression of renal dysfunction has been shown to correlate with serum total cholesterol *(Washio et al, 1996)*. Lipoprotein lipase activity is decreased which may account for the hypertriglyceridemia due to a decrease in lipoprotein clearance *(Olbricht, 1991)*. There is decreased clearance of LDL *(Shapiro, 1991; Vaziri & Liang, 1996)* due to decreased LDL receptor expression *(Portman et al, 1992)*. LDL may also be increased due to an increase in synthesis *(de Sain-van der Velden et al, 1998)*. HMGCoA reductase activity is increased in the liver *(Chmielewski et al, 2003; Szolkiewicz et al, 2002)*, and the increased cholesterol does not up-regulate LDL receptors *(Liang & Vaziri, 1997)*. Reverse cholesterol transport is impaired *(Kes et al, 2002)*, and ACAT activity within the liver is increased with a decrease in LCAT activity *(Liang & Vaziri, 2002)*.

VLDL increases due to decreased catabolism *(de Sain-van der Velden et al, 1998)*, and proteinuria may also stimulate VLDL synthesis by the liver, induced by hypoalbuminemia *(D'Amico, 1991)*. Impaired clearance of VLDL may be due to deficiencies in apoprotein C-II, apoprotein C-III, and apoprotein E, creating smaller VLDL particles that are not cleared efficiently by receptors *(Deighan et al, 2000)*. This altered structure of VLDL results in altered binding to endothelial bound LPL *(Shearer & Kaysen, 2001)*, and proteinuria may also be associated with the urinary loss of heparan sulfate, an important cofactor for LPL *(Kaysen et al, 1986)*. Synthesis of apoprotein A-I by the liver increases in response to proteinuria *(Marsh, 1996)*, and protein catabolism in peripheral tissues is increased.

► Hyperadrenocorticism

Hyperadrenocorticism is uncommon in the cat. In cats with hyperadrenocorticism, hypercholesterolemia may be noted *(Moore et al, 2000)*. Hypercholesterolemia may be more prevalent in cases of pituitary-dependent hyperadrenocorticism than in hyperadrenocorticism caused by adrenal tumors. Many cats with hyperadrenocorticism also have concurrent diabetes mellitus which can also cause an increase in serum cholesterol and other lipid abnormalities. In dogs with hyperadrenocorticism, concentrations of both VLDL and LDL have been noted, but lipoproteins have not been characterized in cats with hyperadrenocorticism.

Lipoprotein lipase activity may be decreased with an increase in hepatic lipase activity *(Berg et al, 1990)*. In addition, hypercortisolism stimulates production of VLDL by the liver *(Taskinen et al, 1983)*. Excess glucocorticoids stimulate lipolysis, and this excess fat breakdown exceeds the liver's capacity for clearance. The occurrence of steroid hepatopathy in hyperadrenocorticism may lead to biliary stasis resulting in further lipid abnormalities.

► Cholestasis

In cats with induced cholestasis, hypercholesterolemia was observed *(Center et al, 1983)*. There may be alterations in the content of lipoproteins *(Danielsson et al, 1977)*, but changes in lipoproteins have not been characterized in cats with cholestasis. Hepatic lipidosis arising from weight of kittens with marked increase in chylomicrons and moderate increase in VLDL. After resolution of hyperlipidemia with the feeding of diets containing 9% fat as-fed (approximately 28 g fat/1000 kcal), LPL activity was only mildly lower in affected kittens as compared to normal kittens. These kittens did not exhibit the LPL gene mutation that has been shown in the inherited hyperchylomicronemia that has been well characterized. This suggests the presence of a separate distinct primary hyperlipidemia.

5 - Effects of persistent hyperlipidemia

Long-term effects of hyperlipidemia in cats are unknown. Cats are resistant to the development of atherosclerosis compared to humans, due to differences in lipoprotein metabolism between the species. Experimental atherosclerosis has been induced in cats by feeding a diet containing 30% fat, 3% cholesterol (as fed) for 2 to 8 months (*Ginzinger et al, 1997*).

► Atherosclerosis

Atherosclerosis is a specific type of arteriosclerosis with deposition of lipid and cholesterol in the arterial tunica intima and tunica media (*Liu et al, 1986*). It is unclear however, whether cats with inherited hyperchylomicronemia are at increased risk for the development of atherosclerosis. Studies of lipoprotein interactions with arterial walls have shown that large lipoprotein molecules such as chylomicrons and VLDL have a low influx into the intima (*Nordestgaard et al, 1992*). Thus inherited hyperchylomicronemia may not be associated with premature atherosclerosis (*Ebara et al, 2001*).

An increased incidence of atherosclerosis has been noted in association with causes of secondary hyperlipidemia in dogs and humans, but has not been reported in cats. This may be due to the low incidence of some causes of secondary hyperlipidemia in the cat, such as hypothyroidism where there has been evidence for associated atherosclerosis in the dog.

► Pancreatitis

There is evidence that persistent hyperlipidemia may lead to pancreatitis (*Dominguez-Munoz et al, 1991*), and pancreatitis often occurs in humans with inherited hyperchylomicronemia and LPL deficiency. A burst of free radical activity in pancreatic acinar cells disrupts glutathione homeostasis and may be the initiating event in pancreatitis (*Guyan et al, 1990*). Increased free radical activity may relate to pancreatic ischemia resulting from sluggish pancreatic microcirculation due to high concentrations of chylomicrons (*Sanfey et al, 1984*). Free radical damage causes leakage of lipase into pancreatic microcirculation. Lipase causes hydrolysis of triglyceride present in excess chylomicrons or VLDL resulting in release of free fatty acids which are intensely inflammatory. Free fatty acids can also cause activation of Hageman factor, or may bind calcium leading to microthrombi and capillary damage. Phospholipid present in chylomicrons and VLDL are also susceptible to free radical attack leading to lipid peroxidation, intensifying inflammation. This results in an increase in release of pancreatic lipase and further lipolysis, leading to pancreatitis (*Havel, 1969*).

► Diabetes mellitus

Persistent hyperlipidemia may also cause diabetes mellitus (*Sane & Taskinen, 1993*), and diabetes mellitus has been noted as a sequel to inherited hyperchylomicronemia in humans. Increased triglyceride and free fatty acids may lead to insulin resistance due to inhibition of glucose oxidation and glycogen synthesis (*Boden, 1997*). Free fatty acids may stimulate glyconeogenesis which contributes to inappropriate glucose production (*Rebrin et al, 1995*). Increased free fatty acids early on act to stimulate insulin production even with low glucose concentrations. In the long term, increased free fatty acids modulate, β-cell gene expression and inhibit insulin secretion (*Prentki &*

Corkey, 1996). By multiple mechanisms, increased serum triglyceride and free fatty acids can lead to hyperglycemia and diabetes mellitus. If hyperlipidemia is corrected, diabetes mellitus caused by hyperlipidemia can be reversed *(Mingrone et al, 1999)*.

6 - Treatment of hyperlipidemia

Because of the clinical signs associated with primary hyperlipidemia, and the potential risks, hyperlipidemia should be treated aggressively in the cat. The underlying disorder in a secondary hyperlipidemia should be treated, but there is no specific therapeutic regimen for cats with inherited hyperchylomicronemia.

▶ Fat restricted-diet

The main therapy of primary hyperlipidemia involves feeding a low-fat diet with moderate protein content. Diets low in protein may cause an increase in serum cholesterol concentration *(Hansen et al, 1992)*, and are therefore not recommended unless the presence of other conditions warrant their use. Human patients with inherited hyperchylomicronemia typically must restrict dietary fat intake to less than 15% of calories to control hyperlipidemia.

Feline diets with less than 10% fat (as-fed) or less than 30g fat/1000 kcal are generally adequate. Protein content should be maintained at about 30% as-fed, or greater than 85g protein/1000 kcal. A diet should not be chosen only on the percent fat present in the diet; the diet should be low in fat based on metabolizable energy (ME). Some diets appear low in fat on a percentage basis, but actually provide a higher fat content than expected when the amount of fiber in the diet and metabolizable energy are taken into account. For example, a diet containing 11% fat with an ME of 4000 kcal/kg provides only 27.5 g fat/1000 kcal, whereas a diet containing 9% fat with an ME of 3000 kcal/kg provides 30 g fat/1000 kcal **(Table 5)**. The presence of a blend of fructo-oligosaccharides and beet pulp in the diet may also be desirable, since this blend has been shown to decrease serum triglyceride and cholesterol concentrations in the dog *(Diez et al, 1997)*.

Obesity in association with familial hyperchylomicronemia is uncommon, so it is usually not necessary to restrict caloric intake. If the cat is not obese, the amount of food offered may need to be increased because of the decreased calories provided by the new diet with decreased fat content. Many cats can continue to be fed free-choice. Treats should be restricted since these are most likely not low in fat content.

After feeding a low-fat diet for approximately 4 weeks, the presence of hyperlipidemia should be re-evaluated. Most cats will show at least partial resolution of hyperlipidemia with consumption of low-fat diets. Body condition should be assessed, and if there has been significant weight loss, the patient should receive an increased amount of diet, or possibly be switched to a different diet with higher caloric density.

If after 4 weeks hyperlipidemia is still present, the diet should be continued, and all other sources of food or treats removed. If there has been good owner compliance, then a switch to a different low-fat diet could be considered. The patient should then be reassessed after another one to two months. If hyperlipidemia still persists at that time, drug therapy could be added.

TABLE 5 - INTERPRETATION OF THE FAT CONTENT IN DIETS		
	Diet A	**Diet B**
Amount of fat g/100g diet	11	9
ME kcal/100 g diet	400	300
Fat content	11 g x 1000 kcal/400kcal = 27.5 g fat/1000 kcal	9 g x 1000 kcal/400kcal = 30.0 g fat/1000 kcal

► Omega-3 fatty acid supplementation

Fish oils are rich in omega-3 fatty acids, and have been the supplement of choice in the treatment of dogs with primary hyperlipidemias. However, little is known about the effectiveness of fish oil therapy in cats. Potential doses range from 10 to 200 mg/kg body weight. The fish oil supplement should contain a high percentage of eicosapentaenoic acid (EPA) and docosahexaenoic acid (DHA), as these are long-chain omega-3 fatty acids. Products containing a high level of linolenic acid (also an omega-3 fatty acid) will not be as effective, as cats have very low delta-6 desaturase necessary for the conversion of linolenic acid to longer chain omega-3 fatty acids (*Sinclair et al, 1979*) **(Figure 11)**.

The use of fish oil in the treatment of hyperlipidemia has been extensively studied in a number of other species. Fish oil supplement has resulted in a decrease in serum triglyceride and cholesterol in humans (*Okumura et al, 2002*), rats (*Adan et al, 1999*), chicks (*Castillo et al, 2000*), dogs (*Brown et al, 2000*), and rabbits (*Mortensen et al, 1998*).

Omega-3 fatty acids act to decrease the synthesis of triglyceride and VLDL in the liver (*Harris et al, 1990; Connor et al, 1993*), stimulate LPL activity (*Levy et al, 1993*), decrease the intestinal absorption of lipid (*Thomson et al, 1993*), and increase cholesterol secretion into bile (*Smit et al, 1991*). Fish oil also decreases the serum concentration of free fatty acids (*Singer et al, 1990*), which may be important in the prevention of pancreatitis and diabetes mellitus.

FIGURE 11 - METABOLISM OF LINOLENIC ACID (OMEGA-3)

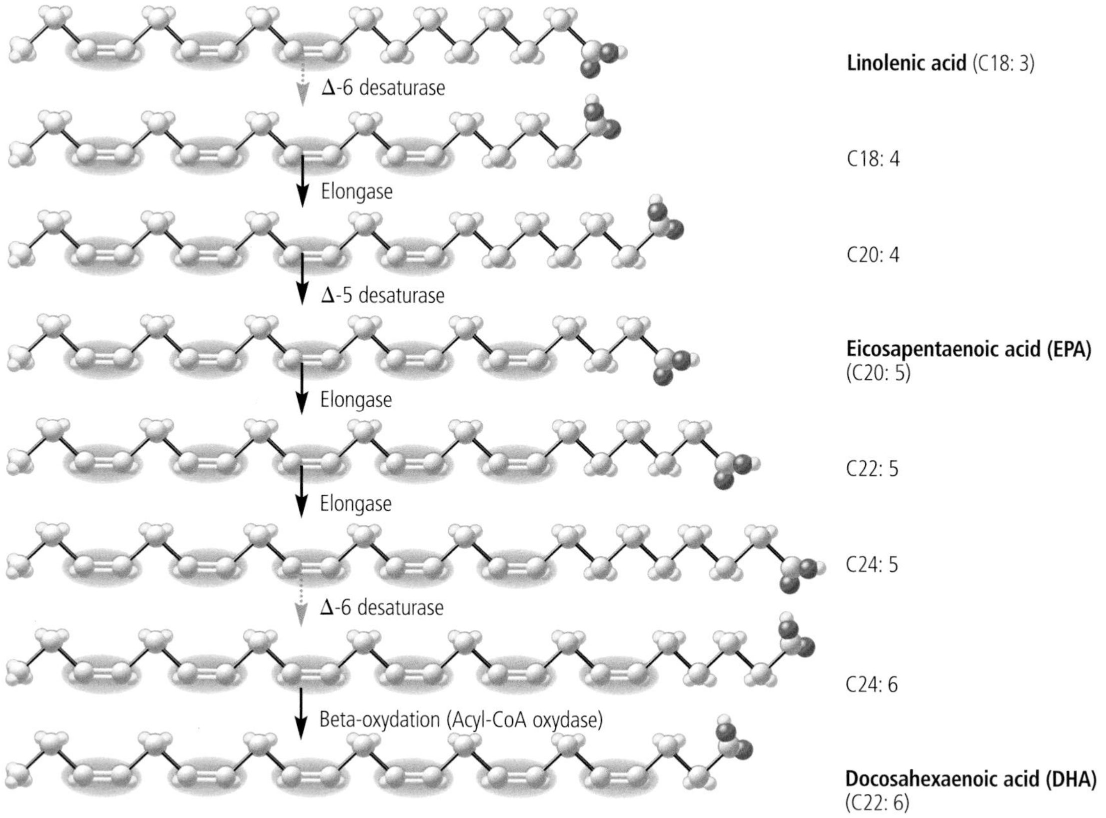

Linolenic acid (C18: 3)

Δ-6 desaturase

C18: 4

Elongase

C20: 4

Δ-5 desaturase

Eicosapentaenoic acid (EPA) (C20: 5)

Elongase

C22: 5

Elongase

C24: 5

Δ-6 desaturase

C24: 6

Beta-oxydation (Acyl-CoA oxydase)

Docosahexaenoic acid (DHA) (C22: 6)

Delta-6 desaturase activity is crucial for the efficient production of long-chain omega-3 fatty acids such as eicosapentaenoic acid (EPA) and docosahexaenoic acid (DHA) from available linolenic acid. In the feline, delta-6 desaturase activity is significantly reduced (dotted arrows), and thus there is little production of EPA and DHA from linolenic acid.

Unfortunately there are no long-term studies to verify the safety and efficacy of any lipid-lowering agent in cats, and any therapy should be used with caution. One concern with fish oil therapy is the evidence that fish oil increases the concentration of lipoperoxides in LDL (*Puiggros et al, 2002*). The addition of vitamin E to the fish oil therapy regimen may enhance beneficial effects by increasing glutathione reductase activity and decreasing peroxide levels (*Hsu et al, 2001*).

▶ Other therapeutic agents

Other therapeutic agents have been used with variable results.

- Gemfibrozil has been used to stimulate LPL activity and decrease VLDL secretion (*Santamarina-Fojo & Dugi, 1994*), and in cats is used at a dosage of 7.5 to 10 mg/kg body weight twice daily.
- Niacin therapy has been used, however adverse effects have been noted (*Bauer, 1995*).
- Garlic extracts have been used to decrease cholesterol in humans (*Steiner et al, 1996*), but have not been evaluated in cats.
- HMGCoA reductase inhibitors reduce cholesterol synthesis and increase the excretion of LDL from the circulation, but their effectiveness in cats has not been studied.
- Thyroxine therapy can decrease serum total cholesterol in humans (*Brun et al, 1980*), and is effective in lowering lipid concentrations in hypothyroid dogs, but its use has not been recommended for cats.

The mutation characterizing the LPL deficiency present in humans and cats with hyperchylomicronemia has been identified, and gene transfer therapy has been attempted. Lipoprotein lipase-deficient cats were given an injection of an adenoviral vector containing the human LPL gene, with disappearance of triglyceride-rich lipoproteins up to day 14, at which time antibodies against the human LPL protein were detected (*Liu et al, 2000*). Concurrent administration of immunosuppressive therapy delayed antibody production, with resolution of hyperlipidemia for three weeks after administration (*Ross et al, 2006*). Gene replacement therapy for inherited hyperchylomicronemia may become a reality in the future.

Conclusion

There are a number of conditions that can cause hyperlipidemia in the feline. Postprandial hyperlipidemia should always be verified, and secondary causes of hyperlipidemia must be ruled out. A number of the causes of secondary hyperlipidemia are uncommon in the cat (hypothyroidism, hyperadrenocorticism), or are fairly evident based on clinical signs or biochemical profile (diabetes mellitus, pancreatitis). If an underlying cause of hyperlipidemia is present, treatment of the primary disease is usually effective at resolving the secondary hyperlipidemia. Primary causes of hyperlipidemia should be aggressively treated because of the potential complications and clinical signs associated with persistent hyperlipidemia.

Frequently asked questions about feline hyperlipidemia

Q	A
What causes serum to be turbid?	Elevated serum triglyceride carried by lipoproteins causes serum to appear turbid. Opacity is seen when triglyceride concentration approaches 600 mg/dL (6.8 mmol/L). Serum may have the appearance of whole milk when triglyceride concentrations reach 2500 – 4000 mg/dL (28.2-45.2 mmol/L).
What conditions cause hyperlipidemia?	The most common cause is a non-fasted animal. If fasting for greater than 12 hours is confirmed, then primary hyperlipidemia, or secondary hyperlipidemia due to hypothyroidism, pancreatitis, diabetes mellitus, hyperadrenocorticism, cholestasis, or nephrotic syndrome may be present.
Are high fat diets harmful to cats?	Not usually. Lipid metabolism in cats is very different from that in humans. Cats carry most of their cholesterol in HDL, and are very resistant to the development of atherosclerosis. However, if certain diseases such as hypothyroidism or diabetes mellitus are present, high fat diets could result in further lipid abnormalities. In addition, high fat diets for neutered and sedentary cats can contribute to obesity with subsequent health issues.
What causes a "cream layer" to separate in some turbid serum samples?	The "cream layer" which floats to the top of serum is due to the presence of chylomicrons. This is normal in a non-fasted animal, but represents an abnormality if the animal has been fasted for greater than 12 hours.
Do cats develop atherosclerosis?	Contrary to humans, cats rarely develop atherosclerosis due to differences in lipid metabolism. Atherosclerosis could develop in some cats that have a concurrent disease that causes chronic hyperlipidemia.
Should persistent fasting hyperlipidemia be treated?	Yes. If the hyperlipidemia is due to a secondary cause, then treatment of the underlying condition may resolve the hyperlipidemia. There is evidence suggesting that chronic hyperlipidemia may lead to the development of pancreatitis, insulin resistance, diabetes mellitus, or atherosclerosis in some cats.

References

Adan Y, Shibata K, Sato M, et al. Effects of docosahexaenoic and eicosapentaenoic acid on lipid metabolism, eicosanoid production, platelet aggregation and atherosclerosis in hypercholesterolemic rats. Biosci Biotechnol Biochem 1999; 63: 111-119.

Alaupovic P, Furman RH, Falor WH, et al. Isolation and characterization of human chyle chylomicrons and lipoproteins. Ann N Y Acad Sci 1968; 149: 791-807.

Albers JJ, Chen CH, Lacko AG. Isolation, characterization, and assay of lecithin-cholesterol acyltransferase. Methods Enzymol 1986; 129: 763-783.

Alberts AW. HMG-CoA reductase inhibitors - the development. In: Stokes J & Mancini M, eds. Atherosclerosis Review. New York: Raven Press Ltd, 1988; 123-131.

Assmann G, Menzel HJ. Apolipoprotein disorders. Ric Clin Lab 1982; 12: 63-81.

Backus RC, Ginzinger DG, Ashbourne Excoffon KJ, et al. Maternal expression of functional lipoprotein lipase and effects on body fat mass and body condition scores of mature cats with lipoprotein lipase deficiency. Am J Vet Res 2001; 62: 264-269.

Baer DM, Paulson RA. The effect of hyperlipidemia on therapeutic drug assays. Ther Drug Monit 1987; 9: 72-77.

Bauer JE, Verlander JW. Congenital lipoprotein lipase deficiency in hyperlipemic kitten siblings. Vet Clin Pathol 1984; 13: 7-11.

Bauer JE. Evaluation and dietary considerations in idiopathic hyperlipidemia in dogs. J Am Vet Med Assoc 1995; 206: 1684-1688.

Bauer JE. Comparative lipid and lipoprotein metabolism. Vet Clin Pathol 1996; 25: 49-56.

Berg AL, Hansson P, Nilsson-Ehle P. Salt resistant lipase activity in human adrenal gland is increased in Cushing's disease. J Intern Med 1990; 228: 257-260.

Blanchard G, Paragon BM, Serougne C, et al. Plasma lipids, lipoprotein composition and profile during induction and treatment of hepatic lipidosis in cats and the metabolic effect of one daily meal in healthy cats. J Anim Physiol Anim Nutr (Berl) 2004; 88: 73-87.

Boden G. Role of fatty acids in the pathogenesis of insulin resistance and NIDDM. Diabetes 1997; 46: 3-10.

Boretti FS, Breyer-Haube I, Kaspers B, et al. [Clinical, hematological, biochemical and endocrinological aspects of 32 dogs with hypothyroidism]. Schweiz Arch Tierheilkd 2003; 145: 149-156, 158-149.

Bossuyt X, Blanckaert N. Evaluation of interferences in rate and fixed-time nephelometric assays of specific serum proteins. Clin Chem 1999; 45: 62-67.

Brooks KD. Idiopathic hyplipoproteinemia in a cat. Companion Animal Practice 1989; 19: 5-9.

Brown SA, Brown CA, Crowell WA, et al. Effects of dietary polyunsaturated fatty acid supplementation in early renal insufficiency in dogs. J Lab Clin Med 2000; 135: 275-286.

Brun LD, Gagne C, Coulombe P, et al. Effects of dextrothyroxine on the pituitary-thyroid axis in hypercholesterolemic children and goitrous adults. J Clin Endocrinol Metab 1980; 51: 1306-1310.

Capurso A, Catapano AL, Mills GL, et al. Formation of HDL-like particles following chylomicron lipolysis. In: Catapano A, Salvioli G, Vergani C, eds. High-Density Lipoproteins: Physiopathological Aspects and Clinical Significance; Atherosclerosis Review. New York: Raven Press, 1987; 19-38.

Carrington SD. Lipid keratopathy in a cat. J Small Anim Pract 1983; 24: 495-505.

Castillo M, Amalik F, Linares A, et al. Fish oil reduces cholesterol and arachidonic acid levels in plasma and lipoproteins from hypercholesterolemic chicks. Mol Cell Biochem 2000; 210: 121-130.

Center SA, Baldwin BH, King JM, et al. Hematologic and biochemical abnormalities associated with induced extrahepatic bile duct obstruction in the cat. Am J Vet Res 1983; 44: 1822-1829.

Chanut F, Colle MA, Deschamps JY, et al. Systemic xanthomatosis associated with hyperchylomicronaemia in a cat. J Vet Med A Physiol Pathol Clin Med 2005; 52: 272-274.

Chapman MJ. Comparative analysis of mammalian plasma lipoproteins. Methods Enzymol 1986; 128: 70-143.

Chmielewski M, Sucajtys E, Swierczynski J, et al. Contribution of increased HMG-CoA reductase gene expression to hypercholesterolemia in experimental chronic renal failure. Mol Cell Biochem 2003; 246: 187-191.

Christophersen B, Nordstoga K, Shen Y, et al. Lipoprotein lipase deficiency with pancreatitis in mink: biochemical characterization and pathology. J Lipid Res 1997; 38: 837-846.

Cobbaert C, Tricarico A. Different effect of Intralipid and triacylglycerol rich lipoproteins on the Kodak Ektachem serum cholesterol determination. Eur J Clin Chem Clin Biochem 1993; 31: 107-109.

Connor WE, DeFrancesco CA, Connor SL. N-3 fatty acids from fish oil. Effects on plasma lipoproteins and hypertriglyceridemic patients. Ann N Y Acad Sci 1993; 683: 16-34.

Cooper AD. The metabolism of chylomicron remnants by isolated perfused rat liver. Biochim Biophys Acta 1977; 488: 464-474.

D'Amico G. Lipid changes in the nephrotic syndrome: new insights into pathomechanisms and treatment. Klin Wochenschr 1991; 69: 618-622.

Danielsson B, Ekman R, Johansson BG, et al. Plasma lipoprotein changes in experimental cholestasis in the dog. Clin Chim Acta 1977; 80: 157-170.

Darras C, Brivet F, Chalas J, et al. Factitious acute hypercalcemia biological interference between calcium and lipids. Intensive Care Med 1992; 18: 131-132.

de Sain-van der Velden MG, Kaysen GA, Barrett HA, et al. Increased VLDL in nephrotic patients results from a decreased catabolism while increased LDL results from increased synthesis. Kidney Int 1998; 53: 994-1001.

Deighan CJ, Caslake MJ, McConnell M, et al. Patients with nephrotic-range proteinuria have apolipoprotein C and E deficient VLDL1. Kidney Int 2000; 58: 1238-1246.

Demacker PN, van Heijst PJ, Hak-Lemmers HL, et al. A study of the lipid transport system in the cat, Felix domesticus. Atherosclerosis 1987; 66: 113-123.

Diez M, Hornick JL, Baldwin P, et al. Influence of a blend of fructo-oligosaccharides and sugar beet fiber on nutrient digestibility and plasma metabolite concentrations in healthy beagles. Am J Vet Res 1997; 58: 1238-1242.

Dimski DS, Buffington CA, Johnson SE, et al. Serum lipoprotein concentrations and hepatic lesions in obese cats undergoing weight loss. Am J Vet Res 1992; 53: 1259-1262.

Dominguez-Munoz JE, Malfertheiner P, Ditschuneit HH, et al. Hyperlipidemia in acute pancreatitis. Relationship with etiology, onset, and severity of the disease. Int J Pancreatol 1991; 10: 261-267.

Ebara T, Okubo M, Horinishi A, et al. No evidence of accelerated atherosclerosis in a 66-yr-old chylomicronemia patient homozygous for the nonsense mutation (Tyr61-->stop) in the lipoprotein lipase gene. Atherosclerosis 2001; 159: 375-379.

Feingold KR, Wilson DE, Wood LC, et al. Diabetes increases hepatic hydroxymethyl glutaryl coenzyme A reductase protein and mRNA levels in the small intestine. Metabolism 1994; 43: 450-454.

Feldman EB, Russell BS, Chen R, et al. Dietary saturated fatty acid content affects lymph lipoproteins: studies in the rat. J Lipid Res 1983; 24: 967-976.

Fettman MJ, Stanton CA, Banks LL, et al. Effects of weight gain and loss on metabolic rate, glucose tolerance, and serum lipids in domestic cats. Res Vet Sci 1998; 64: 11-16.

Field FJ, Albright E, Mathur SN. The effect of hypothyroidism and thyroxine replacement on hepatic and intestinal HMG-CoA reductase and ACAT activities and biliary lipids in the rat. Metabolism 1986; 35: 1085-1089.

Foster SF, Church DB, Watson AD. Effects of phenobarbitone on serum biochemical tests in dogs. Aust Vet J 2000; 78: 23-26.

Garrib A, Griffiths W, Eldridge P, et al. Artifactually low glycated haemoglobin in a patient with severe hypertriglyceridaemia. J Clin Pathol 2003; 56: 394-395.

Gebhard RL, Prigge WF. Thyroid hormone differentially augments biliary sterol secretion in the rat. II. The chronic bile fistula model. J Lipid Res 1992; 33: 1467-1473.

Ginzinger DG, Lewis ME, Ma Y, et al. A mutation in the lipoprotein lipase gene is the molecular basis of chylomicronemia in a colony of domestic cats. J Clin Invest 1996; 97: 1257-1266.

Ginzinger DG, Wilson JE, Redenbach D, et al. Diet-induced atherosclerosis in the domestic cat. Lab Invest 1997; 77: 409-419.

Ginzinger DG, Clee SM, Dallongeville J, et al. Lipid and lipoprotein analysis of cats with lipoprotein lipase deficiency. Eur J Clin Invest 1999; 29: 17-26.

Goldstein JL, Brown MS. Progress in understanding the LDL receptor and HMG-CoA reductase, two membrane proteins that regulate the plasma cholesterol. J Lipid Res 1984; 25: 1450-1461.

Grieshaber RL, McKeever PJ, Conroy JD. Spontaneous cutaneous (eruptive) xanthomatosis in two cats. J Am Anim Hosp Assoc 1991; 27: 509-512.

Groot PH, Jansen H, Van Tol A. Selective degradation of the high density lipoprotein-2 subfraction by heparin-releasable liver lipase. FEBS Lett 1981; 129: 269-272.

Gunn-Moore DA, Watson TD, Dodkin SJ, et al. Transient hyperlipidaemia and anaemia in kittens. Vet Rec 1997; 140: 355-359.

Guyan PM, Uden S, Braganza JM. Heightened free radical activity in pancreatitis. Free Radic Biol Med 1990; 8: 347-354.

Guyard-Dangremont V, Desrumaux C, Gambert P, et al. Phospholipid and cholesteryl ester transfer activities in plasma from 14 vertebrate species. Relation to atherogenesis susceptibility. Comp Biochem Physiol B Biochem Mol Biol 1998; 120: 517-525.

Hansen B, DiBartola SP, Chew DJ, et al. Clinical and metabolic findings in dogs with chronic renal failure fed two diets. Am J Vet Res 1992; 53: 326-334.

Hansson P, Nordin G, Nilsson-Ehle P. Influence of nutritional state on lipoprotein lipase activities in the hypothyroid rat. Biochim Biophys Acta 1983; 753: 364-371.

Harris WS, Connor WE, Illingworth DRet al. Effects of fish oil on VLDL triglyceride kinetics in humans. J Lipid Res 1990; 31: 1549-1558.

Hata Y, Shigematsu H, Tonomo Y, et al. Interference of an anesthetic preparation with plasma triglyceride determinations. Jpn Circ J 1978; 42: 689-694.

Havel RJ. Pathogenesis, differentiation and management of hypertriglyceridemia. Adv Intern Med 1969; 15: 117-154.

Havel RJ. The formation of LDL: mechanisms and regulation. J Lipid Res 1984; 25: 1570-1576.

Hazzard WR, Kushwaha RS, Applebaum-Bowden D, et al. Chylomicron and very low-density lipoprotein apolipoprotein B metabolism: mechanism of the response to stanozolol in a patient with severe hypertriglyceridemia. Metabolism 1984; 33: 873-881.

Hill RC, Van Winkle TJ. Acute necrotizing pancreatitis and acute suppurative pancreatitis in the cat. A retrospective study of 40 cases (1976-1989). J Vet Intern Med 1993; 7: 25-33.

Hoenig M, Wilkins C, Holson JC, et al. Effects of obesity on lipid profiles in neutered male and female cats. Am J Vet Res 2003; 64: 299-303.

Hoenig M, McGoldrick JB, deBeer M, et al. Activity and tissue-specific expression of lipases and tumor-necrosis factor alpha in lean and obese cats. Domest Anim Endocrinol 2006; 30: 333-344.

Holt PR. The roles of bile acids during the process of normal fat and cholesterol absorption. Arch Intern Med 1972; 130: 574-583.

Hsu HC, Lee YT, Chen MF. Effects of fish oil and vitamin E on the antioxidant defense system in diet-induced hypercholesterolemic rabbits. Prostaglandins Other Lipid Mediat 2001; 66: 99-108.

Jaggy A, Oliver JE, Ferguson DC, et al. Neurological manifestations of hypothyroidism: a retrospective study of 29 dogs. J Vet Intern Med 1994; 8: 328-336.

Johnstone AC, Jones BR, Thompson JC, et al. The pathology of an inherited hyperlipoproteinaemia of cats. J Comp Pathol 1990; 102: 125-137.

Jones BR, Wallace A, Harding DR, et al. Occurrence of idiopathic, familial hyperchylomicronaemia in a cat. Vet Rec 1983; 112: 543-547.

Jones BR, Johnstone AC, Cahill JI, et al. Peripheral neuropathy in cats with inherited primary hyperchylomicronaemia. Vet Rec 1986; 119: 268-272.

Jones BR. Inherited hyperchylomicronaemia in the cat. J Small Anim Pract 1993; 34: 493-499.

Kaysen GA, Myers BD, Couser WG, et al. Mechanisms and consequences of proteinuria. Lab Invest 1986; 54: 479-498.

Focus on:
Long-chain omega-3 fatty acids (EPA-DHA)

Omega-3 fatty acids are a separate family of polyunsaturated fatty acids (PUFA). Their precursor is α-linolenic acid (C18:3, n-3), whose chemical structure distinguishes it from linoleic acid (C18:2, n-6), the precursor of the other main family, omega-6 fatty acids.

Linoleic acid is an essential fatty acid for cats, which depend on a dietary intake to cover their requirements. With the exception of docosahexaenoic acid (DHA), the omega-3 series of fatty acids are not considered to be essential, as cats can survive with a food that does not contain them. On the other hand, their health may benefit from their introduction in the diet.

LINOLEIC ACID: C18:2 (N-6); OMEGA-6 FATTY ACID PRECURSOR

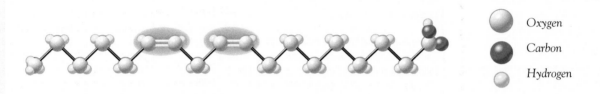

Oxygen
Carbon
Hydrogen

Omega-6 fatty acids are characterized by the first double bond between the 6th and 7th carbon atom, counting from the omega carbon (the carbon atom located opposite the carboxyl–COOH grouping).

α-LINOLENIC ACID: C18:3 (N-3); OMEGA-3 FATTY ACID PRECURSOR

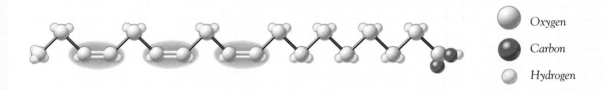

Oxygen
Carbon
Hydrogen

In the omega-3 fatty acid family, the first double bond is located between the 3rd and 4th carbon atom.

Metabolism of unsaturated fatty acids

The synthesis of long-chain fatty acids is triggered by the action of enzymes in the liver (desaturase and elongase), which add to the carbon atoms and the unsaturated double bonds. These are the same enzymes that act in the synthesis of omega-3 and omega-6 fatty acids, which explains the competition between the two families.

In cats, the enzyme responsible for the first desaturation, Δ6 desaturase, has a very low-level of activity *(Sinclair et al., 1979; Pawlosky et al., 1994).*

- In the series of omega-6 fatty acids, Δ6 desaturase produces very low quantities of arachidonic acid. In the absence of dietary intake a healthy adult cat may be able to cover its requirements, but gestating queens will produce no or few viable litters and the proportion of cannibalism appears to be higher *(Morris, 2004).* Arachidonic acid is therefore deemed essential in cats, contrary to dogs.

HEPATIC SYNTHESIS OF LONG-CHAIN OMEGA-3 AND OMEGA-6 FATTY ACIDS FROM THEIR RESPECTIVE PRECURSORS

OMEGA-6 FATTY ACIDS

Linoleic acid C18: 2 (n-6)

↓

γ-linolenic acid C18: 3 (n-6)

↓

Dihydrolipoic acid C20: 3 (n-6)

↓

Arachidonic acid C20: 4 (n-6)

OMEGA-3 FATTY ACIDS

α-linolenic acid C18: 3 (n-3)

↓

Eicosapentaenoic acid C20: 4 (n-3)

↓

Eicosapentaenoic acid **(EPA)** C20: 5 (n-3)

↓

Docosahexaenoic acid **(DHA)** C22: 6 (n-3)

Hyperlipidemia

- With respect to omega-3 fatty acids, the yield from α-linolenic acid (omega-3) is very low. Likewise, the enzyme activity responsible for interconversion from its omega-6 homolog (DHA: C22:5) has only been shown in the brain in cats *(Pawlosky et al., 1994)*. Therefore, when EPA-DHA supplementation is recommended, they should be provided preformed in the food.

Sources of omega-3 fatty acids

Some vegetable oils, such as soy oil and especially linseed oil, contain a non-negligible quantity of α-linolenic acid. In contrast, oils sourced from the sea are the only useful sources of EPA and DHA.

PUFA sourced from the sea are synthesized in the chloroplasts of phytoplankton or micro-algae consumed by fish. Higher up the food chain, some fish incorporate omega-3 PUFA and their metabolism transforms them until the fatty acids contain 20-22 carbon atoms. EPA and DHA are especially concentrated in the adipose tissue of fish. Fish oils (especially cold sea fish like salmon, mackerel, anchovy, halibut and herring) can contain more than 30% EPA-DHA.

COMPARATIVE CONTENT OF OMEGA-3 FATTY ACIDS OF DIFFERENT OILS

Omega-3 fatty acids (% DM)	Soy oil	Linseed oil	Fish oil
α-linolenic acid	6	51	<1
EPA + DHA	–	–	17-34

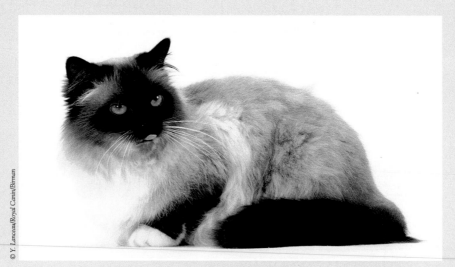

*The adaptation of the cat's metabolism to a carnivorous diet is especially
expressed by the specific requirements of essential fatty acids,
which differ from those of the dog.*

Key points
to remember about:

Nutritional management of hyperlipidemia

1 - **Give the cat a low-fat diet**: < 30 g/1000 kcal or less than 10% fat in a 4000 kcal/kg food:

- in the event of obesity, weight loss is indicated to lower the cholesterol concentration;

- when the body condition is optimal the low-fat diet may need to be supplemented with calories compared with a maintenance food to avoid undesirable weight loss.

2 - When the low-fat diet is inadequate to control hyperlipidemia, fish oil (10-200 mg/kg), which is rich in the long chain omega-3 fatty acids EPA and DHA, can reduce serum lipid concentrations.

3 - Adding a large quantity of unsaturated fatty acids (omega-3) increases the risk of oxidation of the lipid membranes. The administration of biological antioxidants (e.g. vitamin E, vitamin C and beta-carotene) can limit the oxidative reactions.

References

Morris JG. *Do cats need arachidonic acid in the diet for reproduction?* J Anim Physiol Anim Nutr (Berl) 2004; 88: 3-4.

Pawlosky R, Barnes A, Salem N Jr. *Essential fatty acid metabolism in the feline: relationship between liver and brain production of long-chain polyunsaturated fatty acids.* J Lipid Res 1994; 35: 2032-2040.

Sinclair AJ, McLean JG, Monger EA. *Metabolism of linoleic acid in the cat.* Lipids 1979; 14: 932-936.

Kidneys

Jonathan ELLIOTT
MA, Vet MB, PhD,
Cert SAC, Dipl.
ECVPT, MRCVS

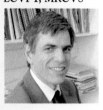

Denise A. ELLIOTT
BVSc (Hons),
PhD, Dipl. ACVIM,
Dipl. ACVN

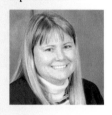

Dietary therapy for feline chronic kidney disease

Kidneys

Introduction 251

1. Kidney physiology 251

2. Staging of kidney disease 253

3. Dietary therapy in detail 256

4. Treating the uremic patient 273

Conclusion 277

Frequently asked questions 278

References 280

Royal Canin nutritional information 282

ABBREVIATIONS USED IN THIS CHAPTER

ACVIM: American College of Veterinary Internal Medicine
ADH: antidiuretic hormone
ADMA: asymmetric dimethylarginine
ASVNU: American Society for Veterinary Nephrology and Urology
CKD: chronic kidney disease
ECF: extracellular fluid

ESVNU: European Society for Veterinary Nephrology and Urology
GFR: glomerular filtration rate
IRIS: International Renal Interest Society
KDOQI ™: The National Kidney Foundation: Kidney Disease Outcomes Quality Initiative
LDL: low density lipoprotein
MCP-1: monocyte chemotractant protein-1

MW: molecular weight
NRC: National Research Council
PRA: plasma renin activity
PTH: parathyroid hormone
PUFA: polyunsaturated fatty acid
RAAS: renin-angiotensin-aldosterone system
UPC: urine protein to creatinine ratio

Dietary therapy for feline chronic kidney disease

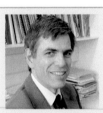

Jonathan ELLIOTT

MA, Vet MB, PhD, Cert SAC, Dipl. ECVPT, MRCVS

Jonathan Elliott graduated from Cambridge University Veterinary School in 1985. After completing a year as an Intern in Small Animal Medicine and Surgery at the Veterinary Hospital, University of Pennsylvania, he returned to Cambridge to undertake his PhD studies in the Department of Pharmacology. He completed his PhD in vascular pharmacology in 1989. In 1990 he was appointed to a lectureship in Veterinary Pharmacology at the Royal Veterinary College in London where he is currently Professor of Veterinary Clinical Pharmacology and has developed research interests in feline chronic renal failure and hypertension and equine laminitis. He was appointed Vice Principal for Research in 2004. He is a Diplomate of the European College of Pharmacology and Toxicology and a member of the Veterinary Products Committee, which advises the UK Government on licensing veterinary medicines. Jonathan Elliott was awarded the Pfizer Academic Award in 1998, the BSAVA Amoroso Award in 2001 and the 2006 Pet Plan Scientific Award for his contributions to companion animal medicine, particularly in the areas of equine laminitis and feline chronic kidney disease.

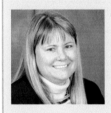

Denise A. ELLIOTT

BVSc (Hons) PhD Dipl. ACVIM, Dipl. ACVN

Denise Elliott graduated from the University of Melbourne with a Bachelor in Veterinary Science with Honors in 1991. After completing an internship in Small Animal Medicine and Surgery at the University of Pennsylvania, Denise moved to the University of California-Davis where she completed a residency in Small Animal Internal Medicine, a fellowship in Renal Medicine and Hemodialysis, and a residency in Small Animal Clinical Nutrition. Denise received board certification with the American College of Veterinary Internal Medicine in 1996 and with the American College of Veterinary Nutrition in 2001. The University of California-Davis awarded a PhD in Nutrition in 2001 for her work on Multifrequency Bioelectrical Impedance Analysis in Healthy Cats and Dogs. Denise is currently the Director of Scientific Affairs for Royal Canin USA.

Kidney disease is extremely prevalent in the aging cat population and is one of the most common medical reasons older cats are seen in veterinary practice. Although good epidemiological data from Europe are lacking, data from the USA suggest that 1 in 3 cats over the age of 12 years have some form of renal insufficiency (Lulich et al, 1992). A study of apparently healthy and biochemically normal cats aged 9 years or older recruited prospectively from primary care practices in central London has demonstrated that, within 12 months, around 1 in 3 cats had biochemical evidence of azotemia (i.e plasma creatinine and/or urea concentrations above upper limits of the reference intervals) (Jepson et al, 2007a).

Introduction

There are a number of well recognized disease processes which damage the kidney in cats and lead to a well defined pathology. In the majority of cats, once the diagnosis of chronic kidney disease (CKD) is made through demonstration of azotemia in association with an inability to produce adequately concentrated urine (see section 2 for further discussion), the underlying disease is often not recognizable, even on renal biopsy. Quite clearly this disease syndrome is not a single entity and a more complete understanding of the pathological processes involved is needed if progress is to be made in the prevention of some forms of CKD in the cat.

Even when azotemia has been detected in cats with clinical evidence suggestive of CKD, progression to the stage where life is not compatible without renal replacement therapy (dialysis or transplantation) is not inevitable in all cases. Progression occurs at different rates in individual cats, emphasizing the heterogeneous nature of chronic kidney disease in the cat. Progress has been made recently on identifying risk factors for progression and evaluating treatments (including diets) in clinical patients against the gold standard of survival.

When CKD has been identified in an individual patient the diagnostic and therapeutic goals are:

1. identify factors that are affecting the quality of life of the cat
2. select treatments (pharmacologic or dietary) that should improve the quality of life of the cat
3. identify factors that increase the risk of progressive renal injury in the individual cat
4. select treatments (pharmacologic and/or dietary) that may reduce the risk of progressive renal injury
5. monitor the response to these treatments and ensure that each treatment is tailored to the individual cat

It is helpful to categorize an individual cat as to the stage of its kidney disease since this will inform the clinician as to the most appropriate treatments and the most likely complications that arise associated with the CKD syndrome.
The aims of this chapter are to:
1. Outline the physiological roles of the kidney that are key to understanding what homeostatic mechanisms fail in CKD
2. Define a staging process for feline CKD
3. Define the management of CKD, making reference to the goals outlined above and to identify the stage at which specific problems will need to be addressed.

1 - Kidney physiology

The nephron (**Figure 1**) is the functional unit of the kidney. Each feline kidney has around 200,000 nephrons. The kidney has the following major roles:
- excretion of water soluble waste products in urine
- homeostasis of the volume and composition of body fluids
- endocrine functions (production of erythropoietin, angiotensin II and calcitriol)

FIGURE 1 - A SCHEMATIC DIAGRAM OF THE NEPHRON

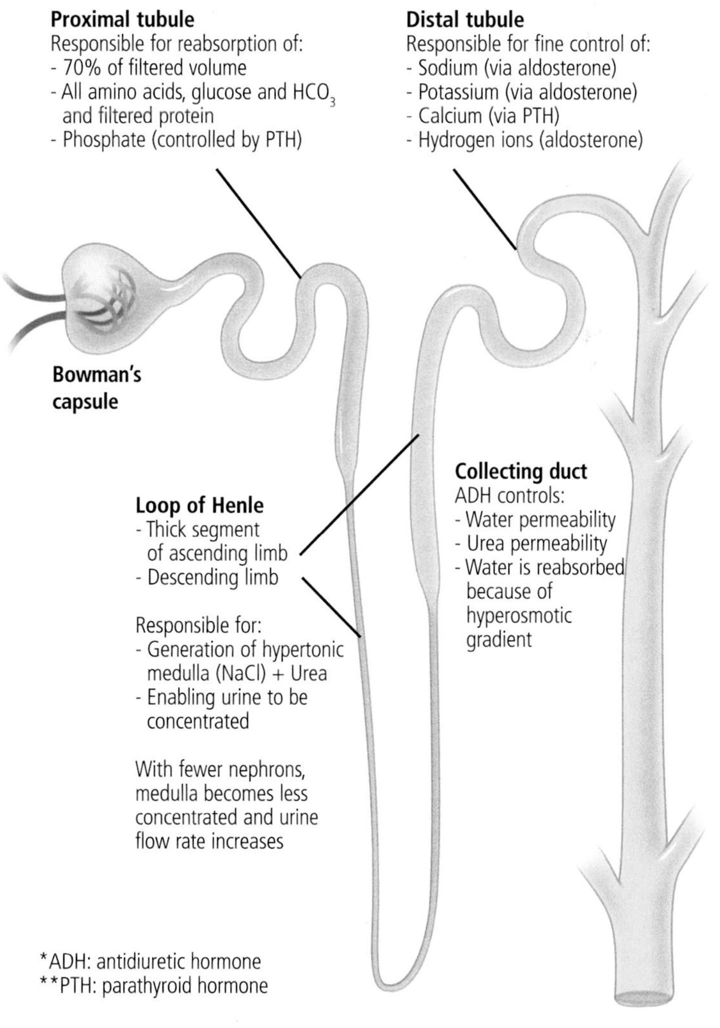

Proximal tubule
Responsible for reabsorption of:
- 70% of filtered volume
- All amino acids, glucose and HCO_3 and filtered protein
- Phosphate (controlled by PTH)

Distal tubule
Responsible for fine control of:
- Sodium (via aldosterone)
- Potassium (via aldosterone)
- Calcium (via PTH)
- Hydrogen ions (aldosterone)

Bowman's capsule

Loop of Henle
- Thick segment of ascending limb
- Descending limb

Responsible for:
- Generation of hypertonic medulla (NaCl) + Urea
- Enabling urine to be concentrated

With fewer nephrons, medulla becomes less concentrated and urine flow rate increases

Collecting duct
ADH controls:
- Water permeability
- Urea permeability
- Water is reabsorbed because of hyperosmotic gradient

*ADH: antidiuretic hormone
**PTH: parathyroid hormone

Each nephron consists of a glomerulus (the filter), a proximal tubule, loop of Henle, distal and cortical collecting tubule and a collecting duct.

The kidney functions by non-specifically filtering the blood such that the water components of plasma appear in the filtrate at the same concentration they are found in plasma. Proteins are excluded from the filtrate progressively as their molecular weight (MW) get higher such that very little protein of MW above 70,000 gets across the normal filter. Approximately 20% of the renal plasma flowing through the kidney appears within the glomerular filtrate. The proximal convoluted tubule then functions to return about 65 to 70% of the filtered load to the blood stream. It ensures that substances the body requires (such as glucose and amino acids) are readily returned whereas water soluble waste products, which are of no use to the body, stay in the filtrate and are excreted in the urine.

The rate of excretion of many water soluble waste products from the body is dependent on the glomerular filtration rate (e.g. creatinine - a waste product of muscle metabolism). Some relatively low molecular weight substances are also actively transported from the plasma into the tubular fluid. Specific transporters are able to secrete organic acids or bases from the peritubular capillaries into the proximal convoluted tubular fluid. There are many examples of these transporters. One of the best known is able to secrete penicillins into the tubular fluid where, due to its high hydrophilicity this drug will stay in the filtrate as water is reabsorbed. Hence the urinary concentration of penicillin G following administration of standard doses rates to a cat can exceed the plasma concentration by more than 300 fold.

Whilst this early part of the nephron (proximal convoluted tubule) is responsible for the bulk return of filtered fluid and electrolytes to the plasma, the later parts are responsible for the fine control of urine composition. The loop of Henle is involved in generating a concentration gradient by trapping sodium chloride and urea in the interstitial area of the kidney. The so called "counter-current multiplier system" is responsible for this function. The descending limb of the loop of Henle is impermeable to sodium chloride but permeable to water whereas the ascending limb is impermeable to water and, the thick ascending limb actively transport sodium chloride into the medullary interstitium.

The cat is supremely adapted to produce concentrated urine having a relatively high proportion of nephrons with long loops of Henle. Cats can produce urine with a specific gravity of in excess of 1.080 and the maximal concentrating capacity of the cat kidney has not been assessed. This means that cats are able to exist with very small amounts of water to drink and, if fed a moist diet, often take in enough water with their food and so do not need to drink very much. The ability to produce concentrated urine and therefore conserve water is highly dependent on the number of functioning nephrons available to generate the gradient of sodium chloride in the medullary interstitium. Dietary sodium (or sodium chloride) and dietary moisture are highly effective in stimulating water consumption and diuresis in cats (_Burger et al, 1980_). Increased diuresis promotes urine dilution (**Figure 2**).

The later parts of the nephron are responsible for the fine control of the urine composition. Primitive urine passing from the loop of Henle to the cortical collecting tubule should be hypotonic (relative to plasma) when entering the cortical collecting tubule. This is because sodium chloride has been removed from the filtrate in excess of water. The early part of the distal tubule continues this process where sodium reabsorption occurs without water (diluting segment). In the later parts of the distal tubule, sodium reabsorption occurs under the regulation of the sodium conserving hormone, aldosterone. Calcium, hydrogen and potassium ion composition of the tubular fluid are all regulated by the action of hormones (parathyroid hormone and aldosterone) in the distal tubule and cortical collecting tubule (also known as the late distal tubule). The later parts of the cortical collecting tubule and the collecting ducts respond to antidiuretic hormone (ADH) which regulates water and urea permeability. ADH secretion from the neurohypophysis is regulated by the osmolality of plasma and water conservation is ensured by the kidney minimizing water losses with the production of maximally concentrated urine when necessary.

FIGURE 2 – INFLUENCE OF DIETARY SODIUM ON URINE VOLUME IN CATS
Biourge et al, 2001

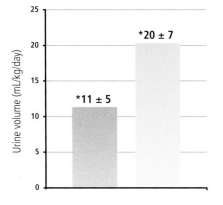

The control diet contains 1.1 g sodium/1000 kcal; the test diet contains 2.5 g sodium/1000 kcal. This study shows that a higher sodium intake significantly (p < 0.05) increases diuresis: urinary volume is almost doubled with a 1% sodium dry diet (4000 kcal/kg) compared with a 0.4% sodium diet.

An important concept to grasp when interpreting clinical laboratory data from cats is that urine composition is highly variable. Physiologically, the kidney is able to vary the composition of urine to ensure that homeostasis is achieved and the following equation balances:
Intake of substance = Non-renal losses + Renal losses

In CKD, as kidney function deteriorates (fewer functioning nephrons present), the homeostatic mechanisms struggle to regulate fluid, electrolyte and mineral balances since either:
- renal losses are limited by the reduced renal mass (limited excretion)
- tubular flow rates increase in the remaining functioning nephrons so fine control of the composition of urine becomes more difficult as the later parts of the nephron are presented with fluid flowing too quickly (hyperfiltration)
- compensatory mechanisms become counter-productive leading to a worsening of the electrolyte or mineral imbalance (**Figure 3**)

Careful regulation of the composition of the diet can help cats with CKD maintain homeostasis, leading to improvements in their quality of life. Possibly, in some cases, it can slow down the progression of CKD to the stage where renal replacement therapy is necessary. The next section of this chapter deals with the staging of CKD and puts forward intrinsic and extrinsic factors that may influence progression of CKD. In subsequent sections manipulation of the different components of the diet for feline CKD patients will be discussed and the rationale for these dietary changes at each stage of CKD explained.

2 - Staging of kidney disease

A comprehensive scheme for staging CKD in cats (and dogs) has been proposed by the International Renal Interest Society (IRIS) and endorsed by the American and European Societies for Veterinary Nephrology and Urology (ASVNU and ESVNU). The staging system should be applied after a diagnosis of CKD. It has been made on the basis of clinical and laboratory tests and only once a clinical case has been shown to be in a stable state rather than acutely deteriorating and requiring supportive therapy to avert a uremic crisis.

The basis for the staging system is the plasma creatinine concentration. The IRIS group is well aware of the limitations of this approach as plasma creatinine concentration is influenced by:
- muscle mass
- hydration status
- diet composition

Plasma creatinine concentration is exponentially and inversely correlated to the gold standard measure of renal function and renal mass, namely the glomerular filtration rate (GFR). At the present time, practical methods that have been validated for use in the cat under primary care practice conditions for the measurement of GFR in the cat are not available. In the fullness of time, these methods will become available and then GFR will replace plasma creatinine concentration as the physiological measurement upon which staging of CKD will be based (*Le Garreres et al, 2007*) (**Figure 4**).

FIGURE 3 - RELATIONSHIP BETWEEN RENAL INJURY, LOSS OF NEPHRONS, RENAL COMPENSATORY ADAPTATIONS, AND PROGRESSION OF RENAL FAILURE

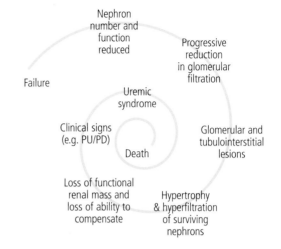

The compensatory changes maintain clinically stable disease until structural and functional damage exceeds a threshold beyond which progression of renal function and clinical signs of uremia occur. Chronic renal disease typically progresses to end-stage renal disease after a critical number of nephrons have been damaged.

FIGURE 4 - PLASMA CREATININE VS TIME CURVES IN 2 CATS AFTER INTRAVENOUS ADMINISTRATION OF EXOGENOUS CREATININE (*dose: 40 mg/kg BW*)
From B. Reynolds, National Veterinary School of Toulouse

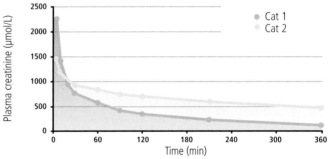

The plasma creatinine clearances (i.e. a GFR estimate) for cat 1 and 2 were 2.6 and 1.3 mL/min/kg, respectively.
Cat 1 *was a 5 year old DSH cat (6.1 kg) with polycystic kidney disease incidentally identified when abdominal ultrasonography was performed for unrelated problems. Plasma creatinine concentration at that time was 158 µmol/L (1.79 mg/dL). Renal function was considered normal after GFR estimation.*
Cat 2 *was a 9 month old DSH cat (2.6 kg) screened for severe polyuria and polydipsia. Both kidneys were abnormal at ultrasonographic examination. Concurrent plasma creatinine concentration was 152 µmol/L (1.72 mg/dL). Renal function was considered impaired after GFR estimation and an appropriate diet prescribed.*
These two cases illustrate the importance of muscle mass influencing the rate of production of creatinine when interpreting plasma creatinine concentration as an indicator of renal function.

TABLE 1 - THE *INTERNATIONAL RENAL INTEREST SOCIETY* (IRIS) STAGING SYSTEM BASED ON PLASMA CREATININE

Stage	Creatinine *	Comments
I	< 140 µmol/L (< 1.6 mg/dL)	Non-azotemic Some other renal abnormality present e.g. inadequate concentrating ability without identifiable non-renal cause; abnormal renal palpation and/or abnormal renal imaging findings; proteinuria of renal origin; abnormal renal biopsy results; increasing plasma creatinine concentrations noted on serial samples
II	140-249 µmol/L (1.6-2.8 mg/dL)	Mild renal azotemia (lower end of the range lies within the reference range for many laboratories but the insensitivity of creatinine as a screening test means that animals with creatinine values close to the upper reference limit often have excretory failure) Clinical signs usually mild or absent
III	250-439 µmol/L (2.8-5.0 mg/dL)	Moderate renal azotemia Many extra-renal clinical signs may be present
IV	> 440 µmol/L (> 5.0 mg/dL)	Severe renal azotemia Many extra-renal clinical signs are usually present

*To convert µmol/L to mg/dL divide by 88.4

Table 1 defines the staging system based on plasma creatinine concentration. The main challenge to the veterinary profession is to identify kidney disease when it is in the non-azotemic stage (stage I and early stage II). The veterinary profession has traditionally identified CKD by the finding of chronically elevated plasma creatinine concentration in conjunction with relatively dilute urine (often inappropriately so for the hydration status of the animal). At this stage (late stage II to IV) the primary cause of the kidney disease is often not evident, even on renal biopsy, and so the opportunity to treat the underlying cause of the kidney disease has been lost. Routine screening of older cats (from 8 years on) for evidence of kidney dysfunction examining serial plasma creatinine concentrations on an annual basis (and eventually measuring GFR) will increase our ability to detect CKD at an earlier stage and perhaps address the primary disease process at a stage where we can treat the primary disease.

Progression is thought to occur through three basic mechanisms:

1. repeated episodes of the primary disease process leading to further damage and loss of functioning nephrons;
2. mal-adaptive mechanisms, intrinsic to the kidney leading to glomerular capillary hypertension, hyperfiltration and hypertrophy. This is thought to occur through local activation of the renin-angiotensin system. The appearance of increasing amounts of protein in the urine may indicate that this process is occurring and there is some evidence that excess filtered protein may damage the tubules and contribute to progressive renal injury;
3. mal-adaptive responses occurring extrinsic to the kidney resulting from reduced renal function which may have detrimental effects on the remaining functioning nephrons:
   - hyperphosphatemia, hyperparathyroidism and nephrocalcinosis
   - systemic arterial hypertension due to an inability to regulate extracellular fluid volume. The diseased kidney's ability to autoregulate and protect itself from systemic arterial hypertension is reduced and this can lead to hypertensive kidney damage.

Progression of CKD in cats, as alluded to above, occurs at different rates such that some cases remain stable in stage II/III CKD and later die of some other problem whereas others progress to stage IV and suffer a renal death. The pattern of progression seems to take at least two forms, namely:
- stepwise progression with a sudden decrement of kidney function leading to a uremic crisis
- gradual linear progression with increases in plasma creatinine occurring steadily over time

Stepwise decrement in kidney function is the more common pattern of progression seen in cats with naturally occurring CKD (*Elliott et al, 2003b; Ross et al, 2006*).

It is clear from evidence in other species that risk factors for rapid progression of chronic kidney disease include proteinuria and systemic arterial hypertension. Thus, the IRIS staging system requires that CKD is sub-staged based on the urine protein to creatinine (UPC) ratio and on the systemic arterial blood pressure. Recent evidence suggests that UPC is an independent risk factor for all cause mortality of cats with CKD (*Syme et al, 2006*) and in cats with systemic hypertension (*Jepson et al, 2007b*). **Table 2** sets out the IRIS sub-staging system based on UPC. The substaging of cases based on UPC refers only to renal proteinuria. Pre-renal and post-renal causes should be ruled out if the substaging system recommended below is to be utilized (*Lees et al, 2005*). Thus, it is imperative to undertake a complete urinalysis and assess the microscopic sediment of a urine sample to ensure evidence of inflammation in the lower tract is absent before assessing the urine protein to creatinine ratio.

Table 3 presents the IRIS sub-staging system based on systemic arterial blood pressure.

The IRIS group recognizes that there is no agreed standard for measuring feline blood pressure. The method used in our practice is the Doppler method which gives readings of systolic pressure only. Cases should not be classified based on measurements taken at a single clinic visit. At least two or more visits should be used to establish their blood pressure status unless significant signs of target organ damage are evident (see above) whereupon specific antihypertensive therapy may be indicated.

TABLE 2 - SUBSTAGING ON URINE PROTEIN TO CREATININE RATIO (UPC)

UPC* value	Interpretation
< 0.2	Non-proteinuric (NP)
0.2 to 0.4	Borderline proteinuric (BP)
> 0.4	Proteinuric (P)

* Calculated using mass units

TABLE 3 - SUBSTAGING ON BLOOD PRESSURE

Risk	Systolic (mm Hg)	Diastolic (mm Hg)	Classification according to evidence of extra-renal complications*
Minimal [N]	< 150	< 95	- Minimal or no risk of end organ damage [N] - Highly unlikely to see evidence of extra-renal damage at this level
Low [L]	150-159	95-99	- Low risk of end organ damage - If no extra-renal complication seen [Lnc] - If evidence of extra-renal complications seen [Lc]
Moderate [M]	160-179	100-119	- Moderate risk of end organ damage - If no extra-renal complications seen [Mnc] - If evidence of extra-renal complications seen [Mc]
High [H]	≥180	≥120	- High risk of end organ damage - If no extra-renal complications seen [Hnc] - If evidence of extra-renal complications seen [Hc]

nc – no extra-renal complications present; c – extra-renal complications detected.
*Extra-renal complications might include:
- left ventricular concentric hypertrophy in the absence of structural/valvular heart problems identified
- ocular abnormalities compatible with damage by high blood pressure such as hyphema or hypertensive retinopathy
- neurological signs - dullness and lethargy, seizures

3 - Dietary therapy in detail

There are many diets available to assist in the management of CKD. These specifically formulated diets are different in several respects from standard diets formulated for feeding adult cats.

- **When dietary changes are introduced in Stages II and III of CKD**, the aim is mainly to address those factors which are likely to contribute to progressive renal injury and further loss of functioning nephrons. In this section the rationale will be reviewed for the manipulation of each element of the diet and published evidence for the efficacy of this treatment in slowing progression, presented.

- **Once late stage III/IV has been reached**, clinical signs of the uremic syndrome are evident and dietary treatment is designed more to improve the quality of life of the patient than to slow disease progression. Section 5 will deal with the approach and the use of renal care diets and supplements to address the problems of the uremic syndrome.

▶ Phosphate restriction and management of secondary renal hyperparathyroidism

Phosphate is freely filtered by the normal kidney but not actively secreted by the tubule. Thus, the amount of phosphate excreted from the body each day is highly dependent on the GFR. Re-absorption of phosphate occurs in the proximal convoluted tubule through a carrier-mediated process (co-transported with sodium ions). The maximum capacity of this system to re-absorb phosphate is influenced by parathyroid hormone (PTH) which reduces phosphate re-absorption and so increases the amount of phosphate excreted in the urine at a given plasma phosphate concentration and a given GFR.

As GFR falls, if dietary phosphate intake remains the same, the daily amount of phosphate excreted in the urine will not match with the daily phosphate intake. Thus, phosphate will start to accumulate in the body. Both intracellular stores and extracellular fluid concentration of phosphate increase. As the plasma phosphate concentration increases, so its rate of excretion will increase until a new steady state is reached at a higher plasma phosphate concentration and higher level of intracellular stores of phosphate. PTH plays a role in this process since increased PTH synthesis and secretion is triggered by a rise in both intracellular stores of phosphate and plasma phosphate concentration. Initially, this adaptive response is helpful as it enhances urinary excretion of phosphate compensating for the effect of the fall in GFR (**Figure 5**).

FIGURE 5 - EFFECTS OF PARATHYROID HORMONE ON CALCIUM HOMEOSTASIS AND THE INVOLVEMENT OF ITS THREE TARGET ORGANS: BONE, KIDNEY AND THE GASTROINTESTINAL TRACT

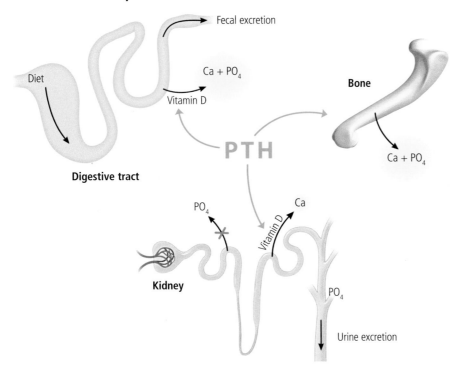

- *Parathyroid hormone (PTH) stimulates calcium and phosphate release from bone into the extracellular fluid (blue in the illustration).*
- *PTH stimulates the kidney to make active vitamin D (1,25 D_3); it inhibits phosphate absorption from the proximal tubule so more phosphate appears in the urine and it increases calcium uptake from the distal tubule, thus conserving calcium.*
- *1,25 D_3 stimulates calcium and phosphate uptake from the small intestine, increasing the proportion of dietary calcium and phosphate that are absorbed.*

Through the action of these hormones, calcium and phosphate homeostasis are achieved by balancing calcium and phosphate intake with urinary excretion of these minerals.

Unfortunately, the adaptive response of increasing PTH secretion to counterbalance the tendency for phosphate retention with loss of functioning nephrons and concomitant fall in GFR is limited by two factors:
1. at least 30% of the filtered load of phosphate has to be re-absorbed in the proximal tubule as part of the reabsorptive process for sodium and hence water
2. as increasing plasma concentrations of PTH are required, the actions of this hormone on bone bring more phosphate from bone stores into the extracellular fluid compartment adding to the problem of hyperphosphatemia.

As the CKD progresses and fewer functioning nephrons remain, secretion of PTH, driven by phosphate retention, becomes counter-productive and so mal-adaptive. Phosphate release from bone adds to the problem by inhibiting renal production of calcitriol and stimulating PTH synthesis and secretion and parathyroid gland growth. In the later stages of CKD (IRIS late stage III and stage IV), calcitriol deficiency (as a result of reduced kidney mass and the inhibitory effects of hyperphosphatemia on calcitriol synthesis) contributes to the problem of hyperparathyroidism in two ways:

- calcitriol inhibits PTH synthesis and secretion by a direct action on the parathyroid gland. This hormone also prevents parathyroid gland hypertrophy
- with a lack of calcitriol, absorption of calcium from the intestine is reduced and hypocalcemia can occur (particularly low ionized calcium) in the more severe stages of CKD. With very high plasma phosphate concentrations, ionized calcium will also decrease due to complexing of calcium with phosphate and other small anions.

The above outline of the pathophysiology of secondary renal hyperparathyroidism is shown schematically in **Figure 6**. Scientific understanding of this process has changed the emphasis from the view that ionized calcium concentration decreases, which were once thought to drive PTH secretion, to recognize that phosphate retention is now central to this process.

That hyperphosphatemia and hyperparathyroidism are important in naturally occurring CKD is clearly evident from published studies (*Barber & Elliott, 1998*). Whether phosphate retention and/or increased parathyroid hormone synthesis and secretion are detrimental to the health and well being of the cat with CKD has been a topic of debate. Evidence from laboratory animal models and from human medicine suggests hyperphosphatemia and hyperparathyroidism are detrimental to the quality of life of the patient and may contribute to progressive renal injury. Direct evidence supporting these conclusions apply to cats is relatively sparse although some data from both an experimental model in the cat (*Ross et al, 1982*) and naturally occurring feline CKD support the conclusions that reduction of phosphate intake to control parathyroid hormone secretion results in:
- reduced mineralization **(Figure 7)** and fibrosis in the remaining functioning kidney tissue (experimental model studies; *Ross et al, 1982*)
- a reduction in all cause mortality in cats with naturally occurring CKD (*Elliott et al, 2000*).

The prospective diet study conducted by *Elliott et al, (2000)* was open label involving cats at stage II and III CKD where the aim was to use phosphate restriction by feeding a renal care diet to con-

FIGURE 6 - PATHOPHYSIOLOGY OF SECONDARY RENAL HYPERPARATHYROIDISM

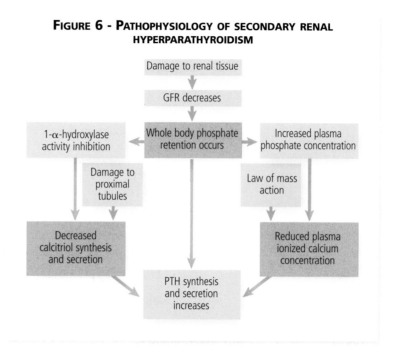

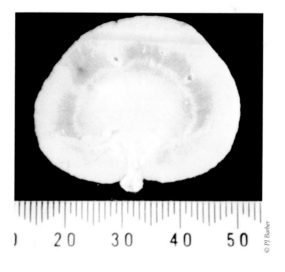

Figure 7 - Renal calcification due to renal hyperparathyroidism in a cat.

A band of calcification can be seen in the inner medulla which was confirmed on histological examinations (scale in mm).

Figure 8 - Radiographic evidence of soft tissue calcification of the vasculature due to hyperparathyroidism in cats with chronic renal failure.

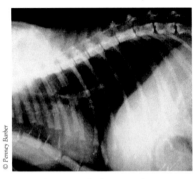

© Penney Barber

A: *Soft tissue calcification of the thoracic aorta in a 20 year old cat with chronic kidney disease (classified as uremic).*

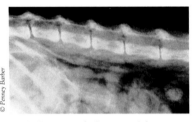

© Penney Barber

B: *Soft tissue calcification of the abdominal aorta and some abdominal vasculature in a 19 year old cat with end stage chronic kidney disease.*

trol plasma PTH and to study the effect this had on survival. The control group were permitted to continue eating their standard maintenance diet after their owners had rejected treatment with the renal care diet. Thus, scientifically the design of this study was not optimal since it was not masked and the control group were self-selecting.

A second study of a renal care diet has been published more recently where the design was a randomized controlled masked clinical trial *(Ross et al, 2006)* and the aim was to determine the benefit of the renal care diet on the time to uremic crises or renal death when fed to cats at stage II and III CKD. The renal care diet tested was compared to a standard maintenance diet that differed in protein, sodium, phosphate and lipid content. The renal care diet contained 0.5% phosphate on an as fed basis (1.2 g/1000 kcal for the dry renal diet, 1.0 g/1000 kcal for the wet renal diet) whereas the maintenance diet contained 0.9 or 1% phosphate on an as fed basis (1.8 g/1000 kcal for the dry maintenance diet, 2.3 g/1000 kcal for the wet maintenance diet). Feeding the renal care diet resulted in a lower plasma phosphate concentration at 12 and 24 months after introduction of the diets although plasma PTH concentrations did not differ significantly. The cats eating the renal care diet suffered significantly fewer uremic crises and there were significantly fewer renal deaths. In both of the above studies, because the renal care diets differed in a number of respects from standard maintenance diets, it is not possible to conclude whether phosphate restriction was responsible for the effect seen but it seems likely to have contributed.

Accumulation of phosphate and calcium in renal tissues will lead to nephrocalcinosis and may contribute to progressive renal injury and these processes are probably ongoing in IRIS stages II and III of CKD. Clearly, in the later stages of CKD (stage IV), extrarenal effects of hyperphosphatemia and hyperparathyroidism are evident with radiographic evidence of renal osteodystrophy and mineralization of soft tissues (**Figure 8**) accompanied by marked parathyroid gland hypertrophy. In human medicine, poor control of phosphate balance in the renal patient on dialysis leads to increased cardiovascular risk as calcium and phosphate accumulate in the vasculature (KDOQI, 2003).

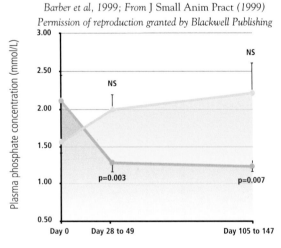

FIGURE 9A - EFFECT OF FEEDING A RENAL CARE DIET TO CATS WITH CKD (STAGES II AND III) ON PLASMA PHOSPHATE CONCENTRATION

Barber et al, 1999; From J Small Anim Pract *(1999)*
Permission of reproduction granted by Blackwell Publishing

Data are mean values from 14 cats (orange) that were fed the renal care diet and 8 cats (blue) maintained on their maintenance diets. Error bars represent 1 SD of the mean. Significant differences compared to day 0 value by a paired t-test are illustrated (NS not significant).

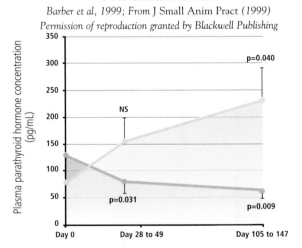

FIGURE 9B - EFFECT OF FEEDING A RENAL CARE DIET TO CATS WITH CKD (STAGES II AND III) ON PLASMA PTH CONCENTRATION

Barber et al, 1999; From J Small Anim Pract *(1999)*
Permission of reproduction granted by Blackwell Publishing

Data are mean values from 14 cats (orange) that were fed the renal care diet and 8 cats (blue) maintained on their maintenance diets. Error bars represent 1 SD of the mean. Significant differences compared to day 0 value by a paired t-test are illustrated (NS not significant).

> Management of secondary renal hyperparathyroidism

From the above discussion of the pathophysiology of hyperphosphatemia and hyperparathyroidism secondary to CKD, the logical way to address these problems is to restrict dietary phosphate intake in the first instance. This can be done by restricting the amount of phosphate in the ration fed and/or adding phosphate binders to reduce phosphate bioavailability in the food that is fed.

Evidence that feeding a commercially formulated renal clinical diet reduces both plasma phosphate concentration and PTH concentrations when fed to cats with naturally occurring CKD has been published (*Barber et al, 1999*; **Figure 9**). The effect on plasma PTH concentration tends to be prolonged with plasma PTH concentrations falling with continued dietary phosphate restriction after the plasma phosphate concentration has stabilized **(Figure 10)**. This probably results from depletion of intracellular stores of phosphate which influence PTH synthesis and secretion. In human medicine, the recommendations regarding control of plasma phosphate concentration have been published based on expert opinion and available clinical research evidence (*KDOQI, 2003*). These guidelines have been adapted by a group of veterinary nephrologists to apply to the cat and have been adopted by the IRIS group as recommendations according to the stage of CKD that is being treated.

- **For stage II CKD**, the post-treatment plasma phosphate concentration should be below 1.45 mmol/L (4.5 mg/dL), but not <0.8 mmol/L (2.5 mg/dL). In our experience, cats where plasma phosphate can be maintained below 1.2 mmol/L (3.72 mg/dL) tend to remain very stable in stage II CKD for prolonged periods of time.
- **For stage III CKD**, the realistic post-treatment target is <1.61 mmol/L (5.0 mg/dL). Intestinal phosphate binders in addition to feeding a diet restricted in phosphate may be necessary to achieve this target in later stage III cases.
- **For stage IV CKD**, the realistic post-treatment plasma phosphate concentration target is 1.93 mmol/L (6.0 mg/dL) and this is unlikely to be achieved with dietary phosphate restriction alone.

FIGURE 10 - EFFECT OF FEEDING A RENAL CARE DIET ON PLASMA PHOSPHATE (BLUE) AND PTH (ORANGE) CONCENTRATIONS IN A CAT WITH CKD

Barber, 1999

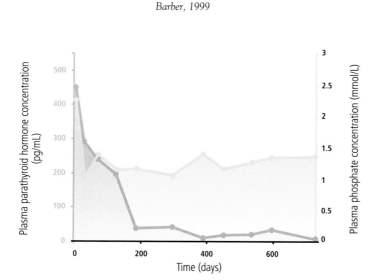

Note that whilst plasma phosphate concentration stabilized very quickly, plasma PTH continued to decrease and finally reached the reference range (2.5 to 20 pg/mL) after almost 400 days of diet therapy.

FIGURE 11 - RELATIONSHIP BETWEEN SURVIVAL TIME AND THE MEAN PLASMA PHOSPHATE CONCENTRATION ACHIEVED IN THE FIRST HALF OF THE SURVIVAL PERIOD

Data re-analyzed from Elliott et al (2000)

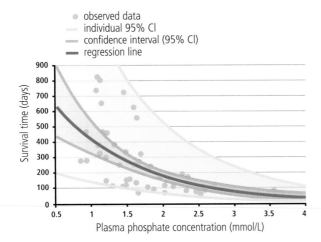

- observed data
- individual 95% CI
- confidence interval (95% CI)
- regression line

Fifty cats were entered into a prospective survival study (Elliott et al, 2000). Blood samples were collected at 2 to 3 month intervals throughout the study. The average plasma phosphate concentration has been calculated for each cat during the first half of their survival period and plotted against their survival time. Linear regression analysis reveals an exponential relationship (R^2 value 0.45).

Unpublished data from our research clinic shows that 55, 90 and 100% of cats presenting in stage II, III and IV CKD respectively have plasma phosphate concentrations above 1.45 mmol/L (4.5 mg/dL) at diagnosis. Re-analysis of the data from the prospective study of the effect of controlling plasma phosphate and PTH on survival of cats with stage II and III CKD (*Elliott et al, 2000*) demonstrated that:

- if the average plasma phosphate concentration was maintained at below 1.45 mmol/L (4.5 mg/dL) for the first half of their survival time (this was achieved in 18 of the 50 cats) their median survival time was 799 (interquartile range 569-1383) days
- for cats where the average plasma phosphate concentration exceeded 1.45 mmol/L (4.5 mg/dL) the median survival time was 283 (interquartile range 193 to 503) days (**Figure 11**).

These data are supportive of the extrapolation of the *KDOQI* (2003) recommendations on the control of plasma phosphate from human to feline medicine. Further prospective studies are necessary which are specifically designed to address the benefit of maintaining plasma phosphate concentrations below 1.45 mmol/L (4.5 mg/dL) in cats with CKD are still required, however, to verify this recommendation.

Adverse effects of restricting phosphate intake are rare. It is recommended that plasma phosphate and calcium (preferably ionized calcium) are measured routinely every 2 to 3 months in cats that have been stabilized on restricted phosphate diets and that hypophosphatemia (plasma phosphate concentration <0.8 mmol/L [2.5 mg/dL]) is avoided. Occasionally, hypercalcemia has been reported (*Barber et al, 1998*). This is a true hypercalcemia since ionized calcium as well as total calcium is outside of the reference range and plasma PTH is below the limit of detection. The underlying cause of the hypercalcemia in these cases is not understood but it appears to result from phosphate restriction since feeding more phosphate in the diet leads to the plasma calcium ion concentration returning to the reference range and the plasma PTH concentration increasing into the measurable range at the same time. Since PTH is important for normal bone turnover it does not seem appropriate to completely suppress PTH secretion in these cases, hence we would recommend feeding more phosphate to these cats. This small proportion of cases clearly do not need the degree of phosphate restriction provided by the commercial diets in order to control PTH and phosphate illustrating the point that any treatment should be tailored to the individual needs of the patient.

▶ Dietary sodium and kidney disease

Sodium is the major determinant of extracellular fluid (ECF) volume and blood pressure being the main ECF cation. Sodium ions are maintained at a stable concentration in ECF and plasma through the osmoreceptor and thirst mechanisms that regulate water balance. Plasma osmolality is maintained at a stable 280 to 290 mOsm/L.

In the normal kidney usually more than 99% of the filtered load of sodium is reabsorbed and returned to the blood stream. The fraction excreted can be reduced considerably under the influence of aldosterone, the salt conserving hormone which acts on the late distal tubule (cortical connecting tubule) to increase sodium reabsorption from this part of the kidney. There is a steep relationship between urinary sodium excretion and systemic arterial blood pressure. Small increases in arterial blood pressure cause a marked increase in sodium excretion in the urine formed by a normal kidney. This occurs through inhibition of aldosterone secretion (reduced activity of the renin-angiotensin system) and through the action of natriuretic factors on the kidney to functionally antagonize aldosterone (e.g. atrial natriuretic peptides, endogenous digitalic like factors).

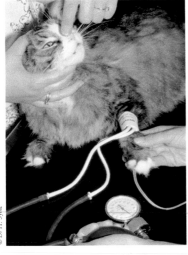

Doppler blood pressure measuring device.

© Dr H. Syme

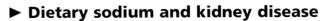

Thus, in cats with normal kidney function, a wide range of sodium intakes can be tolerated without detrimental effects on arterial blood pressure. Indeed, one strategy adopted to reduce the tendency for the formation of uroliths in feline urine is to increase dietary sodium intake. This results in a larger volume of urine being produced and the cats will drink more water to compensate. Hence the urinary calcium and magnesium concentrations are reduced and the tendency for urolith formation also is decreased. Normal cats fed such diets show no tendency for their blood pressures to increase (*Buranakarl et al, 2004; Luckschander et al, 2004*) **(Figure 12)**.

Formulated clinical renal diets tend to have a lower sodium content per calorie than foods designed for healthy cats. The content of the renal diets still provides more than 2 to 4 times the National Research Council (NRC) recommended daily intake of sodium (0.4 to 0.9 mmol/kg/day or 9.2-20.7 mg/kg/day) (*Yu and Morris, 1999*) at around 2 mmol/kg/day (46 mg/kg/day). Standard grocery diets provide between 4 to 6 mmol/kg/day (92-138 mg/kg/day) **(Table 4)**. The rationale for this is that with loss of the number of functioning nephrons, ability to excrete sodium from the body is reduced. If dietary sodium intake remained the same then these cats would be at increased risk of developing hypertension associated with their CKD. There are no controlled studies in the published veterinary literature to demonstrate the benefit of reducing dietary sodium intake on blood pressure in cats with naturally occurring CKD.

In a cross-sectional study of cats presenting at different stages of CKD, we demonstrated that the fractional excretion of sodium increased with decreasing renal function (**Figure 12**; unpublished data taken from cats studied in *Elliott et al, 2003a*). The interpretation of urinary fractional excretion data from an individual case based on a spot urine sample should be made with caution since there appears to be significant intra-animal variability with time (*Adams et al, 1991; Finco et al, 1997*). A 24 hour urine collection would yield more reliable results but is impractical in feline clinical research. In addition, the pattern observed in the data presented in **Figure 13** May well be blurred by the fact these cats were being fed heterogeneous diets. Nevertheless, despite these shortcomings there does appear to be a higher fractional excretion of sodium at the more severe stages of CKD, suggesting an adaptive change of the remaining functioning tubules ensuring more of the filtered load of sodium is excreted from the body. There was no difference in plasma sodium concentrations between the cats at the different stages of CKD in this cross-sectional study although the

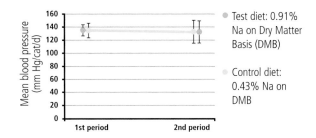

FIGURE 12 - INFLUENCE OF DIETARY SODIUM ON BLOOD PRESSURE IN HEALTHY CATS

(Luckschander et al, 2004)

- Test diet: 0.91% Na on Dry Matter Basis (DMB)
- Control diet: 0.43% Na on DMB

Ten healthy cats were randomly divided into 2 groups. The 1st group was fed the control diet and the 2nd group was fed a diet with a moderately increased sodium content. After a 1-week wash-out period, each group was switched to the opposite diet for 2 weeks.
Follow-up on moderately increased dietary salt intakes failed to show any impact on blood pressure in healthy cats.

FIGURE 13 - BOX AND WHISKER PLOTS SHOWING FRACTIONAL EXCRETION OF SODIUM IN NORMAL CATS AND CATS WITH CKD AT DIAGNOSIS

Data taken from cases included in Elliott et al, 2003a

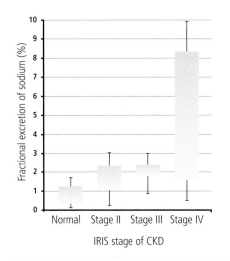

TABLE 4 - SODIUM REQUIREMENT OF ADULT CATS FOR MAINTENANCE
(National Research Council, 2006)

Minimal requirement (mg)			Recommended allowance (mg)			Safe upper limit (g/kg DM)
mg/kg DM	mg/1,000 kcal ME	mg/kg BW [0.67]	mg/kg DM	mg/1,000 kcal ME	mg/kg BW [0.67]	> 15 g
650	160	16	680	170	16.7	

mg/kg DM: amount per kg dry matter, assuming a dietary energy density of 4,000 kcal ME/kg
BW: body weight; the values in mg/BW [0.67] have been calculated for a lean cat with an energy
intake of 100 kcal x BW [0.67]
DM: dry matter
ME: metabolizable energy

plasma chloride ion concentrations were lower in the severe stage (equivalent to IRIS stage IV; *Elliott et al, 2003a*), possibly associated with the development of metabolic acidosis **(see section below)**.

Some cats with naturally occurring CKD do present with severe hypertension. **Figure 14** shows the distribution of blood pressure at initial diagnosis. These data are from 103 consecutive cases of naturally occurring CKD *(Syme et al, 2002a)*. Categorization of these cats according to the IRIS staging system gives the following:
- minimal risk   (<150 mmHg)   – 62/103 or 60%
- mild risk   (150-159 mmHg) – 10/103 or 10%
- moderate risk   (160-179 mmHg) – 15/103 or 14.5%
- severe risk   (>180 mmHg)   – 16/103 or 15.5%

This study was a cross-sectional one and did not address the question as to whether blood pressure rises with time in the feline patient with CKD. If sodium retention occurs over time in the CKD patient due to an inability to excrete the daily quantity of sodium taken in the diet, one might expect blood pressure to increase over time. However, *Syme et al* (2002a) found the plasma creatinine was not a risk factor for high blood pressure – in other words blood pressure did not appear to be higher in cats with more severe CKD. Indeed, the majority of the cats found in the high-risk blood pressure group were in stage II or early stage III CKD according to the IRIS classification system. However, these data are difficult to interpret since cases presenting in stage IV CKD may well have lower blood pressure due to dehydration.

Syme (2003) analyzed data from a population of cats with CKD followed longitudinally to determine whether blood pressure increased from diagnosis of CKD. The inclusion criteria of this retrospective study were carefully defined to avoid extraneous factors that might influence blood pressure other than chronicity of CKD. The study included 55 cats each followed for more than 3 months. Seven of the 55 cats showed an increase in blood pressure to a point where medical treatment was deemed necessary (systolic blood pressure persistently >175 mmHg). Of the 55 cats, 17 showed progression of their CKD (as evidenced by >20% increase in plasma creatinine concentration) over the period of follow-up and 38 cats were classified as non-progressive. The cumulative hazard rate for an increase in blood pressure to a level where treatment was necessary was not significantly different between the progressive and non-progressive groups. Taking the group as a whole, blood pressure increased significantly over time (0.38 [0.2 to 0.56] mmHg/month; P<0.001 by repeated measures linear mixed model approach). These data suggest that blood pressure increases gradually over time in cats with naturally occurring CKD. This phenomenon does not appear to be associated with a decline in kidney function as assessed by repeated measures of plasma creatinine concentrations, although more sensitive measures of kidney function over time (e.g. repeated assessment of glomerular filtration rate) would be necessary to be confident renal function has not changed over time in the non-progressive cases.

Similar findings were reported by *Ross et al* (2006) in their prospective study of the influence of diet on spontaneous CKD. Seven of the 45 cats entered into this study developed hypertension (systolic blood pressure >175 mmHg) and required medical treatment over the 2 year follow-up period despite having normal blood pressure at entry to the study. The overall effect of the renal care diet on the blood pressure of the cats involved in this study was not reported. Nevertheless, the renal care diet did not appear to limit the development of hypertension in this study since 5 of the 7 cats developing hypertension did so despite being fed the renal care diet. The numbers of cats developing hypertension in both these longitudinal studies are too small to conclude anything definitively.

FIGURE 14 - DISTRIBUTION OF SYSTOLIC BLOOD PRESSURE MEASUREMENTS IN 103 CATS WITH CKD

From Syme et al (2002a)

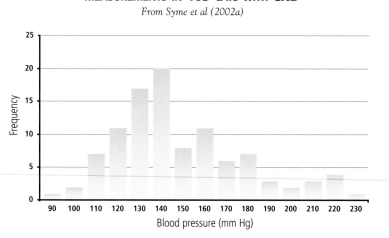

FIGURE 15 - SECONDARY CONSEQUENCES OF SEVERE HYPERTENSION IN CATS WITH NATURALLY OCCURING CHRONIC KIDNEY DISEASE

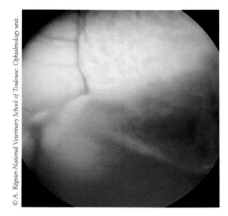

Infundibular retinal detachement and retinal bleeding secondary to systemic arterial hypertension in a cat.

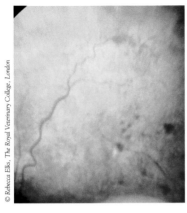

Hypertensive retinopathy in a 15 year old domestic shorthair cat.

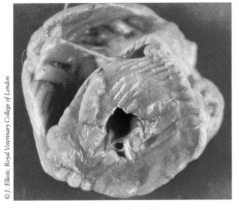

Post-mortem specimen taken from a cat with chronic kidney disease and hypertension demonstrating left ventricular concentric hypertrophy.

From the above theoretical considerations it appears to be logical to restrict sodium intake in cats with naturally occurring CKD. Nevertheless, controlled studies are lacking to determine the benefit of such an intervention on blood pressure control or progressive deterioration in kidney function. *Syme* (2003) reported data on the effect of introduction of a renal care diet on blood pressure in cats with naturally occurring CKD. This was an uncontrolled study as all animals included were fed a standard renal care diet. In addition, this study did not involve cats deemed to be at high risk of end organ damage **(Figure 15)** resulting from high blood pressure as these cases were treated with drugs to control their blood pressure. Systolic blood pressure was measured twice before introduction of the diet and at two time points after the intervention (a minimum of 4 weeks and a maximum of 12 weeks post introduction of the diet) and blood pressure measurements were averaged at the two pre-treatment and two post-treatment time points. Compliance was demonstrated by a significant decline in plasma phosphate concentration (1.55 ± 0.53 mmol/L vs. 1.31 ± 0.32 mmol/L; 4.8 ± 1.64 mg/dl vs. 4.04 ± 0.99 mg/dL; n=28). No changes in plasma sodium or potassium ion concentrations were detected as a result of feeding the renal care diet. Systolic blood pressure did not change in response to introduction of the diet (139 ± 24 mmHg vs. 141 ± 32 mmHg; n=28). The power of the study to detect a 10 mmHg change in systolic blood pressure was calculated to be 90%. A sub-group of cats enrolled in this study had plasma aldosterone and plasma renin activity (PRA) measured before the introduction of the diet and whilst consuming the renal care diet. Plasma aldosterone concentration was higher when the cats were consuming the renal care diet (73 [43, 105] pg/mL vs. 123 [65, 191] pg/mL; pre-diet vs. whilst consuming diet respectively; n=22). Similar changes in PRA were detected following the introduction of the renal care diet (0.53 [0.17, 1.11] vs. 0.75 [0.21, 1.38] ng/mL/h). Both plasma aldosterone concentration and PRA remained in the reference range (derived from aged normal cats fed heterogeneous grocery diets formulated for adult cats) both before and during the renal care diet feeding period.

Results from a study involving the remnant kidney model in cats *(Buranakarl et al, 2004)* suggest that reduction of sodium intake may cause activation of the renin-angiotensin-aldosterone system (RAAS) resulting acutely in a fall in plasma potassium ion concentration and was without beneficial effect on arterial blood pressure. Three diets (with a respective sodium content of: 0.34%, 0.65% and 1.27%) were fed for 7 days sequentially to three groups of cats. The different sodium chloride intake were 50, 100 and 200 mg per kg of body weight (i.e: 0.5 g, 1.4 g and 2.8 g sodium for 1000 kcal), the lowest intake being equivalent to many renal care diets. The three groups of cats involved in this study were:
- control cats with normal kidney function (young adults)

FIGURE 16 - ACTIVATION OF THE RENIN ANGIOTENSIN ALDOSTERONE SYSTEM (RAAS)

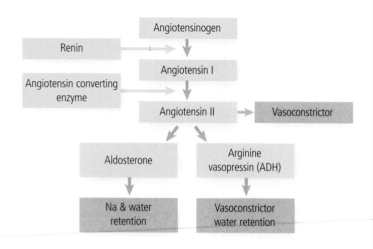

TABLE 5 - OBSERVATIONS THAT HAVE CAST DOUBT ON THE ROUTINE RESTRICTION OF DIETARY SODIUM IN CATS WITH NATURALLY OCCURRING CKD

- Chronic feeding of excess dietary sodium does not lead to hypertension in cats with normal kidney function

- Reduction of sodium intake in experimental models of hypertension (where the RAAS is activated) leads to increased urinary losses of potassium ions and mild hypokalemia with further activation of the RAAS

- The same experimental models of CKD and hypertension tolerate an increase in dietary sodium chloride intake to 200 mg/kg of body weight for 7 days (1.27% sodium diet providing 2.8 g sodium for 1000 kcal) without an increase in blood pressure, a dietary manipulation which inhibited secretion of renin and aldosterone

- Pathological activation of the RAAS can lead to deleterious effects on renal function and exacerbate renal fibrosis in some models of feline kidney disease (*Mathur et al, 2004*) and in other species.

- remnant kidney cats (11/12 nephrectomy model)
- cats which had had a bilateral partial nephrectomy with one kidney wrapped in silk and cellophane (renal wrap model causing severe hypertension) (see *Mathur et al, 2004*). During the feeding trial, these cats received amlodipine besylate treatment to control their blood pressure and prevent development of hypertensive encephalopathy.

Both these models led to renal insufficiency accompanied by elevated arterial blood pressure of the similar order of magnitude as seen in naturally occurring CKD. However, activation of the RAAS (**Figure 16**) with elevated PRA (2 to 6 fold) compared to the control group and markedly elevated aldosterone (4 to 25 fold higher than control cats) was associated with both models (particularly marked in the renal wrap model). Cats with naturally occurring CKD and blood pressures placing them at minimal to moderate risk of end organ damage (up to 175 mmHg) tend to have either normal or suppressed PRAs compared to age-matched control cats fed similar diets. Furthermore, plasma aldosterone concentrations also remain within the reference range and do not differ significantly from age-matched control cats (*Syme et al, 2002b*). Marked activation of the RAAS does occur in unstable naturally occurring CKD patients in stage IV (*Syme, 2003*). Thus, the remnant kidney and renal wrap models of hypertension appear to give rise to significant activation of the RAAS, a finding which is not relevant to naturally occurring CKD at stages II or III with no or only mild to moderate elevations in blood pressure. The relevance of these models to naturally occurring CKD in cats appears to be questionable.

Cats with naturally occurring CKD with marked elevations in arterial blood pressure (systolic pressure >180 mmHg; high risk of target organ damage) tend to have normal or suppressed PRA associated with normal or marginally elevated plasma aldosterone concentrations (*Jensen et al, 1997*; *Syme et al, 2002b*). These cats also tend to have lower plasma potassium ion concentrations at diagnosis and are relatively resistant to the antihypertensive effects of standard doses of angiotensin converting enzyme inhibitors (*Littman, 1994*), both findings suggesting that hypertension in these cases is possibly the result of increased secretion and/or activity of aldosterone but not through activation of the RAAS. It is clear that restriction of sodium chloride intake in these severely hypertensive cats is not sufficient alone to manage their hypertension and pharmacological interventions are required to control blood pressure. Whether dietary sodium restriction helps to achieve control of blood pressure with drugs in these patients has not been studied in feline clinical patients. A clearer understanding of why some cats with naturally occurring CKD develop severe hypertension associated with a high risk of end organ damage remains to be established. Once the reason for this is understood, the role of sodium restriction in managing these patients may become clearer.

In summary, most renal care diets formulated for cats have reduced sodium content compared to standard adult maintenance foods. The logic behind this is that with reduced functional renal mass, maintenance of sodium homeostasis will prove more difficult to achieve and sodium retention could result in increased blood pressure. Hypertension could reduce the quality of life of cats with CKD and lead to further damage to the remaining functioning nephrons and so progressive renal injury. About 20% of cats with naturally occurring CKD do have arterial blood pressures at diagnosis which place them at severe risk of target organ damage (including renal damage) secondary to hypertension. Blood pressure does tend to increase gradually over time in the remaining 80% of cats with CKD where their blood pressure at initial diagnosis does not place them at high risk of target organ damage. However, certain observations have cast doubt on the routine restriction of dietary sodium in cats with naturally occurring CKD (**Table 5**).

Despite these observations, renal care diets, which restrict sodium intake, continue to be routinely used in cats with naturally occurring CKD. Their clinical use does not appear to be associated with worsening of hypokalemia *(Elliott et al, 2000; Ross et al, 2006)* or proteinuria (unpublished data), despite an increase in plasma aldosterone concentration within the physiological range *(Syme, 2003)*. Whether reducing sodium intake is beneficial in limiting the chronic small increase in blood pressure detected over time in cats with naturally occurring CKD remains to be determined by future longitudinal studies, as does their potential benefit in managing severe hypertension in the cat in combination with antihypertensive drug therapy.

▶ Potassium and kidney disease

The cat is somewhat unique in that there appears to be an association between CKD and hypokalemia. Loss of functioning nephrons puts the dog or human patient at increased risk of hyperkalemia. In cats, adaptive changes in the remaining functioning nephrons appear, in some 20 to 30% of cases of CKD, to over compensate and excess loss of potassium in the urine leads to hypokalemia *(DiBartola et al, 1987; Elliott & Barber, 1998)* unless they move into an oliguric stage as part of a uremic crisis. In the face of CKD, hypokalemia also appears to be associated with an increased risk of systemic hypertension *(Syme et al, 2002a)*, possibly also due to the way the kidney responds to loss of functioning nephrons.

Potassium is the major intracellular cation and circulates in plasma at a concentration of around 4 mmol/L. This means measurement of plasma potassium concentration is an indirect assessment of whole body potassium status, particularly as potassium can change its distribution between the cells and ECF, for example in response to acid-base disturbances. Plasma potassium is freely filtered and most of the filtered load is returned to the plasma in the proximal convoluted tubule and the loop of Henle. The cortical connecting tubule is the site of potassium secretion into the tubular fluid **(Figure 17)**. Fractional excretion of potassium will vary depending on various factors **(Table 6)**.

Aldosterone acts on the cortical collecting tubule to increase potassium ion loss in the urine by increasing the number of potassium channels in the apical plasma membrane of the tubular cells through which potassium ions can diffuse. In effect, these potassium ions exchange for sodium ions diffusing from the tubular fluid into the tubular cell through epithelial sodium channels whose synthesis is also under the control of aldosterone. Intracellular potassium is maintained at a high concentration and intracellular sodium is maintained at a low concentration by the action of aldosterone causing the synthesis of basolateral membrane sodium potassium ATPase (pumps) **(Figure 17)**.

Dow and Fettman (1992) hypothesized that potassium depletion may lead to a self-perpetuating cycle of renal damage and further potassium loss. This hypothesis is based on:
- The clinical observation of a strong statistical association between CKD and the occurrence of hypokalemia *(Dow et al, 1989)*.
- Naturally occurring CKD was observed in association with feeding an acidifying diet that was marginally replete in potassium – renal function appeared to improve when the diet was changed and the hypokalemia was corrected *(Dow et al, 1987)*.
- The experimental observation that feeding a diet that was deficient in potassium and supplemented with phosphoric acid (acidifying diet) led to severe hypokalemia and metabolic acidosis accompanied by a decline in glomerular filtration rate *(Dow et al, 1990)*.

FIGURE 17 - CORTICAL COLLECTING TUBULE CELL

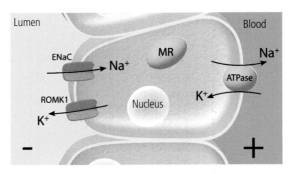

This diagram shows the potassium (ROMK1) and sodium (ENaC) channels on the apical or luminal surface, the mineralocorticoid receptor in the cell cytoplasm (MR) and the Na/K ATPase pump on the basolateral (blood) membrane. This epithelium is negatively charged on the luminal surface.

TABLE 6 – FACTORS INFLUENCING THE FRACTIONAL EXCRETION OF POTASSIUM

- Dietary potassium intake
- Plasma potassium ion concentration (high plasma potassium ion concentration stimulates aldosterone secretion from the adrenal gland)
- Plasma aldosterone concentration
- Number of remaining functioning nephrons and the tubular flow rate
- Acid-base status of the animal (acidosis tends to increase urinary potassium loss)

Kidneys

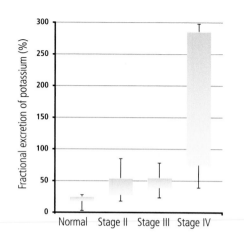

FIGURE 18 - BOX AND WHISKER PLOTS SHOWING FRACTIONAL EXCRETION OF POTASSIUM IN NORMAL CATS AND CATS WITH CKD AT DIAGNOSIS

Data taken from cases included in Elliott et al, 2003a

Support for this hypothesis was provided by demonstration that feeding a similarly formulated diet (marginally replete in potassium but high in protein and acidifying) led to the development of hypokalemia, clinical and laboratory evidence of renal dysfunction and renal lesions in cats over a two-year study period *(DiBartola et al, 1993)*. However, despite a number of small well-controlled and detailed studies, the causal relationship between whole body potassium deficit and progressive renal injury remains to be proven. Whilst it appears possible to induce renal injury by prolonged feeding of acidifying diets marginally replete in potassium, in general it seems most likely that hypokalemia associated with renal disease is mild and occurs as a result, rather than being a major cause of progressive renal disease.

Urinary excretion of potassium (calculated as fractional excretion) increases with increasing severity of renal dysfunction **(Figure 18)**. In some cases, the fractional excretion of potassium can exceed 100%, indicating the capacity of the cortical connecting tubule to up-regulate potassium secretion in adaptation to nephron loss. Hypokalemia is found at all azotemic stages of CKD in our clinical patients with:
- 30% (6 of 20) in stage IV
- 25% (5/20) in stage III
- and 14.3% (3/21) in stage II *(Elliott et al, 2003a)*.

As stated previously, basing the assessment of whole body potassium status solely on plasma potassium concentration may under-estimate the prevalence *(Theisen et al, 1997)*. The higher prevalence at the later stages of CKD is likely to be associated with metabolic acidosis which is more likely to occur at this stage of CKD. In our clinical case-load, the diets consumed by the cats presenting with hypokalemia tend to be standard adult maintenance formulations which are in no way limited in the amount of potassium they supply. Furthermore, hypokalemia in these cases is relatively mild (plasma potassium concentrations usually between 3.0 and 3.4 mmol/L; reference range 3.5 to 5.5 mmol/L) and is not generally associated with overt clinical signs (e.g. severe muscle weakness). Clinical improvements are seen in response to potassium supplementation in these cases, including increased appetite and improved level of activity. However, changes in renal function (as assessed by serial measurements of plasma creatinine concentration) are not seen in response to potassium supplementation alone.

In human medicine, observational studies have shown an inverse relationship between dietary potassium intake and blood pressure in some *(Reed et al, 1985)* but not all studies *(Walsh et al, 2002)*. Randomized controlled clinical trials have shown that potassium supplementation reduces both diastolic and systolic blood pressure in human patients *(Whelton et al, 1997)*. The observation that low plasma potassium concentration increased the risk of hypertension in cats with CKD led us to conduct a randomized controlled clinical trial to determine the effect of potassium supplementation on blood pressure in cats with naturally occurring CKD *(Elliott & Syme, 2003)*. The trial was also designed to determine the benefits on general well-being (as assessed by body weight) and renal function (as assessed by serial plasma creatinine concentration). The supplement used was potassium gluconate at a dose of 2 mEq per cat twice daily as this formulation anecdotally is one of the best tolerated by cats. We chose to evaluate this supplement against corn starch rather than another salt of gluconate. Gluconate is a bicarbonate precursor and might assist in replenishing intracellular stores of potassium by addressing a sub-clinical metabolic acidosis exacerbating potassium loss from the body.

The trial was a prospective, randomized placebo controlled cross-over study with each phase lasting three months. Cases were selected that were in stages II or III CKD that had been on a stable diet for three months prior to enrolment. Cats treated for hypertension were excluded from the study, as were cats with plasma potassium concentrations <3.0 mmol/L. A total of

17 cats were evaluated in this protocol. The plasma potassium concentration (4.35 [4.21, 4.66] vs. 4.16 [3.92, 4.38] mmol/L) and the urine pH (6.08 [5.66, 6.51] vs. 5.63 [5.42, 5.96]) were significantly higher when the cats were taking the potassium supplement indicating at least partial compliance of the cases entered into the study. No beneficial effect of this level of potassium gluconate supplementation was detected on blood pressure or kidney function (as assessed by serial plasma creatinine concentrations and urine protein to creatinine ratio). This study was assessed on the basis of intention to treat. The major reason for owners withdrawing their cats from the study was that their cat would not eat the supplement (potassium gluconate or placebo).

In summary:
- cats with CKD adapt to nephron loss by up-regulating potassium ion excretion. In some cases this can lead to excess urinary potassium loss and hypokalemia
- hypokalemia occurs in about 20% of CKD cases and is found at all stages of this syndrome and clinical benefits are seen from correction of this electrolyte abnormality, particularly when the plasma potassium concentration is less than 3.0 mmol/L
- severe hypokalemia can occur with feeding of acidifying diets which are marginally potassium replete and the feeding of these diets has been associated with the development of renal lesions – this appears to be a relatively uncommon cause of renal damage in cats in the UK
- supplementation of dietary potassium by the addition of potassium gluconate (4 mEq/cat/day) for three months to cats with plasma potassium concentrations of >3.0 mmol/L did not result in any measurable clinical benefit on blood pressure or renal function in cats with naturally occurring stage II and stage III CKD
- ensuring cats with CKD are fed rations which provide potassium in excess of requirements and which are not acidifying should avoid problems of hypokalemic nephropathy in cats. Routine additional supplementation with potassium (over that which is provided in renal care diets) does not appear to be necessary for the majority of cases.

► Dietary management of proteinuria

The intact nephron hypothesis proposed by Hostetter et al, (1981) has shaped research into progression of CKD in the last 20 to 30 years. This hypothesis was based on observations involving experimental rats using surgical reduction of renal mass to mimic the loss of functioning nephrons that occurs in clinical kidney diseases. The observations that with surgical renal mass reduction results in the following adaptations in the remaining functioning nephrons form the basis of the intact nephron hypothesis.

These adaptations to loss of functioning nephrons appear to compensate for the reduction in the number of filtrating nephrons (**Figure 3**). Ultimately, these adaptations are thought of as being mal-adaptive since glomerular hypertension and proteinuria have been shown to lead to glomerulosclerosis and demise of the remaining functioning nephrons, particularly in rat nephrectomy models, where progression is rapid and closely related to the degree of proteinuria.

Similar experimental models can be established using cats. Adaptive changes in feline nephrons following renal mass reduction include glomerular capillary hypertension, associated hyperfiltration and mild proteinuria (*Brown and Brown, 1995*). Functional progression of this feline model to severe end-stage kidney failure is much slower than the rat model and so interventions to slow that progression are more difficult to assess. Proteinuria has been used in the rat model as the hallmark of progressive renal injury, either as a marker of glomerular and/or tubular health or as a mediator of tubular damage.

Hyperfiltration and glomerular capillary hypertension appears to be driven, at least in part, in the surgical reduction models by local activation of the RAAS. In the face of afferent arteriolar vasodilation, this system leads to constriction of the efferent arteriole, glomerular capillary hypertension and exacerbates transglomerular passage of plasma proteins, the most abundant of which is albumin.

Kidneys

INTACT NEPHRON HYPOTHESIS
1. **Hypertrophy** – the remaining nephrons increase in size
2. **Glomerular capillary hypertension** – these nephrons function at a higher glomerular capillary pressure, increasing one of the forces for filtration
3. **Hyperfiltration** – as a result of the increased glomerular capillary pressure the filtration rate per individual nephron increases, partially compensating for the loss of the functional renal mass
4. **Increased** amounts of protein entering the glomerular filtrate and being excreted in the urine (proteinuria)
5. **Increased protein** entering the filtrate is indicative of glomerular hypertension but also overloads the tubular resorptive processes for protein. This stimulates tubular cells to secrete inflammatory and pro-fibrotic mediators into the interstitial compartment, possibly stimulating interstitial fibrosis and inflammation and contributing to progressive renal damage.

FIGURE 19 – PATHOGENESIS OF INTERSTITIAL FIBROSIS

From Remuzzi and Bertani (1998)

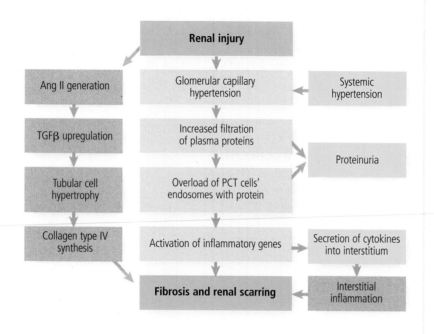

Schematic diagram illustrating how interstitial fibrosis may be triggered by overload of the endosomes of proximal convoluted tubular cells with protein leads to a change in phenotype of these cells stimulating them to secrete cytokines (e.g. MCP-1, RANTES and ET-1) into the interstitial compartment.

Leakage of protein into the glomerular filtrate has been implicated in causing renal pathology. Proteins that transfer across the glomerulus are normally taken back up by the proximal tubule through a process called pinocytosis, whereby the protein molecule is engulfed into a pinocytotic vesicle which buds off from the plasma membrane. This vesicle then fuses with a lysosome inside the cell, containing enzymes which break down the protein to its constituent amino acids which are returned to the plasma. Increasing the traffic through this uptake pathway seem to cause the proximal tubular cell to become overwhelmed with proteins taken up from the filtrate. This stimulates the cell to secrete a number of inflammatory cytokines from its basolateral surface, including endothelin-1, monocyte chemotractant protein-1 (MCP-1) and RANTES, leading to interstitial inflammation and fibrosis as a response to the proteinuria *(Remuzzi & Bertani 1998)* **(Figure 19)**.

Canine and human CKDs tend to be more proteinuric than feline CKDs. For example, in one pathological study, more than 50% of the dogs appear to have primary glomerular pathology *(MacDougall et al, 1986)*. In cats, the pattern of pathology is predominantly interstitial inflammation and fibrosis with glomerulosclerosis occurring as a consequence of the CKD rather than as a primary disease process *(Lucke, 1968)*. Loss of protein in the urine giving rise to urine protein to creatinine ratios greater than 2, usually indicative of primary glomerular pathology, is an uncommon finding in cats with CKD *(Lees et al, 2005)*. Nevertheless, studies have underlined the importance of mild renal proteinuria in cats with CKD as a predictor of all cause mortality *(King et al, 2006; Syme et al, 2006)* and uremic crisis *(Kuwahara et al, 2006)*.

Data from one of these studies *(Syme et al, 2006)* are presented in **Figure 20**. This study involved longitudinal follow-up of 94 cats from initial diagnosis of chronic kidney disease together with 28 aged-matched normal healthy cats and 14 aged cats with hypertension (systolic blood pressure >175 mmHg) but plasma creatinine concentrations within the laboratory reference range. The healthy aged normal cats used in this study defined a reference range for urine protein to creatinine ratio, the upper limit of which was 0.4. Multivariate regression analysis was used to identify risk factors at entry to the study that were associated with proteinuria. The variables identified were plasma creatinine concentration (the higher the creatinine the more likely the cats were to be proteinuric) and blood pressure. Survival analysis was undertaken using Cox's regression analysis. Age, plasma creatinine and proteinuria (assessed by urine protein to creatinine ratio) were significant and independent risk factors associated with reduced survival time. No attempt was made in this study to determine cause of death as this is often difficult to define in aged cats with multiple problems.

The results of this study had been presented in abstract form prior to the full publication and were used to inform the American College of Veterinary Internal Medicine (ACVIM) Consensus Statement on proteinuria *(Lees et al, 2005)*.

It is clear in cats with CKD as the number of functioning nephrons decreases (and plasma creatinine concentration increases) so the proteinuria worsens. This phenomenon has been confirmed by longitudinal studies of progressive CKD in feline patients *(Hardman et al, 2004)*. The increase in UPC with progressive kidney disease probably underestimates the significance of the hyperfiltration that is occurring as progression occurs. This is because as the number of functioning nephrons decreases, so the surface area over which protein can be lost also decreases, tending to offset the amount of protein lost. The ACVIM Consensus statement on proteinuria recommends treatment for renal proteinuria should commence for azotemic cats when UPC exceeds 0.4. It should be accompanied by intensive investigation of factors that might cause or exacerbate proteinuria and extensive monitoring of the proteinuria to determine whether the prescribed treatments are effective.

> Anti-proteinuric therapy

As proteinuria seems to be a significant risk factor for reduced survival in cats with CKD it seems logical that treatments that reduce proteinuria should be prescribed when persistent proteinuria is identified in association with CKD. Specific treatment should be recommended when UPCs >0.4 are documented in an azotemic cat on 2 or more occasions in the absence of evidence of inflammation on urine sediment examination. The anti-proteinuric treatment for which there is greatest evidence of efficacy is ACE inhibitor therapy. Benazepril is authorized for use in the cat in Europe and has been shown to reduce glomerular capillary pressure in a renal reduction model in the cat *(Brown et al, 2001)* and to lower UPC in naturally occurring CKD in a randomized controlled masked clinical trial *(King et al, 2006)*.

Dietary interventions designed to reduce proteinuria include:
• feeding a reduced quantity of high quality protein
• supplementing n-3 polyunsaturated fatty acids to produce a diet enriched in this component relative to n-6 polyunsaturated fatty acids

> Restriction of protein intake

Each time a meal of protein is consumed, renal hemodynamics are altered and glomerular filtration rate increases to an extent which depends on the quantity and nature of the protein fed. Restricting protein intake should limit these feeding related hyperfiltration responses. Much controversy surrounds the efficacy of reducing dietary protein intake as a means of managing proteinuria in both dogs and cats. In experimental models in rats, this approach proved highly successful in limiting proteinuria and slowing the rate of decline of renal function and progression of renal lesions in the renal mass reduction model *(Brenner et al, 1982)* and so was recommended for use in other species. Similar studies were conducted in cats, initially with results suggestive of a beneficial effect of protein restriction on glomerular lesion development in the remnant kidneys *(Adams et al, 1993; 1994)* although the cats fed a reduced amount of protein (2.7 g/kg/day) in these studies also consumed fewer calories (56 calories/kg/day) than the comparator group fed a higher quantity of protein (75 calories/kg/day and 6.8 g protein/kg/day). Furthermore, cats in the low protein group had evidence of protein malnutrition with reduced serum albumin concentration by the end of the study. In a subsequent study addressing the same question, the effect of calorie intake was distinguished from the effect of limiting protein intake and a markedly different pattern of renal lesions resulted with no evidence of a beneficial effect of restricting protein intake *(Finco et al, 1998)*.

> **IRIS** STAGING SYSTEM
> ON PROTEINURIA
> FOR CATS
> - UPCs <0.2 are considered normal,
> - between 0.2 and 0.4 are considered borderline proteinuric
> - >0.4 are considered to be proteinuric

Kidneys

FIGURE 20 - SURVIVAL CURVES DEMONSTRATING THE EFFECT OF URINE PROTEIN TO CREATININE RATIO AND ALL CAUSE MORTALITY IN CATS WITH CKD

Reproduced with permission from Syme et al, (2006); From J Vet Intern Med 2006
Permission of reproduction granted by Blackwell Publishing

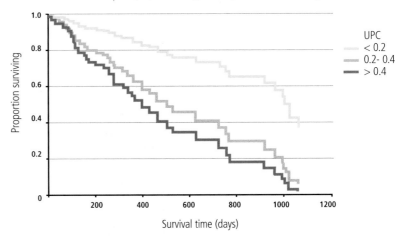

The data have been categorized according the the IRIS classification of non-proteinuric (<0.2); borderline proteinuric (0.2 – 0.4) and proteinuric (>0.4).

One problem with the model used in these two studies is that functional progression (progressive decline in GFR) is not evident over the 12 month post-surgery follow-up period, regardless of the diet that was fed. In the study reported by *Finco et al* (1998), surgical renal reduction caused cats to develop borderline proteinuria (UPC 0.24 to 0.27) whereas pre-surgery they were non-proteinuric (UPC 0.06 to 0.08). No significant difference in UPC was noted between any of the 4 groups of cats used in this study, thus diet had no effect on UPC. Renal histology of the remnant kidneys did, however, reveal a beneficial effect of reducing calorie (but not protein) intake on the severity of renal interstitial (but not glomerular) lesions. Cats in the low calorie intake groups consumed 55 and 58 calories/kg/day and those in the high calorie intake groups consumed 73 and 71 calories/kg/day. Protein consumption was 5.2 and 5.3 g/kg/day in the low protein diet groups and 9 g/kg/day in the high protein diet groups.

The differences between the results of these two studies are striking and are extensively discussed by *Finco et al* (1998), including:
- the source of protein (predominantly animal protein in the *Adams et al*, (1994) study whereas vegetable proteins made a major contribution to the diets fed in the *Finco et al* (1998) study)
- dietary potassium which was lower in the *Adams et al* (1994) study (with cats developing hypokalemia when consuming the high protein diet)
- and dietary lipids which provided a higher proportion of the calories in the *Adams et al* (1994) study.

It is difficult to extrapolate from these two studies recommendations that can be confidently applied to stage II and III cats in terms of diets which will limit proteinuria and therefore possibly slow progressive renal injury by the mechanisms referred to above. Avoidance of diets which deliver a high quantity of animal protein would seem logical. Most renal diets formulated to limit phosphate intake will avoid excessive animal protein in their formulation. Restricting protein intake per se at these stages of kidney failure in the absence of other dietary modifications commonly encountered in renal care diets have not been investigated in the cat. By extrapolation from other species, the cases that are most likely to benefit from the potential renal hemodynamic modifying effects of dietary protein reduction are those with relatively marked proteinuria (UPCs >1.0).

The cats that are most likely to benefit from the potential renal hemodynamic modifying effects of dietary protein reduction are those in stage II and II CKD with relatively marked proteinuria (UPCs >1.0).

> Supplementation of n-3 polyunsaturated fatty acids

Dietary lipids impact a variety of important parameters, including plasma cholesterol concentration and cell membrane structure. In people, hypercholesterolemia and hypertriglyceridemia are important risk factors for cardiovascular and renal disease. This does not appear to be the case in cats, at least partially because they possess only small amounts of low density lipoprotein (LDL) particles, which have been implicated, in their oxidized form, in human cardiovascular and renal disease progression.

However, there is potential in dogs, and possibly cats, for alterations in cell membrane structure through dietary lipid manipulations, specifically by altering the type of polyunsaturated fatty acid (PUFA) present in the diet. The manipulation that has been most well studied in dogs is alteration of the dietary ratio of n-6 PUFA (plant oils) to n-3 PUFA (fish oils). The n-6 and n-3 PUFA are incorporated into cell membrane phospholipids to serve as precursors for eicosanoids of importance in the renal vasculature, such as prostaglandin E_2 and thromboxane A_2. Altering the dietary n-6/n-3 ratio was hypothesized to be a nutritional method for altering renal hemodynamics in an effort to provide renoprotection, limiting the maladaptive hyperfiltration discussed above.

Support for this hypothesis has been provided by studies in dogs using surgical renal reduction as a model of CKD. Feeding a diet markedly enriched in long chain n3-PUFAs lowered glomerular capillary pressure, reduced proteinuria and slowed progres-

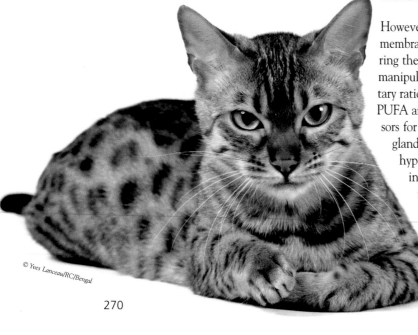

© Yves Lanceau/RC/Bengal

sive decline in GFR seen in this model *(Brown et al, 1998)*. By contrast, feeding a diet markedly enriched in n6-PUFAs raised glomerular capillary pressure, increased proteinuria and caused an accelerated rate of decline in GFR in the same renal reduction model *(Brown et al, 2000)*. These studies used extreme levels of PUFA supplementation but provide the proof of concept for the application of dietary manipulations adopted by some renal care diets where dietary lipids have been manipulated to provide a favorable n6:n3 PUFA ratio, generally achieved by the addition of fish oils. No such data are available in cats, which have somewhat unique PUFA metabolism. Providing long chain n-3 PUFA (eicosapentaenoic acid [EPA] and docosahexaenoic acid [DHA]) is probably even more important in cats than in dogs because the delta 6 desaturase is deficient in feline species. Renal care diets have been produced for cats where dietary lipids have been similarly manipulated.

One such diet has been used in a randomized controlled masked clinical trial in cats with naturally occurring CKD and was shown to be superior to a standardized maintenance diet when fed to cats in stage II and stage III CKD in preventing uremic crises and renal related deaths over a 2 year study *(Ross et al, 2006)*. This positive beneficial effect was not associated with a detectable reduction in UPC in the group receiving the renal care diet. As discussed above, the renal care diet used in this study was also restricted in protein, phosphate and sodium as well as having a different lipid profile when compared to the standard maintenance diet against which it was compared. Further studies are necessary to determine whether n-3 PUFA supplementation to cats is effective in the management of proteinuria in cats and to determine what effect their use has on progression of CKD in the cat.

► Other dietary manipulations designed to slow progressive renal injury

The dietary manipulations discussed above are the main approaches used in the formulation of renal care diets for CKD in cats. There are, however, a number of newer approaches for which a rationale could be put forward based on extrapolation from data derived in other species. Much interest has centered on the phenomenon of endothelial cell dysfunction and the role this plays in progression of CKD in human patients. Endothelial cells line the entire cardiovascular system and they produce a plethora of mediators which in a healthy situation:

- maintain a thromboresistant surface
- produce tonic vasodilation of underlying smooth muscle cells to counter-balance vasoconstrictor mediators produced locally or present in the circulation
- resist leucocyte adhesion and migration in the absence of major inflammatory stimuli
- inhibit inappropriate smooth muscle and fibroblast proliferation

In some disease states, endothelial cell dysfunction is thought to contribute to the chronic and progressive nature of the disease **(Figure 21)**. Examples include congestive heart failure, hypertension, cardiovascular complications that accompany diabetes mellitus and kidney diseases. In human patients and in some experimental models of CKD there is strong evidence to support the role of endothelial cell dysfunction in systemic hypertension, glomerular pathology, progressive proteinuria and tubular interstitial inflammation and fibrosis. In human patients, CKD is a major risk factor for cardiovascular disease and cardiovascular complications are a common cause of mortality.

Endothelial cell dysfunction in renal disease may result from:
- dyslipoproteinemia associated with disturbances in cholesterol metabolism

FIGURE 21 - TYPICAL MICROSCOPIC FEATURES OF FELINE CHRONIC TUBULOINTERSTITIAL NEPHRITIS

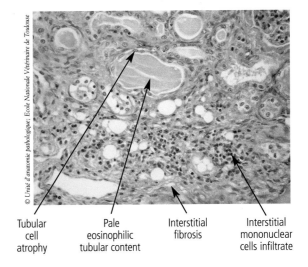

© Unité d'anatomie pathologique; Ecole Nationale Vétérinaire de Toulouse

| Tubular cell atrophy | Pale eosinophilic tubular content | Interstitial fibrosis | Interstitial mononuclear cells infiltrate |

Typical microscopic features of feline chronic tubulointerstitial nephritis are: interstitial mononuclear cells infiltrates, interstitial fibrosis and tubular cell atrophy. Pale eosinophilic tubular content is consistent with concomitant glomerular damage and associated leakage of proteins.

FIGURE 22 - ORIGIN OF FLAVANOLS

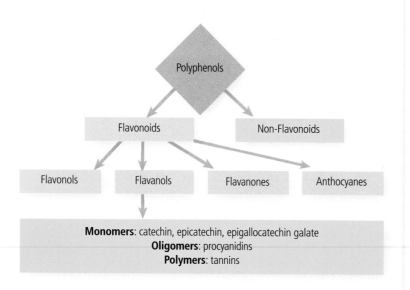

The principal sources of flavanols are cocoa, grapes and especially green tea, where 40 to 50% of flavanols are present as epigallocatechin gallate, which is one of the most active flavanols.

- accumulation of inhibitors of endothelial nitric oxide synthase (principally asymmetric dimethylarginine [ADMA]) as a result of reduced renal excretion of ADMA and reduced catabolism by dimethylarginine dimethylamino-hydrolase as a result of oxidative stress (*Baylis, 2006*)
- reduced renal synthesis of L-arginine, the amino acid substrate required for the synthesis of nitric oxide by the endothelium
- increased oxidative stress which accompanies CKD and results in:
- reduced bioavailability of nitric oxide released from the endothelium
- stimulation of production of profibrotic, promitotic and vasoconstrictor mediators by the endothelium (e.g. endothelin-1, thromboxane A_2 and hydrogen peroxide)

Although there is little published work relating to the relevance of these factors in progressive CKD in cats, some data have been published in abstract form supporting the problems of oxidative stress in naturally occurring feline CKD (*Braun, 2000; personal communication*) and the accumulation of ADMA in stages II, III and IV of CKD (*Jepson et al, 2008*), where the plasma concentration of ADMA correlated closely to the plasma creatinine concentration.

There are a number of dietary therapeutic approaches to correcting endothelial cell dysfunction associated with CKD. None of these approaches have been studied in the cat and their application to cats with CKD remains speculative at present. Possible approaches include:
- supplementation of dietary L-arginine to boost the nitric oxide (NO) system, overcome inhibition induced by ADMA
- dietary supplementation with flavanols (**Figure 22**) which have been shown to boost endothelial production of nitric oxide and improve endothelial cell health generally. By trapping free radicals, flavanols have a protective function in areas of necrosis that occur in the glomeruli following alternating ischemia-reperfusion arising from circulatory disorders that occur in CKD. The anti-hypertensive action of flavanols is due to several combined effects:
- relaxation of smooth muscle fibers (*Duarte et al, 1993; Huang et al, 1998*). This property is beneficial in augmenting the filtration rate in surviving nephrons when functional renal tissue has decreased
- stimulation of endogenous production of NO from arginine (*Chevaux et al, 1999; Duarte et al, 2002*). Nitric oxide is responsible for local vasodilation
- inhibition of angiotensin converting enzyme (ACE), which has an important role in vasoconstriction (*Hara et al, 1987; Cho et al, 1993*)
- use of diets enriched in antioxidants (e.g. vitamin E, vitamin C, taurine, lutein, lycopene, beta-carotene etc.), adressing the balance between pro- and antioxidants and correcting the problem of oxidative stress in CKD.

Effective measures that address the problems of endothelial cell dysfunction are being actively sought for human medicine and some of the approaches listed above have shown promise. Endothelial cell dysfunction clearly complicates both the early stages of CKD as well as the end stage when renal replacement therapy is necessary and cardiovascular complications are a major cause of morbidity and mortality. Whether these measures will prove of benefit in cats with CKD and at what stage of the syndrome they are best applied remains to be determined.

► Role of fiber

Fermentable fiber is a recent addition to the nutritional management of CKD. It is hypothesized that the fermentable fiber provides a source of carbohydrate for gastrointestinal bacteria which consequently utilize blood urea as a source of nitrogen for growth. The increase in bacterial cell mass increases fecal nitrogen excretion and has been suggested to decrease the blood urea nitrogen concentration. However, unlike BUN, the classical uremic toxins (middle-molecules) are too large in molecular size to readily cross membrane barriers. As a consequence, it is highly unlikely that these toxins are reduced by bacterial utilization of ammonia. Fermentable fibers do have beneficial effects for modulating gastrointestinal health in patients with chronic kidney disease.

► Summary

Section 4 of this chapter has dealt with the dietary manipulations commonly used in the production of a renal care diet and discussed them in relation to their application to stage II and early stage III CKD patients. The use of dietary therapy before obvious clinical signs of the uremic syndrome are evident has been somewhat controversial. The main treatment goal in this group of clinical patients is to slow the progression of CKD to stage IV and beyond. The rational basis for dietary modification by:
• limiting phosphate intake
• limiting sodium intake
• supplementing potassium intake
• limiting protein intake and modifying the lipid composition of the diet
has been presented with the evidence for the efficacy of each of these dietary strategies in slowing progressive renal injury reviewed.

Evidence was presented from two prospective trials using renal care diets that clearly indicate that these diets can be beneficial in Stage II and Stage III CKD patients when assessed against the outcome of all cause mortality *(Elliott et al, 2000)* and time to uremic crisis or renal death *(Ross et al, 2006)*. Although these two studies used diets which adopt a combination of the above dietary modifications and it is not possible to conclude precisely which provided the observed benefits, they do provide strong evidence for dietary intervention at stage II and III CKD in the cat.

4 - Treating the uremic patient [Late stage III/stage IV CKD]

In this section use of renal care diets and dietary supplements or additives to treat the uremic syndrome (encountered in late stage III and stage IV CKD) is discussed. The average life expectancy of uremic cats is around 8 months **(Figure 23)**, although cats presenting for the first time suffering from CKD and a uremic crisis often have a much shorter survival time in our experience. In this group of patients the dietary therapeutic goal is to improve the quality of life of the patient rather than trying to address factors which influence progression of CKD.

This group of patients are particularly likely to be unstable and so close attention should be paid to:
1. fluid balance – ensuring these patients receive the right quantity and quality of fluids to ensure they regain an adequate hydration status, particularly if their kidney function has suddenly deteriorated and they face a uremic crisis
2. making any changes to their dietary management slowly and gradually with regular monitoring to ensure they are responding in an appropriate manner.

FIGURE 23 - AVERAGE LIFE EXPECTANCY OF UREMIC CATS
(N = 28 uremic cats)
From Elliott and Barber, 1998

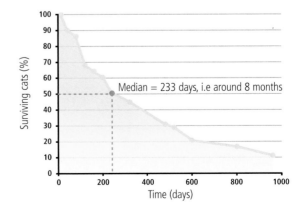

► Management of uremia

Once the nitrogenous waste products reach high levels they start to influence appetite and cause nausea and vomiting due to their irritant effects on mucous membranes. Once plasma urea concentrations exceed 30 mmol/L (84 mg/dL), dietary protein restriction is recommended to limit uremia and counteract these effects on the quality of life of the cat. It is important to ensure adequate calorie intake is maintained in these patients and close monitoring of body weight and body condition score is recommended. The urea to creatinine ratio can be used to factor out the effect of renal dysfunction on plasma urea and to determine the effect of response to dietary protein restriction on nitrogenous waste product formation. Reference ranges have been suggested according to the level of protein intake in dogs but have not been published for cats.

Very high ratios suggest owner noncompliance, dehydration, gastrointestinal bleeding or a hypermetabolic state (e.g. sepsis). Very low values indicate inadequate intake of diet and protein calorie malnutrition, such that body proteins are being used as a source of energy. If this state persists for any length of time, the animal will lose significant amounts of body mass and will exhibit signs of muscle wastage. Such a state can occur if the animal does not find the clinical diet palatable and so consumes inadequate quantities. In these cases, continuing to offer such a diet will be counter-productive and an alternative should be sought. Offering a variety of diets to find the individual animal's preference may well be necessary.

The uremic syndrome is very often accompanied by oral, gastric and intestinal lesions leading to vomiting, diarrhea and anorexia. Incorporation of sodium silico-aluminate into the diet can be very useful to protect the digestive mucosa (Droy et al, 1985).

In the later stages of renal failure (late stage IV) **(Figure 24)**, the animal's voluntary appetite may be inadequate and protein-calorie malnutrition may be unavoidable unless the animal is fed via an enteral feeding device (see chapter 14 about Critical Care). Some owners may find this mode of treatment unacceptable and opt for euthanasia at this point.

In addition to reducing dietary protein to limit the formation of nitrogenous waste products, inclusion of dietary fiber/indigestible polymers that can bind nitrogenous waste and draw these substances into the gastro-intestinal tract is a complementary approach adopted by some renal care diets. Objective data demonstrating the efficacy of such products in lowering plasma urea concentrations and the clinical benefits which ensue following the introduction of such diets to stage IV CKD feline patients have not been published in the peer reviewed literature.

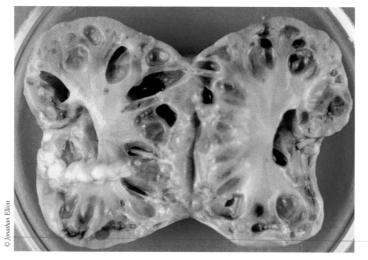

© Jonathan Elliott

Figure 24 - Post-mortem specimen of a kidney taken from a six year old Persian cat euthanazed with end stage kidney disease. *The kidney shows the gross appearance of polycystic kidney disease.*

One practical problem encountered in the later stages of CKD in older cats is constipation. This probably results from a combination of factors:
- dehydration leading to hard dry stools of low volume being formed
- muscle weakness and reduced gastrointestinal motility, exacerbated by hypokalemia
- unwillingness to defecate due to chronic pain on adopting the position to defecate (chronic arthritis; bone pain from renal osteodystrophy)
- use of high doses of intestinal phosphate binders which can cause constipation as an adverse effect
- use of calcium channel blockers as anti-hypertensive agents which may reduce intrinsic gastrointestinal motility.

Constipation can create a vicious cycle of reduced appetite and food intake leading to reduced stimulation of gastrointestinal motility and further problems with potassium balance. Dietary strategies which increase fecal bulk and ensure the production of soft but formed feces and maintain gastrointestinal motility will also be of benefit to the stage IV CKD patient.

► Management of metabolic acidosis and hypokalemia

The stage of CKD at which problems of metabolic acidosis become evident on laboratory testing tends to be late stage III and stage IV. The prevalence of metabolic acidosis was 15% at stage III (3/20) and 52.6% at stage IV (10/19) (*Elliott et al, 2003a*). This suggests that in the earlier stages of CKD, animals are able to excrete the acid ingested in the diet or that small imbalances between intake and excretion are being buffered in the body such that significant changes in plasma bicarbonate concentration are not detectable. The most likely place acid buffering would occur in these animals is in bone, resulting in the leeching of calcium from bone, thus contributing to renal osteodystrophy and increasing the risk of soft tissue mineralization (*Leemann et al, 2003*).

The contribution of metabolic acidosis to bone disease associated with CKD is well recognized in human medicine but has not been studied in cats. Indeed, in a longitudinal study of cats with CKD, the occurrence of metabolic acidosis was not detected on laboratory tests until cases had progressed from stage II to stage III/IV (*Elliott et al, 2003b*). Whether providing alkali supplementation prior to the detection of metabolic acidosis would be beneficial remains to be determined although no effect of three months of potassium gluconate supplementation on bone turnover (assessed by measurement biochemical markers of bone synthesis and degradation) was detectable (*unpublished data*). Clearly, at the later stages of CKD, metabolic acidosis contributes to the uremic syndrome and measures should be taken to treat this problem.

Treatment of metabolic acidosis involves alkali supplementation (**Table 7**). Response to treatment can be monitored by repeated measurements of plasma bicarbonate concentration with the aim to bring this back to the middle of the reference range if possible.

The choice of agent will be dictated by other factors, including palatability when added to the diet, presence of hypertension (when supplementation of sodium should be avoided), presence of hypokalemia (where potassium salts will be chosen) and the presence of hyperphosphatemia, where calcium salts may be considered because of their phosphate binding capabilities (provided hypercalcemia does not become a problem).

Metabolic acidosis tends to exacerbate the likelihood of hypokalemia occurring. Potassium tends to move out of the cells in response to metabolic acidosis and is lost in urine. In addition, reduced food intake and vomiting may accompany metabolic acidosis, both exacerbating loss of potassium ions. As described above, treatment with potassium gluconate or potassium citrate would be appropriate in such circumstances. The use of H_2 blockers, such as famotidine (2.5 mg/cat once daily) can also improve the appetite in these cats by reducing gastric acidity. Hyperacidity occurs in CKD due to hypergastrinemia (*Goldstein et al, 1998*) secondary to reduced renal clearance of gastrin.

► Management of hyperphosphatemia

The degree of dietary phosphate restriction required to attain the post-treatment targets of plasma phosphate concentration will increase with the severity of kidney disease. At late stage III/IV it is unlikely this will be possible by feeding a renal care diet alone and intestinal phosphate binders may be needed to lower the plasma phosphate concentration below the target of 1.9 mmol/L (5.88 mg/dL) (**Table 8**). It is important to recognize that phosphate binders interact with the food and so should be mixed into the food to ensure maximal efficacy. This can create problems in that their addition to the food can reduce the palatability of the diet.

The following are generic recommendations for dosing phosphate binders:
• starting dose 30 to 60 mg/kg should be used
• powered and granular preparations are recommended in preference to liquids and gels which might affect palatability of the diet

FIGURE 25 - RADIOGRAPH OF A CAT WITH SEVERE CKD AND MARKED SECONDARY RENAL HYPERPARATHYROIDISM

Reproduced from Barber (1999)

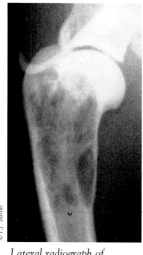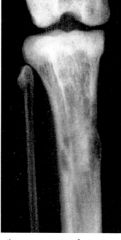

© P.J. Barber

Lateral radiograph of the proximal humerus.

Antero-proximal view of the tibia.

Note the cystic lesions in both long bones leading to thinning of the cortices. This is the same cat shown in Figure 6.

FIGURE 26 - CAUSES OF DEATH IN 50 CATS STUDIED FROM DIAGNOSIS OF STAGE II AND III CKD

- Renal failure
- Cardiovascular disease
- Neoplasia
- Other causes

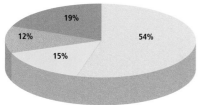

- the binder must be mixed with the diet
- plasma phosphate concentration should be reassessed every 4 weeks
- increase the dose to effect (doubling increments to a maximum tolerable dose), reassess.
- for aluminum containing binders, drug-induced microcytosis, muscular weakness, and encephalopathy are possible
- higher doses of binder will be required if consuming low amounts of clinical renal diets (or a diet which is relatively higher in phosphate) and as the stage of CKD increases
- constipation is a potential complication of higher doses of any of the available intestinal phosphate binding agents
- plasma calcium concentration should be monitored, particularly if using calcium containing phosphate binders to avoid problems of hypercalcemia.

As CKD progresses, achieving control of plasma phosphate concentration and maintaining voluntary consumption of adequate calories per day becomes increasingly difficult. If a gastrostomy tube is placed and food mixed with phosphate binders is administered via this route, control of plasma phosphate is more likely to be achieved. Quality of life is affected by marked hyperphosphatemia as metabolic bone disease becomes more pronounced and radiographically evident (**Figure 25**). Deposition of calcium and phosphate in the vasculature increases the risk of cardiovascular complications of CKD in human patients. Interestingly, the cause of death in cats was attributed to cardiovascular problems in about 20% of cases (**Figure 26**; data from cases presented in *Elliott et al, 2000*).

► Prevention of anorexia and loss of body mass

Sufficient energy needs to be provided to prevent endogenous protein catabolism which will result in malnutrition and exacerbation of azotemia. Cats require 50-60 kcal/kg/day. Energy intake should be individualized to the patient needs based on serial determinations of body weight and body condition score.

Carbohydrate and fat proved the non-protein sources of energy in the diet. Fat provides approximately twice the energy per gram than carbohydrate. Therefore fat increases the energy density of the diet, which allows the patient to obtain its nutritional requirements from a smaller volume of food. A smaller volume of food minimizes gastric distention, which reduces the likelihood of nausea and vomiting.

The efficiency of a renal diet depends upon it being fed exclusively and on a continuing basis. Thus, the diet must be palatable enough to avoid any risk of refusal. Correct energy content and high digestibility of the diet are important to maintain sufficient nutritional intake (**Figure 27**).

At the later stages of CKD, appetite becomes a problem and consumption of sufficient calories to maintain body weight and condition is an issue. Adding flavorings (there are some commercially available products) to the formulated renal care diets can help improve the amount of food consumed. Sometimes warming the food and offering frequent small servings can assist in maintaining daily intake of calories. At the later stages of CKD when voluntary food intake is reduced, it may be necessary to provide additional vitamin supplements, particularly the water soluble vitamins (B and C) may be required since urinary losses of these nutrients may exceed intake. Evidence of vitamin deficiencies associated with CKD have not been documented although many renal care diets are formulated to provide increased amounts of water soluble vitamins when compared to standard maintenance diets.

Conclusion

Diet plays an important role in the management of the feline patient with CKD. It is important to tailor the diet to the needs of the individual patient and to understand the goals in the use of renal care diets at different stages of CKD. These are summarized below.

- **At stages II and III** formulated renal care diets have been shown to be of benefit improving survival and limiting uremic crises. The principles of therapy include:
  - limiting phosphate intake prevents whole body phosphate overload and progressive renal injury induced by nephrocalcinosis
  - reducing protein intake may have some utility to limit hyperfiltration and proteinuria in markedly proteinuric cases (UPC>1.0)
  - the beneficial effects of supplementing n-3 PUFAs remain to be studied in the cat
  - supplementation of potassium is necessary in cats that are hypokalemic but appears to have no detectable benefit in normokalemic cats
  - the benefit of reducing dietary sodium intake on control of blood pressure remains to be determined.

- **At late stage III and stage IV** diet can be used to improve the quality of life of cats entering the uremic phase of CKD. The important principles of therapy at this stage include:
  - limiting protein intake to reduce the build up of nitrogenous waste products, particularly when plasma urea concentration exceeds 30 mmol/L (84 mg/dL). The origin of the protein has to be taken into consideration: very highly digestible protein limits the protein by-products release in the blood
  - the use of dietary components that remain in the gastrointestinal tract and trap urea and other nitrogenous waste products
  - supplementing alkali in the diet to treat metabolic acidosis which contributes to metabolic bone disease, inappetance and malaise
  - supplementing potassium as required to treat hypokalemia which contributes to inappetance, muscle weakness and general malaise
  - further reducing phosphate bioavailability in the diet by the use of intestinal phosphate binding agents to limit the extra-renal effects of hyperphosphatemia and hyperparathyroidism including metabolic bone disease and vascular calcification which affect quality of life.

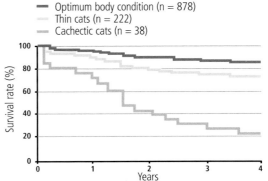

FIGURE 27 - BODY SCORE AND LIFE EXPECTANCY IN CATS

From Doria-Rose & Scarlett, 2000

— Optimum body condition (n = 878)
— Thin cats (n = 222)
— Cachectic cats (n = 38)

TABLE 7 - DIFFERENT FORMS OF ALKALI SUPPLEMENTATION

- Sodium bicarbonate
- Potassium citrate
- Calcium carbonate

Dose rates of 1 to 3 mEq of base per kg per day are usually effective. Animals with a renal tubular acidification defect may require substantially higher dose rates (3 to 9 mEq/kg/day).

TABLE 8 - CURRENTLY AVAILABLE PHOSPHATE BINDING AGENTS

- Aluminium carbonate
- Aluminium hydroxide
- Aluminium oxide
- Calcium carbonate (+/- Chitosan)
- Calcium acetate
- Lanthanum carbonate
- Selevamer hydrochloride

A lanthanum based intestinal phosphate binder has recently been tested for its palatability when mixed with standard maintenance diets of cats *(Schmidt et al, 2006)* and dogs *(Spiecker-Hauser et Schmidt, 2006)*. This product appeared to be acceptable at an inclusion rate of 3g/kg of feed (wet weight) and, in normal cats increased the fecal content of phosphate from 30.7 ± 10.4 mg/day to 66.7 ± 21.0 mg/day. The efficacy and tolerability of this product in cats with advanced CKD remains to be determined.

Frequently asked questions about dietary therapy for feline chronic kidney disease

Q	**A**
Is chronic kidney disease a single disease entity?	No. Chronic kidney disease is a syndrome resulting from the loss of functioning kidney tissue. It is a heterogeneous syndrome. Many disease processes can result in loss of functioning nephrons (infectious, immune-mediated, degenerative, neoplastic, toxicologic, congenital, metabolic, inherited). The response to loss of functioning kidney tissue (whatever the cause) leads to a number of adaptive responses of the remaining function nephrons (intrinsic mechanisms) and of other body systems (extrinsic mechanisms) which can lead to further nephron damage and so are termed mal-adaptive and are common therapeutic targets regardless of the initial underlying cause of the chronic kidney disease.
Why is chronic kidney disease so common in elderly cats?	This is a question, the answer to which is not well understood. The kidney of the cat is adapted to produce a highly concentrated urine enabling this animal to live in climates where water is in short supply. It is possible that the process of generating such a concentrated urine means that nephrons in the cat kidney (of which there are 200,000 per kidney to begin with) 'wear out' over the life-span of the cat. This coupled with other extrinsic insults to the cat's kidneys mean that towards the end of its natural life, less than 25% of its functioning nephrons survive. Hence cats start to show clinical signs of chronic kidney disease as they age. This is certainly not the complete story and is purely a hypothesis since the definitive reason for the high prevalence of chronic kidney disease in the cat is not known.
Why is the composition of urine so variable?	The physiological role of the kidney is to balance dietary intake of substances (water, electrolytes and minerals) with non-renal losses and requirements for growth, lactation and other activities such that homeostasis is achieved. Since dietary and water intake vary from one day to the next, urine composition is highly variable so that body fluid composition remains stable and homeostasis can be achieved.
How do we identify IRIS stage I chronic kidney disease patients if they are not azotemic?	It is important to remember that the IRIS staging system is to be applied only to animals in which a diagnosis of chronic kidney disease has been made. In stage I, kidney disease is not diagnosed based on elevated plasma creatinine so some other clinical/laboratory finding indicates the presence of chronic kidney disease. This may be anatomical abnormality of the kidneys identified on physical examination or imaging confirmed by renal biopsy; a persistent inability to concentrate urine effectively with no evidence of an extra-renal problem as a cause of this renal dysfunction; persistent proteinuria with no evidence of extra-renal disease causing this finding or serial increases in plasma creatinine concentration measured sequentially over time (although these are still within stage I range).
In IRIS stage II chronic kidney disease, there are often no outward clinical signs of chronic kidney disease. Is it necessary to alter the diet at this stage?	The goals in managing the chronic kidney disease patient, if the primary underlying cause of the disease damaging the kidney can not be identified, are to improve the quality of life of the patient and to slow intrinsic progression of the disease towards end stage. There is good evidence from naturally occurring feline chronic kidney disease patients that feeding a specifically formulated renal diet increases long term survival and reduces the occurrence of uremic crises. The patients in these controlled prospective clinical trials were in stage II and early stage III chronic kidney disease according to the IRIS classification where the major benefit of feeding formulated diets is in slowing progressive renal injury.

Q	**A**
Why are clinical diets beneficial to feline patients in stage II chronic kidney disease?	As the clinical trials that have been conducted have involved diets that differ in a number of respects to standard maintenance diets it is not possible to say for certain which dietary manipulation benefits the clinical patient most at which stage of their kidney disease. It is likely that some of the benefit observed is derived from restricting dietary phosphate intake and limiting whole body phosphate overload.
If cats will not eat specifically formulated clinical diets is there anything that can be done?	Restricting phosphate intake is an important part of managing the cat with CKD. It may be possible to achieve appropriate phosphate restriction for the stage of CKD by adding a phosphate binder to a standard maintenance cat food. This is not as desirable as feeding a specially formulated clinical renal diet. The effect of phosphate binding agents can be monitored by measuring plasma phosphate concentration. The dose of phosphate binder to be mixed with the food will depend on the stage of CKD and the phosphate content of the food and should be titrated to effect (starting at 30 to 60 mg/kg) until plasma phosphate concentration is below the target level (i.e. 1.45 mmol/L, 4.5 mg/dL, for stage II).
Should all cats with chronic kidney disease receive an oral potassium supplementation?	No – this is not necessary provided the cat is being fed a non-acidifying diet with an appropriate level of potassium for an adult cat and has a plasma potassium concentration within the laboratory reference range. About 20% of cats with CKD are hypokalemic at diagnosis and require additional potassium by the oral route to correct this. These cats will have an improved appetite and level of activity. These cats can sometimes maintain plasma [K+] within the reference range when fed clinical renal diets, in which case oral supplementation may not need to be continued. Cats with CKD with normal plasma [K+] which are given oral potassium supplementation merely excrete more potassium in their urine to maintain homeostasis.
Why do clinical kidney diets have lower protein content than standard maintenance diets?	Protein restriction was originally thought to benefit the CKD patient by lowering glomerular capillary pressure and so reducing hyperfiltration associated with the intake of food, particularly consumption of a meal high in protein. Whilst this phenomenon clearly slows progressive renal injury in rats with experimental kidney disease, extrapolation to cats and dogs has not proved appropriate. Feeding a diet restricted in protein in stage II and early stage III is usually undertaken because lowering protein enables diets that are restricted in phosphate to be formulated. Clinical benefits of restricting protein are observed in late stage III and stage IV cases where levels of nitrogenous waste products accumulate and restricting protein intake reduces the formation of nitrogenous waste products, thus reducing clinical signs. Such a benefit is not usually evident until the plasma urea concentration approaches 30 mmol/L (87 mg/dL).
What is the most reliable prognostic indicator in a cat with CKD?	CKD in cats tends to progress at very variable rates such that within a given IRIS stage the survival time from diagnosis is highly variable. The most reliable predictor of rapidly progressive CKD is the severity of proteinuria at initial diagnosis. If the UPC is persistently >0.4 (note low level proteinuria is normal for cats with CKD) this is a poor prognostic indicator and survival time is highly likely to be much shorter than cats with UPCs <0.2. Cats with UPCs >0.4 are also likely to benefit most from anti-proteinuric therapies although this remains to be documented by a randomized controlled prospective clinical trial.

Kidneys

References

Adams LG, Polzin DJ, Osborne CA, et al. Comparison of fractional excretion and 24-hour urinary excretion of sodium and potassium in clinically normal cats and cats with induced renal failure. Am J Vet Res 1991; 52: 718-722.

Adams LG, Polzin DJ, Osborne CA, et al. Effects of dietary protein and calorie restriction in clinically normal cats and in cats with surgically induced chronic renal failure. Am J Vet Res 1993; 54: 1653-1662.

Adams LG, Polzin DJ, Osborne CA, et al. Influence of dietary protein/calorie intake on renal morphology and function in cats with 5/6 nephrectomy. Lab Invest 1994; 70: 347-357.

Barber PJ. Parathyroid hormone in the ageing cat. PhD Thesis 1999; University of London.

Barber PJ, Rawlings JM, Markwell PJ, et al. Hypercalcemia in naturally occurring feline chronic renal failure. J Vet Intern Med 1998; 12: 223 (abstract 102).

Barber PJ & Elliott J. Feline chronic renal failure: calcium homeostasis in 80 cases diagnosed between 1992 and 1995. J Small Anim Pract 1998; 39: 108-116.

Barber PJ, Rawlings JM, Markwell PJ, et al. Effect of dietary phosphate restriction on secondary renal hyperparathyroidism in the cat. J Small Anim Pract 1999; 40: 62-70.

Baylis C. Arginine, arginine analogs and nitric oxide production in chronic kidney disease. Nat Clin Pract Nephrol 2006; 2: 209-220.

Biourge V, Devois C, Morice G, et al. Increased dietary NaCl significantly increases urine volume but does not increase urinary calcium oxalate supersaturation in healthy cats. Proc 19th ACVIM, Denver Co, 2001: 866.

Brenner, BM, Meyer TW, Hostetter TH. Dietary protein intake and the progressive nature of kidney disease: the role of hemodynamically mediated glomerular injury in the pathogenesis of progressive glomerular sclerosis in aging, renal ablation and intrinsic renal disease. N Engl J Med 1982; 307: 652-659.

Brown SA, Brown CA. Single-nephron adaptations to partial renal ablation in cats. Am J Physiol 1995; 269: R1002-R1008.

Brown SA, Brown CA, Crowell WA, et al. Beneficial effects of chronic administration of dietary omega-3 polyunsaturated fatty acids in dogs with renal insufficiency. J Lab Clin Med 1998; 13: 447-455.

Brown SA, Brown CA, Crowell WA, et al. Effects of dietary polyunsaturated fatty acid supplementation in early renal insufficiency in dogs. J Lab Clin Med 2000; 135: 275-286.

Brown SA, Brown CA, Jacobs G, et al. Effects of the angiotensin converting enzyme inhibitor benazepril in cats with induced renal insufficiency. Am J Vet Res 2001; 62: 375-383.

Buranakarl C, Mathur S, Brown SA. Effects of dietary sodium chloride intake on renal function and blood pressure in cats with normal and reduced renal function. Am J Vet Res 2004; 65: 620-627.

Burger I, Anderson RS, Holme DW. Nutritional factors affecting water balance in dog and cat. In: Anderson RS (ed). Nutrition of the Cat and Dog. Pergamon Press, Oxford 1980: 145-156.

Chevaux KA, Schmitz HH, Romanczyk LJ. Products containing polyphenol(s) and L-arginine to stimulate nitric oxide production. PCT/US99/05545; WO 99/45797, 1999.

Cho YJ, An BJ, Choi C. Inhibition effect against angiotensin converting enzyme of flavanols isolated from Korean green tea. Korean J Food Sci Technol 1993; 25: 238-242.

DiBartola SP, Rutgers HC, Zack PM, et al. Clinicopathologic findings associated with chronic renal disease in cats: 74 cases (1973-1984). J Am Vet Med Assoc 1987; 190: 1196-1202.

DiBartola, SP, Buffington CA., Chew DJ, et al. Development of chronic renal disease in cats fed a commercial diet. J Am Vet Med Assoc 1993; 202: 744-751.

Doria-Rose VP, Scarlett JM. Mortality rates and causes of death among emaciated cats. J Am Vet Med Assoc 2000; 216: 347-351.

Dow SW, Fettman SJ, LeCouteur RA, et al. Potassium depletion in cats: renal and dietary influences. J Am Vet Med Assoc 1987; 191: 1569-1575.

Dow SW, Fettman MJ, Smith KR, et al. Effects of dietary acidification and potassium depletion on acid-base balance, mineral metabolism and renal function in adult cats. J Nutr 1990; 120: 569-578.

Dow SW, Fettman MJ. Chronic renal disease and potassium depletion in cats. Semin Vet Med Surg (Small Anim) 1992; 7: 198-201.

Dow SW, Fettman MJ, Curtis CR, et al. Hypokalemia in cats: 136 cases (1984-1987). J Am Vet Med Assoc 1989; 194: 1604-1609.

Droy M.T, Drouet Y, Géraud G, et al. La filance: nouvelle approche de l'agression intestinale et de sa thérapeutique. Gastroenterol Clin Biol 1985; 9: 119-121.

Duarte J, Perez Vizcaino F et al. Vasodilatory effects of flavonoids in rat smooth muscle. Structure-activity relationships. Gen Pharmacol 1993; 24: 857-862.

Duarte J, Jimenez R, O'Valle F et al - Protective effects of the flavonoid quercetin in chronic nitric oxide deficients rats. J Hyperten 2002; 20: 1843-1854.

Elliott J, Barber PJ. Feline chronic renal failure: clinical findings in 80 cases diagnosed between 1992 and 1995. J Small Anim Pract 1998; 39: 78-85.

Elliott J, Syme HM. Response of cats with chronic renal failure to dietary potassium supplementation. J Vet Intern Med 2003; 17: 418 (abstract 156).

Elliott J, Rawlings JM, Markwell PJ, et al. Survival of cats with naturally occurring renal failure: effect of conventional dietary management. J Small Anim Pract 2000; 41: 235-242.

Elliott J, Syme HM, Reubens E, et al. Assessment of acid-base status of cats with naturally occurring chronic renal failure. J Small Anim Pract 2003a; 44: 65-70.

Elliott J, Syme HM, Markwell PJ. Acid base balance of cats with naturally occurring chronic renal failure: effect of deterioration in renal function. J Small Anim Pract 2003b; 44: 261-268.

Finco DR, Brown SA, Barsanti JA, et al. Reliability of using random urine samples for 'spot' determination of fractional excretion of electrolytes in cats. Am J Vet Res 1997; 58: 1184-1187.

Finco DR, Brown SA, Brown CA, et al. Protein and calorie effects on progression of induced chronic renal failure in cats. Am J Vet Res 1998; 59: 575-582.

Goldstein RE, Marks SL, Kass PH, et al. Gastrin concentration in plasma of cats with chronic renal failure. J Am Vet Med Assoc 1998; 213: 826-828.

Hara Y, Matsuzaki T, Suzuki T et al. Angiotensin-I converting enzyme inhibiting activity of tea components. Nippon Nogeikagaku Kaishi 1987; 61, 803.

Hardman R, Cariese S, Syme HM, et al. Effect of deterioration in renal function on urine protein excretion in cats with chronic renal failure, in Proceedings. British Small Animal Veterinary Association Congress 2004; Birmingham.

Hostetter TH, Olsen JL, Rennke HG, et al. Hyperfiltration in remnant nephrons: a potentially adverse response to renal ablation. Am J Physiol 1981; 241: F85-F93.

Huang, Yu, Zhang A, Lau CW et al. Vaso-relaxant effects of purified green tea epicatechin derivatives in rat mesenteric artery. Life Sciences 1998; 63 (4):275-283.

Jensen J, Henik RA, Brownfield M, et al. Plasma renin activity and angiotensin I and aldosterone concentrations in cats with hypertension associated with chronic renal disease. Am J Vet Res 1997; 58: 535-540.

Jepson RE, Elliott J, Syme HM. Evaluation of plasma asymmetric dimethylarginine (adma), symmetric dimethylarginine (sdma) and l-arginine in cats with renal disease. J Vet Intern Med 2008; 22: 317-324.

Jepson RE, Syme HM, Vallance C, et al. Proteinuria, albuminuria, creatinine concentration and urine specific gravity as prospective predictors for the development of azotemia in cats. J Vet Intern Med 2007a; abstract submitted for presentation at ACVIM forum 2007.

Jepson RE, Elliott J, Brodbelt D, et al. Evaluation of the effects of control of systolic blood pressure on survival in cats with systemic hypertension. J Vet Intern Med 2007b; 3:402-409.

Kidney Disease Outcomes Quality Initiative (KDOQI). Clinical practice guidelines for bone metabolism and disease in chronic kidney disease. Am J Kidney Dis 2003; 42: Suppl 3: S1-S201.

King JN, Gunn-Moore DA, Tasker S, et al. Benazepril in renal insufficiency in cats study group: tolerability and efficacy of benazepril in cats with chronic kidney disease. J Vet Intern Med 2006; 20:1054-1064.

Kuwahara Y, Ohba Y, Kitih K, et al. Association of laboratory data and death within one month in cats with chronic renal failure. J Small Anim Pract 2006; 47: 446-450.

Leemann J, Bushinsky DA, Hamm LL. Bone buffering of acid and base in humans. Am J Physiol 2003; 285: F811-F832.

Lees GE, Brown SA, Elliott J, et al. Assessment and Management of Proteinuria in Dogs and Cats; 2004 ACVIM Forum Consensus Statement (Small Animal). J Vet Intern Med 2005; 19(3): 377-385.

Le Garreres A, Laroute V, De La Farge F, et al. Disposition of plasma creatinine in non-azotaemic and moderately azotaemic cats. J Feline Med Surg 2007; 9: 89-96.

Littman M. Spontaneous systemic hypertension in 24 cats. J Vet Intern Med 1994; 8: 79-86.

Lucke VM. Renal disease in the domestic cat. J Pathol Bacteriol 1968; 95: 67-91.

Luckschander N, Iben C, Hosgood G, et al. Dietary NaCl does not affect blood pressure in healthy cats. J Vet Intern Med 2004; 18: 463-467.

Lulich JP, Osborne CA, O'Brien TD, et al. Feline renal failure: questions, answers, questions. Compendium on Continuing Education for the Practising Veterinarian 1992; 14:127-152.

MacDougall DF, Cook T, Steward AP, et al. Canine chronic renal disease: prevalence and types of glomerulonephritis in the dog. Kidney Int 1986; 29: 1144-1151.

Mathur S, Brown CA, Dietrich UM, et al. Evaluation of a technique of inducing hypertensive renal insufficiency in cats. Am J Vet Res 2004; 65: 1006-1013.

Reed D, McGee D, Yano K, et al. Diet, blood pressure and multicolinearity. Hypertension 1985; 7: 405-410.

Remuzzi G, Bertani T. Pathophysiology of progressive nephropathies. N Engl J Med 1998; 339: 1448-1456.

Ross LA, Finco DR, Crowell WA, et al. Effect of dietary phosphorus restriction on the kidneys of cats with reduced renal mass. Am J Vet Res 1982;43:1023-1026.

Ross SJ, Osborne CA, Kirk CA, Lowry, et al. Clinical evaluation of dietary modification for treatment of spontaneous chronic kidney disease in cats. J Am Vet Med Assoc 2006; 229: 949-957.

Schmidt B, Delport P, Spiecker-Hauser U. Bay 78-1887, a novel lanthanum-based phosphore binder, decreases intestinal phosphorus absorption in cats. J Vet Pharmacol Ther 2006;29:206-7

Spiecker-Hauser U, Schmidt B. Dose-dependent effect of BAY 78-1887, a novel lanthanum-based phosphore binder, on intestinal phosphorus absorption in dogs. J Vet Pharmacol Ther 2006;29:207-8.

Syme HM. Studies of the epidemiology and aetiology of hypertension in the cat. PhD thesis 2003; University of London.

Syme HM, Barber PJ, Rawlings JM, et al. Incidence of hypertension in cats with naturally occurring chronic renal failure. J Am Vet Med Assoc 2002a; 220: 1799-1804.

Syme HM, Markwell PJ, Elliott J. Aldosterone and plasma renin activity in cats with hypertension and/or chronic renal failure. J Vet Int Med 2002b; 16: 354. (Abstract 109).

Syme HM, Markwell PJ, Pfeiffer DU, et al. Survival of cats with naturally occurring chronic renal failure is related to severity of proteinuria. J Vet Intern Med 2006; 20: 528-35.

Theisen SK, DiBartola SP, Radin J, et al. Muscle potassium and potassium gluconate supplementation in normokalaemic cats with naturally occurring chronic renal failure. J Vet Intern Med 1997; 11: 212-217.

Walsh CR, Larson MG, Leip EP, et al. Serum potassium and risk of cardiovascular disease: the Framingham heart study. Archives Internal Medicine 2002; 162: 1007-1012.

Whelton PK, He J, Cutler JA, et al. Effects of oral potassium on blood pressure. Meta-analysis of randomised controlled clinical trials. J Am Vet Med Assoc 1997; 227: 1624-1632.

Yu S, Morris JG. Sodium requirements of adult cats based on plasma aldosterone concentrations. J Nutr 1999; 129: 419-423.

Focus on:

Phosphorus

Etymologically speaking, the word phosphorus means 'light-bringing.' It was discovered in 1669 by a German alchemist, Hennig Brandt. By evaporating urine and calcifying the residue, he obtained phosphorus in gas form that shone in the dark.

In the form of phosphates, phosphorus enters into the composition of bone. Eighty-six percent of the phosphorus in the organism is stored in the structure of the skeleton.

Phosphorus is also incorporated into large molecules such as DNA, RNA and membrane phospholipids. In addition, it is an active constituent of the adenosine triphosphate molecule (ATP), which stores the energy living organisms need to function properly.

Following the reduction of the glomerular filtration rate (GFR), phosphorus accumulates in the organism that responds by increasing the secretion of parathyroid hormone (PTH). This response initially helps maintain the phosphorus within normal thresholds, but also leads to the release of phosphate and calcium from bone reserves.

In time, even this compensatory response is not enough to restore homeostasis. Phosphorus and calcium accumulate, leading to the mineralization of soft tissue (kidney, heart). In the kidney, this phenomenon accelerates the loss of functional nephrons.

While it is vital to limit the phosphorus content in the food, the difficulty lies in the necessity of finding raw ingredients that are low in phosphorus. Animal protein sources traditionally used in dog food are fairly high in phosphorus. For example, there is 1.6-2.5% phosphorus on a a dry matter basis in dehydrated poultry proteins. This level is dependent on the overall content of remaining mineral matter after sieving. Vegetable protein sources that are lower in phosphate concentration (wheat or corn gluten, soy protein isolate hydrolysate) are an interesting alternative

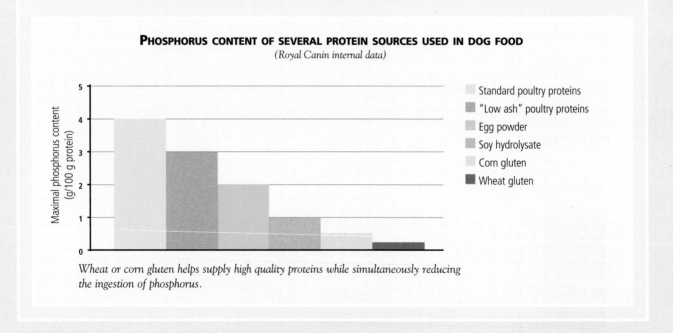

PHOSPHORUS CONTENT OF SEVERAL PROTEIN SOURCES USED IN DOG FOOD

(Royal Canin internal data)

- Standard poultry proteins
- "Low ash" poultry proteins
- Egg powder
- Soy hydrolysate
- Corn gluten
- Wheat gluten

Wheat or corn gluten helps supply high quality proteins while simultaneously reducing the ingestion of phosphorus.

References

Brown SA, Brown CA, Crowell WA, et al. Effects of dietary polyunsaturated fatty acid supplementation in early renal insufficiency in dogs. J Lab Clin Med 2000; 135: 275-286.

Ross SJ, Osborne CA, Kirk Ca, et al. Clinical evaluation of dietary modification for treatment of spontaneous chronic kidney disease in cats. J Am Vet Med Assoc 2006; 229: 949-957.

Key points

Treatment and prevention of chronic kidney disease in cats

Diet composition plays an important role in maintaining homeostasis in cats suffering from chronic kidney disease (CKD). The recommendations with respect to nutritional treatment must be tailored to the patient, based on the clinical and laboratory results. CKD is a progressive disease and so examinations must be conducted regularly if treatment is to be efficient.

The priority dietary modifications have the following objectives:
- combating against anorexia and maintaining sufficient energy consumption
- preventing secondary renal hyperparathyroidism by controlling hyperphosphatemia
- limiting azotemia and/or uremia
- preventing hypokalemia
- combating the risk of metabolic acidosis
- strengthening the antioxidant defenses

Combating anorexia and maintaining sufficient energy consumption

The palatability of the food is a key factor in stimulating food consumption in cats with CKD and promoting observance of the nutritional treatment.

A high-energy food permits the volume of the meal to be reduced, which facilitates the feeding of animals whose appetites are affected by the disease.

Preventing secondary renal hyperparathyroidism by controlling hyperphosphatemia

The aim is to limit the phosphorus level of foods to 0.7-1.0 g/1000 kcal (around 0.3-0.4% of a dry food of 4000 kcal/kg). This restriction helps double the life expectancy of cats with renal insufficiency (*Ross et al., 2005*). If such a low level does not stabilize the phosphatemia at the desired level **(Figure 1)**, the use of phosphorus binders must be considered.

Limiting azotemia and/or uremia

When CKD leads to uremia, it is recommended to reduce the protein intake to prevent the uremia altering the cat's well being to too great a degree. Measurement of the protein/creatinine ratio in the urine is helpful to appreciate the response to protein restriction (reduced production of nitrogenous waste).

It is also important to provide the cat suffering from renal insufficiency with long-chain omega-3 polyunsaturated fatty acids (eicosapentaenoic acid [EPA] and docosahexaenoic acid [DHA]). In dogs with CKD, the administration of a diet with a high-fish oil content slows down the deterioration of GFR (*Brown et al., 2000*).

Preventing metabolic acidosis and hypokalemia

Metabolic acidosis requires oral alkaline treatment. Metabolic acidosis increases the risk of hypokalemia: potassium gluconate or potassium citrate treatment is therefore indicated.

Preventing metabolic acidosis and hypokalemia in cats with CKD entails avoiding acidifying foods and make sure the potassium intake exceeds the requirement. The systematic prescription of potassium supplements will generally be redundant if a food tailored to the needs of the kidneys is used.

Strengthening the antioxidant defenses

Enriching the levels of vitamin E, vitamin C, taurine, lutein, lycopene, beta-carotene, etc. in the food helps limit the oxidative stress that aggravates CKD lesions.

The nutritional diet is the cornerstone in the treatment of renal insufficiency. In cats, it has been proven to contribute to a significant increase in life expectancy by slowing down the progression of the kidney disease.

FIGURE 1 - THERAPY BASED ON THE PLASMA PHOSPHATE CONCENTRATION MEASUREMENT

From F. Hebert, 2008

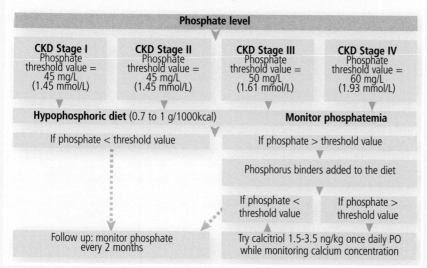

FLUTD

**Doreen
M. HOUSTON**
DVM, DVSc,
Dipl. ACVIM

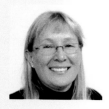

Denise A. ELLIOTT
BVSc (Hons),
PhD, Dipl. ACVIM,
Dipl. ACVN

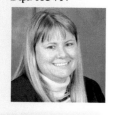

Nutritional management of feline lower urinary tract disorders

1. Epidemiology **287**

2. Etiology **287**

3. Pathophysiology **289**

4. Diagnosis **290**

5. Specific diseases **295**

Conclusion **312**

Frequently asked questions 313

References 314

Royal Canin nutritional information 318

FLUTD

Nutritional management of feline lower urinary tract disorders

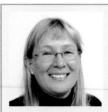

Doreen M. HOUSTON
DVM, DVSc, Dipl. ACVIM

Dr. Houston graduated from the Ontario Veterinary College in 1980, spent 4 years in private practice in Thunder Bay, Ontario and then returned to the OVC for further education (Internship, Residency and DVSc in Internal Medicine). She became a Board Certified Diplomate of the American College of Veterinary Internal Medicine (ACVIM) in 1991. Doreen joined the Western College of Veterinary Medicine at the University of Saskatchewan in 1990 and climbed the ranks to Full Professor in 1995. During her tenure in academia, Doreen received numerous teaching awards. In July 1996, Doreen left academia to become part of the team at Veterinary Medi-Cal (Royal Canin) Diets in Guelph, Ontario. She is currently the Clinical Trial Research Director for Medi-Cal Royal Canin Veterinary Diets in Canada. Dr. Houston is the author of several published papers, book chapters and a textbook.

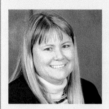

Denise A. ELLIOTT
BVSc (Hons), PhD, Dipl. ACVIM, Dipl. ACVN

Denise Elliott graduated from the University of Melbourne with a Bachelor in Veterinary Science with Honors in 1991. After completing an internship in Small Animal Internal Medicine and Surgery at the University of Pennsylvania, Denise moved to the University of California-Davis where she completed a residency in Small Animal Internal Medicine, a fellowship in Renal Medicine and Hemodialysis, and a residency in Small Animal Clinical Nutrition. Denise received board certification with the American College of Veterinary Internal Medicine in 1996 and with the American College of Veterinary Nutrition in 2001. The University of California-Davis awarded a PhD in Nutrition in 2001 for her work on Multifrequency Bioelectrical Impedance Analysis in Healthy Cats and Dogs. Denise is currently the Director of Scientific Affairs for Royal Canin USA.

Feline lower urinary tract disease (FLUTD) refers to a heterogeneous group of disorders all characterized by similar clinical signs including hematuria (macroscopic and microscopic), dysuria, stranguria, pollakiuria, inappropriate urination (periuria or signs of irritative voiding outside of the litter box), and partial or complete urethral obstruction *(Kruger et al, 1991; Osborne et al, 1996a).*

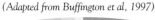

FIGURE 1 - CONDITIONS RESPONSIBLE FOR THE CLINICAL SIGNS OF NON-OBSTRUCTIVE FELINE LOWER URINARY TRACT DISEASE IN CATS

(Adapted from Buffington et al, 1997)

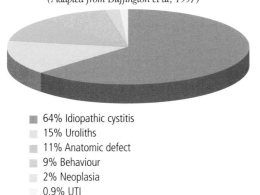

- 64% Idiopathic cystitis
- 15% Uroliths
- 11% Anatomic defect
- 9% Behaviour
- 2% Neoplasia
- 0.9% UTI

FIGURE 2 - CONDITIONS RESPONSIBLE FOR THE CLINICAL SIGNS OF LOWER URINARY TRACT DISEASE IN EUROPEAN CATS

(Adapted from Gerber et al, 2005)

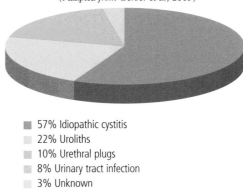

- 57% Idiopathic cystitis
- 22% Uroliths
- 10% Urethral plugs
- 8% Urinary tract infection
- 3% Unknown

1 - Epidemiology

Incidence, prevalence and proportional morbidity rate are all terms used to describe the frequency of disease.

- **The incidence** rate of FLUTD is defined as the number of new cases of FLUTD occurring in the population during a defined time interval (often annual). The incidence of disease is useful to epidemiologists because it is used as a measure of the risk of disease. The incidence rate of FLUTD has been estimated at approximately 0.85% in the USA *(Lawler et al, 1985)*. In the United Kingdom, the incidence rate was estimated at 0.34 to 0.64% *(Fennell, 1975; Walker et al, 1977; Willeberg, 1984)*.
- **The prevalence** of FLUTD is defined as the total number of pets with FLUTD in the population at a specific time. Prevalence differs from incidence in that it does not convey information about risk.
- The ratio of FLUTD cases to all cases seen in a clinic or hospital in a given time period is the **proportional morbidity rate** (PMR). The PMR of FLUTD in North America has been estimated at 1.5-8% *(Bartges, 1997; Lund et al, 1999; Lekcharoensuk et al, 2001a)*.

2 - Etiology

Worldwide, idiopathic cystitis is by far the most common cause of FLUTD reported in male and female cats *(Kruger et al, 1991; Buffington et al, 1997; Osborne et al, 2000; Lekcharoensuk et al; 2001a; Gerber et al, 2005)* **(Figures 1, 2, 3)**.

Urolithiasis is the second leading cause of FLUTD. Uroliths can form anywhere in the urinary tract but the vast majority in cats occur in the bladder *(Cannon et al, 2007)*. The majority of uroliths in the bladder are composed of magnesium ammonium phosphate (struvite) or calcium oxalate. Conversely, nephroliths are typically composed of calcium oxalate *(Lulich et al, 1994)*.

The prevalence of struvite and calcium oxalate uroliths in cats has changed over the last 20 years **(Table 1)**. Struvite uroliths analyzed at two laboratories in the USA performing quantitative analysis far outnumbered calcium oxalate uroliths before the late 1980s *(Cannon et al, 2007)*. Between 1984 and 1995, the proportion of calcium oxalate uroliths submitted to the University of Minnesota Urolith Center increased from 2% to 40% *(Osborne et al, 1996b)*. By the mid 1990's, struvite urolith submissions began to decline and calcium oxalate became the number one sub-

FIGURE 3 - FREQUENCY OF DISORDERS IN MALE AND FEMALE CATS IN THE UNITED STATES WITH SIGNS OF FLUTD

(Adapted from Osborne et al, 2000)

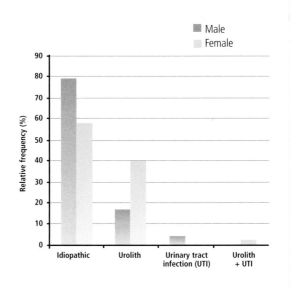

Year	1984	1986	1989	1990	1993	1995	1997-98	2001	2002	2003	2004	2005
TABLE 1 - CHANGE IN STRUVITE AND CALCIUM OXALATE UROLITH SUBMISSIONS IN THE USA OVER THE LAST TWO DECADES *(Adapted from Osborne et al, 1986; 1992a; 1995a,b; 2000; Forrester, 2006; Cannon et al, 2007)*												
Struvite (%)	88-90	85	70-80	65	54	50	42	34	40	42.5	44.9	48
Calcium oxalate (%)	2.4	3	10.6	19	27	37	46	55	50	47.4	44.3	41
Urate (%)	2		5.6[+]	6.3[+]		6.80[+]	5.60[+]					4.60[+]

Struvite predominated throughout the 1980's and early 1990's.
Calcium oxalate predominated through the latter part of the 1990's and early 2000's.
Struvite predominates again in 2005.
+includes data from 1984 and 1986

mission in North America and other parts of the world *(Lekcharoensuk et al, 2001a; Cannon et al, 2007; Forrester, 2006; Houston et al, 2003; 2006; Gerber et al, 2005)*. However, since 2002, struvite uroliths have been on the rise and have surpassed calcium oxalate as the number one urolith submission in the USA **(Figure 4)**. Based on 9221 feline uroliths analyzed at the Minnesota Urolith Center in 2005, the most common mineral types were struvite (48%), calcium oxalate (41%) and purine (4.6%) *(Forrester et al, 2006)*. In Canada, equal numbers of struvite and calcium oxalate uroliths were submitted in 2005 *(Houston et al, 2006)*. In Hong Kong, Italy and Great Britain, struvite uroliths were the most common submission in the time period studied (1998-2000) with calcium oxalate second *(Stevenson, 2001)*. In the Netherlands, calcium oxalate was the most common submission in the same time period with struvite uroliths second *(Stevenson, 2001)*. Less frequently reported uroliths include ammonium urate, cystine, silica, xanthine, calcium phosphate, pyrophosphate and dried solidified blood uroliths.

In male cats with obstructive FLUTD, urethral plugs are the number one cause followed by idiopathic cystitis **(Figure 5)** *(Kruger et al, 1991)*. Less common causes of FLUTD in both male and female cats are those caused by anatomical defects, neoplasia, urinary tract infections and neurological disorders *(Kruger et al, 1991)*. In cats older than 10 years, idiopathic cystitis is uncommon and urinary tract infection is the leading cause of FLUTD followed by urolithiasis **(Figure 6)** *(Bartges, 1997)*. Bacterial cystitis is typically identified in cats less than one year of age, in older cats, and in cats with compromised host factors (perineal urethrostomies, diabetes mellitus, chronic kidney disease etc).

FIGURE 4 - CHANGING PREVALENCE OF CALCIUM OXALATE AND STRUVITE UROLITHS FROM 2001 TO 2005
(Adapted from Forrester, 2006)

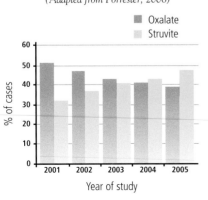

FIGURE 5 - PERCENTAGE OF OBSTRUCTIVE CAUSES OF FLUTD IN 51 MALE CATS IN THE UNITED STATES
(Adapted from Osborne et al, 2000)

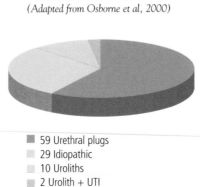

59 Urethral plugs
29 Idiopathic
10 Uroliths
2 Urolith + UTI

FIGURE 6 - CONDITIONS RESPONSIBLE FOR THE CLINICAL SIGNS OF FLUTD IN CATS OLDER THAN 10 YEARS OF AGE
(Adapted from Bartges 1997)

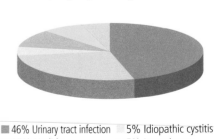

46% Urinary tract infection   5% Idiopathic cystitis
27% Uroliths   5% Incontinence
7% Urethral plugs   3% Neoplasia
7% Trauma

3 - Pathophysiology

▶ Feline idiopathic cystitis

Feline idiopathic (or interstitial) cystitis (FIC) is thought to be a noninfectious, inflammatory, psychoneuroendocrine disorder with abnormalities in the bladder, central nervous system and hypothalamic-pituitary-adrenal response system **(Figure 7)**. It is hypothesized that decreased levels of glycosaminoglycans (GAG) reduce the protective effect of the uroepithelium permitting urine constituents such as calcium and potassium ions to penetrate the epithelium and cause inflammation *(Buffington et al, 1994; 1999a; Buffington & Pacak, 2001; 2002; 2004; Westropp et al, 2002; 2003; Pereira et al, 2004)*. In addition, the ions may stimulate the sensory neurons (C-fibers) in the submucosa, which, via the spinal cord and brain, are perceived as pain. Stressors in a sensitive cat's environment may precipitate clinical signs by activation of the efferent sympathetic nervous system, which stimulates the dorsal root ganglia. The dorsal root ganglia cause the peripheral release of neuropeptides and mediators responsible for inflammation and pain *(Buffington et al, 1994; 1999a; Buffington & Pacak, 2001; Westropp et al, 2002; 2003; Pereira, 2004)*.

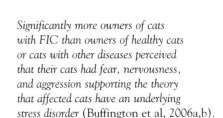

© Yves Lanceau/Royal Canin/Singapura

Significantly more owners of cats with FIC than owners of healthy cats or cats with other diseases perceived that their cats had fear, nervousness, and aggression supporting the theory that affected cats have an underlying stress disorder (Buffington et al, 2006a,b).

Cats may be born with a predisposition to FIC and clinical signs of FLUTD are manifested if such a cat is placed in a "provocative or stressful" environment. FIC is a chronic, waxing and waning disease characterized by periods of remission interspersed with relapse precipitated by stress. Some affected cats have been shown to have small adrenal glands *(Westropp et al, 2003)*.

▶ Urethral plugs

Urethral plugs are disorganized precipitates typically composed of sloughed tissues, blood or inflammatory cells, mixed with large quantities of matrix. Crystalline material may or may not be present. Struvite is the predominate mineral type in those urethral plugs that contain a mineral component. There are physical differences and probably etiological differences between uroliths and urethral plugs however, the actual cause of the matrix-crystalline plugs has not been clearly determined. It has been suggested, but not definitively established that Tamm-Horsfall mucoprotein is the predominant matrix compound which has been hypothesized to be a local host defense

FIGURE 7 - SCHEMATIC REPRESENTATION OF THE PROPOSED PATHOPHYSIOLOGICAL ALTERATIONS IN CATS WITH FELINE IDIOPATHIC/INTERSTITIAL CYSTITIS

(Adapted from Buffington et al, 1999a)

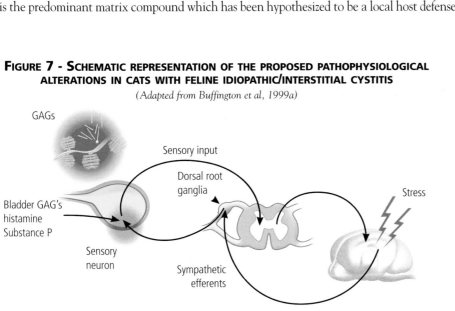

mechanism. *(Kruger et al, 1991; Osborne et al, 1992b; 1996c; 1996d; Houston et al, 2003; Forrester, 2006).* Urethral plugs are much more common in male cats and cause partial or complete urinary tract obstruction. FIC may predispose some cats to forming urethral plugs.

► Uroliths

A urolith (commonly referred to as a stone) is defined as the formation of sediment, consisting of one or more poorly soluble crystalloids, in the urinary tract. Microscopic sediment is referred to as crystals, and macroscopic precipitates are called uroliths.

Urinary crystals form when the urine is supersaturated with respect to a specific mineral or mineral compound. Precipitation is a result of increasing supersaturation. The initial phase, or nucleation, of urolith formation involves the formation of a crystal nidus. This phase is dependent on supersaturation of urine with calculogenic crystalloids and is influenced by the extent of renal excretion of the crystalloid, the urine pH, urine temperature, the presence or absence of various inhibitory factors (e.g., citrate, pyrophosphate), and the presence of promoters of crystallization (e.g., dead cells, cellular debris, protein, bacteria or other crystals). Crystal growth depends on the ability of the nidus to remain within the urinary tract, the duration of supersaturation of the urine and the physical ultra structure of the crystal. The actual rate of growth of the urolith depends on numerous factors including mineral composition and risk factors such as infection *(Osborne et al, 1996a,b; 2000).*

4 - Diagnosis

► History and clinical signs

Regardless of cause, cats with FLUTD present with hematuria (macroscopic and/or microscopic), dysuria, stranguria, pollakiuria, inappropriate urination (periuria or signs of irritative voiding outside of the litter box), or partial or complete urethral obstruction *(Kruger et al, 1991; Osborne et al, 1996a).* Male cats may be observed to lick the tip of the penis. Cats are often observed to spend longer amounts of time than normal in the litter box attempting to urinate or are observed to pass small amounts of urine frequently. Restless behavior or excessive grooming of the caudal abdomen may indicate discomfort.

Urinary tract obstruction may occur suddenly or over a period of weeks. Complete obstruction is characterized by depression, anorexia, lethargy, dehydration, hypothermia, and vomiting. In severe cases the bladder may rupture providing a transient relief of signs followed rapidly by the development of peritonitis and death.

► Physical examination

A complete physical examination should be performed in any cat presenting with FLUTD. Special attention should be paid to the hydration status, bladder, and external urethral orifice. The bladder should be palpated to evaluate its size (degree of distension), shape, contours, thickness of the bladder wall, intramural or intraluminal masses (tumors, uroliths, clots), or grating within the bladder lumen. Most uroliths cannot be detected by abdominal palpation *(Osborne et al, 2000).* Palpation frequently elicits an expression of pain such as crying, resistance to further abdominal palpation, straining to urinate, or passage of a few drops of blood-tinged urine. The penis, prepuce, or vulvar area should be examined for urethral abnormalities and evidence of blood, mucus, or mineral crystals.

In cats with obstructive FLUTD, the bladder is distended, turgid, and painful. In obstructed cats, the tip of the penis may appear discolored because of inflammation and trauma from licking or because of the presence of a urethral plug **(Figure 8)**. Urethral obstruction is a medical emergency that requires immediate relief of the urethral obstruction. The patient's fluid, electrolyte (especially hyperkalemia), and acid-base status should be assessed and appropriate therapeutic maneuvers initiated **(see below in treatment section)**.

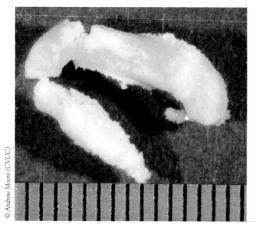

© Andrew Moore (CVUC)

Figure 8 - Feline urethral plug.
A cream to straw-colored urethral plug may be visualized protruding from the urethra. Struvite crystals are the predominant crystals found.

► Laboratory evaluation

In the non obstructed cat, the initial evaluation should include a urinalysis with sediment examination, urine culture, and abdominal imaging. A complete blood count can be conducted; however, it is nearly always normal. A comprehensive biochemical profile should be obtained from cats that are sick or have urethral obstruction. In cats with urate urolithiasis, serum urea nitrogen may be low in cases of portosystemic shunts or liver failure; some cats with calcium oxalate urolithiasis have hypercalcemia.

Urine for analysis may be collected by the owner using a special litter or in the clinic by obtaining a midstream sample during natural voiding, catheterization, or cystocentesis. Manual expression should be avoided as iatrogenic hemorrhage/trauma can be a significant consequence. In addition, in the rare occasion where infection is present, retrograde ascension from the bladder to the kidney and the development of pyelonephritis is possible.

The method of collection will influence the diagnostic results and their interpretation. Cystocentesis is preferred because it prevents contamination of the urine sample by the urethra or genital tract. It is minimally invasive, well tolerated, and safe so long as proper technique is used to prevent iatrogenic urinary tract trauma or infection. The main contraindications to cystocentesis are insufficient volume of urine in the urinary bladder, patient resistance to restraint and abdominal palpation, and coagulopathy or bleeding disorders. Cystocentesis should not be performed if the bladder cannot be palpated.

Urinary catheterization may be performed for:
• **diagnostic indications:** collection of urine for analysis, detection of urethral obstacles (e.g. uroliths, tumors), and instillation of contrast medium for radiographic studies
• **therapeutic indications:** relief of urethral obstruction and facilitation of surgery of the bladder, urethra, or surrounding structures.

The time of day at which the urine is collected should be recorded. In addition, the owner should be questioned on when the cat last ate and how stressed the cat was coming into the hospital. The urine pH is generally the most acidic first thing in the morning, prior to the animal eating. The pH may be higher if the urine is collected in the post prandial period (anywhere from 2-6 hours after a meal). Once the urine pH is above 6.5, struvite crystals can form. If the cat was stressed by transportation to the clinic, hyperventilation may have occurred and this too can raise the urine pH above 6.5 resulting in the appearance of struvite crystals (*Buffington & Chew, 1996a*).

The urine sample should be collected into a sterile collection container. If culture is to be performed, a portion of the urine should be refrigerated immediately in an airtight sterile container. For sediment analysis, the urine should not be refrigerated but is kept at room temperature and covered to avoid light exposure. Analysis should be performed on fresh urine (within 15-60 minutes of collection); otherwise struvite and calcium oxalate crystals can form (*Albasan et al, 2003*). Physical properties of the urine, chemical properties of the urine and examination of urinary sediment should all be determined. Abnormalities consistent with FLUTD that may be noted on urinalysis and sediment examination include hematuria, proteinuria, pyuria, and crystalluria (struvite, amorphous phosphates, urate, calcium oxalate, cystine and xanthine **(Figures 9-12)**.

The identification of crystals in the urine is dependent on the urine pH, temperature, and specific gravity. However, it is important to note that the presence of struvite or calcium oxalate crystals in the urine does not necessarily signify a problem. A few crystals in highly concentrated urine generally have less significance than a few crystals in dilute urine (*Laboto, 2001*). Absolutely fresh urine must be examined as crystals may form in urine that is allowed to stand and cool prior to examination (in-vitro crystallization) **(Table 2)**. The presence of crystals observed in stored samples should be validated by reevaluation of fresh urine (*Albason et al, 2003*).

Quantitative bacterial culture of the urine is indicated to conclusively diagnosis urinary tract infection. Urine should be obtained by cystocentesis to prevent iatrogenic bacterial contamination and submitted for culture within 30 minutes of collection. If this is not possible, urine should be refrig-

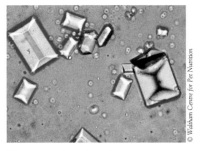

Figure 9 - *Struvite urinary crystals.*

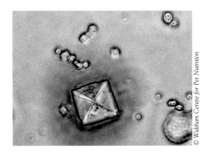

Figure 10 - *Calcium oxalate urinary crystals.*

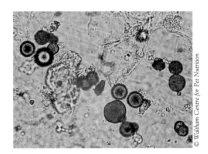

Figure 11 - *Ammonium urate urinary crystals.*

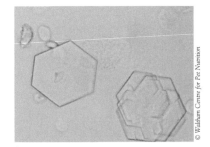

Figure 12 - *Cystine urinary crystals.*

FLUTD

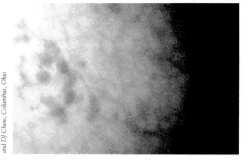

Figure 13 - Lateral radiograph of a male cat with urolithiasis.
The image indicates numerous small, radio-dense uroliths in the urethra of a male cat presenting with obstructive feline lower urinary tract disease.

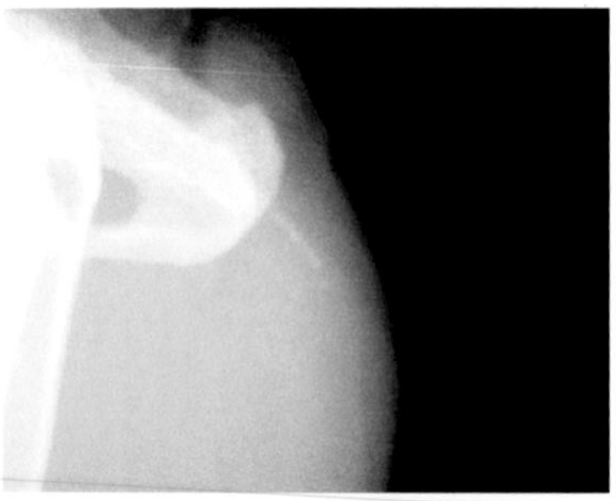

© Dr Brian Crabbe, Port Elgin, Ontario, Canada

Figure 14 - Lateral radiograph of a two year old cat with feline idiopathic/interstitial cystitis.
Note the bladder wall appears thickened and non-distensible.

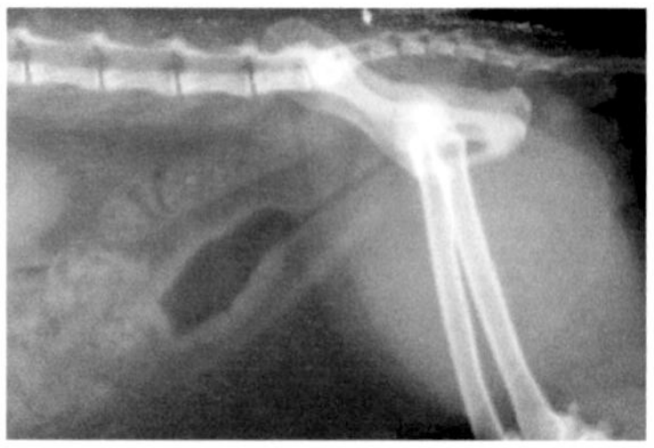

© Gagemount Animal Hospital, Hamilton, Ontario, Canada.

TABLE 2 - TIPS TO HELP INTERPRET CRYSTALLURIA

- Crystals must be evaluated in absolutely fresh urine.
- Crystals observed in stored or refrigerated urine may be artifactual and urine should be restored to room temperature before examination.
- Struvite and/or calcium oxalate crystals may be a normal finding in some cat's urine, especially if the urine is highly concentrated; it is abnormal when they appear in large numbers or are clumped together.
- The presence of crystals in urine indicates that the urine is able to support crystal growth.
- The presence of crystals in urine does not necessarily indicate urolithiasis.
- Crystals may be absent in cats with urolithiasis.
- Cats may pass crystals that are different than the urolith they may have.
- Cats with cystine crystals have cystinuria and this predisposes them to cystine uroliths.

erated. Once positive identification of the organism is obtained, antimicrobial sensitivity should be performed to guide appropriate antimicrobial therapy.

▶ Diagnostic imaging

Diagnostic imaging techniques include survey radiographs, ultrasound, contrast radiography (excretory urography, cystography, urethrography), computed tomography, and magnetic resonance imaging (Samii, 2003).

- **Survey radiographs** are used to screen for changes in the size, shape, position, or radiodensity of the urinary tract. It is important to radiograph the entire urinary system including the perineal urethra to ensure no abnormalities are overlooked **(Figure 13)**. In some cases, a cleansing enema may be needed to ensure adequate visualization of the urinary system. In cats with FIC, the bladder may appear thickened and non-distensible on radiographic examination **(Figure 14)**.

- **Ultrasound** allows assessment of intra-luminal abnormalities not seen on survey radiographs, determines what area is affected and to what extent, and provides information regarding tissue composition, i.e. solid versus cystic lesions.

- **Positive contrast cystography** is used to determine bladder location, rupture, diverticulae, and fistulas.

- **Double contrast cystography** is used to evaluate the mucosal surface of the bladder and luminal contents. A good quality double contrast study requires only a small volume (1-2 mL) of positive contrast medium. It is important to palpate the bladder as it is being filled with contrast in order to monitor the degree of distension and to avoid over inflation. The bladder should

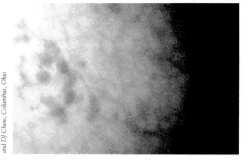

Figure 15 - Endoscopic appearance of the bladder mucosa in a cat with lower urinary tract disease.
The endoscopy demonstrates glomerulations consistent with feline idiopathic/interstitial cystitis.

© Compliments CA Buffington and DJ Chew, Columbus, Ohio

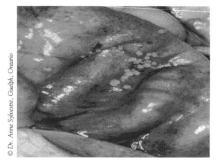

Figure 16A - Multiple calcium oxalate calculi in a cat bladder.
Note the bladder has been opened fully to allow for complete removal of all uroliths, a number of which are embedded in the bladder mucosa.

© Dr. Anne Sylvestre, Guelph, Ontario

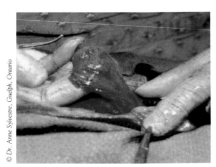

Figure 16B - Surgical removal of uroliths in the bladder.
The bladder of the cat has been entirely opened and the mucosal surface everted to ensure complete removal of uroliths. A post operative radiograph confirmed the complete removal of all of the uroliths.

© Dr. Anne Sylvestre, Guelph, Ontario

be well distended with the negative contrast medium and a small volume of positive contrast (the so called contrast puddle) should lie on the dependant surface of the bladder lumen. Radiolucent uroliths are identified as filling defects in the contrast puddle. Blood clots are identified as irregular filling defects either at the margin of the contrast puddle or adherent to the mucosal surface. Recognition of small alterations of the contour of the mucosal surface is an important clue in the diagnosis of both cystitis and tumor, but can be artifactual as a result of incomplete filling of the bladder. Urethrography is used to examine the urethra.

▶ Uroendoscopy

Endoscopy of the urethra and bladder is now possible using a flexible fiber optic scope in male cats and a rigid human pediatric cystoscope in female cats *(Chew et al, 1996; McCarthy 1996)*. The mucosal surface of the bladder of cats with FIC displays characteristic findings of submucosal petechial hemorrhages (glomerulations) during cystoscopy following bladder distension to 80 cm H_2O *(Chew et al, 1996; Buffington et al, 1999a)* **(Figure 15)**.

▶ Surgery

When surgery is performed for exploration, biopsy or urolith removal, the bladder should be fully opened **(Figure 16)**. Because many feline uroliths are very small, complete surgical removal of all uroliths may be difficult and post surgical radiography should always be performed to ensure all uroliths have been removed *(Lulich et al, 1993a)*. Failure to remove all uroliths at the time of cystotomy is common and seems to be more likely with calcium oxalate uroliths. *Lulich et al* (1993a) reported that calcium oxalate uroliths were incompletely removed in 20% of cats.

▶ Histopathology

Biopsies of the bladder mucosa of cats with FIC may show relatively normal epithelium and muscularis with submucosal edema and vasodilation; infiltration of inflammatory cells is mild to moderate **(Figure 17)**. Some cats have increased numbers of mast cells; others have erosions, ulcerations or fibrosis of the bladder wall.

▶ Analysis of urolith composition

Uroliths may be collected by spontaneous voiding (use an aquarium fishnet to catch the urolith), voiding urohydropropulsion, aspiration into a urethral catheter, via cystoscopy, or surgical removal *(Lulich et al, 1992,1993b; Osborne et al, 2000)*. Uroliths need to be submitted in a clean dry container without preservatives or additional fluids. In many cases, uroliths cannot be identified simply by visual characteristics. All uroliths retrieved should be quantitatively analyzed by specialized laboratories to determine mineral composition of any/all of the 4 layers that may be present **(Figure 18)**. There are

© Compliments CA Buffington and DJ Chew, Columbus, Ohio

Figure 17 - Histological appearance of the bladder mucosa of a cat with lower urinary tract disease.
Submucosal edema and erosions consistent with feline idiopathic/interstitial cystitis.

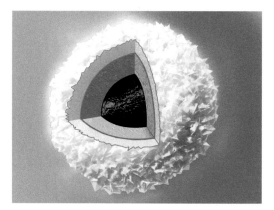

Figure 18 - Illustration of the layers of a urolith.
Quantitative analysis allows accurate determination of the mineral composition of any of the four layers that may be present: nidus, stone, shell and surface crystals.

TABLE 3 - AGE, SEX AND BREED PREDISPOSITIONS AND OTHER POTENTIAL RISK FACTORS FOR UROLITHS IN CATS

Urolith Type	Breed	Age	Sex	Other
Struvite	- **USA:** Foreign Shorthair, Ragdoll, Chartreux, Oriental Shorthair, DSH, Himalayan *(Lekcharoensuk et al, 2000; 2001a)*; Himalayan and Persian *(Cannon et al, 2007)*, DSH, DLH *(Ling et al, 1990)*; No breed predilection *(Osborne et al, 1995a; 1995b; 2000)* - **Canada:** DSH, DLH, DMH, Himalayan, Persian *(Houston et al, 2004; 2006)* - **Great Britain:** DSH, Persian *(Stevenson, 2001)*	- Sterile: 3 months-22 years; average 7.2 + 3.5 years *(Osborne et al, 2000)* - Infection induced-any age *(Osborne et al, 1995a)* - Average 5 years for females and <2 years for males *(Ling et al, 1990)* - 1-2 years *(Thumachai et al, 1996)* - 6.8 + 3.7 years *(Stevenson, 2001)*	- Female slightly > male *(Ling et al, 1990; Osborne et al, 2000; Houston et al, 2004; 2006)* - Male <2 more common than female <2 years *(Ling et al, 1990)* - Male slightly >female *(Lekcharoensuk et al, 2000)* - Male = female *(Stevenson, 2001)*	- Overweight/inactive - Low water intake *(Osborne et al, 1995)* - Alkaline urine *(Osborne et al, 1995)* - Indoor housing *(Kirk et al; 1995)*
Calcium oxalate	- **USA:** Himalayan, Persian *(Kirk et al, 1995; Cannon et al, 2007)*; Himalayan, Persian, Ragdoll, Shorthair, Foreign Shorthair, Havana brown, Scottish fold, Exotic shorthair *(Lekcharoensuk et al, 2000; 2001a)*; Burmese, Persian and Himalayan *(Thumachai et al, 1996; Osborne et al, 1995b; 1996b; Kirk et al, 1995)* - **Canada:** Himalayan, Persian *(Houston et al, 2004; 2006)* - **Great Britain:** DSH, Persian *(Stevenson, 2001)*	- 7 years; 3 months -22 years *(Osborne et al, 2000)* - Older cats and greatest risk at 10-15 years *(Thumachai et al, 1996)* - Bimodal peaks at 5 and 12 years *(Kirk et al, 1995)* - 7-10 years *(Lekcharoensuk et al, 2000)* - 6.8 + 3.5 years *(Stevenson, 2001)*	- Male > female *(Ling et al, 1990; Kirk et al; 1995, Thumachai et al, 1996; Lekcharoensuk et al; 2000; 2001a; Osborne et al, 2000; Houston et al, 2004; 2006; Cannon et al, 2007)* - Male = female *(Stevenson, 2001)*	- Overweight/inactive - Low water intake - Indoor housing *(Kirk et al, 1995)* - Serum hypercalcemia *(Osborne et al, 1996b; McClain et al, 1995; Savary et al, 2000; Midkiff et al, 2000)*
Urate	- **USA:** None *(Osborne et al, 2000; Ling & Sorenson, 1995)* - **Canada:** Siamese and Egyptian mau *(Houston, 2006)*	- 5.8 years (5 months-15 years) *(Osborne et al, 1996b)* - 4.4 + 2 years *(Stevenson, 2001)*	- Male = female *(Osborne et al, 2000; 1995b; Westropp et al, 2006)* - Male slightly > female *(Ling et al, 1990; Houston et al, 2004; 2006)*	- Low water intake - Portovascular shunts - Urinary tract infections *(Hostutler et al, 2005)*
Cystine	- **USA:** None *(Osborne et al, 1995)* SH, Siamese *(Osborne et al, 2000)* - **Canada:** None *(Houston et al, 2004; 2006)*	- > 3.6 years (4 months-12 years) *(Osborne et al, 2000)*	- Male = female *(Osborne et al, 2000)* - Male slightly > female *(Osborne et al, 2000)*	- Low water intake - Indoor housing - Inborn error of metabolism *(Dibartola et al, 1991; Osborne et al, 1992a)*
Xanthine	- **USA:** None *(Osborne et al, 2000)*	- 2.8 + 2.3 years (4 months to 10 years) *(Osborne et al, 1992a)*	- None *(Osborne et al, 1992a)*	- Inborn error of purine metabolism? *(Osborne et al, 1992; White et al, 1997)*
Silica	- **USA:** None *(Osborne et al, 2000)*	?	- None *(Osborne et al, 2000)* - Male? *(Houston, 2006)*	- Low water intake
Calcium phosphate (brushite)	- **USA:** None *(Osborne et al, 2000)* - **Canada:** None *(Houston et al, 2004; 2006)*	- 8 + 5 years (5 months-19 years) *(Osborne et al, 2000)* - 7.1 + 3.6 years *(Stevenson, 2001)*	- Female >male *(Osborne et al, 2000)* - Male > female *(Houston, 2006)*	- Low water intake - Primary hyperparathyroidism *(Osborne et al, 1995; 1996b)*
Pyro-phosphate	- **Canada:** None *(Houston, 2006)* - **Europe:** Persians? *(Frank et al, 2002)*		- None *(Houston, 2006)*	
Dried solidified blood calculi	- **USA:** None *(Westropp et al, 2006)*			

4 techniques available for quantitative analysis including polarizing light microscopy, x-ray diffraction, infrared spectroscopy, and scanning electron microscopy. Accurate identification of the type or types of minerals present in a urolith is paramount in order to apply the appropriate therapeutic and preventative regime.

► Predicting urolith type

Effective treatment and prevention of uroliths depends on knowledge of their mineral composition. Ideally, a urolith should be retrieved and quantitatively analyzed, however, there are a number of factors that can help in predicting urolith composition including signalment (age, sex, breed, **Table 3**), history of underlying disorders, radiodensity of the uroliths and urine parameters (pH, specific gravity, crystalluria, **Table 4**). It is important to remember that crystals may or may not be present in the urine sample and the urine sample may contain crystals that differ from the underlying urolith composition (*Buffington & Chew, 1999b*).

5 - Specific diseases

► Feline idiopathic cystitis

The diagnosis of FIC requires documentation of signs of chronic irritative voiding (dysuria, hematuria, pollakiuria, inappropriate urination), sterile urine, negative imaging studies, and cystoscopic observation of submucosal petechial hemorrhages (glomerulations). In addition, there may be increased urinary bladder permeability, decreased urine concentrations of glycosaminoglycans, increased mucosal vascularity, erosions, ulcerations, edema, fibrosis, and neurogenic inflammation (*Buffington et al, 1994; 1996b; 1999a; Buffington & Chew 1999b; Buffington & Pacak, 2001; Buffington, 2002; 2004; Westropp et al, 2002; 2003; Pereira et al, 2004*).

> Epidemiology

Cats with FIC tend to be young to mid-age (<10 years) and otherwise healthy. Male and females are affected and many of the predisposed cats eat dry food exclusively (*Buffington et al, 1997; Jones et al, 1997; Markwell et al, 1998; Buffington, 2002*). A significant number have high urine specific gravities.

> Management

One of the cornerstones of therapy is to identify and relieve the stressors in the cat's environment. Potential sources of stress include environmental aspects such as other cats, changes in weather, lack of activity, litter box placement, litter type, diet, owner work schedule, and the addition or removal of people or animals. Stress can be managed by providing the cat with hiding places and equipment such as climbing posts and toys that can be chased and caught which allow the cat to express predatory behavior (*www.indoorcat.org/: The Indoor Cat Initiative 2006, Buffington et al, 1994; 1999b; 2006a,b; Buffington, 2002; Cameron et al, 2004*).

Diet plays an important role in the pathophysiology and treatment of interstitial cystitis. An abrupt change or frequent changes in diet has been associated with the recurrence of clinical signs. Therefore, it is reasonable to limit the frequency of diet changes in sensitive cats (*Buffington et al, 1994; 1996b; 2006a,b; Jones et al, 1997*).

Urine dilution is thought to help cats with FIC because it decreases the concentration of substances in urine that may be irritating to the bladder mucosa. In one study, cats with FIC were significantly more likely to eat dry pet food exclusively (59%) compared with cats in the general population (19%) (*Buffington et al, 1997*). In a one year, non-randomized

	Radiodensity	Urine pH
Struvite	++ - ++++	> 6.5
Calcium oxalate	++++	Variable
Calcium phosphate	++++	Alkaline to neutral (apatite forms)
Ammonium urate	0 - ++	Acid to neutral
Cystine	+ à ++	Acid to neutral
Xanthine	0 - ++	Acid to neutral
Silica	++ - ++++	Acid to neutral
Pyrophosphates	++ - ++++	Unknown
Dried solidified blood clots	0 - ++	Unknown

TABLE 4 - RADIODENSITY AND URINE pH OF FELINE UROLITHS
(*Adapted from Osborne et al, 2000; Frank et al, 2002; Westropp et al, 2006*).

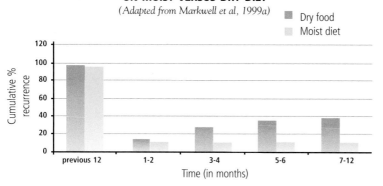

FIGURE 19 - RECURRENCE RATES OF FELINE IDIOPATHIC CYSTITIS ON MOIST VERSUS DRY DIET

(Adapted from Markwell et al, 1999a)

prospective study of 46 cats with FIC, feeding a moist therapeutic food specifically designed to promote lower urinary tract health was associated with significant improvement compared with feeding a dry diet. At the end of the one year study, the recurrence of clinical signs in cats eating the moist food was significantly less (11% of 18 cats), compared with cats eating the dry food (39% of 28 cats) (*Markwell et al, 1999a*) **(Figure 19)**. Compared with the cats consuming the dry food, the urine specific gravity was significantly less in the cats eating the moist food. The mean urine specific gravity ranged from 1.032-1.041 in the cats eating the moist food compared to 1.051-1.052 in the cats eating the dry food.

Highly acidifying diets are not recommended as highly acid urine may increase sensory nerve fiber transmission in the bladder and increase pain perception (*Chew & Buffington, 2003*).

In some cases, additional therapy may be indicated. Cats naturally release pheromones during facial rubbing when they feel content in their environment. A synthetic analogue of a naturally occurring feline facial pheromone may help decrease anxiety-related behaviors in some cats (*Chew et al, 1998; Mills & Mills, 2001; Gunn-Moore & Cameron, 2004*). Although a number of additional treatments have been advocated over the years, none, except diet, have been clinically proven to make a significant difference. Additional therapeutic options will likely evolve to decrease central noradrenergic drive and normalize the responsiveness of the stress response system in these sensitive cats (*Buffington et al, 1999a; 2006a,b; Buffington, 2004*). In the interim, a number of drugs have been suggested including amitriptyline and pentosan polysulfates (glycosaminoglycan or GAG replenishment agents) (*Chew et al, 1998; Buffington et al, 1999a; 2006a,b; Buffington & Chew, 1999b; Buffington, 2002; Kraiger et al, 2003; Kruger et al, 2003; Gunn-Moore & Shenoy, 2004; Mealey et al, 2004*).

Clinical signs resolve spontaneously in as many as 85% of cats with FIC within 2-3 days, regardless of therapy. However, about 40-50% of these cats will relapse within 12 months, and some will have multiple recurrences (*Markwell et al, 1998; 1999a; Kruger, 2003*).

▶ Urethral plugs

Relief of urinary tract obstruction and reestablishment of urine flow is mandatory in a cat with urethral obstruction. In addition, correction of fluid, electrolyte and acid-base imbalances associated with the obstruction and post-renal azotemia are needed. A number of excellent references are available on the emergency management of uretheral obstruction (*Osborne et al, 2000; Westropp et al, 2005*).

▶ Uroliths

> Universal risk factors: relative supersaturation

Urine supersaturation is the driving force for the formation of crystals within the urinary tract. More than 40 years ago, human researchers began exploring ways of evaluating urine parameters and predicting urolithiasis risk. This led to a research methodology called Relative Supersaturation (RSS) ratio, a technique first introduced in human medicine in 1960's by Dr. W.G. Robertson (*Nordin & Robertson, 1966*). The measurement of the RSS predicts the crystallization potential of that urine. This technique has become the gold standard for urine evaluation in human patients (*Pak et al, 1977*).

The ability to predict the crystallization potential of urine is a useful tool for clinicians and researchers who wish to develop therapeutic interventions for patients with urolithiasis. In the late 1990's, Dr Robertson began collaborative work with scientists at the Waltham Centre for Pet Nutrition (WCPN) to validate the relative supersaturation ratio for use in dog and cat urine and a number of publications have now appeared in the veterinary literature on the technique and interpretation thereof (*Smith et al, 1998; Markwell et al, 1999b; Robertson et al, 2002*).

FLUTD

In order to study urine parameters using RSS, it is necessary to obtain complete urine collections over a 2 to 5 day-period. The urine is analyzed for the concentration of 10 solutes (calcium, magnesium, sodium, potassium, ammonium, phosphate, citrate, sulfate, oxalate and uric acid) and the urine pH *(Robertson et al, 2002)*. The number of interactive complexes that could occur between these ions, together with activity coefficients of the salts is calculated and the activity product determined. The activity product is an indicator of the likelihood of a urolith forming. The activity product is divided by the thermodynamic solubility product of the crystal and the resultant RSS ratio is produced. (The thermodynamic solubility product is the activity product at which a urolith will remain static and not grow or dissolve.)

The RSS is unique for each crystal type. RSS can be used to define three different zones of urine saturation: undersaturated, metastable or oversaturated. Each of these zones has different implications for the risk of urolith formation **(Figure 20)**. The higher the RSS, the greater the risk of crystal formation, and with low RSS values, the risk of crystal formation is much less likely *(Robertson et al, 2002)*.

A RSS less than one means that the urine is undersaturated and that crystals will not form. In a complex media such as urine, it is possible to have a RSS above one without spontaneous precipitation of crystals *(Markwell et al, 1999b)*. This is due to electrical fields (ionic strength) induced by the numerous ions in solution and the presence of inhibitors of crystallization. Both prevent the free fractions of minerals (e.g. calcium and oxalate) to interact to form crystals. This level of supersaturation is qualified as metastable supersaturation. At this level of saturation, calcium oxalate crystals will not spontaneously form, but might occur in the presence of a nucleus. In the zone of metastable supersaturation, crystals, and thus uroliths, will not dissolve.

At higher levels of minerals in the urine, crystals will form spontaneously within minutes to hours. This is the labile supersaturation zone. The limit between metastable and labile supersaturation is called the formation product. Kinetic precipitation studies in urine have shown that the RSS for the formation product for struvite is 2.5 and for calcium oxalate is 12 **(Tables 5 & 6)**.

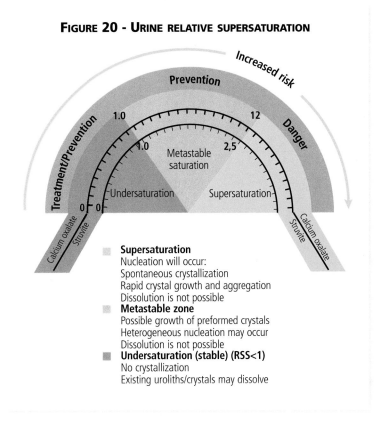

FIGURE 20 - URINE RELATIVE SUPERSATURATION

Supersaturation
Nucleation will occur:
Spontaneous crystallization
Rapid crystal growth and aggregation
Dissolution is not possible

Metastable zone
Possible growth of preformed crystals
Heterogeneous nucleation may occur
Dissolution is not possible

Undersaturation (stable) (RSS<1)
No crystallization
Existing uroliths/crystals may dissolve

TABLE 5 - USING RSS TO ASSESS THE RISK OF STRUVITE UROLITH FORMATION		
If a diet has an RSS for struvite of:	**The urine produced by cats fed that diet is**	**The risk for struvite formation is**
Less than 1	Under-saturated	• New struvite uroliths will not form. • Existing struvite uroliths will dissolve.
Between 1 and 2.5	Metastable	• New struvite uroliths will not form. • Any existing struvite uroliths will not dissolve and may grow.
Over 2.5	Over-saturated	• New struvite uroliths may form. • Any existing struvite uroliths will grow.

TABLE 6 - USING RSS TO ASSESS THE RISK OF CALCIUM OXALATE UROLITH FORMATION		
If a diet has an RSS for calcium oxalate of:	**The urine produced by pets fed that diet is said to be**	**The risk for calcium oxalate formation is**
Less than 1	Undersaturated	• New calcium oxalate uroliths will not form. • Existing calcium oxalate uroliths will not grow.
Between 1 and 12	Metastable	• New calcium oxalate uroliths will not form. • Any existing calcium oxalate uroliths may grow.
Over 12	Oversaturated	• New calcium oxalate uroliths may form. • Any existing calcium oxalate uroliths will grow.

TABLE 7 - METHODS TO ENCOURAGE WATER INTAKE

Increase water consumption by feeding increased amounts of canned food or feeding a dry diet formulated to stimulate diuresis. It has been shown that salt significantly increases water intake and urine production *(Hawthorne & Markwell, 2004)*. Salt has not been shown to contribute to hypertension or renal disease in healthy cats *(Devois et al, 2000a; Buranakarl et al, 2004; Luckschander et al, 2004; Cowgill et al, 2007)*.

Multiple small meals may help. It has been suggested that, for a given energy level, the water intake significantly increases by increasing meal frequency *(Kirschvink et al, 2005)*.

Provide easy access to fresh water at all times. Cats are nocturnal and may prefer to drink in the evening.

Provide a bowl with a wide surface area. Cats have very sensitive whiskers and many seem to prefer a large bowl in which the whiskers do not touch the sides of the bowl. The water bowl should be kept full at all times.

A variety of water types: (Brita, distilled, bottled, warm tap water, cold tap water) can be offered.

Do not sweeten the water as cats lack sweet taste receptors (defective Tas 1r2) *(Li et al, 2006)*

Flavoring the water or providing ice cubes flavored by tuna or clam juice may help encourage water consumption. Some companies provide different flavors to add to the drinking water to encourage water consumption.

Some cats prefer a source of running water (water fountains are available for cats).

It is important **to keep water bowl away from the litter box area.** The water bowl must be clean (cats have a very keen sense of smell and are easily turned off by odors on the edge of the bowl).

Some cats prefer a clear glass bowl; others stainless steel or ceramic.

Some cats prefer not to share their bowl (especially with dogs).

TABLE 8 - WATER INTAKE SIGNIFICANTLY INCREASES WHEN CATS WERE FED THREE MEALS VERSUS ONE MEAL PER DAY.
(Adapted from Kirschvink et al, 2005).

	Daily energy intake (kcal/kg BW)	Na intake (mg/kg BW)	Water intake (mL/cat/day)
1 meal	71	103	72 ±10
2 meal	71	103	89 ± 4
3 meal	71	103	95 ± 6

BW: *body weight*
Na: *sodium*

TABLE 9 - POORLY DIGESTIBLE DIETS ARE ASSOCIATED WITH INCREASED FECAL WATER LOSS
(internal data from the Waltham Centre of Pet Nutrition)

	Diet A	Diet B
Digestibility	79.5%	50.6%
Fecal water loss (per 1000 kcal)	89 g	330 g

> Universal management

Stimulate diuresis

The easiest way of reducing supersaturation and indeed, one of the simplest and most effective treatments for all causes of FLUTD, is to increase urine volume and promote diuresis. There is a great deal of evidence in cats that low urine volume as well as urine concentration are risk factors for urolith formation. High urine volumes will actually reduce the risk of urolith formation by increasing the frequency of micturition, which helps remove any free crystals, proteinaceous material and debris from the urinary tract. In addition, urine dilution and increased urinary flow is known to help cats with urolithiasis and urethral plugs as it reduces the concentration of lithogenic substances and reduces the time available for urinary solutes to form crystals or stones.

To stimulate diuresis, drinking must be encouraged **(Table 7)**. Cats when fed two identical diets except for their moisture content tend to consume less water, to urinate less frequently and to produce less, but more concentrated urine on the lower moisture diet *(Burger et al, 1980)*. An increase in water turnover can be achieved by feeding diets that contain 70-85% moisture (canned, pouch, tray), by increasing feeding frequency (increasing number of meals/day), by increasing the sodium chloride content of the diet, or by adding water to the diet *(Dumon et al, 1999)*.

The water intake of a cat is significantly influenced by the number of meals per day. *Kirschvink et al* (2005) reported that that water intake increased from 72 mL/cat/day to 95 mL/cat/day by feeding three meals rather than one meal per day **(Table 8)**.

The digestibility of the diet will influence the absolute amount of water available to dilute urine. Less digestible diets have been associated with increased fecal water loss **(Table 9)**. The increased loss of water into the feces decreases the amount of water absorbed and subsequently excreted in the urine. The risk of urolithiasis increases the more concentrated the urine. Therefore, cats with

FIGURE 21 - INFLUENCE OF THE DIETARY SODIUM CONTENT ON MEAN DAILY WATER INTAKE AND URINE VOLUME IN CATS

(Data adapted from Hawthorne & Markwell, 2004).

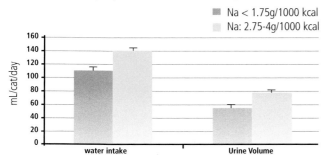

The sodium content is either < 1.75 g/1000 kcal or included in the 2.75-4.0 g/1000 kcal range. Increasing dietary sodium content resulted in a significant (p < 0.001) increase in water intake and urine volume.

FIGURE 22 - INFLUENCE OF THE DIETARY SODIUM CONTENT ON MEAN DAILY URINE SPECIFIC GRAVITY IN CATS

(Data adapted from Hawthorne & Markwell, 2004)

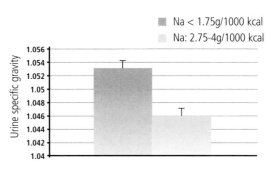

The sodium content is either < 1.75 g/1000 kcal or included in the 2.75-4.0 g/1000 kcal range. Increasing dietary sodium content resulted in a significant (p = 0.003) decrease in urine specific gravity.

lower urinary tract disease should be fed highly digestible diets to minimize fecal water loss.

Increased dietary sodium content has been used to increase water intake and cause subsequent urine dilution in cats. The effectiveness of dietary sodium on increasing urine volume was clearly shown in a study by *Biourge et al* (2001). Healthy cats fed 1.1 g NaCl/1000 kcal had a mean urine volume of 11 ± 5 mL/kg/day. Urine volume increased significantly to 20 ± 7 mL/kg/day when the dietary sodium intake was increased to 2.5 g NaCl/1000 kcal.

Effect of dietary sodium on urinary calcium excretion

Historically, there has been controversy about the use of sodium chloride to stimulate thirst and diuresis, as it could also potentially affect urinary calcium excretion, blood pressure and renal disease *(Osborne et al, 2000)*. However, recent studies in cats have refuted this theory, and support the use of moderate increases in sodium to help maintain urinary tract health.

In studies by *Devois et al* (2000a, b), it was shown that a sodium intake of 1.04% DMB was associated with an increase in 24 hour calcium excretion and urine output. However, as urinary output increased by 100%, the sodium intake resulted in similar calcium and lower oxalate urinary concentrations compared with a sodium intake of 0.30-0.39% DMB. Due to the significant effect of sodium on urine volume, increasing dietary NaCl does not increase the urinary calcium oxalate RSS and therefore does not increase the risk for calcium oxalate urolith formation. The results of this study is supported by epidemiological studies that report that diets with a salt content of 1.43-3.70 g/1000 kcal have a decreased risk of calcium oxalate urolith formation compared with diets containing 0.48-0.77 g/1000 kcal *(Lekcharoensuk et al, 2001b)*.

Hawthorne & Markwell (2004) evaluated the effect of the dietary sodium content of 23 commercially available extruded diets on water intake and urine composition in 55 healthy adult cats. Cats fed diets containing higher levels of dietary sodium content had significantly higher water intake and urine volume **(Figure 21)**, and significantly lower urine specific gravity **(Figure 22)**, and calcium oxalate RSS values **(Figure 23)** compared to cats fed lower sodium diets. Urinary

FIGURE 23 - INFLUENCE OF THE DIETARY SODIUM CONTENT ON MEAN CALCIUM OXALATE RSS IN CATS

(Data adapted from Hawthorne & Markwell, 2004)

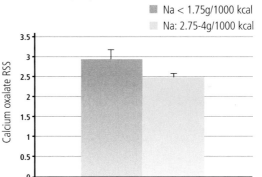

The sodium content is either < 1.75 g/1000 kcal or included in the 2.75-4.0 g/1000 kcal range. Increasing dietary sodium content resulted in a significant (p = 0.04) decrease in calcium oxalate RSS.

FLUTD

FIGURE 24 - DIETARY SODIUM CONTENT IS VERY EFFECTIVE AT REDUCING THE RSS FOR STRUVITE IN HEALTHY CATS

*(Royal Canin Research Center 2005;
internal data collected during a 2 year-period)*

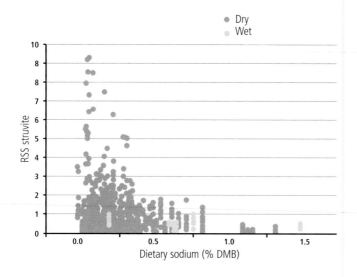

Individual data collected with 125 different diets fed to a group of 7 cats. Each point represents one cat fed one diet.

FIGURE 25 - RELATIONSHIP BETWEEN DIETARY SODIUM AND CALCIUM OXALATE (CaOx) RSS IN HEALTHY CATS

(Biourge, 2007)

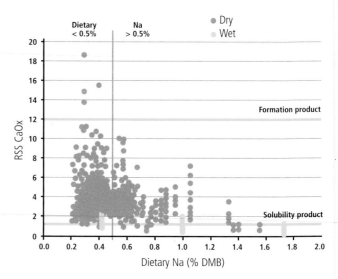

Dietary sodium content is very effective at reducing the RSS for calcium oxalate in healthy cats.

calcium concentration did not differ significantly between cats fed the moderate and lower sodium diets. The results of this study indicate that dietary sodium concentrations up to 4 g/1000 kcal did not increase the urine calcium concentrations in cats, but did however, increase water turnover and urine volume compared to cat foods with sodium content less than 1.75 g/1000 kcal.

Zu et al (2006) evaluated the effect of dietary sodium content on water intake, urine volume, urine specific gravity, mineral excretion, relative supersaturation and activity product ratios of calcium oxalate and struvite in nine healthy cats. Increasing sodium content from 0.4 to 1.2% DMB was associated with a significant increase in urine volume. Increased dietary sodium did not increase calcium excretion in these healthy cats.

Effect of dietary sodium on urinary RSS values

The calculation of RSS from the urine of cats fed a specific diet can be used to study the effect of that diet on the crystallization potential of urine (*Markwell et al, 1999b; Robertson, 2002*). Studies have confirmed that increasing the dietary intake of sodium significantly reduces the RSS of struvite and calcium oxalate in healthy cats (**Figure 24-25**) (*Tournier et al, 2006a; Xu et al, 2006*). *Tournier et al* (2006a) evaluated 11 extruded diets with a sodium content ranging from 0.44% to 1.56% DMB on urinary parameters in healthy cats. A significant linear correlation was found between dietary sodium and calcium oxalate RSS, demonstrating that increasing dietary sodium content significantly decreases calcium oxalate RSS in cats by increasing urine volume and thus urine dilution. Increased moisture intake has also been shown to reduce calcium oxalate RSS in urolith former cats (*Lulich et al, 2004*).

Effect of dietary sodium on blood pressure and renal function

As in humans, the long term risks of increased (1.75 to 3.25 g/1000 kcal) dietary NaCl intake on the health of cats are controversial. The levels of dietary NaCl that will stimulate diuresis do not appear to affect blood pressure in healthy pets, in cats with early renal disease as well as in feline models of renal failure (*Buranakarl et al, 2004; Luckschander et al, 2004; Cowgill et al, 2007*). More-

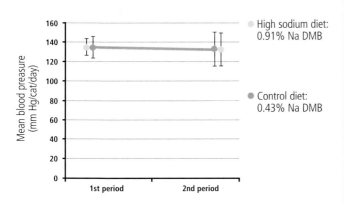

FIGURE 26 - THE EFFECT OF SODIUM CHLORIDE ON SYSTOLIC BLOOD PRESSURE IN HEALTHY ADULT CATS.

(Data adapted from Luckschander et al, 2004)

High sodium diet: 0.91% Na DMB

Control diet: 0.43% Na DMB

The study was a cross-over design. 10 European cats (4 males, 6 females, 2.6 +/- 0.5 years, 4.5 +/- 0.89 kg) received a control diet for 14 days. The diets contained respectively 0.46% sodium DMB (control diet) and 1.02% DMB sodium (study diet). The systolic blood pressure was not affected by altering the dietary sodium intake.

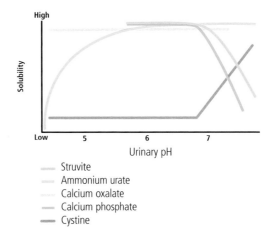

FIGURE 27 - SOLUBILITY AND pH

(personnal communication with Dr WG Robertson)

- Struvite
- Ammonium urate
- Calcium oxalate
- Calcium phosphate
- Cystine

Urinary pH can have a marked influence on the solubility of certain crystals and calculi. Struvite crystals are sensitive to changes in urine pH. Acidification of urine increases the solubility of struvite crystals, reducing the risk of struvite urolithiasis. Calcium oxalate is less sensitive to urine pH.

over, an epidemiological study concluded that feeding cats' higher level of Na among other nutrients reduced the odds of suffering from chronic renal failure *(Hughes et al, 2002)*.

Short-term feeding of high-sodium foods (1.02% Na versus 0.46% DMB) to young, healthy cats for 14 days was associated with a significantly increased water intake and decreased urine specific gravity without increasing systolic blood pressure **(Figure 26)**. Blood pressure measurements remained within the reference range throughout the study in all 10 cats *(Luckschander et al, 2004)*. The results of this study suggests that feeding a diet with moderately increased salt content increases water intake and causes diuresis without increasing systolic blood pressure in healthy adult young cats.

Cowgill et al (2007) evaluated the effect of dietary sodium concentration on renal function in adult cats. There were no differences in plasma creatinine, BUN or glomerular filtration rate (GFR, assessed by 10-hour pharmacokinetic analysis of exogenous plasma creatinine clearance) when cats were fed 0.22% versus 1.3% sodium diets. These data suggest that extremes of dietary salt have no short-term effect on renal function in healthy cats.

Buranakarl et al (2004) evaluated the effect of salt intake on blood pressure in cats with induced azotemia similar in degree to IRIS Stages II and III in cats. Salt intake had no effect on blood pressure. Further, the lowest level of salt intake was associated with the lowest values for GFR, inappropriate hypokalemic kaliuresis and activation of the renin-angiotensin-aldosterone system. The results of this study suggest that, similar to healthy cats, cats with induced renal disease are not salt sensitive.

Adjusting urine pH

Adjusting urine pH via dietary manipulation or medical means can be very effective in the management of some but not all uroliths **(Figure 27)**. Urine acidification markedly increases struvite solubility and is essential in the medical dissolution of these uroliths *(Stevenson et al, 2000; Smith et al, 2001)*. In contrast, urine alkalinization is important in increasing the solubility of metabolic uroliths including some urate uroliths and cystine uroliths. Alkalinization above 7.5 is not recommended as this may contribute to calcium phosphate urolithiasis. Calcium oxalate uroliths appear at any urine pH and to date, medical dissolution is impossible.

The effect of urine pH on the risk of forming crystals, and as a method of treatment or prevention will be discussed further as it relates to individual uroliths.

> Struvite

Risk factors

Unlike dogs, the majority of struvite (magnesium ammonium phosphate hexahydrate; $Mg\,NH_4\,PO_4\,6H_2O$) uroliths in cats are sterile (*Buffington et al, 1997; Lekcharoensuk et al, 2000; 2001a; Cannon et al, 2007*). Struvite uroliths form when the urine becomes supersaturated with magnesium, ammonium, and phosphorus and when the urine pH is greater than 6.5. Struvite crystals are more soluble when the urine pH is less than 6.5 and crystallization is unlikely to occur when the pH is less than 6.3. However, pH is less critical when food promotes diuresis and urine dilution as it is the case with wet food (**Figure 28**).

A case-control study reported that diets with the highest magnesium, phosphorus, calcium, chloride and fiber, moderate protein and low fat content were associated with an increased risk of struvite urolithiasis (*Lekcharoensuk et al, 2001b*).

Magnesium

Diets containing 0.15 to 1.0% magnesium on a dry matter basis were associated with the formation of struvite uroliths (*Lekcharoensuk et al, 2001b*). However, the magnesium effect depends on the form of magnesium and on the urine pH (*Tarttelin, 1987; Buffington et al, 1990; Reed et al, 2000a*). Buffington et al. (1990) reported that cats fed 0.5% magnesium as $MgCl_2$ did not form struvite uroliths whereas cats that were fed 0.5% magnesium as MgO did form struvite uroliths (**Table 10**). The difference in susceptibility to struvite formation was due to magnesium oxide promoting the formation of alkaline urine whereas magnesium chloride promoted the formation of a protective acidic urine.

Phosphorus

Cats fed diets high in phosphorus (3.17-4.70 g/1000 kcal) were almost four times as likely to develop struvite uroliths compared to cats fed diets with 0.85-1.76 g/1000 kcal phosphorus (*Lekcharoensuk et al, 2001b*). High dietary intake of phosphorus enhances urinary phosphorus excretion and therefore, promotes superaturation of urine with magnesium, ammonium, and phosphate (*Finco et al, 1989*).

Management

Elimination of the urinary tract infection

Although not common, infection-induced struvite uroliths require a combination of an appropriate antimicrobial and dissolution dietary therapy (see below).

FIGURE 28 - THE ASSOCIATION BETWEEN URINE pH AND RSS FOR STRUVITE IN FELINE URINE
(*Royal Canin Research Center 2005; internal data collected during a 2 year-period*)

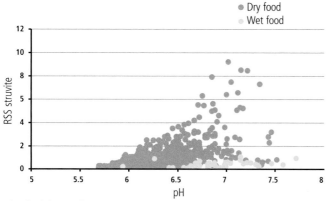

Individual data collected with 125 different diets fed to a group of 7 cats. Each point represents one cat fed one diet. The more alkaline the urine, the higher the risk of struvite formation.

TABLE 10 - THE RISK OF FORMING STRUVITE DEPENDS ON THE URINE pH AND FORM OF MAGNESIUM
(*Adapted from Buffington et al, 1990*)

	Basal diet 0.05% Mg	MgCl₂ diet 0.5% Mg	MgO diet 0.5% Mg
pH	7.2 ± 0.3	5.8 ± 0.1	7.9 ± 0.3
Magnesium (mMol)	7.3 ± 2.8	53.1 ± 16.3	49.1 ± 14.4
Calcium (mMol)	4.7 ± 1.5	15.5 ± 8.2	8.1 ± 3.6
RSS struvite	24.7	0.7	87.1
RSS calcium oxalate	41.3	12.8	8.6

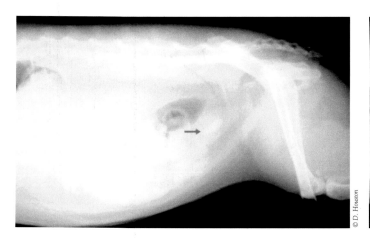

Figure 29A - Lateral radiograph of the abdomen of a cat. *The arrow points to a large, single urolith.*

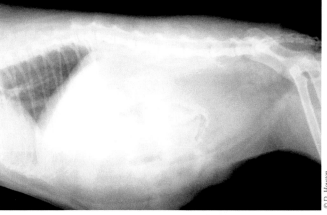

Figure 29B - Lateral radiograph of the abdomen of a cat four weeks after institution of a struvite dissolution diet. *The previously noted urolith (Figure 29A) has completely dissolved.*

Antibiotic therapy should be based on culture and sensitivity determination of urine obtained by cystocentesis. Antibiotic therapy should be continued for one month following radiographic resolution of the urolith/s, as viable bacteria may remain in the urolith and uroliths may be too small or too lucent to see on radiographs post dissolution.

Calculolytic diets to dissolve struvite uroliths

Pure struvite uroliths can be dissolved by the administration of a diet that promotes an increased urine volume and a urine pH less than 6.3 (*Osborne et al, 1990a; Houston et al, 2004*). The diet should have a controlled magnesium level and create an RSS value less than one (undersaturated zone). The diet should contain adequate quantities of sodium to promote water intake and the formation of dilute urine. Sterile struvite uroliths do not need adjunctive antibiotic therapy.

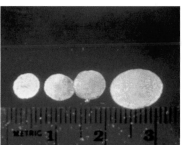

Figure 30 - Four struvite uroliths removed from the bladder of a cat. *Typical round to wafer or disc-shaped struvite uroliths.*

The efficacy of a canned, magnesium-restricted, urine acidifying, salt-supplemented diet designed to dissolve struvite urolithiasis was shown in 1990 (*Osborne et al, 1990a*). More recently, the efficacy of a canned and dry moderately magnesium restricted diet specifically designed to promote the formation of acidic urine, with a RSS value less than one for the dissolution of feline struvite urolithiasis has been reported by *Houston et al* (2004). In this study of 30 cats, the mean time required for dissolution of struvite uroliths was 26 days on the canned diet and 34 days on the dry diet (**Figure 29**).

It is recommended that dissolution therapy should continue for 1 month after radiographic documentation of struvite dissolution. If the urolith does not dissolve, the wrong mineral type or a complex mineral type may be involved.

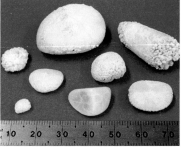

Figure 31 - A collection of feline struvite uroliths showing variability in appearance.

Prevention of recurrence

The recurrence rate for struvite uroliths has been reported as 2.7% with a mean recurrence time of 20 months (*Albasan et al, 2006*). Therefore, following dissolution or mechanical removal of struvite uroliths, a diet designed to help prevent recurrence is recommended. The diet should have a RSS in the undersaturated to metastable range, a urine pH less than 6.5 and should either be high in moisture (canned, pouch, or tray product) or designed to encourage diuresis (enhanced with sodium chloride).

Drug therapy

Urinary acidifying agents such as ammonium chloride or DL methionine are not necessary provided an appropriate urine acidifying diet is used.

Monitoring

The efficacy of therapy should be monitored with urinalysis (pH, urine specific gravity, sediment examination) at two weeks, four weeks and then every three to six months. Not all cats with uroliths shed crystals, therefore abdominal radiography should be obtained every three to six months to monitor for early urolith recurrence.

> Calcium oxalate (Figure 32)

Risk factors

The mean age at diagnosis of calcium oxalate urolithiasis in cats is 7.8 years, with a range of 2-18 years. The risk for calcium oxalate urolith formation increases with age. One study reported a bimodal age distribution peaking at 5 and 12 years. The highest risk for developing calcium oxalate uroliths appears to be from 7-10 year of age. *Smith et al* (1998), reported that senior cats (mean age 10.6 ± 1.3 years) produced urine that had significantly lower struvite RSS values (0.72 ± 0.58 vs. 4.98 ± 4.03) and significantly higher calcium oxalate RSS values (3.45 ± 1.62 vs. 0.91 ± 0.87) when compared to a group of younger (4.1 ± 1.0 years) cats. The senior cats had a significantly lower urine pH, compared to the younger cats (6.1 ± 0.2 vs. 6.4 ± 0.2, respectively). The decrease in urine pH in the senior cats may partially explain the increased risk for forming calcium oxalate uroliths with age (*Smith et al, 1998*).

Genetic and gender differences, inactivity, obesity, and environment have been associated with an increased risk for developing calcium oxalate uroliths (*Lekcharoensuk et al, 2001b*). Male cats (55%) are more commonly affected and are 1.5 times more likely to develop calcium oxalate uroliths compared to female cats. The Burmese, Himalayan, and Persian breeds have an increased risk of developing calcium oxalate urolithiasis, suggesting that genetic factors may contribute to the formation of calcium oxalate uroliths. Indoor housing has been reported as a risk factor for calcium oxalate urolithiasis (*Kirk et al, 1995; Jones et al, 1997; Gerber et al, 2005*).

In humans, hyperoxaluria occurs as a result of at least two types of inherited errors of metabolism, both resulting in increased oxalate production and recurrent calcium oxalate urolithiasis (*Williams & Wilson, 1990*). Inherited primary hyperoxaluria (L-glyceric aciduria), a deficiency of hepatic d-glycerate dehydrogenase, an enzyme required for metabolism of oxalic acid precursors, has been reported in cats but the clinical manifestations of this metabolic disorder have been related to weakness and acute onset of renal failure, not calcium oxalate urolithiasis (*McKerrell et al, 1989; De Lorenzi et al, 2005*).

The explanation for the increased risk of calcium oxalate uroliths in cats from 1984 to 2002 is not clear although the widespread use of severely magnesium-restricted, urine-acidifying diets to control struvite uroliths has been implicated (*Kirk et al, 1995; McClain et al, 1995; Thumachai et al, 1996; Osborne et al, 1996c; Lekcharoensuk et al, 2000; 2001a,b*). However, many cats are fed acidifying diets and yet few appear to develop hypercalcemia, metabolic acidosis, and calcium oxalate urolithiasis. Therefore additional factors such as gastrointestinal hyperabsorption or increased renal excretion of calcium and/or oxalate may be important in susceptible cats.

Acidosis

Lekcharoensuk et al (2000) reported that cats fed diets formulated to produce a urine pH between 5.99 and 6.15 were three times as likely to develop calcium oxalate uroliths. Persistent aciduria may be associated with low-grade metabolic acidosis, which promotes bone mobilization of carbonate and phosphorus to buffer hydrogen ions **(Figure 33)**. Simultaneous mobilization of calcium coupled with inhibition of renal tubular reabsorption of calcium, results in increased urinary excretion of calcium. Increased urinary calcium excretion has been reported in clinically normal cats fed diets supplemented with urinary acidifiers (*Fettman et al, 1992*). In five cats with hypercalcemia and calcium oxalate uroliths, discontinuation of the acidifying diets or urinary acidifiers was associated with normalization of serum calcium concentration (*McClain et al, 1999*).

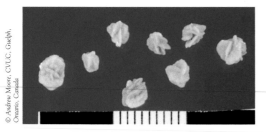

Figure 32 - Typical appearance of feline calcium oxalate uroliths.

FIGURE 33 - THE EFFECT OF METABOLIC ACIDOSIS ON URINARY CALCIUM EXCRETION.

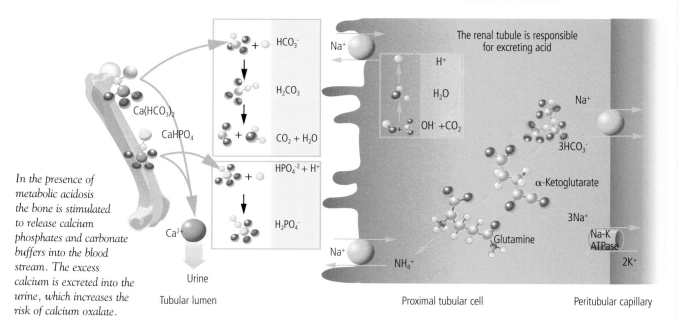

In the presence of metabolic acidosis the bone is stimulated to release calcium phosphates and carbonate buffers into the blood stream. The excess calcium is excreted into the urine, which increases the risk of calcium oxalate.

In one study on cats, the addition of an acidifier to a canned food was associated with a small but significant increase in calcium oxalate RSS. However, this higher RSS was still well below the formation product of 12 (*Stevenson et al, 2000*). Furthermore, this study demonstrated that it is possible to formulate a very acidifying diet (mean urine pH=5.8) that will both minimize struvite and calcium oxalate crystallization **(Figure 34)**. When comparing urinary pH and calcium oxalate RSS values associated with various commercial and experimental feline diets, urinary pH appears to be a very poor predictor of calcium oxalate RSS **(Figure 35)** (*Tournier et al, 2006b*).

Calcium

Hypercalciuria was a consistent abnormality in ten cats with calcium oxalate uroliths (*Lulich et al, 2004*). Increased intestinal absorption of calcium may occur due to excess dietary calcium, excess vitamin D, or hypophosphatemia. Increased renal excretion of calcium may occur with decreased renal tubular reabsorption (furosemide and corticosteroids), or increased mobilization of calcium from body stores (acidosis, hyperparathyroidism, hyperthyroidism, excessive vitamin D) (*Ling et al, 1990; Osborne, 1995a; 1996b; 2000*).

Protein

Diets high in animal protein have been associated with acidosis, increased urinary calcium and oxalate excretion, and decreased urinary citric acid excretion in humans (*Holmes et al, 2001; Borghi et al, 2002; Pietrow & Karellas, 2006*). Consumption of animal protein by both healthy cats and cats with calcium oxalate urolithiasis is associated with increased water consumption, urine volume, and urinary phosphorus excretion, while calcium excretion is not increased (*Funaba et al, 1996; Lekcharoensuk et al, 2001; Lulich at al 2004*). High protein diets (105-138 g/1000 kcal) were less than half as likely to be associated with calcium oxalate urolith formation as diets low in protein (52 - 80 g/1000 kcal) (*Lekcharoensuk et al, 2001b*). A case-control study reported that cats fed diets low in moisture and low in protein had an increased risk of calcium oxalate urolithiasis (*Lekcharoensuk et al,*

FIGURE 34 - INFLUENCE OF URINARY pH ON CALCIUM OXALATE AND STRUVITE RSS

(Adapted from Stevenson et al, 2000)

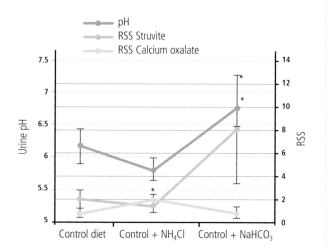

*p < 0.05

Mean ± SE urine pH, calcium oxalate and struvite RSS in six cats fed a control diet (C), the control diet with NH$_4$Cl or the control diet with NaHCO$_3$. Urine pH does significantly affect both RSS CaOx (NH$_4$Cl diet) and RSS Struvite (NaHCO$_3$ diet). However, even increased, the RSS CaOx is still well below the formation product.

FIGURE 35 - URINE pH IS A POOR PREDICTOR OF THE RISK OF CALCIUM OXALATE IN FELINE URINE

Data from 125 individual diets (from Tournier et al, 2006b)

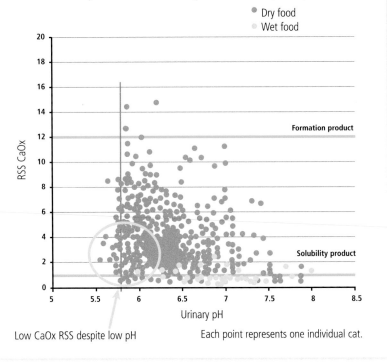

Low CaOx RSS despite low pH

Each point represents one individual cat.

2001b). Protein type has also been shown to influence urinary oxalate excretion in cats (*Zentek & Schultz, 2004*).

Water consumption

Intravascular volume depletion and concentration of urine volume increases the risk of urine supersaturation with calcium and oxalate. Cats fed diets high in moisture content are about one third as likely to develop calcium oxalate uroliths compared to cats fed diets low in moisture.

Oxalate

Excessive dietary oxalate (e.g., broccoli, spinach, rhubarb, nuts, strawberries) will increase the renal clearance of oxalate and the risk of urolithiasis in humans and such foods are to be avoided in pets (*Lulich et al, 1994; Holmes et al, 2001*).

Vitamin C

In humans, although controversial, calcium oxalate uroliths have been associated with excessive consumption of vitamin C and low levels of vitamin B_6 (*Hughes et al, 1981; Mitwalli, 1989; Curhan et al, 1999*). Vitamin C is metabolized to oxalic acid and excreted in urine. The effect of dietary vitamin C supplement on urinary oxalate concentration has been studied in 48 adult American Domestic Short Hair cats (*Yu et al, 2005*). Cats were fed a nutritionally complete and balanced dry control food for two weeks before they were fed for four weeks, one of four diets containing 40 mg/kg, 78 mg/kg, 106 mg/kg, or 193 mg/kg of vitamin C, respectively. Vitamin C supplementation up to 193 mg/kg did not affect urinary oxalate concentration in the healthy cats.

Vitamin B_6

Vitamin B_6 increases the transamination of glyoxylate, an important precursor of oxalic acid, to glycine. Therefore pyridoxine deficiency increases the endogenous production and subsequent excretion of oxalate. Experimentally induced vitamin B_6 deficiency resulting in increased urinary oxalate concentrations and oxalate nephrocalcinosis has been reported in kittens (*Bai et al, 1989*). However, a naturally occurring form of this syndrome has not yet been reported. Supplementation with vitamin B_6 does not decrease urinary oxalic acid excretion compared with a diet containing adequate levels of vitamin B_6 (*Wrigglesworth et al, 1999*). Consequently, the ability of supplemental vitamin B_6 to reduce urinary oxalic acid excretion in cats with calcium oxalate uroliths consuming diets with adequate quantities of vitamin B_6 is unlikely.

Citrate

Urinary citrate deficiency has been suggested to increase the risk of calcium oxalate in humans by increasing the availability of calcium ions to bind with oxalate (*Allie-Hamdulay & Rodgers, 2005; Pietrow & Karellas, 2006*). Citrate deficiency may be an inherited defect or be secondary to acidosis, which promotes the renal tubular utilization of citrate. If consumption of dietary acid precursors is associated with hypocitraturia in cats, the risk of calcium oxalate uroliths may increase as citrate is an inhibitor of calcium oxalate urolith formation (*Lekcharoensuk et al, 2001b*).

Magnesium

Magnesium has been reported to be an inhibitor of calcium oxalate urolithiasis in other species (*Johansson et al, 1980*). In cats, diets with low magnesium content (0.09-0.18 g/1000 kcal) are associated with an increased risk of calcium oxalate urolith formation, compared with diets with moderate magnesium content (0.19-0.35 g/1000 kcal) (*Lekcharoensuk et al, 2001b*). Conversely, diets with magnesium contents more than 0.36 g/1000 kcal were associated with an increased risk of calcium oxalate urolithiasis (*Lekcharoensuk et al, 2001b*). Magnesium contributes to increased urinary calcium loss by increasing blood-ionized calcium concentration and suppressing PTH secretion.

Phosphate

Hypophosphatemia may increase the risk of calcium oxalate urolithiasis in cats. The risk of calcium oxalate urolith formation was five times higher in cats fed a diet with 0.85-1.76 g/1000 kcal of phosphorus compared with a diet containing 1.77-3.16 g/1000 kcal of phosphorus (Lekcharoensuk et al, 2001b). Hypophosphatemia will result in the activation of Vitamin D_3 to calcitriol by 1-alpha-hydroxylase in the kidney and cause increased intestinal absorption and renal excretion of calcium. In addition, urinary pyrophosphate has been suggested to be an inhibitor of calcium oxalate urolith formation (*Osborne et al, 1995b; Reed et al, 2000b,c*). Conversely, diets higher in phosphorus (>3.17 g/1000 kcal) were associated with an increased risk of calcium oxalate urolith formation compared with diets containing moderate levels (1.77-3.16 g/1000 kcal) (*Lekcharoensuk et al, 2001b*).

Sodium

Supplemental sodium chloride has long been suggested to increase urinary calcium excretion in humans. Similar observations have been made in cats. The link between dietary Na and urinary Ca excretion led to the assumption that high salt diets could promote calcium oxalate formation in cats, and thus lead to the recommendation that diets designed for the management of FLUTD should be low in sodium. However, although increased sodium intake increases calcium excretion, calcium concentration does not increase because of the concomitant increase in urine volume and a significant decrease in CaOx RSS is observed (see above, Effect of dietary sodium on urinary calcium excretion). Furthermore, a recent epidemiological study found that increasing dietary sodium reduces the risk of calcium oxalate uroliths in cats (*Lekcharoensuk et al, 2001b*).

Potassium

Diets low in potassium have been shown to contribute to the risk for calcium oxalate uroliths (*Lekcharoensuk et al, 2001b*). Potassium-rich diets may be protective against calcium oxalate urolith formation by altering urinary calcium excretion. This has been shown to be true in humans (*Lemann et al, 1991*).

Management and prevention of recurrence

Calcium oxalate uroliths do not respond to medical dissolution. Consequently, cystouroliths must be mechanically removed by voiding urohydropropulsion or surgery. Once removed, preventive measures are indicated as the risk of recurrence is high.

Recurrence rates have been reported as 10.9% with a mean recurrence time of 20 months. The recurrence rate was 1.8 times higher in male compared to female cats (*Albasan et al, 2006*). Medical protocols are therefore essential to reduce urolith recurrence following removal.

Eliminate risk factors

If the cat is hypercalcemic, a complete medical work up is indicated to identify and treat the underlying cause. In many cases, an underlying cause for the hypercalcemia can not be determined.

If the cat is normocalcemic, risk factors for urolithiasis should be identified and controlled. Dry acidifying diets that have not been formulated to increase urine production and drugs that promote excessive urinary calcium excretion (urinary acidifiers, furosemide, etc.) should be avoided. No treats or dietary supplements containing calcium, vitamin D or excessive amounts of vitamin C should be given, as these may promote increased excretion of calcium and/or oxalate (*Osborne et al, 1995a*).

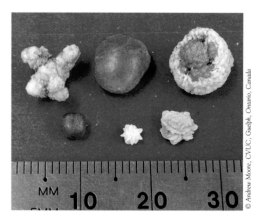

© Andrew Moore, CVUC, Guelph, Ontario, Canada

A collection of feline calcium oxalate uroliths indicating variability in appearance.
Most often, calcium oxalate dehydrate has a speculated appearance (bottom right corner); calcium oxalate monohydrate is often round (bottom left corner).

Dietary modification

Crystallization of calcium oxalate, the first step in the formation of this urolith cannot occur unless the urine is supersaturated with these crystalloids. Therefore, diets promoting the production of urine that is metastable or undersaturated with calcium oxalate should help prevent reoccurrence. The diet should produce an RSS value significantly less than 12 (ideally less than 5). Augmenting water intake remains a major factor in managing and preventing calcium oxalate urolithiasis (see above: Stimulate diuresis)

Calcium and oxalate

Studies have clearly shown that the concentrations of dietary calcium and dietary oxalate influence the urinary calcium oxalate RSS (*Smith et al, 1998; Markwell et al, 1998a; 1999a,b; Stevenson et al, 2000*). Excessive dietary calcium and dietary oxalate should be avoided but calcium oxalate preventive diets should not be calcium or oxalate restricted to any significant degree. Reducing consumption of either one of these constituents could increase the availability of the other constituent for intestinal absorption. In one study of ten cats, reduction in dietary calcium was not associated with increased urinary oxalic acid concentration (*Lulich et al, 2004*) but in other studies (*Lekcharoensuk et al, 2001b*), a decreased risk of calcium oxalate urolithiasis was observed in cats fed diets containing moderate quantities of dietary calcium.

Phosphorus, Magnesium, Potassium

Dietary phosphorus should not be restricted or supplemented (*Lekchareonesuk et al, 2001b*). The severe phosphate restriction may increase urinary calcium excretion, which contributes to urolith formation. Low protein/renal diets are not recommended because they are the lowest phosphorus containing diets.

As both dietary magnesium restriction and magnesium supplementation have been associated with an increased risk of calcium oxalate urolithiasis in cats; diets should neither be severely restricted nor supplemented with magnesium (*Osborne et al, 1995a; Lekcharoensuk et al, 2001b*).

Urinary pH

Recent work in our facility suggests that urine pH is not a good predictor of calcium oxalate saturation in healthy cats **(Figure 35)**. . Even though metabolic acidosis will increase urinary calcium concentration (*Kirk et al, 1995; McClain et al, 1995; Thumachai et al, 1996; Lekcharoensuk et al, 2000; 2001*), it is possible to formulate a diet that will induce a urine pH between 5.8-6.2 and still induce a RSS CaOx well below 5, thus allowing to prevent both struvite and calcium oxalate crystal formation.

Drug therapy and monitoring

Adjunct medical therapies with citrate, thiazide diuretics, and vitamin B_6 have been recommended in some cases of persistent calcium oxalate crystalluria or recurrent urolithiasis. Potassium citrate has been useful in humans to prevent recurrent calcium oxalate urolithiasis, via its ability to form soluble salts with calcium (*Pietrow & Karellas, 2006*). Oral potassium citrate increases the urine pH and may be of use in cases where the urine pH is more acidic than desired, a state that could contribute to hypocitraturia (*Osborne et al, 1995b; Lekcharoensuk et al, 2001b*).

Hydrochlorothiazide diuretics are used to treat people with calcium oxalate urolithiasis. Hydrochlorothiazide has been shown to decrease the calcium oxalate RSS in healthy adult cats (*Hezel et al, 2006*). However hydrochlorothiazide administration was associated with increased excretion of potassium, sodium, magnesium, phosphorus and chloride, which could result in whole body depletion with long term administration.

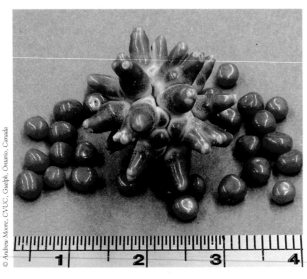

A collection of feline calcium oxalate uroliths.
The "Jackstone" like appearance may easily be mistaken for a silica urolith on radiograph.

The efficacy and safety of hydrochlorothiazide have not evaluated in cats with calcium oxalate uroliths, hence its use can not be recommended at this time.

Efficacy of therapy should be monitored with urinalysis (pH, urine specific gravity and sediment examination) at two weeks, four weeks and then every three to six months. As not all cats with calcium oxalate uroliths shed crystals, abdominal radiography should be completed every three to six months to reveal urolith recurrence at a time when the uroliths are small enough that voiding urohydropropulsion may be possible.

Managing renal and ureteral uroliths

Controversy exists as how to most effectively manage renal and ureteral uroliths. *Kyles et al* (2005) reported that 92% of cats with ureterolithiasis were azotemic at the time of presentation, 67% of cats had multiple uroliths, and 63% were affected bilaterally. The high probability of bilateral involvement, concurrent renal insufficiency, and likelihood of reoccurrence limit nephrectomy as a surgical option. Nephrotomy results in the unavoidable destruction of nephrons, hence, this surgery is not recommended unless it is clearly established that the renal uroliths are causing clinically significant disease. Ureterotomy may be indicated for those cats with progressive hydronephrosis and an identifiable ureterolith. Post-operative complications include uroabdomen and ureteral stricture. Alternatively, partially obstructing uroliths can be managed conservatively. The ureterolith will pass into the bladder in 30% of cats managed conservatively (*Kyles et al, 2005*). Although commonly used in human medicine, lithotripsy has not been established as a routine procedure in the cat.

> Calcium phosphate

Recognition and management of underlying contributing conditions is the first and most important step in the prevention of calcium phosphate urolithiasis. The cat should be assessed for evidence of primary hyperparathyroidism, hypercalcemia, excessive urine concentrations of calcium and/or phosphate, and an inappropriately alkaline urine pH (>7.5). There may also be a previous history of dietary therapy and administration of alkalinizing agents to prevent another urolith type. If a specific underlying disorder is not diagnosed, calcium phosphate uroliths are generally managed similar to strategies used for calcium oxalate urolithiasis. One should, however, be very careful to avoid excessive urine alkalinization, which may occur with some diets used for the prevention of calcium oxalate uroliths.

> Urate (Figure 36)

Risk factors

Urate uroliths are the third most common type of urolith reported in cats. They are composed of uric acid and the monobasic ammonium salt of uric acid (ammonium acid urate). Compared to struvite and calcium oxalate, the prevalence is less than six percent (*Osborne et al, 2000; Houston et al, 2004; 2006*) and this has not changed significantly in the last two decades. In Canada, ten of 321 (3.1%) ammonium urate submissions were from Siamese cats and nine of 321 (2.8%) were from Egyptian Maus (*Houston et al, 2006*).

Urate uroliths may occur in cats with portosystemic shunts or any form of severe hepatic dysfunction. This may be associated with reduced hepatic conversion of ammonia to urea resulting in hyperammonemia. Urate uroliths in cats with portosystemic shunts often contain struvite. Urate uroliths may also occur:
• in cats with urinary tract infections that result in increased urinary ammonia concentrations,
• in cats with metabolic acidosis and highly acidic urine,
• and when cats are fed diets high in purines, such as liver or other organ meats (*Osborne et al, 1992a; Ling 1995; Ling & Sorenson, 1995*).
In the majority of cases, the exact pathogenesis remains unknown (*Cannon et al, 2007*).

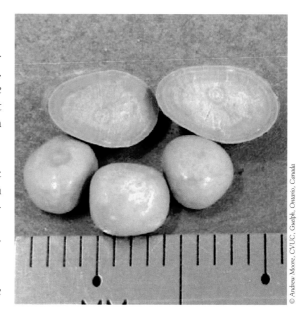

Figure 36 - Urate urolith.

309

FLUTD

Treatment

Urate uroliths may be amenable to dietary dissolution, however, there are no published clinical trials on the efficacy of diet for the medical dissolution of feline urate uroliths.

The dietary strategy aims at decreasing the purine content of the diet. As with all urolith types, encouraging water intake and urine dilution by feeding a moist (canned, pouch, tray) diet or adding supplemental water or sodium to the food can help to lower urinary saturation.

Alkalinization of urine

Alkaline urine contains low levels of ammonia and ammonium ions, and thus alkalinizing the urine will decrease the risk of ammonium urate urolithiasis. Low protein, vegetable based diets have an alkalinizing effect but additional potassium citrate may be needed. The dose should be individualized to maintain a urine pH in the range of 6.8-7.2. Alkalinizing the urine above 7.5 should be avoided as this may promote formation of secondary calcium phosphate crystals. If a vegetable based diet is used in a cat, care must be taken to ensure it is adequately balanced to meet the unique needs of the cat.

Xanthine oxidase inhibitors

Allopurinol, an inhibitor of xanthine oxidase, the enzyme responsible for catalyzing the conversion of xanthine and hypoxanthine to uric acid has been used in other species to help lower urinary urate excretion. Although a dosage of 9 mg/kg PO per day has been suggested for cats (*Plumb, 2002*), the efficacy and potential toxicity of allopurinol in cats is unknown and consequently, it's use in cats is not recommended.

Monitoring

During dissolution, the size of the urolith(s) should be monitored by survey and/or double contrast radiography or ultrasonography every four to six weeks. Following complete dissolution, ultrasound examination (or double contrast cystography) is recommended at least every two months for one year as the risk of recurrence is high. The efficacy of preventative therapy should be also be monitored with urinalysis (pH, urine specific gravity, sediment examination) every three to six months.

> Cystine (Figure 37)

Risk factors

Cystine uroliths occur in cats with cystinuria, an inborn error of metabolism characterized by a defective proximal tubular reabsorption of cystine and other amino acids (ornithine, lysine, arginine) (*DiBartola et al, 1991; Osborne et al, 1992a; Ling, 1995; Osborne et al, 1996*). No obvious gender or breed predisposition has been reported but the Siamese breed may be at risk (*Ling et al, 1990; Osborne et al, 2000; Cannon, 2007*). Most cats are middle to older aged (*Kruger et al, 1991*).

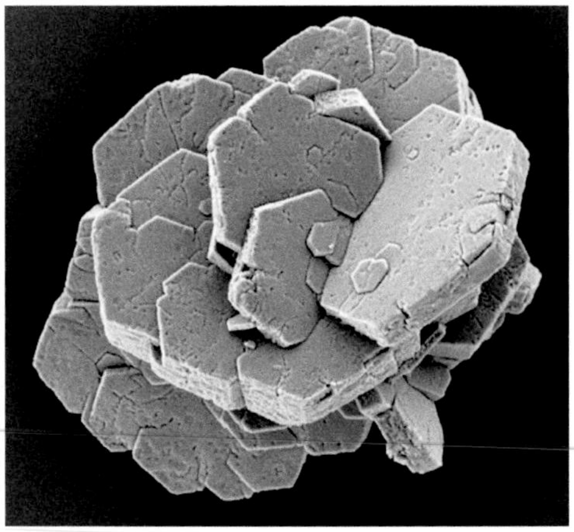

Management

Medical protocols that consistently promote the dissolution of cystine uroliths in cats have not yet been developed (*Osborne et al, 2000*). Small uroliths may be removed by voiding urohydropulsion (*Lulich et al, 19993b*). Cystotomy is required to remove larger uroliths.

If medical dissolution is attempted, the aim of therapy is to reduce the concentration of cystine in the urine and to increase cystine solubility. This usually requires dietary modification with a methionine-cystine reduced protein diet in combination with a thiol-containing drug.

Thiol-containing drugs

These drugs react with cystine by a thiol disulfide exchange reaction, resulting in the formation of a complex that is more soluble in urine than cystine. N-2-mercaptopropionyl-glycine (2-MPG) is recommended at a dosage of 12-20 mg/kg q 12 hours (*Osborne et al, 2000*).

© Andrew Moore, CVUC, Guelph, Ontario, Canada

Figure 37 - *Scanning electron microscope image of a cystine urolith from a cat.*

Alkalinization of urine

The solubility of cystine is pH dependent, being markedly more soluble in alkaline urine. Urine alkalinization may be achieved using a diet that contains potassium citrate or additional potassium citrate may be administered.

Monitoring

During dissolution, the size of the urolith(s) should be monitored by survey and double contrast radiography or ultrasonography every four to six weeks. Following complete dissolution, ultrasound examination (or double contrast cystography) is recommended at least every two months for one year as risk of recurrence is high. Efficacy of therapy should be also be monitored with urinalysis (pH, urine specific gravity, sediment examination) every two to three months.

> Xanthine (Figure 38)

Xanthine uroliths are rare and may be due to an inborn error of purine metabolism or arise secondary to the administration of allopurinol. In most cases, no identifying risk factors are observed. There is no apparent breed, age or sex predisposition reported (*Osborne et al, 1992a; 1996b; White et al, 1997*).

The dietary strategy aims at decreasing the purine content of the diet. As with all urolith types, encouraging water intake and urine dilution by feeding a moist (canned, pouch, tray) diet or adding supplemental water or sodium to the food can help to lower urinary saturation. Allopurinol therapy must be discontinued in the management of urate urolithiasis as it is a contributing factor to xanthine urolith formation.

> Silica (Figure 39)

Silica uroliths are uncommon. Based on limited numbers, there is no breed predisposition. In Canada, males outnumbered females in submission (*Houston et al, 2006*). The pathogenesis, at least in dogs, may involve consumption of an absorbable form of silica in various foods, resulting in urinary silica hyperexcretion. There may be some relationship to the increased use of plant-derived ingredients such as fibers and bran in pet foods (*Osborne et al, 1995a,b*).

Silica uroliths may be an incidental findings in cats. Surgical removal is indicated if clinical signs of FLUTD are thought to be due to the urolith. Because the initiating and precipitating causes of silica urolithiasis are unknown, only nonspecific dietary recommendations can be made. Empiric recommendations are to change the diet to one with high quality protein and if possible, reduced quantities of plant ingredients. Increased water intake and urine dilution is to be encouraged.

> Miscellaneous uroliths

Potassium magnesium pyrophosphate uroliths have been reported in four Persian cats (*Frank et al, 2002*). In Canada, a total of 15 potassium magnesium pyrophosphate uroliths have been analyzed at the Canadian Veterinary Urolith Center. Two thirds were identified in male cats. The majority occurred in domestic cats (66.7%). There was one male and one female Himalayan, one male and one female Persian, and one male Maine Coon cat. There were an additional nine uroliths with a nidus of either calcium oxalate (eight) or struvite (one) surrounded by pyrophosphate uroliths or shells. Although the etiology is not definitively known, it is postulated that it is related to some temporary or permanent enzyme dysfunction causing pyrophosphate supersaturation of the urine, which leads to crystallization of the urolith (*Frank et al, 2002*).

Dried solidified blood uroliths (**Figure 40**) have been reported in cats in North America (*Westropp et al, 2006*). Their etiology remains unknown. These uroliths usually do not contain any mineral material and a large number are radio-transparent.

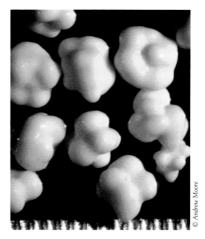

© Andrew Moore

Figure 38 - Xanthine urolith (scale: 0.1 mm markings). *Small xanthine calculi from a 9 month male siamese cross cat. The pale color is atypical; usually they are green or yellow.*

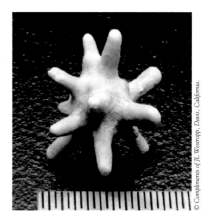

© Compliments of JL Westropp, Davis, California.

Figure 39 - *Silica urolith.*

FLUTD

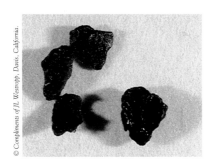

Figure 40 - A collection of dried solidified blood uroliths from the bladder of a cat.

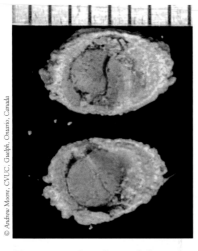

Figure 41 - Complex urolith removed from a cat. The urolith was submitted for quantitative analysis: once opened, the nidus was analyzed as ammonium acid urate. The shell was determined to be struvite.

Because the initiating and precipitating causes of both potassium magnesium pyrophosphate uroliths and dried solidified blood uroliths are unknown, only nonspecific dietary recommendations can be made. Empiric recommendations are to change the diet to one that is highly digestible and low in fiber with high quality protein. Increased water intake and urine dilution is to be encouraged.

> Compound uroliths

Compound uroliths consist of a nidus of one mineral type and a urolith or shell of another mineral type **(Figure 41)**. They form because factors promoting precipitation of one type of urolith supersede earlier factors promoting precipitation of another mineral type. Some mineral types may also function as a nidus for the deposition of another mineral type; for instance, all urolith types predispose to urinary tract infections, which in turn, may result in secondary struvite precipitation *(Osborne et al, 2000)*.

The possibility of compound uroliths highlights the need to submit uroliths for quantitative analysis so that the appropriate dietary and medical strategy can be implemented. The dietary strategy aims at managing the factors that lead to the formation of the nidus. As with all urolith types, encouraging water intake and urine dilution by feeding a moist (canned, pouch, tray) diet or adding supplemental water or sodium to the food can help to lower urinary saturation.

Conclusion

Encouraging water intake to enhance urine volume and diuresis is paramount for the management of all cats with clinical signs of lower urinary tract disease. For FIC, urine dilution decreases noxious, irritating substances in the bladder. For urethral plugs, urine dilution and enhanced urine volume will also help decrease the concentration of proteinaceous material and urinary tract debris. For urolithiasis, urine dilution enhances urine volume for a given solute load, reduces saturation, and decreases the concentrations of crystalloids. In addition, increasing urine volume may influence crystal transit time through the urinary tract, thus reducing the potential for crystal growth.

Dietary modification is an important part of the management regimen for cats with urolithiasis, regardless of the cause. Specific dietary recommendations for individual uroliths are dependent on the mineral composition of the urolith. For cats with struvite urolithiasis, control of magnesium and reduction of urine pH through dietary manipulation are necessary to achieve urine which is undersaturated with struvite. For cats with calcium oxalate urolithiasis, attention is paid to the amount of calcium and oxalate precursors in the diet and the goal is to achieve an RSS in the metastable range. Manipulating urinary pH is not effective for the management of calcium oxalate uroliths. For metabolic uroliths (cystine, xanthine, urate), reduced quantities of dietary protein are recommended and urine pH is adjusted to be in the neutral to alkaline range.

Frequently asked questions
about nutritional management
of feline lower urinary tract disorders

Q	**A**
A cat presents with hematuria and inappropriate urination. There are no bacteria seen on the urinalysis. Should I treat the cat with antibiotics and see if he responds to therapy or should I recommend radiographs or other diagnostic procedures?	Urinary tract infections (UTIs) are very uncommon (<1%) in healthy cats and the routine use of antibiotics is not recommended. Idiopathic cystitis or urolithiasis is more common than UTIs in cats and a radiograph is indicated. Struvite and calcium oxalate uroliths are the two most common uroliths in cats and they are both radiodense. Note: urate and cystine stones are usually radiolucent, and require positive contrast studies or ultrasound for determination.
If I see a urolith on a radiograph, is it most likely to be struvite or calcium oxalate?	In some regions of the world, struvite predominates in cats; in other regions, calcium oxalate uroliths are more common. Therefore, rather than predict what the urolith is, it is appropriate to retrieve a urolith and perform quantitative analysis. The urolith can be retrieved via free catch using an aquarium net, via catheter assistance, voiding urohydropropulsion, cystoscopy or cystotomy. Urine pH and sediment examination may or may not be helpful as crystals may not be passed at all or the crystals that are present could be different than the underlying urolith that is present. If struvite is suspected, dissolution therapy may be attempted. Failure to dissolve the uroliths within six weeks suggests the urolith is of a different mineral composition and surgical removal is indicated.
Are kidney stones in cats more likely to be struvite or calcium oxalate?	In cats, approximately 70% of nephroliths are calcium oxalate. Calcium oxalate nepholiths are present in up to 50% of cats with renal disease. Therefore, all cats that have renal disease should have abdominal radiographs. It is important to recognize if nephroliths are present and to monitor for obstruction and a decline in renal function.
How should nephroliths and ureteroliths be managed in cats?	If the nephroliths are causing complete obstruction or progressive deterioration in renal function, surgical removal is indicated. However, because of the unavoidable destruction of nephrons during nephrotomy, surgical removal is not recommended unless it can be established that the uroliths are the cause of clinically significant disease. If not, the patient should be monitored for indications of disease progression or ureteral obstruction. In many cases, ureteroliths will migrate into the bladder so it is appropriate to obtain serial radiographs to monitor for urolith movement.
How often should the cat be reexamined after a urolith has been removed? What diagnostic tests are recommended to monitor the patient?	Because many uroliths have a high risk of recurrence, it is recommended to obtain radiographs every three to six months. For metabolic uroliths (urate, cystine), contrast radiography or ultrasound examination may be necessary as these stones are typically radiolucent. Urine pH and urine specific gravity should be performed every three months to ensure owner compliance and diet efficacy.

References

Albasan H, Lulich JP, Osborne CA, et al. *Effects of storage time and temperature on pH, specific gravity, and crystal formation in urine samples from dogs and cats.* J Am Vet Med Assoc 2003; 222: 176-179.

Albasan H, Osborne CA, Lulich JP, et al. *Urolith recurrence in cats.* J Vet Intern Med 2006; 20: 786-787.

Allie-Hamdulay S, Rodgers AL. *Prophylactic and therapeutic properties of a sodium citrate preparation in the management of calcium oxalate urolithiasis: randomized, placebo-controlled trial.* Urol Res 2005; 33: 116-124.

Bai SC, Sampson DA, Morris JG, et al. *Vitamin B-6 requirement of growing kittens.* J Nutr 1989; 119: 1020-27

Bartges JW. *Lower urinary tract disease in geriatric cats.* Proceedings of the 15th American College of Veterinary Internal Medicine Forum, Lake Buena Vista, Florida, 1997: 322-324.

Borghi L, Schianchi T, Meschi T, et al. *Comparison of two diets for the prevention of recurrent stones in idiopathic hypercalciuria.* N Engl J Med 2002; 346: 77-84.

Biourge V. *Urine dilution: a key factor in the prevention of struvite and calcium oxalate uroliths.* Veterinary Focus 2007; 17: 41-44.

Biourge V, Devois C, Morice G, et al. *Dietary NaCl significantly increases urine volume but does not increase urinary calcium oxalate supersaturation in healthy cats.* J Vet Intern Med 2001; 15: 866.

Buffington CA, Rogers QR, Morris JG. *Effect of diet on struvite activity product in feline urine.* Am J Vet Res 1990; 151: 2025-2030.

Buffington CA, Chew DJ, DiBartola SP. *Lower urinary tract disease in cats: Is diet still a cause?* J Am Vet Med Assoc 1994; 205: 1524-1527.

Buffington CA, Chew DJ. *Intermittent alkaline urine in a cat fed an acidifying diet.* J Am Vet Med Assoc 1996a; 209: 103-104.

Buffington CA, Blaisdell JL, Binns SP. *Decreased urine glycosaminoglycan excretion in cats with interstitial cystitis.* J Urol 1996b; 155: 1801-1804.

Buffington CA, Chew DJ, Kendall MS, et al. *Clinical evaluation of cats with nonobstructive lower urinary tract diseases.* J Am Vet Med Assoc 1997; 210: 46-50.

Buffington CA, Chew DJ, Woodworth BE. *Feline interstitial cystitis.* J Am Vet Med Assoc 1999a; 215: 682-687.

Buffington CA, Chew DJ. *Diet therapy in cats with lower urinary tract disorders.* Vet Med 1999b; 94: 626-630.

Buffington CA, Pacak K. *Increased plasma norepinephrine concentration in cats with interstitial cystitis.* J Urol 2001; 165: 2051-2054.

Buffington CA. *External and internal influences on disease risk in cats.* J Am Vet Med Assoc 2002; 220: 994-1002.

Buffington CA. *Comorbidity of interstitial cystitis with other unexplained clinical conditions.* J Urology 2004; 172: 1242-1248.

Buffington CA, Westropp JL, Chew DJ, et al. *Risk factors associated with clinical signs of lower urinary tract disease in indoor-housed cats.* J Am Vet Med Assoc 2006a; 228: 722-725.

Buffington CAT, Westropp JL, Chew DJ, et al. *Clinical evaluation of multimodal environmental modification (MEMO) in the management of cats with idiopathic cystitis.* J Feline Med Surg 2006b; 8: 261-268.

Buranakarl C, Mathur S, Brown SA. *Effects of dietary sodium chloride intake on renal function and blood pressure in cats with normal and reduced renal function.* Am J Vet Res 2004; 65: 620-627.

Burger I, Anderson RS, Holme DW. *Nutritional factors affecting water balance in dog and cat.* In: Anderson RS (ed) Nutrition of the Cat and Dog. Oxford. Pergamon Press, 1980: 145-156.

Cameron ME, Casey RA, Bradshaw JW, et al. *A study of environmental and behavioural factors that may be associated with feline idiopathic cystitis.* J Small Anim Pract 2004; 45: 144-147.

Cannon AB, Westropp JL, Ruby AL, et al. *Evaluation of trends in urolith composition in cats: 5,230 cases (1985-2004).* J Am Vet Med Assoc 2007; 231: 570-576.

Chew DJ, Buffington T, Kendall MS, et al. *Urethroscopy, cystoscopy, and biopsy of the feline lower urinary tract.* Vet Clin North Am 1996; 26: 441-462.

Chew DJ, Buffington CA, Kendall MS. *Amitriptyline treatment for severe recurrent idiopathic cystitis in cats.* J Am Vet Med Assoc 1998; 213: 1282-1286.

Chew DG, Buffington CA. *Diagnosis and management of idiopathic cystitis/interstitial cystitis in cats.* Proceedings of the North American Veterinary Conference, Orlando, Florida; 2003: 556-560.

Cowgill LD, Sergev G, Bandt C, et al. *Effects of dietary salt intake on body fluid volume and renal function in healthy cats.* J Vet Intern Med 2007; 21: 600

Curham GC, Willett WC, Speizer FE, et al. *Intake of vitamins B6 and C and the risk of kidney stones in women.* J Am Soc Nephrol 1999; 10: 840-845.

De Lorenzi D, Bernardini M, Pumarola M. *Primary hyperoxaluria (L-glyceric aciduria) in a cat.* J Feline Med Surg 2005; 7: 357-361.

Devois C, Biourge V, Morice G, et al. *Influence of various amounts of dietary NaCl on urinary Na, Ca, and oxalate concentrations and excretions in adult cats.* Proceedings of the 10th Congress of the European Society of Veterinary Internal Medicine, Neuchâtel, Suisse; 2000a: 85.

Devois C, V Biourge, Morice G, et al. *Struvite and oxalate activity product ratios and crystalluria in cats fed acidifying diets.* Urolithiasis, Cape Town; 2000b: 821-823.

DiBartola SP, Chew DJ, Horton ML, et al. *Cystinuria in a cat.* J Am Vet Med Assoc 1991; 198: 102-104.

Dumon H, Nguyen P, Martin L, et al. *Influence of wet vs. dry food on cat urinary pH: preliminary study.* J Vet Intern Med 1999; 13: 726.

Fennell C. *Some demographic characteristics of the domestic cat population in Great Britain with particular reference to feeding habits and the incidence of the Feline Urological Syndrome.* J Small Anim Pract 1975; 16: 775-783.

Fettman MJ, Coble JM, Hamar DW, et al. *Effect of dietary phosphoric acid supplementation on acid-base balance and mineral and bone metabolism in adult cats.* Am J Vet Res 1992; 53: 2125-2135.

Finco DR, Barsanti JA, Brown SA. *Influence of dietary source of phosphorus on fecal and urinary excretion of phosphorus and other minerals by male cats.* Am J Vet Res 1989; 50: 263-266.

Forrester SD. *Evidence-based nutritional management of feline lower urinary tract disease.* Proceedings of the 24th American College of Veterinary Internal Medicine Forum, Louisville, Kentucky, 2006: 510-512.

Frank A, Norrestam R, Sjodin A. A new urolith in four cats and a dog: composition and crystal structure. J Biol Inorg Chem 2002; 7: 437-444.

Funaba M, Hashimoto M, Yamanaka C, et al. Effects of high-protein diet on mineral metabolism and struvite activity product in clinically normal cats. Am J Vet Res 1996; 57: 1726-1732.

Gerber B, Boretti FS, Kley S, et al. Evaluation of clinical signs and causes of lower urinary tract disease in European cats. J Small Anim Pract 2005; 46: 571-577.

Gunn-Moore DA, Cameron ME. A pilot study using feline facial pheromone for the management of feline idiopathic cystitis. J Feline Med Surg 2004; 6: 133-138.

Gunn-Moore DA, Shenoy CM. Oral glucosamine and the management of feline idiopathic cystitis. J Feline Med and Surg 2004; 6: 219-225.

Hawthorne AJ, Markwell PJ. Dietary sodium promotes increased water intake and urine volume in cats. J Nutr 2004; 134: 2128S-2129S.

Hezel A, Bartges J, Kirk C, et al. Influence of hydrochlorothiazide on urinary calcium oxalate relative supersaturation in healthy adult cats. J Vet Intern Med 2006: 20: 741.

Holmes RP, Goodman HO, Assimos DG. Contribution of dietary oxalate to urinary oxalate excretion. Kidney Int 2001; 59: 270-276.

Hostutler RA, Chew DJ, DiBartola SP. Recent concepts in feline lower urinary tract disease. Vet Clin North Am Small Anim Pract 2005; 35: 147-170.

Houston DM, Moore AE, Favrin MG, et al. Feline urethral plugs and bladder uroliths: a review of 5484 submissions 1998-2003. Can Vet J 2003; 44: 974-977.

Houston DM, Rinkardt NE, Hilton J. Evaluation of the efficacy of a commercial diet in the dissolution of feline struvite bladder uroliths. Vet Therap 2004; 5: 187-201.

Houston DM, Moore AE, Favrin MG, et al. Data on file, Canadian Veterinary Urolith Centre, University of Guelph, Lab Services, Guelph, Ontario, Canada; 2006.

http://www.indoor/www.indoorcat.org/: The Indoor Cat Initiative 2006.

Hughes C, Dutton S, Stewart-Truswell A. High intakes of ascorbic acid and urinary oxalate. Human Nutrition 1981; 35: 274-280.

Hughes KL, Slater MR, Geller S, et al. Diet and lifestyle variable as risk factors for chronic renal failure in cats. Prev Vet Med 2002; 10: 1-15.

Johansson G, Backman U, Danielson BG, et al. Biochemical and clinical effects of the prophylactic treatment of renal calcium stones with magnesium hydroxide. J Urol 1980: 124: 770-774.

Jones BR, Sanson RL, Morris RS. Elucidating the risk factors of feline lower urinary tract disease. NZ Vet J 1997; 45: 100-108.

Kirk CA, Ling GV, Franti CE, et al. Evaluation of factors associated with development of calcium oxalate urolithiasis in cats. J Am Vet Med Assoc 1995; 207: 1429-1434.

Kirschvink N, Lhoest E, Leemans J, et al. Effects of feeding frequency on water intake in cats. J Vet Intern Med 2005; 19: 476.

Kraiger M, Fink-Gremmels J, Nickel RF. The short term clinical efficacy of amitriptyline in the management of idiopathic feline lower urinary tract disease: a controlled clinical study. J Feline Med Surg 2003; 5: 191-196.

Kruger JM, Osborne CA, Goyal SM, et al. Clinical evaluation of cats with lower urinary tract disease. J Am Vet Med Assoc 1991; 199: 211-216.

Kruger JM, Conway TS, Kaneene JB, et al. Randomized controlled trial of the efficacy of short-term amitriptyline administration for treatment of acute, nonobstructive, idiopathic lower urinary tract disease in cats. J Am Vet Med Assoc 2003; 222: 749-758.

Kyles AE, Hardie EM, Wooden BG, et al. Management and outcome of cats with ureteral calculi: 153 cases (1984-2002). J Am Vet Med Assoc 2005; 226: 937-944.

Laboto MA. Managing urolithiasis in cats. Vet Med 2001; 96: 708-718.

Lawler DF, Sjolin DW, Collins JE. Incidence rates of feline lower urinary tract disease in the United States. Feline Pract 1985; 15: 13-16.

Lekcharoensuk C, Lulich JP, Osborne CA, et al. Association between patient-related factors and risk of calcium oxalate and magnesium ammonium phosphate urolithiasis in cats. J Am Vet Med Assoc 2000; 217: 520-525.

Lekcharoensuk C, Osborne CA, Lulich JP, et al. Epidemiologic study of risk factors for lower urinary tract diseases in cats. J Am Vet Med Assoc 2001a; 218: 1429-1435.

Lekcharoensuk C, Osborne CA, Lulich JP, et al. Association between dietary factors and calcium oxalate and magnesium ammonium phosphate urolithiasis in cats. J Am Vet Med Assoc 2001b; 219: 1228-1237.

Lemann J Jr, Pleuss JA, Gray RW, et al. Potassium administration increases and potassium deprivation reduces urinary calcium excretion in healthy adults. Kidney Int 1991; 39: 973-983.

Li X, Li W, Wang H, et al. Cats lack a sweet taste receptor. J Nutr 2006; 136; 1932S-1934S.

Ling GV, Franti CE, Ruby AL, et al. Epizootiologic evaluation and quantitative analysis of urinary calculi from 150 cats. J Am Vet Med Assoc 1990; 196: 1459-1462.

Ling GV, Sorenson JL. CVT Update: Management and prevention of urate urolithiasis. In: Bonagura JD, Kirk RW (eds). Kirk's Current Veterinary Therapy XII Small Animal Practice. Philadelphia: WB Saunders Co, 1995: 985-989.

Ling GV. Lower Urinary Tract Diseases of Dogs and Cats. Diagnosis, medical management, prevention. St. Louis: Mosby, 1995: 143-177.

Luckschander N, Iben C, Hosgood G, et al. Dietary NaCl does affect blood pressure in healthy cats. J Vet Intern Med 2004; 18: 463-467.

Lulich JP, Osborne CA. Catheter assisted retrieval of urocystoliths from dogs and cats. J Am Vet Med Assoc 1992; 201: 111-113.

Lulich JP, Osborne CA, Polzin DJ, et al. Incomplete removal of canine and feline urocystoliths by cystotomy. Proceedings of the 11th American College of Veterinary Internal Medicine Forum, Washington, DC, 1993a: 397.

Lulich JP, Osborne CA, Carlson M, et al. Nonsurgical removal of urocystoliths in dogs and cats by voiding urohydropropulsion. J Am Vet Med Assoc 1993b; 203: 660-663.

Lulich JP, Osborne CA, Felice L. Calcium oxalate urolithiasis: cause, detection and control. In: August JR (ed). Consultations in Feline Internal Medicine. Philadelphia: WB Saunders, 1994: 343-349.

FLUTD

Lulich JP, Osborne CA, Lekcharoensuk C, et al. Effects of diet on urine composition of cats with calcium oxalate urolithiasis. J Am Anim Hosp Assoc 2004; 40: 185-191.

Lund EM, Armstrong PJ, Kirk CA, et al. Health status and population characteristics of dogs and cats examined at private veterinary practices in the United States. J Am Vet Med Assoc 1999; 214: 1336-1341.

Markwell PJ, Buffington CT, Smith BH. The effect of diet on lower urinary tract disease in cats. J Nutr 1998; 128: 2753S-2757S.

Markwell PJ, Buffington CA, Chew DJ, et al. Clinical evaluation of commercially available acidification diets in the management of idiopathic cystitis in cats. J Am Vet Med Assoc 1999a; 214: 361-365.

Markwell PJ, Smith BHE, McCarthy K. A non-invasive method for assessing the effect of diet on urinary calcium oxalate and struvite supersaturation in the cat. Animal Technology 1999b; 50: 61-67.

McCarthy TC. Cystoscopy and biopsy of the feline lower urinary tract. Vet Clin North Am 1996; 26: 463-482.

McClain HM, Barsanti JA, Bartges JW. Hypercalcemia and calcium oxalate urolithiasis in cats: a report of 5 cases. J Am Anim Hosp Assoc 1999; 35: 297-301.

McKerrell RE, Blakemore WF, Heath MF, et al. Primary oxaluria (L-glyceric aciduria) in the cat: a newly recognized inherited disease. Vet Rec 1989; 125: 31-34.

Mealey KL, Peck KE, Bennett BS, et al. Systemic absorption of amitriptyline and buspirone after oral and transdermal administration to healthy cats. J Vet Intern Med 2004; 18: 43-46.

Midkiff AM, Chew DJ, Randolph JF, et al. Idiopathic hypercalcemia in cats. J Vet Intern Med 2000; 14: 619-626.

Mills DS, Mills CB. Evaluation of a novel method for delivering a synthetic analogue of feline facial pheromone to control urine spraying by cats. Vet Rec 2001; 149: 197-199.

Mitwalli A. Control of hyperoxaluria with large doses of pyridoxine in patients with kidney stones. Annals of Saudi Medicine 1989; 541-546.

Nordin BEC, Robertson WG. Calcium phosphate and oxalate ion-products in normal and stone forming urines. Br Med J 1966; 1: 450-453.

Osborne CA, Kruger JM, Polzin DJ, et al. Medical dissolution and prevention of feline struvite uroliths. In: Kirk RW (ed). Current Veterinary Therapy IX. Philadelphia: WB Saunders 1986: 1188-1195.

Osborne CA, Lulich JP, Kruger JM, et al. Medical dissolution of feline struvite urocystoliths. J Am Vet Med Assoc 1990a; 196: 1053-1063.

Osborne CA, Lulich JP, Bartges JW, et al. Feline metabolic uroliths: risk factor management. In: Kirk RW, Bonagura JD (eds). Current Veterinary Therapy XI. Philadelphia: WB Saunders, 1992a: 905-909.

Osborne CA, Kruger JM, Lulich JP, et al. Feline matrix-crystalline urethral plugs: a unifying hypothesis of causes. J Small Anim Pract 1992b; 33: 172-177.

Osborne CA, Kruger JM, Lulich JP, et al. Feline lower urinary tract diseases. In: Ettinger SJ, Feldman EC (eds). Textbook of Veterinary Internal Medicine 4th ed. Philadelphia: WB Saunders 1995a: 1805-1832.

Osborne CA, Kruger JM, Lulich JP, et al. Disorders of the feline lower urinary tract. In: Osborne CA and Finco DR (eds). Canine and Feline Nephrology and Urology. Baltimore: Williams and Wilkins 1995b; 625-680.

Osborne CA Kruger JM, Lulich JP. Feline lower urinary tract disorders. Definition of terms and concepts. Vet Clin North Am Small Anim Pract 1996a; 26: 169-179.

Osborne CA, Lulich JP, Thumchai R et al. Feline Urolithiasis. Vet Clin North Am Small Anim Pract 1996b; 10: 217-232.

Osborne C, Polzin D, Kruger JM, et al. Relationship of nutritional factors to the cause, dissolution and prevention of feline uroliths and urethral plugs. Vet Clin North Am Small Anim Pract 1996c; 10: 561-581.

Osborne CA, Lulich JP, Kruger JM, et al. Feline urethral plugs-etiology and pathophysiology. Vet Clin North Am Small Anim Pract 1996d; 26: 233-253.

Osborne CA, Kruger JM, Lulich JP, et al. Feline Lower Urinary Tract Diseases. In: Ettinger SJ, Feldman EC (eds). Textbook of Veterinary Internal Medicine 5th ed. Philadelphia: WB Saunders Co, 2000: 1710-1747.

Pak CYC, Hayashi Y, Finlayson B, et al. Estimation of the state of saturation of brushite and calcium oxalate in urine: A comparison of three methods. J Lab Clin Med 1977; 89: 891-901.

Pereira DA, Aguiar JAK, Hagiwara MK, et al. Changes in cat urinary glycosaminoglycans with age and in feline urologic syndrome. Biochimica et Biophysica Acta 2004; 1672: 1-11.

Pietrow PK, Karellas ME. Medical management of common urinary calculi. Am Family Physician 2006; 74: 86-94.

Plumb DC. Veterinary Drug Handbook, 4th ed. Ames, Iowa, Iowa State University Press, 2002.

Reed CF, Markwell PJ, Jones CA, et al. The effects of oral magnesium salt administration on urinary calcium oxalate crystallization and agglomeration in cats. J Vet Intern Med 2000a; 14: 383.

Reed CF, Markwell PJ, Jones CA, et al. In vitro pyrophosphate supplementation in cat urine, and its effect on calcium oxalate formation and agglomeration. J Vet Intern Med 2000b; 14: 384.

Reed CF, Markwell PJ, Jones CA, et al. Oral orthophosphate salt administration and its effect on feline urinary calcium oxalate formation and agglomeration. J Vet Intern Med 2000c; 14: 351.

Robertson WG, Jones JS, Heaton MA, et al. Predicting the crystallization potential of urine from cats and dogs with respect to calcium oxalate and magnesium ammonium phosphate (struvite). J Nutr 2002; 132: 1637S-1641S

Samii VF. Urinary Tract Imaging. Proceedings of the 27th Waltham/OSU Symposium 2003; 15-17.

Savary KC, Price GS, Vaden SL. Hypercalcemia in cats: a retrospective study of 71 cases (1991-1997). J Vet Intern Med 2000; 14: 184-189.

Smith BH, Stevenson AE, Markwell PJ. Urinary relative supersaturations of calcium oxalate and struvite in cats are influenced by diet. J Nutr 1998; 128: 2763S-2764S.

Smith BHE, Moodie S, Markwell PJ. Longterm feeding of an acidifying diet to cats. J Vet Intern Med 2001; 15: 305.

Stevenson AE, Wrigglesworth DJ, Markwell PJ. Urine pH and urinary relative supersaturation in healthy adult cats. Urolithiasis 2000: 818-820.

FLUTD

Discussion and conclusion

With saturated urine (diet A - RSS = 7.3), little dissolution was observed over the duration of the study **(Figure 4)** possibly due to the abrasion of the stones during agitation.

When the RSS is < 1 (undersaturation zone), urine dissolves struvite stones efficiently **(Figure 4)** and the lower the RSS, the faster the dissolution kinetics **(Table 2)**. RSS is thus a good predictor of the potential of urine to dissolve struvite.

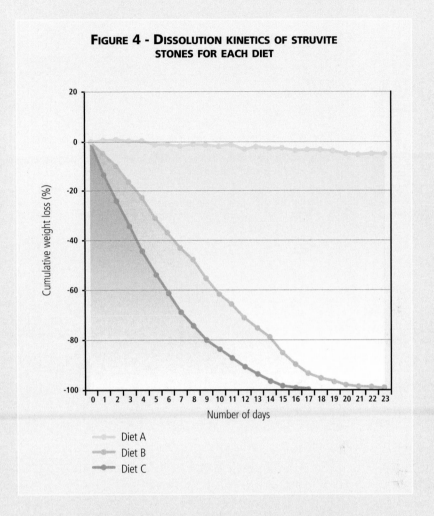

FIGURE 4 - DISSOLUTION KINETICS OF STRUVITE STONES FOR EACH DIET

— Diet A
— Diet B
— Diet C

TABLE 2 – DISSOLUTION SPEED OF STRUVITE STONES FOR EACH DIET			
	Diet A	Diet B	Diet C
Struvite RSS	7.30	0.45	0.19
Number of days before complete dissolution	-	23	17
Dissolution speed (mg/day)	0.01	8.52	11.59

Reference

Robertson WG, Jones JS, Heaton MA, et al. Predicting the crystallisation potential of urine from cats and dogs with respect to calcium oxalate and magnesium ammonium phosphate (struvite). J Nutr 2002; 132: 1637s-1641s.

Heart

Valérie CHETBOUL
DMV, PhD, Dipl.
ECVIM-CA (cardiology)

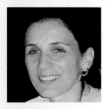

Vincent BIOURGE
DMV, PhD, Dipl. ACVN
& ECVCN

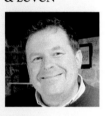

Acquired cardiovascular diseases in cats: the influence of nutrition

Introduction 325

1 - Systemic hypertension in cats 325

2 - Feline cardiomyopathies 332

3 - Nutritional recommendations for the management of feline cardiopathy 339

Conclusion 345

Frequently asked questions 346

References 348

Royal Canin nutritional information 352

Heart

ABBREVIATIONS USED IN THIS CHAPTER		
ACEI: angiotensin-converting enzyme inhibitors	**HCM**: hypertrophic cardiomyopathy	**SH**: systemic hypertension
BID: twice daily	**HR**: heart rate	**SID**: once daily
BP: blood pressure	**ME**: metabolizable energy	**TID**: three times a day
CKD: chronic kidney disease	**NRC**: National Research Council	**TPR**: total peripheral resistance
DCM: dilated cardiomyopathy	**RAAS**: renin-angiotensin-aldosterone system	
DMB: dry matter basis	**RCM**: restrictive cardiomyopathy	

Acquired cardiovascular diseases in cats: the influence of nutrition

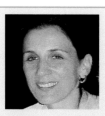

Valérie CHETBOUL
DVM, PhD, Dipl. ECVIM-CA (cardiology)

A qualified veterinarian since 1984 with a degree from the Alfort National Veterinary School (France), Professor Valérie Chetboul has taken training courses, obtained diplomas and carried out research projects in her favourite field, cardiology, in both Europe and the United States. In 1986, in collaboration with Professor Pouchelon, she opened the first echocardiography clinic for domestic carnivores. The growth of her field of specialization is illustrated by the creation of the Alfort Cardiology Unit and the first French Holter veterinary center (2000) and by an active collaboration with a cardiovascular surgical research unit in Paris (2002). Her involvement in the field of cardiovascular research was translated into her participation in the establishment of a National Health and Medical Research Institute center on the Alfort National Veterinary School campus (2005), attached to the University of Paris XII and dedicated to cardiology. She has published numerous articles in scientific referred journals with an international readership and has written several works, among which an 'An Echo-Doppler Colour Atlas of Dogs and Cats', which in 2002 earned her the Groulade Prize by the Veterinary Academy of France. She was editor-in-chief of the Journal of Veterinary Cardiology (2002-2006) and she is still editor of this journal. She has also given numerous papers at different international conferences, both in human and veterinary medicine. Her competence has been recognized by her peers, who in 2001 granted her the prestigious Award of the American College of Veterinary Internal Medicine.

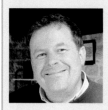

Vincent BIOURGE
DVM, PhD, Dipl. ACVN, Dipl. ECVCN

Vincent Biourge graduated from the Faculty of Veterinary Medicine of the University of Liège (Belgium) in 1985. He stayed as an assistant in the nutrition department for 2 more years before moving to the Veterinary Hospital of the University of Pennsylvania (Philadelphia, USA) and to the Veterinary Medical Teaching Hospital of the University of California (Davis, USA) as a PhD/resident in clinical nutrition. In 1993, he was awarded his PhD in Nutrition from the University of California and became a Diplomate of the American College of Veterinary Nutrition (ACVN). In 1994, he joined the Research Center of Royal Canin in Aimargues (France) as head of scientific communication and then as manager of the nutritional research program. Vincent is now Scientific Director of Health Nutrition at the Research Center of Royal Canin. He has published more than 30 papers, and regularly present scientific papers as well as guest lectures at International Veterinary Medicine and Nutrition meetings. He is also a Diplomate of the European College of Veterinary Comparative Nutrition (ECVCN).

Diet has a major impact on the etiology and the therapy of feline cardiovascular diseases. As in humans and dogs, sodium intake in the diet can help modify cardiovascular function. More specifically, cats are dependent on a diet that provides sufficient taurine. Contrary to dogs, taurine is an essential amino acid for cats. The synthesis of bile acids in the cat is exclusively dependent on taurine, and the hepatic activity of the enzymes responsible for its synthesis from the sulfur amino acids, methionine and cysteine is extremely weak.

Introduction

Essentially, acquired cardiovascular disease in cats is due to either systemic hypertension (SH) or a cardiomyopathy (including more specifically taurine deficiency). This chapter will review separately and successively each of these pathological entities. An epidemiological, etiological, pathophysiological and diagnostic review will be conducted for and the potential etiological or therapeutic influence of the diet will be considered. While cardiomyopathies (especially hypertrophic forms) are the most commonly found cardiopathies in practice, it would appear justified to first consider SH, due to the key role dietary sodium plays in the development of cardiovascular diseases in general. Additional points of the nutritional management of cardiopathies will be handled in the third part of this chapter.

1 - Systemic hypertension in cats

SH is defined as the chronic systolic and/or diastolic increase in systemic blood pressure (BP). It is now a well-recognized clinical phenomenon in domestic carnivores, especially cats older than ten years (*Chetboul et al, 2003; Brown, 2006; Brown et al, 2007*). Most clinicians consider a diagnosis of SH in cats when the systolic BP and diastolic BP is at least 160 and 100 mmHg respectively, measured in a calm animal and according to current recommendations (*Stepien, 2004; Brown et al, 2007*).

► Etiology and pathogenesis

BP is the lateral force the blood exercises on each surface unit of the arterial vascular wall (*Guyton & Hall, 1996*). BP depends on heart rate (HR) and total peripheral resistance (TPR).

$$BP = HR \times TPR$$

The increase in BP can therefore result in a higher HR (due to an increase in the heart inotropism or blood volume) or a rise in TPR (during vasoconstriction, structural modification of the vessels or blood hyperviscosity). The circumstances that may lead to SH are therefore multiple.

Contrary to humans, in which primary or essential SH is the most common form, feline SH is most often secondary to another disorder **(Figure 1)**, most commonly renal or endocrine dysfunction (hyperthyroidism) (*Kobayashi et al, 1990; Syme et al, 2002; Chetboul et al, 2003*). Essential SH is rare in the feline species. However, more routine measures of BP in veterinary medicine associated with the aging of the animal population suggest a greater frequency. At the moment it is difficult to establish, but SH may affect up to 18-20% of cats (*Elliott et al, 2001; Maggio et al, 2000*). Just like in humans, BP tends to rise with age in normal cats (*Samson et al, 2004*).

The main cause of feline SH **(Figure 1)** is chronic kidney disease (CKD). Studies show that 20-60% of feline renal patients are hypertensive (*Kobayashi et al, 1990; Stiles et al, 1994*). There are many pathogenic mechanisms linking the kidneys and SH to varying

FIGURE 1 - ETIOLOGY OF SYSTEMIC ARTERIAL HYPERTENSION IN CATS

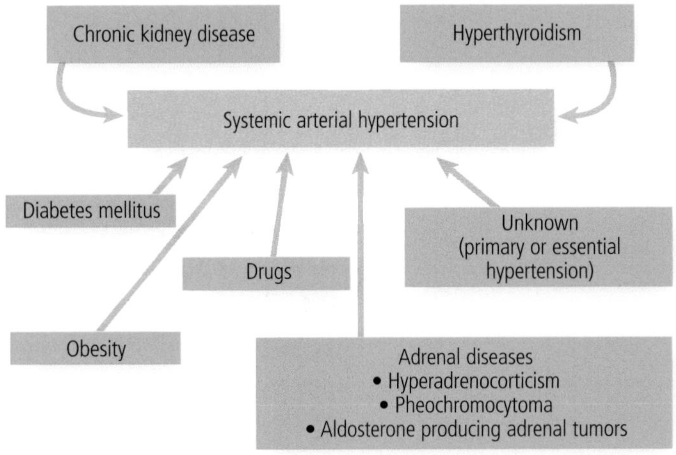

- Chronic kidney disease
- Hyperthyroidism
- Systemic arterial hypertension
- Diabetes mellitus
- Drugs
- Unknown (primary or essential hypertension)
- Obesity
- Adrenal diseases
  - Hyperadrenocorticism
  - Pheochromocytoma
  - Aldosterone producing adrenal tumors

degrees of sodium and water retention and hyperactivity of the renin-angiotensin-aldosterone system, as evidenced by:
- hormonal alterations (plasma renin activity, aldosteronema, plasma aldosterone/renin ratio)
- histological and immunohistochemical analysis of the kidneys of animal patients (*Taugner et al, 1996; Jensen et al, 1997; Mishina et al, 1998; Pedersen et al, 2003*).

SH in cats is also a frequent complication of untreated or poorly controlled hyperthyroidism, affecting a highly variable proportion of animals according to the studies. Between 20% and almost 90% of cats with hyperthyroidism are reported to be hypertensive in the literature (*Kobayashi et al, 1990; Stiles et al, 1994*). The true prevalence of pathologic SH is probably over-estimated due to the sensitivity of the cat to stress. SH in cats with hyperthyroidism is most often moderate and reversible with the treatment of the underlying endocrinopathy. The origin of SH in the event of hyperthyroidism (*Feldman & Nelson, 1997*) is multifactorial, including an increase in heart rate induced by the thyroidal hormones, an inotropic and chronotropic action directly and indirectly mediated by the receptors coupled to adenylate cyclase, and hyperactivation of the renin-angiotensin-aldosterone system via stimulation of the β juxta-glomerular receptors that initiate increased synthesis of renin.

Other less common causes of SH in cats include diabetes mellitus or more rarely obesity, hyperadrenocorticism, pheochromocytoma, hyperaldosteronemia, or even drugs such as glucocorticoids, phenylpropanolamine, erythropoietin and cyclosporine A (*Maggio et al, 2000; Chetboul, 2003; Senello et al, 2003; Brown, 2006; Brown et al, 2007*). Predisposing factors include (*Brown, 2006*) rapid sodium chloride infusion (classic example of a cat with CKD), which may accelerate the expression of subclinical SH or lead to a sharp increase in BP that was initially within the upper limits of normal.

▶ Role of sodium

> In rodents

An excess in dietary sodium (Na) is well known in some animal species to be directly responsible for SH or at least a predisposing factor to its expression. A diet with a very high salt content [8% Na on a dry matter basis (DMB)]; (by comparison, commercially available diets for cats do not exceed 2% Na DMB) for a period of eight weeks leads to increased BP not only in spontaneously hypertensive rats but also in the initially normotensive Wistar-Kyoto rat (*Yu et al, 1998*). In the abovementioned rats, these changes were accompanied by the development of interstitial fibrotic lesions in the kidneys (glomeruli, tubules) and the arteries of the left myocardium (*Yu et al, 1998*). These changes paralleled the increased tissue expression of the gene coding for transforming growth factor-beta 1 (TGFβ1). Likewise, in a murine model of renal failure induced by nephron reduction, it has been shown that excessive sodium intake is accompanied by a rise in systemic BP (*Cowley et al, 1994*).

The genetic models of SH include the salt-sensitive Dahl rat, which develops SH as well as disproportionate fibrotic and hypertrophic lesions in the arteries and left myocardium after the administration of a salt-enriched diet (2-8% Na DMB) (*Zhao et al, 2000; Siegel et al, 2003; Charron et al, 2005*).

> In humans

It has been demonstrated that excessive salt intake in humans can also be deleterious and a direct cause of increased BP, although there is great heterogeneity in responses depending on the individual (*Weinberger et al, 1986; 1996; 2001*). Thus, in people who are said to be sensitive to salt – less than 25% of the normotensive population (*Weinberger et al, 1986, 1996*) – the increase in dietary salt intake (from 230 mg (10 mmol)/day to 34.5 g

(1500 mmol) over a period of 15 days) is accompanied by an abnormally large rise in BP that may exceed 30% of the baseline value *(Luft et al, 1979; Weinberger et al, 1996; 2001)*. This abnormal sensitivity to salt is said to be a mortality factor independent of the BP value *(Weinberger et al, 2001)*. Inversely, in some hypertensive diseases, sodium restriction may help reduce BP in a manner comparable to that of an anti-hypertensive drug *(Weinberger et al, 1986; Luft & Weinberger, 1997)*. The effect on BP of salt intake in humans is however highly variable, depending on various factors including genetic context, age, consumption of other electrolytes or even the concomitant intake of some drugs *(Luft & Weinberger, 1997)*. The genetic predisposition to salt sensitivity is said to play a major role in humans, as demonstrated in African American people or people with non-insulin dependent diabetes mellitus.

> In healthy cats

Compared with humans or rats, there are fewer data on the influence of dietary sodium in the genesis of SH in cats. To the authors' knowledge no case of salt-sensitivity has been truly described comparable to those depicted in humans or rats. In the feline species, it has even been shown that a relatively high sodium level in a normotensive animal is accompanied by an increase in water consumption and urine output *(Devois et al, 2000; Luckschander et al, 2004)*. Thus, in healthy young cats (average age 2.5 years, n=10) the administration of a diet with a moderate sodium chloride (NaCl) content (1.02% Na and 2.02% Cl DMB) for a period of two weeks does not change the systolic BP value (measured with the Doppler method), which remains within reference intervals comparable to what is obtained with a control diet (0.46% Na and 1.33% Cl DMB). In the same study, compared with the control diet, the diet with the higher salt content resulted in only a significant increase in water consumption (in excess of 50%) and urinary osmolarity associated with a reduction in urine density.

While supplementary data (high-salt diet given over a longer period to several animals) are needed to complete the results, the National Research Council (NRC) has estimated that there is now sufficient scientific evidence to conclude that a value of 1.5% Na DMB in a dry food providing 4000 kcal/kg could be considered as being risk-free, in healthy cats *(NRC 2006)*. This level equates to an intake of 3.75 g of sodium per 1000 kcal.

> What about cats whose renal function is impaired?

Six different studies of healthy dogs and cats as well as animals with renal failure (presenting maximum azotemia equivalent to stage III CKD according to the IRIS classification) show no influence of a moderate rise in sodium ingestion (up to 3.2 g of sodium per 1000 kcal of metabolizable energy (ME)) on BP *(Greco et al, 1994; Buranakarl et al, 2004; Luckschander et al, 2004; Kirk et al, 2007)*.

▶ Pathophysiological consequences

Most of the organic consequences of SH appear for systolic BP values in excess of 180 mmHg *(Brown, 2006)*, more particularly during the sharp rise in pressure (30 mmHg or more in less than 48 hours).

- **The kidneys** are one of the preferred targets of SH *(Brown, 2006)*. Untreated SH can lead to the development of nephroangiosclerotic lesions, which themselves have the potential to accentuate the initial hypertension.

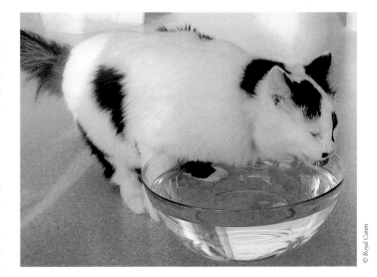

According to the available scientific information, blood pressure in healthy cats or cats with moderate CKD is not affected by the sodium levels required to stimulate water consumption and urine output in cats.

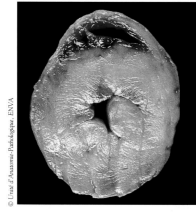

Figure 2 - Example of marked symmetrical concentric hypertrophy of the left ventricle in a cat with renal failure and systemic arterial hypertension.

© Unité d'Anatomie-Pathologique, ENVA

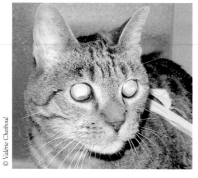

© Valérie Chetboul

Figure 4 - Sudden blindness in a cat, caused by hypertensive retinopathy.

- **The heart**, and specifically the left ventricle, is another main target organ of SH. In a study conducted in association with Toulouse National Veterinary School on 58 hypertensive cats *(Chetboul et al, 2003)*, 85 % presented with an abnormal echocardiograph. In 59% of the cases, the alteration was concentric hypertrophy of the left ventricular wall **(Figures 2 & 3A)**, symmetric or not. There was no correlation between the degree of parietal hypertrophy and blood pressure values nor the age of the animals. Eccentric hypertrophy and septal hypertrophy localized in the subaortic region **(Figures 3B & 3C)** were found in a lower but similar proportion (13% each). Dilatation of the left atrium was associated with the left ventricular remodelings in less than one third of cases (28%). Feline SH has also been shown to accompany modification of the proximal aorta (dilatation, twisting contours) *(Nelson et al, 2002)*.

- **Ocular lesions** are common in hypertensive animals *(Maggio et al, 2000; Chetboul et al, 2003; Samson et al, 2004)*, affecting up to 50% of hypertensive cats and 80% of hypertensive cats with renal failure. These lesions mainly correspond to alterations in the vascularization of the fundus termed 'hypertensive retinitis' **(Figure 4)**: abnormal twisting and dilatation of blood vessels in the retina, localized or diffuse preretinal or retinal hemorrhages, and partial or total detachment of the retina potentially leading to permanent blindness in the absence of early treatment. SH may also cause hyphema, anterior uveitis due to vasculopathy of the ciliary bodies or even glaucoma caused by an obstruction of the iridial angle by blood.

- A sharp and marked rise in BP may lead to the appearance of **cerebral lesions** (edema or hemorrhage) classified as hypertensive encephalopathy *(Brown et al, 2005; Brown, 2006)*. Hypertensive encephalopathy causes various nervous problems ranging from simple behavioral modifications (hypernervosity, anxiety, complaining mewing), ataxia and disorientation, to more serious signs (torpor **(Figure 5)**, convulsions or coma). For reasons that are not yet apparent, cats suffer from hypertensive encephalopathy more often than dogs.

FIGURE 3 - THE THREE MAIN TYPES OF LEFT VENTRICULAR REMODELING ASSOCIATED WITH SYSTEMIC ARTERIAL HYPERTENSION IN CATS

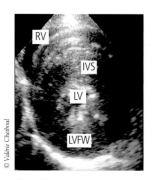

© Valérie Chetboul

3A - Concentric hypertrophy.

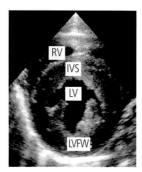

3B - Eccentric hypertrophy.

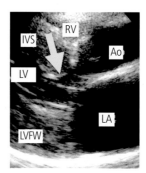

3C - Localized hypertrophy.

2D echocardiographic image, right parasternal route, images taken at the end of the diastole, transventricular short axis views (3A and 3B) and long-axis 5-chamber view (3C).

Symmetrical parietal hypertrophy is concentric in the animal in Figure 3A and eccentric in the animal in Figure 3B with very reduced and normal left ventricular diameter respectively. Note the large deformation of the localized interventricular septum in the subaortic region in Figure 3C (marked).

LVFW: left ventricular free wall
IVS: interventricular septum
RV: right ventricle

LV: left ventricle
Ao: aorta
LA: left atrium

► Diagnosis

> Diagnostic step n°1: suspicion

In practice, SH must be suspected when the cat has a disorder that is a known cause of SH (especially CKD or hyperthyroidism). Other suspicious circumstances include:
a) when one or more (physical or functional) symptoms are suggestive of SH (**Table 1**).
b) identification of left cardiomegaly or left ventricular remodeling by radiograph or ultrasound imaging, respectively.

The diagnosis of SH can also be established during the routine measurement of BP despite the absence of other signs based on clinical observation, etiology, radiograph or ultrasound. However, an increase in BP alone, should be carefully interpreted (do not hesitate to repeat the BP measurement in the absence of clinical signs or biochemical modifications).

> Diagnostic step n°2: confirmation via BP measurement

The Doppler method (**Figures 6 & 7**) is currently recommended by the majority of authors due to its speed and simplicity compared with oscillometry (*Jepson et al, 2005*). In addition, the Doppler method is strongly correlated with the values obtained by the gold standard reference method of direct catheterization (*Binns et al, 1995*). The only drawback of this technique is the occasional difficulty determining the diastolic BP value, which is negated by experienced operators. Several rules must however be followed to ensure that the values measured are as repeatable and reproducible as possible and to limit anxiety-induced hypertension ("white coat effect"), which can lead to the erroneous diagnosis of pathological SH.

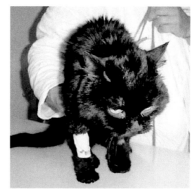

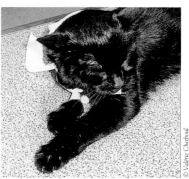

Figure 5 - *Exhaustion and torpor in a cat with systolic arterial hypertension (systolic arterial pressure = 290 mmHg).*

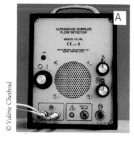

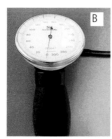

Figure 6 - *Example of equipment used to measure blood pressure by the Doppler method.* 6A: machine - 6B: manometer - 6C: occlusive cuff - 6D: transducer (8-10 MHz).

FIGURE 7 - BLOOD PRESSURE MEASUREMENT BY THE DOPPLER METHOD IN A CAT

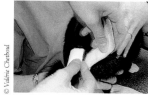

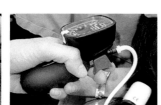

7A: *Positioning of the cuff at the base of the tail and distal application of gel.*

7B: *Inflation of the cuff after location of the blood flow. The animal is lying on its sternum (measurement taken at heart level).*

TABLE 1 - COMPARATIVE DISTRIBUTION OF CLINICAL SIGNS IN HYPERTENSIVE CATS (N=58) AND NORMOTENSIVE CATS (N=113). ALL ANIMALS WERE REFERRED WITH SUSPECTED SYSTEMIC ARTERIAL HYPERTENSION

(*Chetboul et al, 2003*)

Clinical signs	Hypertensive cats (n=58)	Normotensive cats (n=113)
Heart murmur	62%	72%
Polyuria-polydipsia	53%*	29%
Retinal lesions (detachment, hemorrhage)	48%**	3%
Anorexia- fatigue	45%	71%
Gallop rhythm	16%**	0%
Vomiting	15%	16%
Nervous symptoms	13%	13%
Dyspnea – Coughing	12%	17%
Weight loss	12%	14%
Other	1%	17%

*The most specific symptoms (albeit not pathognomonic) of SH were retinal lesions**, galloping sound** and polyuria-polydipsia*, the only ones to be significantly more common in hypertensive cats than in normotensive cats (**: p<0.001; *: p<0.01).*

Heart

329

RULES TO BE FOLLOWED TO MEASURE BLOOD PRESSURE IN CATS

(Stepien et al, 2004; Snyder et al, 2006; Brown et al, ACVIM consensus statement, 2007)

1) The following recommendations help limit "white coat hypertension" and avoid erroneous diagnosis of pathological hypertension.

- Conduct the test in a separate room that is calm, in the presence of the owner.
- Wait until the heart rate is stable or the cat calms down before conducting a test or registering the results.
- Eliminate the first BP values, then take 3-5 additional measures, if possible at 30-60 seconds intervals to calculate the average.
- Do not hesitate to repeat the test within 48 hours, in the event of clinical or etiological suspicion, or 15-30 days, in less urgent circumstances in borderline cases (cat showing stress and BP values above the upper limits: 160 mmHg in systole, 100 mmHg in diastole).

2) The following rules help increase the reliability of the technique.

- The same people, trained in the technique and the use of the equipment should always conduct BP tests at any given clinic or in any given team.
- The ambient temperature in the room should not be too low, to avoid the appearance of peripheral vasoconstriction, which could cause the BP value to be higher than expected or even make it difficult to get a measurement.
- Use the appropriate cuff (if it is too small BP may be overestimated; if it is too big the BP may be underestimated).
- The average BP value, the name of the tester, the test site and the number of measurements taken should be noted, to ensure maximum rigor in longitudinal monitoring.

TABLE 2 - COMMON HYPERTENSIVE AGENTS RECOMMENDED FOR CATS WITH SYSTEMIC ARTERIAL HYPERTENSION

Classes	Substances	Doses
Diuretic	Hydrochlorothiazide	2-6 mg/kg/day PO BID
Calcium inhibitor	Amlodipine: highly effective in cats	0.625-1.25 mg/cat/day (or 0.18-0.3 mg/kg PO SID)
Angiotensin conversion enzyme inhibitors *(in the event of very moderate SH with proteinuria, or if nephroprotective effect is desired or in association with amlodipine (if amlodipine alone does not work)*	Benazepril Enalapril Imidapril Ramipril	0.25-0.5 mg/kg/day SID PO 0.25-0.5 mg/kg SID to BID PO 0.5 mg/kg/day SID PO 0.125 mg/kg/day (up to 0.25 mg/kg if necessary) SID PO
β-blockers	Propranolol Atenolol	0.1-1 mg/kg 2-3 x/day PO or 2.5-5 mg/cat BID to TID PO or 6.25-12.5 mg/cat SID to BID PO
Other	Spironolactone	1-2 mg/kg/day PO (little documented in cats)

By far the best anti-hypertensive documented in the feline species is amlodipine.
PO: per os
The use of these agents in cats can be restricted according to the licence applicable in each country.

> Diagnostic step n°3: determination of the cause

When SH is identified in a cat the veterinarian must begin with a simple blood test (urea, creatinine and T_4 measurement) to confirm or rule out CKD and hyperthyroidism. If the results are normal, a complete medical evaluation must be conducted before concluding primary SH. This examination includes a CBC, biochemical profile, urine analysis and even an abdominal ultrasound to check for an adrenal mass. Finally, it also advised to analyse the urine protein to creatinine ratio (UPC) as proteinuria can be a negative pronostic factor *(Jepson et al, 2007)*.

► Medical treatment

Anti-hypertensive drugs that can be administered to cats are listed in **Table 2**. Amlodipine besylate is by far the anti-hypertensive of choice in cats. It is a documented drug in the species with efficacy in most cases without the additional need of other anti-hypertensive treatments *(Henik et al, 1997; Elliott et al, 2001; Snyder et al, 2001; Tissier et al, 2005)*. Amlodipine is a long-action calcium inhibitor of the dihydropyridine group that acts against the opening of the voltage-dependant slow calcium channels. Its long action (contrary to that of nifedipine) limits the secondary effects of sudden hypotension (tachycardia, exhaustion, malaises). Amlodipine also has few negative effects on inotropism and conduction. Amlodipine is not recommended in cats with hepatic failure.

Treatment of the primary disorder, when known, is a priority. In cats with hyperthyroidism, normalization of BP may be achieved in association with the restoration of euthyroidism without use of anti-hypertensives (*Snyder & Cooke, 2006*). In an emergency (sudden blindness or major tachyarrhythmia), it will be necessary to quickly reduce BP with the administration of amlodipine (calcium inhibitor) or β blockers (propranolol, atenolol), which have the advantage of directly targeting the action sites of thyroidal hormones on the cardiovascular system (**Table 2**).

► Adapting the sodium content in food

Based on the data on excess dietary sodium from animal SH models or human medicine (see above), it is often accepted that the ingestion of sodium must be severely reduced in hypertensive cats. While excessive and sudden sodium intake (1.3%/DMB or more) must be avoided in the event of feline SH (*Snyder & Cooke, 2006*), no study has yet shown the benefit of sodium restriction in cats in terms of blood pressure values or life expectancy.

Contrary to preconceived ideas, too low an intake of dietary sodium in cats can be rather harmful, as shown by *Buranakarl et al (2004)*. For one week, three groups of cats were given the same dry food differentiated only by sodium content: 0.34%, 0.65% and 1.27% as fed, (0.5 g, 1.4 g and 2.8 g per 1000 kcal, respectively). One group of healthy cats (control group, n=7) was compared with two groups of cats with experimental renal disease by renal infarct (ligature of the branches of the renal artery) associated either with contralateral nephrectomy ('remnant kidney (RK) model', n=7) or contralateral 'wrapping' (wrapping or WA model, n=7).

In the two groups of cats with renal failure, in spite of the prescription of amlodipine (0.25 mg/kg/24 hours PO) systemic, systolic, diastolic and average BP (measured by radiotelemetry) were higher than in the control group, significantly in the RK group and to a lesser degree in the WA group. However, no influence of dietary sodium was observed in the three groups of cats, on heart rate, blood pressure variability (shown by a retained baroreflex also in sick animals) or the systemic BP value (systolic, diastolic and mean). In other terms, and contrary to the data published in rats (*Cowley et al, 1994*), the high sodium diet characterized by 2.8 g Na/1000 kcal was not responsible for a rise in BP in either the healthy control cats, which concurs with the data obtained for healthy dogs (*Krieger et al, 1990; Greco et al, 1994*) or cats with renal failure. Likewise, the lower sodium diet did not induce a lower systemic BP in the two groups of sick cats nor in the control group. This latter diet was shown to have no beneficial anti-hypertensive protector effect in cats with renal disease.

In the same study (*Buranakarl et al, 2004*), the lowest sodium intake (0.5 g/1000 kcal) was also associated with:
- a significant reduction in the glomerular filtration rate in control cats compared with the values obtained in the same group with the other two diets. The same observation was made in the WA group;

- activation of the renin-angiotensin-aldosterone system (RAAS) in cats with renal disease which was greater in the WA group than in the RK group. This activation was characterized by aldosteronemia and a higher serum aldosterone/renin ratio compared with the control group. These hormonal modifications were reduced with NaCl supplementation. This diet was also associated with an increase in the arginine-vasopressin plasma concentration in the RK group;

- hypokalemia in healthy cats and even more in cats with renal disease, associated with an increase in the excreted potassium fraction (very marked in the WA model) linked to a large degree to hyperaldosteronism, which is potentially harmful (risk of hypokalemic nephropathy and progressive renal lesions).

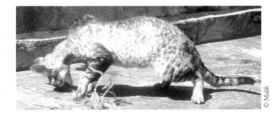

This cat shows a typical posture signifying general muscle weakness, with drooping of head and neck, that may be encountered with severe hypokalemia in patients with CKD, as well as in hypokalemia due another cause.

FIGURE 8 - EXAMPLE OF HYPERTROPHIC CARDIOMYOPATHY IN A CAT

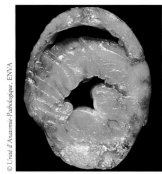

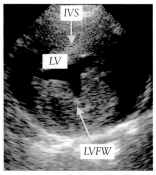

8A: Marked systemic concentric hypertrophy of the left ventricle visually similar to that of Figure 3A.

8B: The concentric hypertrophy in Figure 8A was initially identified on echocardiographicexamination (2D, right parasternal route, image obtained at the end of diastole, transventricular short axis view).

LVFW: left ventricular free wall; IVS: interventricular septum; LV: left ventricular cavity.

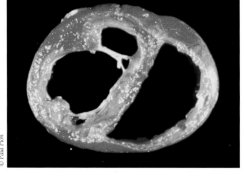

Figure 9 - Example of taurine deficiency dilated cardiomyopathy.

To summarize, the data presented above demonstrate that major restriction of sodium is not recommended in hypertensive cats or in cats with CKD that have hypertensive tendencies. Excessive restriction risks stimulating the renin-angiotensin-aldosterone system, a pressure system par excellence. This aggravates the reduction in the glomerular filtration rate and favors hypokalemia due to increased kaliuresis. The same recommendation applies to healthy cats.

Lastly the prescription of a low calorie diet has not been shown to have a hypotensive effect in obese cats (*Snyder & Cooke, 2006*), although few data are available on this subject.

2 - Feline cardiomyopathies

Cardiomyopathy designates all the disorders of the myocardium not secondary to a disease of another part of the cardiovascular system (valvular disease, alteration of the pericardium or the conducting system). These disorders are described as primary when their cause is undetermined or poorly identified. They are secondary when their origin is identified (hormonal, dietary, toxic, infectious or infiltrative cause). The importance of cardiomyopathies in cats is linked to the fact that they represent more than 90% of acquired cardiopathies in this species and are found in around 10% of cats at post mortem (*Fox, 1999*).

▶ Classification – Main characteristics

Cardiomyopathies are very heterogenous and can be classified according to different criteria. The most commonly used classification in practice is one that combines morphological, functional and lesional characteristics. There are four main groups of cardiomyopathy: hypertrophic (HCM), dilated (DCM), restrictive (RCM) and 'unclassified' also known as intermediate.

- **Hypertrophic forms (Figure 8)** are characterized by myocardial hypertrophy, most often of the free wall of the left ventricle and/or the interventricular septum. This hypertrophy may be symmetrical, asymmetrical or localized in the subaortic region, at the mainstays or the apex, which is described as segmentary hypertrophy (*Fox, 2003; Häggström, 2003*). HCM includes the primary forms, some of which have been shown to be genetically determined. These are handled in the next section. There are also secondary HCM, especially associated with hyperthyroidism, SH (see chapter 2), acromegaly and inflammatory or cancerous myocardial infiltration (particularly lymphoma).

- **Dilated forms** are rare compared with hypertrophic forms. They may be primary or secondary. Secondary forms are either due to the cardiotoxicity of adriamycin (now uncommon), a sequela of myocarditis or taurine deficiency. Taurine deficiency cardiomyopathy **(Figure 9)**, which is now very rare due to the supplementation of taurine in commercial foods, is discussed further in the text (*Pion et al, 1992 a,b*). DCM is characterized by a drop in inotropism concerning the left ventricle only or both ventricles simultaneously. Dilated cardiomyopathies that affect only the right heart have also been described (*Fox et al, 2000*).

- **Restrictive forms**, of varying phenotypical expression, are characterized by a diastolic myocardial dysfunction caused by endocardial fibrosis or most often major endomyocardial fibrosis. The origin of these restrictive forms remains unclear *(Fox, 2004)*. Fibrosis may be cicatricial, secondary to an immune process, a viral infection or inflammation.

- **Intermediate cardiomyopathies** cover all myocardial modifications not strictly dilated, hypertrophic or restrictive. They include primary cardiomyopathies associating hypertrophy and dilatation as well as various infiltrations (e.g. myocardial mineralization in the event of hypervitaminosis D or hyperparathyroidism).

One study *(Gouni et al, 2006)* has been conducted on acquired feline cardiovascular diseases (primary cardiomyopathies, SH and degenerative valve lesions) diagnosed by echo Doppler at the Cardiology Unit at Alfort (UCA) between 2001 and 2005. Primary HCM was by far the most common disease among the 305 cats in the study (197/305 or 65% of cases), representing more than 85% of all primary cardiomyopathies. The second cardiomyopathy was RCM, followed by DCM and 'unclassified' cardiomyopathies, accounting for only 9%, 2% and 1.3% of all 305 cardiopathies respectively.

► Current knowledge on primary hypertrophic cardiomyopathy

> Genetic determinism

Breed predispositions to HCM have been described, especially the Maine Coon, American Shorthair and Persian. HCM on the other hand is fairly rare in the Siamese, Burmese and Abyssinian *(Kittleson et al, 1998)*. A hereditary form of the disease was recently proven in a colony of Maine Coon cats in the United States *(Meurs et al, 2005)*. The mutation is in the gene coding for myosin binding protein C (MYBPC3) and the described mode of transmission is dominant autosomal with variable expression. A different mutation of the same gene was recently found in the Ragdoll *(Meurs et al, 2007)*.

Sex is also a factor in the expression of HCM. Most cats (up to 90% according to the studies) affected by HCM are toms. Age on the other hand does not appear to have so great an influence on the disease, which can affect cats aged 3 months to 17 years, with an average between 4 and 7 years *(Fox, 2000)*.

> Pathophysiological consequences

Left myocardial hypertrophy characterizing HCM mainly causes alteration of the diastolic function, at least initially, both at the very start of diastole (relaxation phase or active phase necessitating energy) and in the second and final phase of diastole (compliance phase). Due to myocardial hypertrophy and especially the fibrotic lesions frequently associated with HCM, the elasticity of the myocardium is reduced and the compliance phase is altered. Furthermore, due to coronary alterations and myocardial ischemia connected with a "relative" reduction in the coronary/myocardial mass ratio, the relaxation phase is also altered.

This diastolic myocardial dysfunction leads eventually to dilatation of the left atrium because of the problems of diastolic emptying of the atrium, followed by the development of left heart failure and finally to the terminal phase of overall heart failure. Left atrial dilatation is frequently accentuated by the presence of mitral layers that cause mitral systolic reflux, which in turn is aggravated by the abnormal movement of the mitral layers – mitral anterior systolic motion – accompanying the obstructive hypertrophies (the extremity of the mitral layers move in the left ventricular outflow tract during systole).

Recent studies using modern ultrasound imaging technology (tissue Doppler imaging (TDI)) have shown that systolic dysfunction associated with diastolic dysfunction occurs much earlier than previously thought. This may contribute to the earlier development of congestive heart failure *(Carlos Sampedrano et al, 2006; Chetboul et al, 2006a b)*.

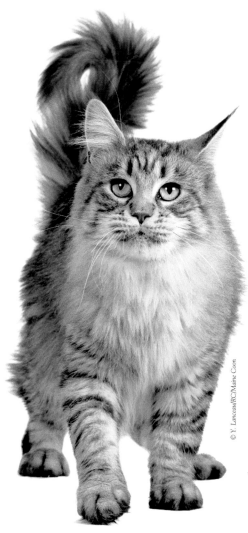

The Maine Coon is predisposed to primary hypertrophic cardiomyopathy.

Heart

Arterial thromboembolism, defined as the partial or total obliteration of an artery by a distally formed blood clot, constitutes another potential complication of HCM. According to a retrospective study of 100 cases of arterial thromboembolism in cats, the most common cause of this complication is HCM (*Laste & Harpster, 1995*). The primary thrombus forms most often in the left atrium (especially during atrial dilatation), sometimes in the left ventricle and much less frequently in the right cavities unless they are dilated themselves (*Laste & Harpster, 1995; Smith et al, 2003*). In the majority of cases (on average 90%), the embolized thrombus ends in the aortic trifurcation, causing ischemic neuropathy of the two posterior limbs. Other localizations are sometimes observed (brachial, cerebral, mesenteric, pulmonary and renal arteries). Congestive heart failure and cardiac arrhythmias (*Smith et al, 2003*) are commonly associated with arterial thromboembolism (more than 40% of cases for each).

Fatty acid metabolism

Fatty acids (FA) are the heart's main source of energy. Abnormalities in the metabolism of FA are sometimes associated with some cardiopathies, including some forms of HCM in humans (*Kelly & Strauss, 1994*). A deficiency of CD36 has been described in human DCM. CD36 is a FA transporter that helps provide energy to the myocardium (*Okamoto et al, 1998; Watanabe et al, 1998; Nakata et al, 1999; Hirooka et al, 2000*).

In spontaneously hypertensive rats, in which SH is associated with insulin resistance and dyslipidemia, the administration of short- and medium-chain fatty acids (SMCFA) at 21.5 g/100 g diet permits restoration of normoglycemia and limits the consequences of hyperinsulinemia and cardiac hypertrophy (*Hajri et al, 2001*). These results suggest that insufficient provisioning of energy to the myocardial cells could contribute to the development of HCM.

Additional studies will be needed to confirm the positive role of SMCFA in cats with HCM.

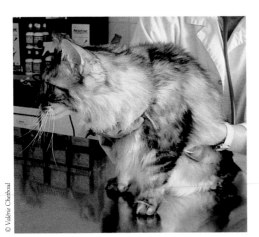

Figure 10 - *Auscultation (here a Maine Coon) is a fundamental part of the clinical cardiovascular examination, even in asymptomatic animals.*

FIGURE 11 - EARLY SCREENING FOR HYPERTROPHIC CARDIOMYOPATHY IN A MAINE COON USING ECHOCARDIOGRAPHY
(Chetboul et al, 2006b).

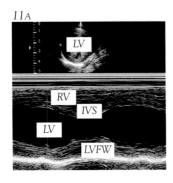
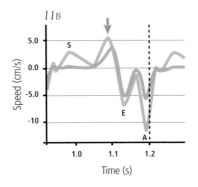

The conventional echocardiograph image, especially in M mode (11A), fails to show any anomaly. Tissue Doppler imaging on the other hand (11B) (2D color mode) shows major diastolic dysfunction characterized by abnormal inversion of E and A waves (normally E/A>1), with the presence of a post-systolic contraction (marked). The left and septal myocardial walls hypertrophied one year later.
LVFW: left ventricular free wall
IVS: interventricular septum
RV: right ventricular cavity
LV: left ventricular cavity

> Diagnosis

The first step in the diagnosis of HCM is a careful clinical examination, with special attention for auscultatory abnormalities (**Figure 10**): tachyarrhythmia, systolic murmur in the left apex, often also audible in the sternal region, systolic murmur in the left basal region during sub-valvular aortic obstruction, and a gallop rhythm. However, the absence of a heart murmur does not exclude the presence of HCM, as around 40% of cats are exempt (*Rush et al, 2002*). Almost half of cats with HCM have congestive heart failure characterized by restrictive dyspnea (pulmonary edema and pleural effusion), ascites or much more rarely coughing. Syncope is a rare expression of the disease, found in less than 5% of cases (*Rush et al, 2002*).

An echocardiographic examination permits the direct confirmation of myocardial hypertrophy (precise quantification and location) as well as its consequences for the cavities (dilatation of the left atrium) and hemodynamics (sub-valvular aortic obstruction, pulmonary arterial hypertension). An earlier diagnosis of HCM can be obtained by tissue Doppler imaging (**Figure 11**), which may sometimes reveal a diastolic or systo-diastolic myocardial dysfunction even before parietal hypertrophy is detectable by conventional ultrasound imaging (*Chetboul et al, 2005; Chetboul et al, 2006a, b*). This technique can be especially useful for animals destined for breeding or 'doubtful' cases, whose myocardial walls are at the higher end of the thickness limit.

A DNA test is now available to look for the gene mutation in the Maine Coon coding for MYBPC3. This test enables differentiation of wild homozygote animals from heterozygote animals or animals with mutated homozygotes. However, this genetic status does not predict myocardial disease (presence or absence, quantitative importance). Data collected over more than two years (unpublished UCA data) from complete clinical, ultrasound and TDI data in Maine Coons (more than 100) show that some heterozygote animals may remain asymptomatic for many years, when they undergo conventional ultrasound examinations or even normal TDI. Conversely, some rare cats genetically tested 'normal' (wild homozygotes) can present signs of HCM in an ultrasound examination and/or TDI, implying that HCM is not linked to a single gene, at least in this breed. In practice, if owners have the resources, the ideal scenario is a precautionary DNA test together with ultrasound imaging.

> Prognosis and therapeutic principles

HCM is a serious cardiopathy due to the potential complications, which include congestive heart disease (46% of cases), arterial thromboembolic accidents (16.5%) and arrhythmia potentially causing sudden death *(Rush et al, 2002)*. In a retrospective study by *Rush et al* (2002), which included 260 cats with HCM, the median survival time in animals that survived more than 24 hours was 709 days with a large variability (2-4418 days). Animals whose disease was not clinically expressed had a better survival (median of 1129 days). Conversely, those presenting with an arterial thromboembolic accident had a lower survival rate (median of 184 days). The seriousness of thromboembolic complications in the cat is shown in other studies, including a study by *Smith et al* (2003) that reported a median survival rate of 117 days, and only 77 days if associated with heart failure.

The treatment of HCM is based on the different classes of drugs **(Table 3)**: angiotensin-converting enzyme inhibitors, calcium inhibitors of the benzothiazepine family and beta-blockers. In the event of congestive heart failure, angiotensin-converting enzyme inhibitors will be preferred due to preliminary results of the study by *Fox et al* (Multicenter Feline Chronic Failure Study) *(Fox, 2003)*. Studies are however necessary to improve understanding of the comparative position of each of these classes in the treatment of feline HCM.

► Taurine deficiency cardiomyopathy

Until the end of the 1980s, dilated cardiomyopathy (DCM) was more common than HCM in the feline population *(Fox, 1999)*. Improved knowledge of the taurine requirements of cats has since reduced its incidence considerably.

Taurine was discovered in 1827 as a constituent of ox bile *(Bos taurus)*, which is where the name is derived from. It is a sulfur-containing amino acid.

$$(H_3^+ N - CH_2 - CH_2 - SO_3^-)$$

Taurine cannot be linked by peptide bonds and thus cannot be part of a protein. In its free form, it is mainly found in the striated muscles (including the myocardium), the central nervous system, the retina and the liver *(Zelikovic et al, 1989)*. Taurine plays a membrane protection role in the myocardium and regulates contractile function. An inadequate taurine intake can thus cause myocardial dysfunction, which in turn may be complicated by congestive heart failure *(Pion et al, 1992a,b)*.

TABLE 3 - CATEGORIES OF THERAPEUTIC AGENTS USED TO TREAT FELINE HYPERTROPHIC CARDIOMYOPATHY

Drugs	Properties	Dose, administration method
ACEI (enalapril, benazepril, ramipril, imidapril)	- Reduction of pre- and post-load resulting in lessening of symptoms of cardiac failure - Anti-ischemic effects via reduction of the post-load (so reduction of systolic constraints of the myocardium) and coronary vasodilatation - Anti-hypertrophy effects and reduction of remodeling	- Benazepril (with amylodipine in the cat with CKD): 0.5 mg/kg (SID) PO (palatable form available) - Imidapril, only ACEI in liquid form: 0.5 mg/kg (SID) PO or directly in the mouth or in the food (very advantageous in cats). Long-term innocuousness documented - Enalapril: 0.5 mg/kg SID to BID PO - Ramipril: 0.125 mg/kg (up to 0.25 mg/kg) SID PO
Calcium inhibitors of the benzothiazepine family (diltiazem)	- Direct improvement in the diastolic function - Moderate chronotrope <0 effect, beneficial for diastolic alteration and ischemia - Anti-ischemic effects via coronary vasodilatation and drop in myocardium's O_2 consumption - Anti-hypertrophic effects - Possible drop in subaortic gradient	Reconditioned diltiazem: - short-action form: 1.75-2.5 mg/kg TID or 7.5 mg/cat TID PO - slow-release form: 5-10 mg/kg/day (SID) PO
β-blockers (atenolol, propranolol)	- Indirect beneficial effect on diastolic alteration and ischemia, mainly via increase in ventricular and coronary refilling time (chronotrope <0) - Indicated in the event of MCH with major tachyarrhythmia or major systolic subaortic gradient - Propranolol not recommended in the event of heart failure due to inhibition of β2 receptors	- Propranolol: 0.1-1 mg/kg BID to TID PO or 2.5-5 mg/cat/day BID to TID (starting with low doses); - Atenolol: 0.2-1 mg/kg SID to BID PO or 6.25-12.5 mg/cat/day SID to BID (starting with low doses).

The use of these agents in cats can be restricted according to the licence applicable in each country.
ACEI: angiotensin-converting enzyme inhibitors

> Genetic determinism

Taurine is primarily synthesized in the liver from sulfur-containing amino acids, methionine and cysteine **(Figure 12)**, and the action of several enzymes, including cysteine dioxygenase and cysteine sulphinic acid decarboxylase. In cats, the biosynthesis of taurine from its precursors is inadequate to cover the needs, as the activity of the hepatic enzymes is very low (especially compared with dogs). A dietary intake of taurine is therefore essential.

Moreover cats waste large amounts of taurine. Indeed, as dogs, they use only taurine for the conjugation of bile acids, whereas humans and rats can also use glycine *(Morris et al, 1987)*. This represents a continual loss of taurine, as a substantial part is not recovered by the entero-hepatic circulation and is lost in the feces **(Figure 13)**.

Why has the cat lost its ability to synthesize a nutrient as essential as taurine? Taurine is one of the most abundant amino acids in animal tissues, so cats are not at risk of taurine deficiency when on their natural diet. Under those circumstances producing taurine is a waste of energy whereas the deamination and desulfurization of cysteine is an alternative metabolic pathway that allows cats to produce energy rather than taurine from sulfur amino acid catabolism.

> Pathophysiological consequences of taurine deficiency

When a cat is deficient, the body's taurine concentrations fall in a few days to a few months depending on the tissue: the plasma is affected first, followed by the whole blood, then the muscles and lastly the retina and the nervous tissue *(Pacioretty et al, 2001)*.

The requirement of taurine in cats is a unique example of a nutritional need that varies according to the influence of the diet on the intestinal flora *(Backus et al, 2002)*. The measurement of breath hydrogen in cats (a measure of the level of intestinal fermentations) shows that wet food favors the proliferation of a flora that consumes larger quantities of taurine than the flora associated with dry expanded kibbles *(Morris et al, 1994; Backus et al, 1994; Kim et al, 1996a,b)*. Taurine losses are linked to the level of protein in the diet as well as the heat processing applied in canning. This explains why wet food requires higher levels of taurine supplementation (1.7 g/kg DMB) compared to dry food (1 g/kg DMB).

FIGURE 12 - GENERAL PATHWAY OF TAURINE SYNTHESIS IN THE LIVER FROM SULPHUR AMINO ACIDS

From Morris, 2002

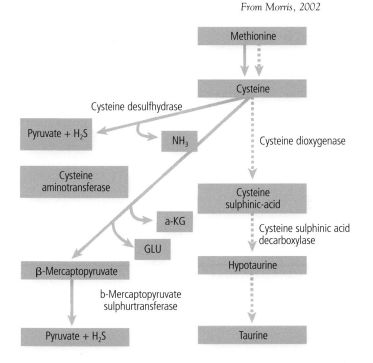

The activities of the enzymes cysteine dioxygenase and cysteinesulphinic acid decarboxylase are low in cats, which severely restricts synthesis of taurine. Cysteine is metabolized to pyruvate, which provides an energy substrate.

Taurine deficiency has been shown to be the main cause of DCM in cats (*Pion et al, 1987*). If identified in time, this disease can be reversed by the oral administration of taurine. Deficient cats present anatomical abnormalities of the heart but there are no histological lesions that would suggest an organic disease of the cardiac tissue. The pathophysiological mechanisms by which taurine deficiency affects cardiac function remain poorly understood. Taurine affects ionic flow of calcium and sodium in the myocardium and thus plays a role in regulating systolic and diastolic myocardial activity (*Novotny et al, 1991*). The interaction between taurine and calcium (characterized by the spontaneous release of calcium by the reticulum and increased sensitivity of the myofilaments to calcium) contributes to its positive inotrope effects.

FIGURE 13 - ENTEROHEPATIC CIRCULATION OF TAURINE

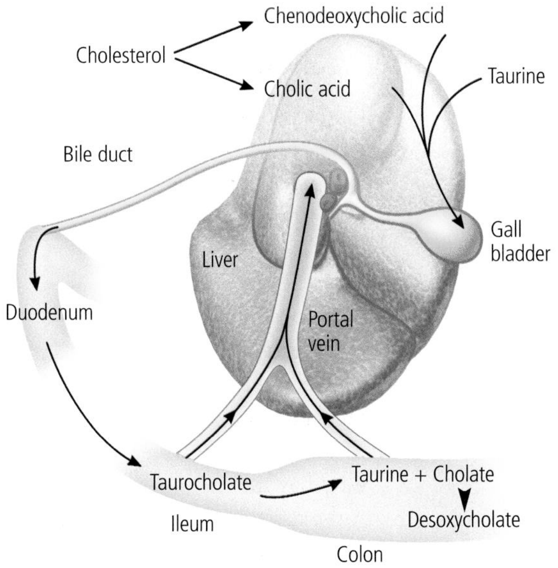

> Diagnosis

The role of taurine in feline DCM has been known for twenty years (*Pion et al, 1987*). Clinical signs vary widely depending on the individual. Experimental taurine deficiency often produces the simultaneous appearance of irreversible central retinal degeneration **(Figure 14)** (within six months and inducing total blindness within less than two years) and DCM of varying degrees within two to four years. Not all cats fed taurine deficient diets will develop ultrasonographic or clinical signs of DCM during this time frame.

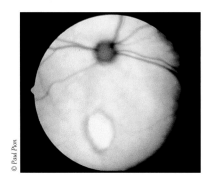

© Paul Pion

Figure 14 - *Central retinal degeneration in a cat suffering from taurine deficiency.*

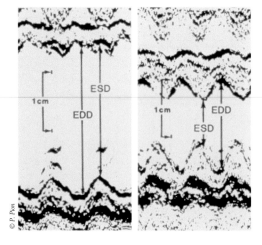

© P. Pion

Figure 15 - Echocardiograph of taurine-deficiency associated dilated cardiomyopathy (time-movement mode) before (on the left) and after (on the right) taurine supplementation.
In this patient, the echocardiography shows a reduced shortening fraction and a dilatation of the left cavities (left picture). These alterations are reversible after taurine administration (right picture).

ESD: end systolic diameter of the left ventricle
EDD: end diastolic diameter of the left ventricle

Taurine deficiency also affects reproduction (reduced fertility in both males and females, fetal resorption, abortions and malformations of newborn kittens) as well as poor growth.

When taurine-deficiency DCM develops, owners are often alerted by the sudden appearance of dyspnea caused by the development of congestive heart failure. Echocardiography shows a reduced shortening fraction **(Figure 15)** as well as an increased systolic diameter of the left ventricle. Later on a left ventricular dilatation that is both systolic and diastolic, associated with thinning of the cardiac walls occurs. In well-developed forms, all four heart chambers are dilated.

In healthy cats, the plasma taurine concentration is greater than 50 nmol/mL (*Pacioretty et al, 2001*) but the plasma concentration reflects recent taurine intake only. It is affected by fasting and does not provide any information on the body's reserves. The result may be artificially high in cats with systemic thromboembolism. As white blood cells and platelets contains high levels of taurine, plasma concentration will be affected by hemolysis or poor separation of the buffy coat.

Establishing a conclusive diagnosis of taurine deficiency requires measurement of the whole blood taurine level because it better reflects taurine concentrations in the myocardium and skeletal muscles. In healthy cats, the whole blood taurine concentration should be higher than 250 nmol/mL (*Pacioretty et al, 2001*). If lower, taurine deficiency is confirmed.

> Treatment

In addition to feeding a diet containing adequate taurine, it is generally recommended to supplement the cat with 250 mg of taurine twice daily (*Freeman, 2000*). If the cat's heart failure can be controlled initially the prognosis is good and clinical signs should clearly improve within one to two weeks. This delay corresponds to the recovery of a normal plasma concentration. Improvements in radiographic and echocardiographic signs will take at least 3-6 weeks. Even if clinical signs improve rapidly supplementation should be pursued for several months.

Some cases of taurine-deficiency associated DCM do not respond to the administration of taurine. The reason for this remains unclear. Nevertheless, taurine supplementation is still recommended for these 'resistant' animals at 250 mg twice daily (*Freeman, 2000*).

> Prevention

Prior to 1987 the taurine levels found in commercial wet cat foods were commonly inadequate to maintain plasma and whole blood concentrations. As the role of taurine in the pathogenesis of DCM has been better understood, manufacturers have increased taurine levels in their diets and the incidence of feline DCM is now very low (*Pion et al, 1992a,b*).

To maintain plasma and whole blood taurine concentrations within the physiological range, feline dry expanded diets must contain at least 1 g taurine/kg DMB and wet diets at least 1.7 g/kg DMB (*NRC 2006*). Taurine supplementation is very safe and no harmful effect on health has been found, even at doses in excess of 10 g/kg DMB in diets with energy concentrations around 4500 kcal/kg (*NRC, 2006*).

3 - Nutritional recommendations for the management of feline cardiopathy

While little information is available in the literature on the specific nutritional requirements of cats with cardiac diseases, several general recommendations can be provided by extrapolating from other species and considering the metabolic peculiarities of cats.

▶ Equate energy density of the diet to the cat's body condition

The body condition score of cats with cardiopathy is highly variable. Maintaining optimal condition in these patients is one of the major goals of dietary treatment.

> Cachexia

Severe weight loss and muscle wasting is less common in cats than in dogs with cardiopathy. (*Freeman, 2000*). "Cardiac cachexia" does not generally appear until advanced stages of heart failure and can be associated with very rapid muscle atrophy. The myocardium is not protected from general protein catabolism, in addition to lower immune defenses and generalized weakness, "cardiac cachexia" may also contribute to the progression of heart failure.

"Cardiac cachexia" is multifactorial: anorexia, increased energy requirements, metabolic alterations, poor blood perfusion of the tissues, as well as complication of renal failure, either primary or secondary to cardiovascular disease all contribute **(Figure 16)**.

Spontaneous food consumption must thus be encouraged in cats with cachexia, by feeding palatable diets (see below recommendations on protein and sodium levels), presenting frequent small meals and warming wet foods to name a few. In order to reduce the volume of the meals, the energy density of the diet should be increased (e.g. higher fat and lower fiber levels).

> Overweight cats

Around 35% of the cats presented to veterinarians are overweight (*Lund et al, 2006*). Whatever the species, obesity is associated with an increased cardiovascular risk. Caloric restriction to induce weight loss in obese cardiac cats is desirable and more so if the cat is exercise intolerant.

Studies in rodents have found that long term energy restriction reduces oxidative stress and protects against several degenerative diseases including cardiomyopathies (*Kemi et al, 2000; Guo et al, 2002*). To our knowledge, such a study has not been conducted on cats.

▶ Provide protein and amino acids to fight cachexia and promote food intake

It has long been recommended that animals with heart failure should be fed diets with reduced protein levels to protect renal function, as renal and cardiac diseases are often linked (*McClellan et al, 2004; Nicolle et al, 2007*). Those recommendations are now clearly outdated (see chapter 7). Moreover cats, because of their true carnivorous nature, have high protein requirements and their metabolism cannot adapt to low protein intakes. Restricting protein simply increases the risk of "cardiac cachexia" and exercise intolerance. Food for cats with cardiac disease must therefore contain at least the minimum protein requirement (60-70 g protein/1000 kcal) (*Freeman, 2002*).

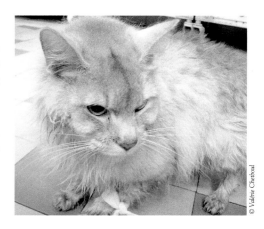

© Valérie Chetboul

Figure 16 - Cachexic cat with chronic kidney disease and systemic arterial hypertension.
(*systolic BP = 170 mmHg*)
Cats with cardiac disease have many reasons for not eating. Aside of the weaknesses associated to the disease, drugs prescribed in this condition may induce nausea and the dietary restrictions commonly found in therapeutic diets (e.g. low protein and low sodium) may produce a diet that is not very palatable.

> Taurine supplementation

The essential requirement for taurine to insure normal cardiac as well as other functions in cats has been discussed above.

Studies have shown that dietary taurine supplementation increases the taurine concentration in the myocardium of both healthy cats and cats with heart failure (Fox & Sturman, 1992). Bearing in mind taurine's protective and positive inotrope roles with respect to cardiac function, taurine supplementation may thus be encouraged, whatever the type of cardiopathy. The recommendation is in the range of 625 mg/1000 kcal (Freeman, 2002).

There is a reciprocal relationship between taurine and potassium requirements. Taurine slows the loss of potassium through the cell, while potassium prevents the loss of taurine by the myocardium. Taurine supplementation (> 625 mg/1000 kcal) could therefore be beneficial to cats with potassium deficiency, e.g. those with impaired renal function (Dow et al, 1992).

> Dietary arginine

Contrary to other species, cats are unable to synthesize arginine. Arginine must therefore be provided by the diet. Furthermore, the cat's high-protein requirement necessitates high arginine requirements due to its involvement in the urea cycle for ammonia detoxification.

Arginine is a nitric oxide (NO) precursor **(Figure 17)**. NO is produced by the vascular endothelium and acts as a blood vessel myorelaxant. NO thus helps regulate blood pressure. In humans and rodents, arginine supplementation has been shown to increase NO production (Lerman et al, 1998).

NO also has an antithrombotic effect (Moncada et al, 1991). A study reported that cats with HCM and associated thromboembolism presented with lower levels of circulating arginine than healthy cats or cats with an uncomplicated cardiomyopathy (McMichael et al, 2000). Arginine supplementation may therefore have beneficial effects in this condition although this has yet to be proven. The NRC recommends a level of at least 1.93 g/1000 kcal in healthy cats. The optimum range required in patients with heart disease has yet to be determined.

▶ Benefits of long-chain omega-3 fatty acids (EPA/DHA)

The composition of dietary fats (especially the ratio of unsaturated omega-6 to omega-3 fatty acids) influences membrane fluidity as well as other hemodynamic factors. In cardiology, many studies have been conducted on the potential role of omega-3 fatty acids. In humans and dogs, much lower plasma concentrations of eicosapentaenoic acid (EPA; 20:5n-3) and docosahexaenoic acid (DHA; 22:6n-6) have been shown, regardless of the underlying cardiac disease (Freeman et al, 1998). While few studies have been conducted on cats, the properties of omega-3 fatty acids deserve some attention.

Linseed oil contains high levels of α-linolenic acid but this is only a precursor of EPA and DHA, and the ability of cats to convert α-linolenic acid to EPA/DHA is very limited **(Figure 18)**. Only fish oils are good sources of EPA and DHA. Cod liver oil should not be used due to its high levels in vitamins A and D.

On usual diets, cell membranes contain very low concentrations of long chain omega-3 fatty acids, but these can be increased with a food that is supplemented with fish oil. For example, with a supplementation of 180 mg DHA and 117 mg EPA/cat/day over a 4 week period, the level of EPA in the plasma phospholipids increases by 70% while the DHA levels increased by a factor of 3.4 (Filburn & Griffin, 2005). Dietary enrichment with EPA and DHA can

FIGURE 17 - ORIGIN OF NITRIC OXIDE

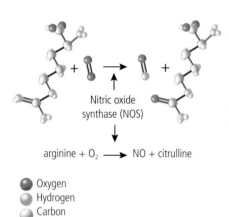

Nitric oxide synthase (NOS)

arginine + O₂ ⟶ NO + citrulline

- ⬤ Oxygen
- ⬤ Hydrogen
- ⬤ Carbon
- ⬤ Hydrogen

The reaction is catalyzed by the enzyme, nitric oxide synthase (NOS). There are three forms of NOS:
Endothelial NOS (eNOS):
eNOS is required for maintenance of normal vascular tone
Neuronal NOS (nNOS):
eNOS and nNOS are constitutive forms and are always produced in low levels
Inducible NOS (iNOS): *iNOS is inducible by a variety of inflammatory mediators including the cytokines, tumor necrosis factor (TNF), and interleukin-1 (IL-1), and free radicals.*

facilitate membrane peroxidation by free radicals (*Meydani et al, 1991*) but this adverse phenomena can be minimized by adjusting the levels of dietary vitamin E.

> Antithrombotic action

Long chain omega-3 fatty acids are known for their antithrombotic activity. This could be highly beneficial for cats, a species in which platelet activation is easily triggered (*Welles et al, 1994*). Increasing the omega-3 fatty acids (1.03 g/kg diet vs 0.07 g/kg in the control diet) and decreasing the omega-6 fatty acids (1.20 g/kg vs 1.34 g/kg in the control diet) reduces platelet aggregation and activation in healthy cats by day 112 (*Saker et al, 1998*). This benefit has yet to be confirmed in cats with HCM.

> Anti-inflammatory effect

In rodents, increasing the level of long chain omega-3 fatty acids in the fat content of food reduces the production of 2 and 4 series eicosanoids from arachidonic acid, which have a pro-inflammatory action (*Broughton & Wade, 2001*). On the other hand the production of anti-inflammatory 5 series leukotrienes (LT) is stimulated.

In humans with heart failure, long chain omega-3 fatty acids reduce the production of "inflammatory cytokines", TNFα and IL-1 (*Levine et al, 1990*). These cytokines contribute to cardiac cachexia by increasing energy requirement and muscle catabolism (*Mahoney & Tisdale, 1988*). Moreover, by regulating the expression of proteosomes, EPA inhibits the loss of lean mass (*Whitehouse et al, 2001*).

In dogs with cardiac disease, supplementation of EPA (27 mg/kg weight/day) and DHA (18 mg/kg weight/day) improves dietary consumption, reduces the production of inflammatory cytokines and so reduces cachexia (*Freeman et al, 1998*). To our knowledge, no information with respect to cats with cardiac disease is available at this time.

> Anti-arrhythmogenic effect

Several studies have shown a benefit of EPA and DHA in the management of cardiac arrhythmia in rodents and dogs (*Kang & Leaf, 1996; Charnock, 2000; Smith et al, 2007*). The mode of action relies on the ability of long chain omega-3 fatty acids to modulate the sodium and calcium flows inside the myocytes (*Gerbi et al, 1997*).

Arrhythmia is often one of the first signs of feline HCM. Based on observations in other species EPA and DHA supplementation could thus be recommended at early stages of cardiopathy but, to our knowledge, no information on this subject is available at this time.

> Regulating endothelial function

EPA and DHA are involved in the regulation of endothelial function, probably by modulating NO production (*Kristensen et al, 2001*). In humans, supplementation induces a vasodilatation effect (*Kenny et al, 1992*). Very high doses (>3 g/day) even led to a fall in BP in hypertensive individuals (*Kris-Etherton et al, 2002*). Studies in cats with cardiac disease are thus needed.

FIGURE 18 - GENERAL PATHWAY OF LONG CHAIN OMEGA-3 AND OMEGA-6 FATTY ACIDS SYNTHESIS

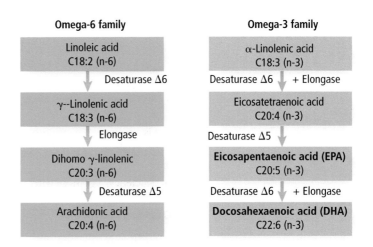

Cats present an increased risk for PUFAs C_{20} deficiency due to a low activity of the desaturase $\Delta 6$ if the diet does not contain enough of these fatty acids.

Heart

341

> Omega-3 fatty acids, ratio versus absolute intake and doses

There is an ongoing debate about whether the dose of omega-3 fatty acids or rather the omega-6 to omega-3 ratio is most important to producing the beneficial effects of omega-3 fatty acids (NRC, 2006). Some results suggest that the total dose of omega-3 is important, although the ratio (n-6/n-3) must also be kept as low as possible to promote the anti-inflammatory effect of omega-3 fatty acids (Grimm et al, 2002). In light of the results obtained in humans, it appears reasonable to recommend tripling the traditional recommended quantity of omega-3 fatty acids in healthy cats to at least 0.06 g/day, corresponding to a concentration in the food of 0.10-0.35 g/1000 kcal (Freeman, 2002).

▶ Monitor mineral balance

> Sodium and chloride

It is usually recommended to feed cardiac patients a very low sodium diet. There is evidence in dogs, however, that this restriction would not be beneficial especially at early stages of heart disease. Indeed, low Na diets will activate the renin-angiotensin-aldosterone system, while the purpose of medical treatments for heart disease is to inhibit it. Sodium restriction (up to 0.5 g/1000 kcal) is thus only justified when an advanced stage of congestive heart failure is reached.

Studies on the influence of sodium in cardiac patients use salt (NaCl) as the source of dietary sodium. It is therefore impossible to differentiate between the respective influences of those two elements. Some data in rats indicate that chloride can also influence plasma renin activity (Kotchen et al, 1980). Therefore, current knowledge does not go further than recommending observance of a moderate dietary chloride level.

> Potassium

Potassium is an intracellular electrolyte whose plasma concentration must be monitored in cardiac animals undergoing medical treatment (although the plasma level is not a good reflection of body reserves). Hypokalemia can occur when diuretics are prescribed (e.g. furosemide) and in the event of CKD. The symptoms associated with hypokalemia are muscle weakness and bradycardia (Linder, 1991). Hypokalemia will also potentialize digoxin toxicity. As mentioned before, there is a reciprocal relationship between taurine and potassium. Thus, it appears sensible to advise both potassium and taurine supplementation in cats with hypokalemic cardiopathy.

Angiotensin-converting enzyme inhibitors (ACEI) are often used in the management of cardiopathy in both humans and animals. In theory they could promote hyperkalemia by stimulating potassium renal reabsorption (Lefebvre et al, 2007). In practice, hyperkalemia, is minimized by the prescription of furosemide and appears negligible in animals (Lefebvre et al, 2007). Extended administration of ACEI has not been associated with hyperkalemia in dogs (Pouchelon et al, 2004). Dietary potassium levels in cats with cardiac disease should thus be similar to those for adult maintenance (1.5-2 g/1000 kcal) even when treated with ACEI.

> Magnesium

Magnesium is a cofactor in hundreds of enzymatic reactions involving carbohydrate and lipid metabolism. The activity of the heart muscle is dependant on the right balance between magnesium and calcium. Magnesium therefore plays an important role in normal cardiac function and magnesium deficiency is implicated in many cardiopathies across species (Rush et al, 2000; Gottlieb et al, 1990).

Diuretics may promote urinary losses of magnesium, and thus the risks of low magnesium status causing arrhythmias and reduced cardiac output. Plasma magnesium is a poor indicator of body reserves and hypomagnesemia is rare in practice (*Freeman, 2000*). A study on hospitalized cats found no significant alteration of magnesium status associated with cardiopathies (*Toll et al, 2002*). Magnesium supplementation in HCM cats did not result in clear clinical benefit (*Freeman et al, 1997*). There is thus no evidence to date to recommend dietary magnesium levels above those necessary for adult maintenance (0.12-0.25 g/1000 kcal) for cats with cardiac disease.

> Phosphorus-calcium balance

Due to the common association between cardiopathy and renal disease (*McClellan et al, 2004; Nicolle et al, 2007*), dietary phosphorus levels should be limited to minimize secondary hyperparathyroidism (see chapter 7).

▶ Reverse any deficiencies

> B group vitamins

Cats naturally have high B vitamin requirements (*Burger, 1993*). B vitamin deficiencies (**Table 4**) in cardiac patients result from anorexia and increased urinary losses secondary to the use of diuretics (*Rieck et al, 1999*).

Plasma vitamin B_6 and B_{12} concentrations are significantly lower in cats with HCM than in healthy cats (*McMichael et al, 2000*). A correlation was found between plasma B_6, B_{12} and folic acid concentrations and the size of the left atrium. The role of these vitamins in the development of HCM (primary or secondary) has yet to be clarified, however.

Based on the evidence, cats with cardiac disease probably have higher B vitamin requirements than healthy cats. Diet for cats with cardiac disease should thus contain two to three times the levels recommended for adult maintenance.

> L-carnitine

L-carnitine is a quaternary amine synthesized in the liver from lysine and methionine (**Figure 19**). It is present in all striated muscles, but the myocardium contains 95% of the body reserves. Its main role is transporting long-chain fatty acids into the mitochondria, where they are oxidized to produce energy.

DCM associated with carnitine deficiency has been described in humans and some dog breeds such as the Boxer, Doberman and Cocker Spaniel (*Brevetti et al, 1991; Helton et al, 2000; Keen et al, 1991*).

It has been suggested that HCM could be associated with abnormal fatty acid metabolism. Therefore, L-carnitine could be beneficial in avoiding the intracellular accumulation of fatty acids in the myocardium (*Lango et al, 2001*). In humans, L-carnitine supplementation (3-4 g/day) in combination with lower long-chain fatty acid intakes improves the clinical status of HCM patients (*Bautista et al, 1990*). This has yet to be demonstrated in cats.

▶ To strengthen the antioxidant defenses

The role of antioxidants in the prevention and treatment of human heart diseases has been extensively studied. Free radicals are the by-products of oxygen metabolism, against which the body defends itself by producing endogenous antioxidants. An imbalance between oxidants and antioxidants (oxidative stress) may increase the risk of cardiopathy (**Figure 20**). Antioxidants can also be provided in the diet. The main antioxidants are enzymes (superoxide dismutase and its cofactor copper, catalase, as well as glutathione peroxidase and its cofactor selenium) and free radical

TABLE 4 - B GROUP VITAMINS	
Name	**Abbreviations**
Thiamin	B_1
Riboflavin	B_2
Pantothenic acid	B_5
Pyridoxine	B_6
Biotin	B_8
Folic acid	B_9
Cobalamin	B_{12}
Niacin	PP
Choline	Ch

FIGURE 19 - CARNITINE MOLECULE

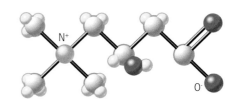

Discovered in 1905, L-carnitine is synthesized from lysine and methionine, if vitamin C and pyridoxine (vitamin B_6) are present. It is a quaternary amine that acts as a water soluble vitamin. Carnitine can be synthesized in D or L forms, but L-carnitine is the only one of relevance for cats with cardiac disease.

Heart

FIGURE 20 - ORIGIN OF OXIDATIVE STRESS

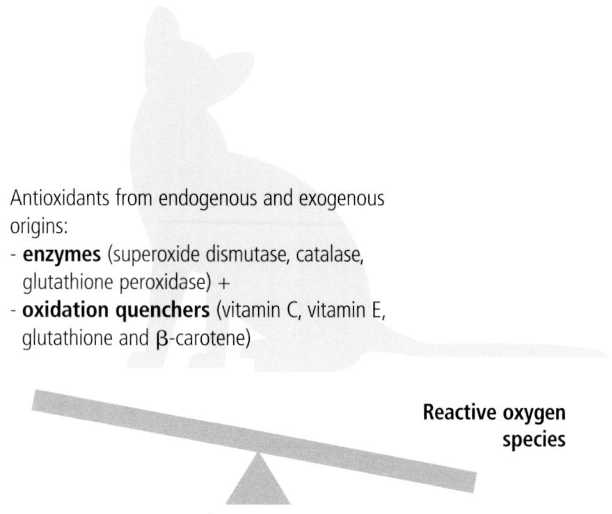

Antioxidants from endogenous and exogenous origins:
- **enzymes** (superoxide dismutase, catalase, glutathione peroxidase) +
- **oxidation quenchers** (vitamin C, vitamin E, glutathione and β-carotene)

Reactive oxygen species

Oxidative stress occurs when there is an imbalance between the production of free radicals and antioxidant defenses.

scavengers (vitamin E, vitamin C, glutathione, taurine, carotenoid pigments). Current research is also focused on new classes of antioxidant such as polyphenols.

Some antioxidants will now be reviewed but it is important to remember that synergy can be observed by using a mixture of antioxidants. Different antioxidants will also be located in different areas of the cell (membrane, intracellular organelles and nucleus).

> Vitamin E

The antioxidant effect of vitamin E (α-tocopherol) has been the subject of studies for many years. In the cardiovascular domain many studies show its beneficial role, especially via two particular effects:
- It maintains endothelial tissue relaxation through NO (*Plotnick et al, 1997*)
- It reduces platelet adhesion and aggregation (*Mower & Steiner, 1982; Calzada et al, 1997*). Its role is especially clear in human atheroma patients.

An imbalance between oxidant and antioxidant production has been shown in DCM dogs with heart failure (*Freeman et al, 1999*). As the cardiopathy develops, the animals increasingly produce quantities of oxidants (malondialdehyde is used as a marker for lipid peroxidation) and present lower levels of vitamin E (*Freeman et al, 1999*). Oxidative stress is thus said to play a role in the development of DCM. Similar observations were made within the framework of a recent study of dogs with heart failure secondary to degenerative valve disease or DCM.

In the light of the data obtained on humans and dogs, vitamin E supplementation is not expected to have any negative effects in cats with cardiac disease. In fact, such supplementation is expected to be beneficial, although this is yet to be confirmed as no studies have been conducted in this species. The optimal supplementation level depends on the quantity of unsaturated fatty acids in the food.

> Vitamin C

Vitamin C is water-soluble. In addition to preventing oxidation of LDL lipoprotein, it is known to facilitate the regeneration of vitamin E. Studies on humans show that a single dose of vitamin C (2000 mg) or administration of 500 mg/day for four weeks promotes vasodilatation in coronary disease patients (*Kugiyama et al, 1998*). However, no specific data are available for cats and unlike humans, cats can synthetize vitamin C.

> Copper

In cats deficient in copper and genetically sensitive to HCM, a high saturated fat content compared with omega-3 fatty acids (2:1) exacerbates the cardiac anomalies induced by copper deficiency (*Jalili et al, 1995*). This suggests that copper could be involved in HCM, although there is nothing to warrant changing the usual recommendations for copper (1.25-7 mg/1000 kcal in the cat). Furthermore, excess copper can act as a pro-oxidant.

> Coenzyme Q10 (CoQ10)

Coenzyme Q10 (also known as ubiquinone) is an antioxidant that is naturally present in the mitochondria. It is found throughout the electron transport chain that produces energy, improving energy production by shunting defective elements from the respiratory chain *(Rosen-feldt et al, 2002)*. Some studies on humans show its potential benefit in the event of cardiovascular pathology.

> Flavonoids

Flavonoids are substances belonging to the family of plant-extracted polyphenols. Epidemiological studies on humans show an inverse relationship between the consumption of fruits and vegetables, which are rich in flavonoids, and cardiovascular risk *(Steinmetz & Potter, 1996)*.

A very high number of in vivo and in vitro cardiovascular pathology studies show the benefit of consuming diverse sources of flavonoids: black and green tea *(Duffy et al, 2001a,b; Geleijnse et al, 2002)*, grape juice *(Keevil et al, 2000)* and red wine *(Rimm et al, 1996; Rein et al, 2000a)*.

Flavonoids have several modes of action. In addition to their antioxidant action, they have an antithrombotic action *(Rein et al, 2000b)* and, by increasing endothelial production of NO, a vasodilative action *(Karim et al, 2000)*. Their beneficial role in cats with cardiac disease is yet to be determined.

> Selenium

Selenium is an essential trace element that is an integral part of glutathione peroxidase, an antioxidant enzyme. It works in synergy with vitamin E. Selenium intake must be carefully dosed as tolerable minimum and maximum levels are fairly close to each other. An adequate intake of selenium goes hand in hand with the fulfillment of glutamate, cysteine and glycine requirements; these three compounds are necessary for glutathione synthesis.

> Taurine

Besides its major role in cardiac inotropism, taurine also has an antioxidant action that protects the myocardium membrane.

Conclusion

The first dietary goal in the event of cardiac disease in cats is to combat the occurrence of cachexia, which can in turn contribute to the progression of the disease. This can be achieved in several ways: increasing level of dietary protein, increasing levels of omega-3 fatty acids and promoting food intake.

Taurine supplementation is necessary in the event of DCM (especially taurine-deficiency DCM). It is also indicated in the event of hypokalemia.

Low-sodium foods should be restricted to symptomatic animals (with signs of heart failure). When used too early in the stage of the disease, sodium restriction may induce undesired side-effects, such as stimulation of the renin-angiotensin-aldosterone system.

Unfortunately, no data is available concerning the benefits of long chain omega-3 fatty acids in the feline cardiac patient. Their antithrombotic and anti-arrhythmic roles as demonstrated in other species would be very beneficial in cats. The same can be said of antioxidants.

Heart

Frequently asked questions about the influence of diet on cardiovascular diseases

Q	**A**
My cat suffers from compensated hypertrophic cardiomyopathy. Should its diet have a low sodium content?	The traditional recommendation for cats with cardiac disease is a diet that is very low in sodium. The current data, on the other hand, suggest that such a restriction will be beneficial only when the heart disease is decompensated. Too low a sodium content stimulates the renin-angiotensin-aldosterone system (RAAS), which can have harmful effects on the cat's heart and renal functions.
My cat suffers from decompensated hypertrophic cardiomyopathy (history of pulmonary edema). Should its diet have a low sodium content different than for compensated hypertrophic cardiomyopathy?	Sodium restriction (up to 0.5 g/1000 kcal) is justified when the cardiopathy has reached the stage of congestive heart failure. Some results obtained in rats suggest that insufficient intake of energy by the cells may contribute to the development of hypertrophic cardiomyopathy. The administration of short- and medium-chain fatty acids is said to limit the consequences of cardiac hypertrophy. The benefit for cats has yet to be evaluated.
My cat suffers from systemic arterial hypertension. Should its diet have a low sodium content?	Large sodium intake (> 2 g/1000 kcal) must be avoided but clinical studies fail to determine whether a low-sodium diet facilitates medical treatment to control arterial pressure. Major sodium restriction is not recommended in hypertensive cats. Excessive restriction will stimulate the renin-angiotensin-aldosterone system (RAAS), a classic pressure regulator, and promote hypokalemia by increasing potassium loss through the urine.
My cat suffers from systemic arterial hypertension secondary to chronic kidney disease. Is a food specifically formulated for cats with chronic kidney disease indicated or are additional nutritional measures needed?	Diets for cats with chronic kidney disease contain low or moderate levels of sodium (0.5-1 g/1000 kcal) (see chapter 7). In cats with chronic kidney disease showing a clear increase in arterial pressure, restricting the consumption of sodium chloride is not sufficient to prevent arterial hypertension, which must be treated medically. Other nutrients that may help control arterial pressure include: - Arginine: precursor of nitric oxide (NO•), which helps regulate arterial pressure - Omega-3 fatty acids, EPA and DHA: in humans, very high doses (>3 g/day) produce a vasodilator effect and a reduction in arterial pressure. This effect has not been established in cats.
My cat suffers from decompensated hypertrophic cardiomyopathy and chronic kidney disease. What type of food is best recommended?	Food with a sodium content of around 0.5 g/1000 kcal is recommended for cats with chronic kidney disease. Reducing the phosphorus content in this food will slow down the progression of the renal disease. Furthermore, foods formulated for cats with chronic kidney disease are enriched in omega-3 fatty acids, which is also beneficial in the event of cardiopathy.
My cat is obese and suffers from hypertrophic cardiomyopathy. What type of food should be prescribed?	The priority is implementing medical treatment and a diet that best supports cardiac function. Restricting energy intake will then be desirable, as obesity is associated with increased cardiovascular risk. Some studies on rodents show that dietary restriction reduces the level of oxidative stress and protects against some degenerative diseases, especially cardiomyopathies. This has not been studied in cats.

Q	**A**
When should taurine deficiency be suspected during dilated cardiomyopathy?	Taurine deficiency in cats has been uncommon since the end of the 1980s, because commercial foods are now supplemented with taurine. This deficiency may however be suspected if the cat is fed a home-prepared ration, a vegetarian diet or poor quality foods. Measuring the taurine level in the whole blood (>250 nmol/mL) will help establish a definitive diagnosis. As central retinal degeneration is irreversible, it can be used to determine whether the cat has been fed with a taurine-deficient food for several months during the course of its life, but not whether its current diet is taurine-deficient.
Should cats with cardiac disease be prescribed potassium supplements?	Hypokalemia may appear with the use of diuretics (e.g. furosemide). Hypokalemia also occurs in 20% of cats with chronic kidney disease, and it increases the risk of hypertension (see chapter 7). Hypokalemia potentializes the toxicity of digoxin as well. In cardiopathic cats, the correction of hypokalemia through the supplementation of potassium is therefore strongly recommended. Supplementation, on the other hand, is not necessary in the absence of hypokalemia. In cats treated with an angiotensin converting enzyme inhibitor, which stimulates reabsorption of potassium by the kidneys, the potassium content of the food must not be different from that of a maintenance food (1.5-2 g/1000 kcal).

Heart

References

Backus RC, Morris JG, Rogers QR. Microbial degradation of taurine in fecal cultures of cats given commercial and purified diets. J Nutr 1994; 124: 2540S-2545S.

Backus RC, Puryear LM, Crouse BA, et al. Breath hydrogen concentrations of cats given commercial canned and extruded diets indicate gastrointestinal microbial activity vary with diet type. J Nutr 2002; 132: 1763S-1766S.

Bautista J, Rafel E, Martinez A, et al. Familial hypertrophic cardiomyopathy and muscle carnitine deficiency. Muscle Nerve 1990; 13: 192-194.

Binns SH, Sisson DD, Buoscio DA, et al. Doppler ultrasonographic, oscillometric sphygmomanometric, and photoplethysmographic techniques for noninvasive blood pressure measurement in anesthetized cats. J Vet Intern Med 1995; 9: 405-414.

Brevetti G, Angelini C, Rosa M, et al. Muscle carnitine deficiency in patients with severe peripheral vascular disease. Circulation 1991; 84: 1490-1495.

Brown SA. Pathophysiology of systemic hypertension. In: Ettinger S ed. Textbook of Veterinary Internal Medicine. Philadelphia, 6th ed. Elsevier 2006: 472-476.

Brown S, Atkins C, Bagley R, et al. ACVIM consensus statement. Guidelines for the identification, evaluation, and management of systemic hypertension in dogs and cats. J Vet Intern Med 2007; 2: 542-58.

Brown CA, Munday JS, Mathur S, et al. Hypertensive encephalopathy in cats with reduced renal function. Vet Pathol 2005; 42: 642-649.

Broughton KS, Wade JW. Total fat and (n-3):(n-6) fat ratios influence eicosanoid production in mice. J Nutr 2001; 132: 88-94.

Buranakarl C, Mathur S, Brown SA. Effects of dietary sodium chloride intake on renal function and blood pressure in cats with normal and reduced renal function. Am J Vet Res 2004; 65: 620-627.

Burger I. The Waltham book of companion animal nutrition. Pergamon Press, Oxford; 1993.

Carlos Sampedrano C, Chetboul V, Gouni V, et al. Systolic and diastolic myocardial dysfunction in cats with hypertrophic cardiomyopathy or systemic hypertension. J Vet Intern Med 2006; 20: 1106-1115.

Calzada C, Bruckdorfer KR, Rice-Evans CA. The influence of antioxidant nutrients on platelet function in healthy volunteers. Atheroscl 1997; 128: 97-105.

Charnock JS. Gamma linolenic acid provides additional protection against ventricular fibrillation in aged rats fed linoleic acid rich diets. Prostaglandins Leukot Essent Fatty Acids 2000; 62: 129-134.

Charron S, Lambert R, Eliopoulos V, et al. A loss of genome buffering capacity of Dahl salt-sensitive model to modulate blood pressure as a cause of hypertension. Hum Mol Genet 2005; 14: 3877-3884.

Chetboul V, Lefebvre HP, Pinhas C, et al. Spontaneous feline hypertension: clinical and echocardiographic abnormalities, and survival rate. J Vet Intern Med 2003; 17: 89-95.

Chetboul V, Blot S, Carlos Sampedrano C, et al. Tissue Doppler imaging for detection of radial and longitudinal myocardial dysfunction in a family of cats affected by dystrophin-deficient hypertrophic muscular dystrophy. J Vet Intern Med 2006a; 20: 640-647.

Chetboul V, Carlos Sampedrano C, et al. Two-dimensional color tissue Doppler imaging detects myocardial dysfunction before occurrence of hypertrophy in a young Maine Coon cat. Vet Radiol Ultrasound 2006b; 47: 295-300.

Cowgill LD, Sergev G, Bandt C, et al. Effects of dietary salt intake on body fluid volume and renal function in healthy cats. J Vet Intern Med 2007; 21: 600 (abst 104).

Cowley AW Jr, Skelton MM, Papanek PE, et al. Hypertension induced by high salt intake in absence of volume retention in reduced renal mass rats. Am J Physiol 1994; 267(5 Pt 2): H1707-712.

Devois C, Biourge V, Morice G, et al. Influence of various amount of dietary NaCl on urinary Na, Ca oxalate concentrations and excretions in adult cats. Congress of the ECVIM, Neuchatel, Suisse, September 2000.

Dow SW, Fettman MJ, Smith KR, et al. Taurine depletion and cardiovascular disease in adult cats fed a potassium depleted acidified diet. Am J Vet Res 1992; 53: 402-405.

Duffy SJ, Keaney JF, Holbrook M, et al. Short and long term black tea consumption reverses endothelial dysfunction in patients with coronary artery disease. Circulation 2001a; 104: 151-156.

Duffy SJ, Vita JA, Holbrook M, et al. Effect of acute and chronic tea consumption on platelet aggregation in patients with coronary artery disease. Art Throm Vasc Biol 2001b 21: 1084-1092.

Elliott J, Barber PJ, Syme HM, et al. Feline hypertension: clinical findings and response to antihypertensive treatment in 30 cases. J Small Anim Pract 2001; 42: 122-129.

Feldman EC, Nelson RW. Feline hyperthyroidism (thyrotoxicosis). In: Feldman EC, Nelson RW, eds. Canine and Feline Endocrinology and Reproduction. Philadelphia, WB Saunders Co, 1996, 118-166.

Filburn CR, Griffin D. Effects of supplementation with a docosahexaenoic acid-enriched salmon oil on total plasma and plasma phospholipids fatty acid composition in the cat. Intern J Appl Res Vet Med 2005; 3: 116-123.

Fox PR. Feline cardiomyopathies. In: Fox PR, Sisson D, Moïse NS, eds. Textbook of canine and feline cardiology. Philadelphia, WB Saunders Co, 1999, 621-678.

Fox PR, Maron BJ, Basso C, et al. Spontaneously occurring arrhythmogenic right ventricular cardiomyopathy in the domestic cat: A new animal model similar to the human disease. Circulation 2000; 102: 1863-1870.

Fox PR. The Multicenter Feline Chonic Failure Study. Proceedings of the 21st Annual ACVIM Forum, Charlotte, USA, June 2003.

Fox PR. Endomyocardial fibrosis and restrictive cardiomyopathy: pathologic and clinical features. J Vet Cardiol 2004; 6: 25-31.

Fox PR. Hypertrophic cardiomyopathy. Clinical and pathologic correlates. J Vet Cardiol 2003; 5: 39-45.

Fox PR, Sturman JA. Myocardial taurine concentrations in cats with cardiac disease and in healthy cats fed taurine modified diets. Am J Vet Res 1992; 53: 237-241.

Freeman LM. Personal communication to Waltham Centre For Pet Nutrition, 2002.

Freeman LM. Nutritional modulation of cardiac disease. Waltham Focus 2000; 10: 19-24.

Freeman LM, Brown DJ, Rush JE. Assessment of degree of oxidative stress and antioxidant concentrations in dogs with idiopathic dilated cardiomyopathy. J Am Vet Med Assoc 1999; 215: 644-646.

Freeman LM, Rush JE, Kehayias JJ et al. Nutritional alterations and the effect of fish oil supplementation in dogs with heart failure. J Vet Intern Med 1998; 12: 440-448.

Freeman LM, Brown DJ, Smith FW, et al. Magnesium status and the effect of magnesium supplementation in feline hypertrophic cardiomyopathy. Can J Vet Res 1997; 61: 227-231.

Geleijnse JM, Launer LJ, vander Kulp DA, et al. Inverse association of tea and flavonoid intakes with incident of myocardial infarction: the Rotterdam Study. Am J Clin Nutr 2002; 75: 880-886.

Gerbi A, Barbey O, Raccah D, et al. Alteration of Na, K-ATPase isoenzymes in diabetic cardiomyopathy: effect of dietary supplementation with fish oil (n-3 fatty acids) in rats. Diabetologia 1997; 40: 496-505.

Gottlieb SS, Baruch L, Kukin ML. Prognostic importance of the serum magnesium concentration in patients with congestive heart failure. J Am Coll Cardiol 1990; 16: 827-831.

Gouni V, Chetboul V, Pouchelon JL, et al. Prevalence of azotemia in 305 cats with acquired heart diseases: a retrospective study (2001-2005). Congress of the ECVIM, Amsterdam, the Netherlands, September 2006.

Greco DS, Lees GE, Dzendzel G, et al. Effects of dietary sodium intake on blood pressure measurements in partially nephrectomized dogs. Am J Vet Res 1994; 55: 160-165.

Grimm H, Mayer K, Mayser P, et al. Regulatory potential of n-3 fatty acids in immunological and inflammatory processes. Br J Nutr 2002; 87: S59-S67.

Guo Z, Mitchell-Raymundo F, Yang H, et al. Dietary restriction reduces atherosclerosis and oxidative stress in the aorta of apolipoprotein E-deficient mice. Mech Ageing Dev 2002; 123: 1121-1131.

Guyton AC, Hall JE. Vascular distensibility, and functions of the arterial and venous systems. In: Guyton AC, ed. Textbook of Medical Physiology. 9th ed. Philadelphia, WB Saunders Co, 1996, 171-181.

Häggström J. Hypertrophic cardiomyopathy in cats: it used to be so simple!. J Feline Med Surg 2003; 5: 139-141.

Hajri T, Ibrahimi A, Coburn CT, et al. Defective fatty acid uptake in the spontaneously hypertensive rat is a primary determinant of altered glucose metabolism, hyperinsulinemia and myocardial hypertrophy. J Biol Chem 2001; 276: 23661-23666.

Helton E, Darragh R, Francis P, et al. Metabolic aspects of myocardial disease and a role for L-carnitine in the treatment of childhood cardiomyopathy. Pediatrics 2000; 105: 1260-1270.

Henik RA, Snyder PS, Volk LM. Treatment of systemic hypertension in cats with amlodipine besylate. J Am Anim Hosp Assoc 1997; 33: 226-234.

Hirooka K, Yasumura Y, Ishida Y, et al. Improvement in cardiac function and free fatty acid metabolism in a case of dilated cardiomyopathy with CD36 deficiency. Jpn Circ J 2000; 64: 731-735.

Jalili T, Medeiros DM, Wildman REC. Aspects of cardiomyopathy are exacerbated by elevated dietary fat in copper restricted rats. J Nutr 1995; 126: 807-816.

Jensen J, Henik RA, Brownfield M, et al. Plasma renin activity and angiotensin I and aldosterone concentrations in cats with hypertension associated with chronic renal disease. Am J Vet Res 1997; 58: 535-540.

Jepson RE, Elliott J, Brodbelt D, et al. Effect of control of systolic blood pressure on survival in cats with systemic hypertension. J Vet Intern Med 2007; 21: 402-409.

Jepson RE, Hartley V, Mendl M, et al. Comparison of CAT Doppler and oscillometric Memoprint machines for non-invasive blood pressure measurement in conscious cats. J Feline Med Surg 2005; 7: 147-152.

Kang JX, Leaf A. Antiarrhythmic effects of polyunsaturated fatty acids. Recent studies. Circulation 1996; 94: 1774-1780.

Karim M, McCormick K, Kappagoda CT. Effects of cocoa extracts on endothelium dependent relaxation. J Nutr 2000; 130: 2105S-2109S.

Keen BW, Panciera DP, Atkins CE, et al. Myocardial L-carnitine deficiency in a family of dogs with dilated cardiomyopathy. J Am Vet Med Assoc 1991; 198: 647-650.

Keevil JG, Osman HE, Reed JD, et al. Grape juice, but not orange or grapefruit juice inhibits human platelet aggregation. J Nutr 2000; 130: 53-56.

Kelly DP, Strauss AW. Inherited cardiomyopathies. N Engl J Med 1994; 330: 913-919.

Kemi M, Keenan KP, McCoy C, et al. The relative protective effects of moderate dietary restriction versus dietary modification on spontaneous cardiomyopathy in male Sprague-Dawley rats. Toxicol Pathol 2000; 28: 285-296.

Kenny D, Warltier DC, Pleuss JA, et al. Effect of omega-3 fatty acids on the vascular response to angiotensin in normotensive men. Am J Cardiol 1992; 70: 1347-1352.

Kim SW, Rogers QR, Morris JG. Maillard reaction products in purified diets induce taurine depletion in cats which is reversed by antibiotics. J Nutr 1996a; 126: 195-201.

Kim SW, Rogers QR, Morris JG. Dietary antibiotics decrease taurine loss in cats fed a canned heat-processed diet. J Nutr 1996b; 126: 509-515.

Kirk CA, Jewell DE, Lowry SR. Effects of sodium chloride on selected parameters in cats. Vet Ther 2007; 7: 333-346.

Kobayashi DL, Peterson ME, Graves TK, et al. Hypertension in cats with chronic renal failure or hyperthyroidism. J Vet Intern Med 1990; 4: 58-62.

Kotchen TA, Krzyzaniak KE, Anderson JE, et al. Inhibition of renin secretion by HCl is related to chloride in both dog and rat. Am J Physiol 1980; 239: F44-F49.

Krieger JE, Liard JF, Cowley AW Jr. Hemodynamics, fluid volume, and hormonal responses to chronic high-salt intake in dogs. Am J Physiol 1990; 259(6 Pt 2): H1629-1636.

Kris-Etherton PM, Etherton TD, Carlson J, Gardner C Recent discoveries in inclusive food-based approaches and dietary patterns for reduction in risk for cardiovascular disease. Curr Opin Lipidol 2002; 13: 397-407

Kristensen SD, Iverson AMB, Schmidt EB. n-3 polyunsaturated fatty acids and coronary thrombosis. Lipids 2001; 36: S79-82.

Kugiyama K, Motoyama T, Hirashima O, et al. Vitamin C attenuates abnormal vasomotor reactivity in spasm coronary arteries in patients with coronary spastic angina. J Am Coll Cardiol, 1998; 32: 103-109.

349

Lango R, Smoleski RT, Narkiewicz M, et al. Influence of L-carnitine and its derivatives on myocardial metabolism and function in ischemic heart disease and during cardiopulmonary bypass. Cardiovasc Res 2001; 51: 21-29.

Laste NJ, Harpster NK. A retrospective study of 100 cases of feline distal aortic thromboembolism: 1977-1993. J Am Anim Hosp Assoc 1995; 31: 492-500.

Lefebvre HP, Brown SA, Chetboul V, et al. Angiotensin-converting enzyme inhibitors in veterinary medicine. Curr Pharm Des 2007; 13: 1347-1361.

Lerman A, Burnett JC, Higano ST. Long term arginine supplementation improves small vessel coronary endothelial function in humans. Circulation 1998; 97: 2123-2128.

Levine B, Kalman J, Mayer L, et al. Elevated circulating levels of tumour necrosis factor in severe chronic heart failure. N Engl J Med 1990; 323: 236-241.

Linder MC. Nutritional Biochemistry and Metabolism. Elsevier, London. 2nd Ed: 1991.

Luckschander N, Iben C, Hosgood G, et al. Dietary NaCl does not affect blood pressure in healthy cats. J Vet Intern Med 2004; 18: 463-467.

Luft FC, Rankin LI, Bloch R, et al. Cardiovascular and humoral responses to extremes of sodium intake in normal black and white men. Circulation 1979; 60: 697-706.

Luft FC, Weinberger MH. Heterogeneous responses to changes in dietary salt intake: the salt-sensitivity paradigm. Am J Clin Nutr 1997; 65: 612S-617S.

Lund EM, Armstrong PJ, Kirk CA, et al. Prevalence and risk factors for obesity in adult dogs from private US veterinary practices. Intern J Appl Res Vet Med 2006; 4: 177-186.

Mahoney SM, Tisdale MJ. Induction of weight loss and metabolic alterations by human recombinant tumour necrosis factor. Br J Cancer 1988; 58: 345-349.

McClellan WM, Langston RD, Presley R. Medicare patients with cardiovascular disease have a high prevalence of chronic kidney disease and a high rate of progression to end-stage renal disease. J Am Soc Nephrol 2004; 15: 1912-1919.

McMichael M, Freeman L, Selhub J, et al. Plasma homocysteine, B vitamins, and amino acid concentrations in cats with cardiomyopathy and arterial thromboembolism. J Vet Intern Med. 2000; 14: 507-512.

Maggio F, DeFrancesco TC, Atkins CE, et al. Ocular lesions associated with systemic hypertension in cats: 69 cases (1985-1998). J Am Vet Med Assoc 2000; 217: 695-702.

Meurs KM, Sanchez X, David RM, et al. A cardiac myosin binding protein C mutation in the Maine Coon cat with familial hypertrophic cardiomyopathy. Human Molecular Genetic 2005; 14: 3587-3593.

Meurs KM, Norgard MM, Ederer MM, et al. A substitution mutation in the myosin binding protein C gene in ragdoll hypertrophic cardiomyopathy. Genomics 2007; 90: 261-264.

Meydani SN, Endres S, Woods MM. Oral (n-3) fatty acid supplementation suppresses cytokine production and lymphocyte proliferation. J Nutr 1991; 121: 547-555.

Mishina M, Watanabe T, Fujii K, et al. Non-invasive blood pressure measurements in cats: clinical significance of hypertension associated with chronic renal failure. J Vet Med Sci 1998; 60: 805-808.

Moncada S, Palmer RM, Higgs EA. Nitric oxide: physiology, pathophysiology, and pharmacology. Pharmacol Rev 1991; 43: 109-142.

Morris JG. Nutrition Research Reviews 2002, 15,153-168.

Morris JG, Rogers QR. Comparative aspects of the nutrition and metabolism of dogs and cats. In: Waltham Symposium #7 "Nutrition of the Dog and Cat" Edited I.H. Burger and J.P.W. Rivers. Cambridge University Press; 1987: 35-66.

Morris JG, Rogers QR, Kim SW, et al. Dietary taurine requirement of cats is determined by microbial degradation of taurine in the gut. Adv Exp Med Biol 1994; 359: 59-70.

Mower R, Steiner M. Synthetic byproducts of tocopherol oxidation as inhibitors of platelet function. Prostaglandins 1982; 24: 137-147.

Nakata T, Nakahara N, Sohmiya K, et al. Scintigraphic evidence for a specific long chain fatty acid transporting system deficit and the genetic background in a patient with hypertrophic cardiomyopathy. Jpn Circ J 1999; 63: 319-322.

National Research Council of the National Academies. Nutrient requirements of dogs and cats. The National Academies Press, Washington, D.C., 2006.

Nelson L, Reidesel E, Ware WA, et al. Echocardiographic and radiographic changes associated with systemic hypertension in cats. J Vet Intern Med 2002; 16: 418-425.

Nicolle AP, Chetboul V, Allerheiligen T, et al. Azotemia and glomerular filtration rate in dogs with chronic valvular disease. J Vet Intern Med 2007; 21:943-949.

Novotny MJ, Hogan PM, Paley DM, et al. Systolic and diastolic dysfunction of the left ventricle induced by dietary taurine deficiency in cats. Am J Physiol 1991; 26: H121-H127.

Okamoto F, Tanaka T, Sohmiya K, et al. CD36 abnormality and impaired myocardial long chain fatty acid uptake in patients with hypertrophic cardiomyopathy. Jpn Circ J 1998; 62: 499-504.

Pacioretty L, Hickman MA, Morris JG, et al. Kinetics of taurine depletion and repletion in plasma, serum, whole blood and skeletal muscle in cats. Amino Acids 2001; 21: 417-427.

Pedersen KM, Pedersen HD, Häggström J, et al. Increased mean arterial pressure and aldosterone-to-renin ratio in Persian cats with polycystic kidney disease. J Vet Intern Med 2003; 17: 21-27.

Pion PD, Kittleson MD, Rogers QR et al. Myocardial failure in cats associated with low plasma taurine: a reversible cardiomyopathy. Science 1987; 237: 764-768.

Pion PD, Kittleson MD, Thomas WP, et al. Clinical findings in cats with dilated cardiomyopathy and relationship of findings to taurine deficiency. J Am Vet Med Assoc 1992 a; 201: 267-274.

Pion PD, Kittleson MD, Thomas WP, et al. Response of cats with dilated cardiomyopathy to taurine supplementation. J Am Vet Med Assoc 1992 b; 201: 275-284.

Plotnick GD, Corretti MC, Vogel RA. Effect of antioxidant vitamins on the transient impairment of endothelial dependent brachial artery vasoactivity following a single high fat meal. J Am Med Assoc 1997; 278: 1682-1686.

Pouchelon JL, King JN, Martignoni L, et al. Long-term tolerability of benazepril in dogs with congestive heart failure. J Vet Cardiol 2004; 6: 7-13.

Rein D, Lotito S, Holt RR, et al. Epicatechin in human plasma: In vivo determination and effect of chocolate consumption on plasma oxidation status. J Nutr 2000a; 130: 2109S-2115S.

Rein D, Paglieroni TG, Pearson DA, et al. Cocoa and wine polyphenols modulate platelet activation and function. J Nutr 2000b; 130: 2120S-2126S.

Rieck J, Halkin H, Almog S, et al. Urinary loss of thiamine is increased by low doses of furosemide in healthy volunteers. J Lab Clin Med, 1999; 134: 238-243

Rimm EB, Katan MB, Ascherio A, et al. Relation between intake of flavonoids and risk for coronary heart disease in male health professionals. Ann Intern Med 1996; 125: 384-389.

Rosenfeldt FL, Pepe S, Linnane A, et al. Coenzyme Q10 protects the aging heart against stress: studies in rats, human tissues, and patients. Ann N Y Acad Sci 2002; 959: 355-359.

Rush JE, Freeman LM, Brown DJ et al. Clinical, echocardiographic, and neurohumoral effects of a sodium-restricted diet in dogs with heart failure. J Vet Intern Med 2000; 14: 513-520.

Rush JE, Freeman LM, Fenollosa NK, et al. Population and survival characteristics of cats with hypertrophic cardiomyopathy: 260 cases (1990-1999). J Am Vet Med Assoc 2002; 220: 202-207.

Saker KE, Eddy AL, Thatcher CD, et al. Manipulation of dietary (n-6) and (n-3) fatty acids alters platelet function in cats. J Nutr 1998; 128: 2645S-2647S.

Samson J, Rogers K, Wood JL. Blood pressure assessment in healthy cats and cats with hypertensive retinopathy. Am J Vet Res 2004; 65: 245-252.

Sennello KA, Schulman RL, Prosek R, et al. Systolic blood pressure in cats with diabetes mellitus. J Am Vet Med Assoc 2003; 223: 198-201.

Siegel AK, Planert M, Rademacher S, et al. Genetic loci contribute to the progression of vascular and cardiac hypertrophy in salt-sensitive spontaneous hypertension. Arterioscler Thromb Vasc Biol 2003; 23: 1211-1217.

Smith SA, Tobias AH, Jacob KA, et al. Arterial thromboembolism in cats: acute crisis in 127 cases (1992-2001) and long-term management with low-dose aspirin in 24 cases. J Vet Intern Med 2003; 17: 73-83.

Smith CE, Freeman LM, Rush JE, et al. Omega-3 fatty acids in Boxer dogs with arrhythmogenic right ventricular cardiomyopathy. J Vet Intern Med 2007; 21: 265-273.

Snyder PS, Cooke KL. Management of hypertension. In: Ettinger S ed. Textbook of Veterinary Internal Medicine. 6th ed. Elsevier copyright 2006, 477-479.

Snyder PS, Sadek D, Jones GL. Effect of amlodipine on echocardiographic variables in cats with systemic hypertension. J Vet Intern Med 2001; 15: 52-56.

Steinmetz KA, Potter JD. Vegetables, fruit and cancer prevention: a review. J Am Diet Assoc 1996; 96: 1027-1039.

Stepien RL. Blood pressure measurement: equipment, methodology and clinical recommendations. Proceedings of the 22nd ACVIM forum, Minneapolis, MN, USA, 2004.

Stiles J, Polzin DJ, Bistner SI. The prevalence of retinopathy in cats with systemic hypertension and chronic renal failure or hyperthyroidism. J Am Anim Hosp Assoc 1994; 30: 564-572.

Syme HM, Barber PJ, Markwell PJ, et al. Prevalence of systolic hypertension in cats with chronic renal failure at initial evaluation. J Am Vet Med Assoc 2002; 220: 1799-1804.

Taugner F, Baatz G, Nobiling R. The renin-angiotensin system in cats with chronic renal failure. J Comp Pathol 1996; 115: 239-252.

Tissier R, Perrot S, Enriquez B. Amlodipine: One of the main antihypertensive drugs in veterinary therapeutics. J Vet Cardiol 2005; 7: 53-58.

Toll J, Erb H, Birnbaum N, et al. Prevalence and incidence of serum magnesium abnormalities in hospitalized cats. J Vet Intern Med 2002; 16: 217-221.

Watanabe K, Toba K, Ogawa Y, et al. Hypertrophic cardiomyopathy with type I CD36 deficiency. Jpn Circ J 1998; 62: 541-542.

Weinberger MH, Fineberg NS, Fineberg SE, et al. Salt sensitivity, pulse pressure, and death in normal and hypertensive humans. Hypertension 2001; 37: 429-432.

Weinberger MH. Salt sensitivity of blood pressure in humans. Hypertension 1996; 27: 481-90.

Weinberger MH, Miller JZ, Luft FC, et al. Definitions and characteristics of sodium sensitivity and blood pressure resistance. Hypertension 1986; 8: II127-134.

Welles EG, Boudreaux MK, Crager CS, et al. Platelet function and antithrombin, plasminogen and fibrinolytic activities in cats with heart disease. Am J Vet Res 1994; 55: 619-627.

Whitehouse AS, Smith HJ, Drake JL, et al. Mechanism of attenuation of skeletal muscle protein catabolism in cancer cachexia by eicosapentanoic acid. Cancer Res 2001; 61: 3604-3609.

Xu H, Laflamme DP, Riboul C, et al. High sodium has no adverse effects on blood pressure or renal function in healthy cats. J Vet Intern Med 2007; 21: 600 (abst 105).

Yu HC, Burrell LM, Black MJ, et al. Salt induces myocardial and renal fibrosis in normotensive and hypertensive rats. Circulation 1998; 98: 2621-2628.

Zelikovic I, Chesney RW. Taurine in biology and nutrition. In: Friedman M, ed. Absorption and utilization of amino-acids, vol I. Boca Raton, FL: CRC Press Inc, 1989: 199-228.

Zhao X, White R, Van Huysse J, et al. Cardiac hypertrophy and cardiac renin-angiotensin system in Dahl rats on high salt intake. J Hypertens 2000; 18: 1319-1326.

Heart

Nicolas GIRARD
DMV

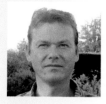

Eric SERVET

MEng, Royal Canin
Research Center in
Aimargues, France

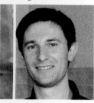

Nutrition and oral health in cats

1 - Dietary behavior in cats **359**

2 - Common oral diseases **362**

3 - Preventing oral diseases **372**

Conclusion **375**

Fallacies regarding oral diseases in cats 376

References 377

Royal Canin nutritional information 379

Oral Health

ABBREVIATIONS USED IN THIS CHAPTER

C: canine
DR: dental resorption (type 1 or 2)
FORL: feline odontoclastic resorptive lesion
I: incisor
M: molar
PM: premolar
PRN: plaque reduction nutrient
TMJ: temporo-mandibular joint

Nutrition and oral health in cats

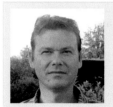

Nicolas GIRARD

DVM

Nicolas Girard graduated from the National Veterinary School of Alfort in 1987. After practicing general veterinary medicine for small animals for approximately twelve years. Nicolas is now a practicing veterinary dentist and ear, nose and throat specialist in the southwest of France.

Nicolas is in charge of the dentistry consultation at the National Veterinary School of Alfort. He is also responsible for the scientific committee of the Veterinarian Dentistry Study and Research Group Office (GEROS), a component of the French Association of Veterinarians for Companion Animals (AFVAC). Nicolas is also a member of the European Veterinary Dental Society (EVDS).

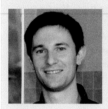

Eric SERVET

MEng, Royal Canin Research Center in Aimargues, France

Eric Servet graduated in engineering from ENITIAA in Nantes, specializing in dietary ingredients and technologies. In 1999-2001 he worked on the pilot development and formulation of commercial dairy products. He subsequently spent a year in the United States at Royal Canin USA, working in product stability and palatability. Since 2002 he has been a research engineer at the Royal Canin Research and Development Center in Aimargues, France. His main fields of feline and canine research are dental hygiene, joint cartilage nutrition, and obesity.

Oral Health

The teeth have an essential influence on the cat's general health. They have a role to play in many different functions, such as hunting, grasping and breaking food, self-defense and competition. There are few precise epidemiological studies describing the oral health of cats. Data on cats are mostly extrapolated from dogs, although the oral-dental pathology of cats in all their diversity has special particularities that veterinarians need to know.

Periodontal diseases are common in cats but are often underrated by veterinarians and treated superficially. Recent advancements in feline veterinarian dentistry have provided new tools for their evaluation and diagnosis, as well as more effective prevention tools. All this information must be at the center of the care agreement between the clinic and the owner and aimed at minimizing pain and associated infections.

1 - Dietary behavior in cats

► Anatomical and pathological specificities

Cats are genuine carnivores and their dentition is the same as the major Felidae **(Figure 1)**. They have four types of teeth [incisors (I), canines (C), premolars (PM) and molars (M)] but unlike dogs and other carnivores, cats do not have any chewing teeth – upper molars **(Figures 1 and 2)**.

In the various sequences of dietary behavior, the role of teeth is to capture and dismember small prey, using groups of differentiated teeth.
- The shape of the incisors enables them to cut, hollow out and hack.
- The canines are profiled to pierce and grasp prey.
- The premolars serve to transport the food and to break it into small pieces.

FIGURE 1 - PROFILE VIEW OF THE DENTITION OF AN ADULT CAT

FIGURE 1 - PROFILE VIEW OF THE DENTITION OF AN ADULT CAT

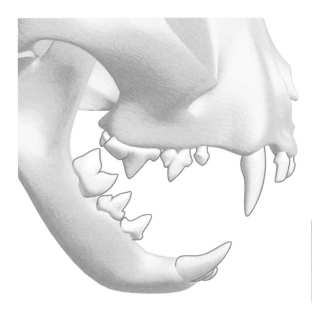

The four largest cutting teeth at the back of the upper and lower jaws are called carnassials (PM4 upper and M1 lower).

Dental formula of an adult cat (per quadrant):
I 3/3; C 1/1; PM 3/2; M 1/1
Collectively, there are 30 teeth in the oral cavity of the adult cat.

The oral cavity of cats can be opened wide to enable the canines to grasp the prey, while facilitating the powerful action of the carnassials. Once the prey has been broken up into pieces, it is swallowed *(Wiggs & Lobprise, 1997)*.

The movements of the jaws are limited sagittally (no transversal masticatory movement). This extreme specialization of the jaws and the temporomandibular joints in cats guarantees great efficiency with respect to the forces exercised when prey is grasped and broken down *(Orsini & Hennet, 1992)*. In domesticated cats, the canines apply around 23 kg of pressure, the carnassials around 28 kg *(Buckland, 1975)*. Joint integrity is maintained by powerful lateral ligaments covered by an effective jaw musculature. Typically, while the carnassials break the food up, the temporomandibular joints twist and rotate it, doubling the effect. The fibrous symphysis connecting the two branches of the mandible enables the distinct movements of the right and left jaw according to the needs and the side used by the cat *(Harvey & Emily, 1993)*.

► Varied oral prehension techniques

In nature, the diet of a wild cat comprises mostly of small rodents, rabbits, birds and some lizards. After catching its prey, step-by-step the cat cuts and swallows it in small pieces.

While domestication has changed their behavior to a degree, domesticated cats still have the ability to return to their wild life, as they retain the hunting instinct, separate from the feeding function. Only 13% of tracked prey is actually caught *(Kays & DeWan, 2004)*. A study shows that, even properly fed housecats with outdoor access will continue to hunt and eat prey, although the proportion of such prey in the total ration is clearly lower than in that of cats that permanently live outdoors (66 g/day vs. 294 g/day) *(Liberg, 1984)*.

FIGURE 2 - FRONT VIEW OF DENTAL OCCLUSION IN THE CAT

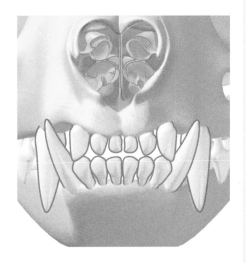

When the oral cavity is closed, the incisors of the lower jaw rest directly behind the incisors of the upper jaw, and the lower canine is between the upper canine and the third upper incisor.

Oral Health

Oral Health

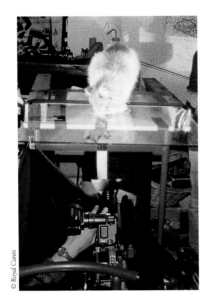

Figure 3 - Video analysis of the oral prehension method of Persian cats.

Analysis conducted in association with Royal Canin, École Nationale des Arts et Métiers d'Angers (ENSAM) and Ecole des Mines d'Alès (EMA).

FIGURE 4 - DIFFERENT ORAL PREHENSION METHODS OBSERVED IN CATS

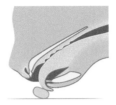 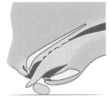 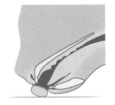 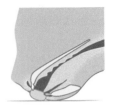

Supra-lingual mode
First point of contact with the kibble is the upper side of the tongue.

Sub-lingual mode
First point of contact with the kibble is the lower side of the tongue.

Labial mode
First point of contact with the kibble is the lips.

"Shovel" mode
First point of contact with the kibble is the incisors.

The palatability of commercial food has been studied in detail to continually improve product quality. Dry kibbles in various shapes, sizes, textures and densities are given to cats to evaluate their reaction. Analyzing videos of the feeding behavior of different breeds of domesticated cats **(Figure 3)** has enabled the characterization of how cats grasp their food in general, while also identifying several kibble prehension methods **(Figure 4)**:
- *supra-lingual mode*: using the upper side of the tongue
- *labial mode*: using the lips and jaws
- *"shovel" mode*: using the incisors
- *sub-lingual mode*: using the lower side of the tongue

The kibble prehension method varies with the breed. A certain degree of adaptability in terms of prehension and mastication behavior is observed depending on the kibble shape and size *(unpublished internal Royal Canin studies, 2002)*.

Observing brachycephalic breeds (e.g. Persians), it is clear that they have difficulty grasping standard-sized, round kibbles, particularly with the incisors. Persians use the tongue to trap a standard kibble in 80% of cases (60% lower tongue **(Figure 5)** and 20% upper tongue). They use their lips just 20% of time, while the "shovel" method is not observed.

FIGURE 5 - COMPARATIVE JAW CONFORMATION BETWEEN A BRACHYCEPHALIC CAT (PERSIAN) AND A MESOCEPHALIC CAT

Source: Royal Canin Research Center, 2002

Lower tongue prehension method

Persian cat
Upper jaw

2.75 cm
2.95 cm
2.50 cm
2.60 cm

Lower jaw

European cat
Upper jaw

3.45 cm
3.50 cm
2.89 cm
3.12 cm

Lower jaw

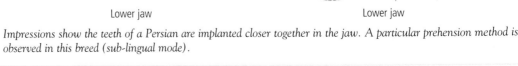

Impressions show the teeth of a Persian are implanted closer together in the jaw. A particular prehension method is observed in this breed (sub-lingual mode).

- Dolichocephalic cats (e.g. Siamese) like to use their incisors **(Figure 6)**. The "shovel" method is observed in 30% of cases, which is more efficient when the kibble bowl is full. Prehension tends to progress towards the upper tongue method as the bowl empties (to ensure the tongue grasps the kibble). Siamese cats use the upper tongue method in 70% of cases.

- Mesocephalic cats (e.g. Maine Coon) make almost equal use of upper tongue and lips at the start of the meal (in 57% and 42% of cases respectively) **(Figure 7)**. The upper tongue method may become more prevalent during the course of the meal or if the kibbles are smaller (83% tongue vs. 17% lips).

The influence of anatomical particularities related to breed also affects others aspects of feeding behavior. After grasping a standard kibble, Persians chew in only around 10% of cases, whereas the chewing percentage is 90% among Maine Coons and Siamese cats (*unpublished internal Royal Canin studies, 2002*).

Hence, prehension methods differ significantly from one breed to the other, and especially from one maxillofacial biometric to another.

▶ Feeding rhythm in domesticated cats

Domesticated cats habitually divide up much of their daily food. When different types of dry food are offered, the frequency and average duration of meals varies according to the breed and the food (*internal Royal Canin studies, 2006*).

On average, a cat fed ad libitum will feed a dozen or so times a day. Each session lasts about two minutes, with the cat consuming around 6 g of food. In one 24-hour period, the cat therefore devotes an average of 20 minutes to eating and digesting 50-60 g of kibbles **(Table 1)**. Nocturnal consumption accounts for 30% of all food ingested. At night, meals are generally larger and take longer. A strong correlation between breed and feeding rhythm **(Figure 8)** and the quantities ingested at each meal has been shown.

The influence of maxillofacial biometric variations on the feeding method of the domesticated cat is accordingly self-evident. The significant differences observed between facial morphologies provide more proof of different prehension methods, feeding rhythms and quantities of food ingested. The low adaptability of jaw movements (see above) requires them to adapt the natural sequences of prehension and ingestion to suit the food.

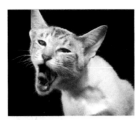
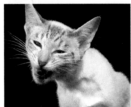
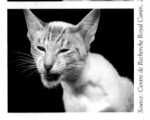

Source: Centre de Recherche Royal Canin, 2002

Figure 6 - Traditional food prehension method used by the Siamese cat.
The sequential analysis of 4800 prehension sessions shows that the Siamese uses its incisors in 30% of cases. The jaws open at a very wide angle.

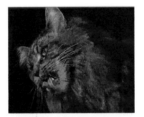
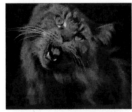
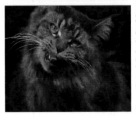

Source: Centre de Recherche Royal Canin, 2002

Figure 7 - Traditional food prehension method used by the Maine Coon cat
The sequential analysis of 7200 prehension sessions shows that the Maine Coon uses the lower tongue and labial method almost equally.

TABLE 1 – FOOD CONSUMPTION INDEXES IN CATS FED DRY FOOD AD LIBITUM
(Data from 16 cats fed ad libitum one of four foods consecutively – internal Royal Canin studies, 2006)

	Food 1	Food 2	Food 3	Food 4	Average
Number of meals/24 h	9.5	8.4	10.0	10.1	**9.5**
Size of meal (g)	6.7	6.7	5.6	5.3	**6.1**
Total consumption/24 h (g)	57.1	53.1	53.7	52.8	**54.2**
Average duration of meal (min' sec")	1'48"	2'16"	2'16"	2'09"	**2'07"**
Total consumption time/24 h (min' sec")	16'39"	18'35"	22'28"	21'46"	**19'53"**
Speed of consumption (g/min)	4.1	3.3	2.9	2.7	**3.2**

FIGURE 8 - INFLUENCE OF BREED ON THE AVERAGE DURATION OF MEALS IN CATS FED WITH A DRY FOOD

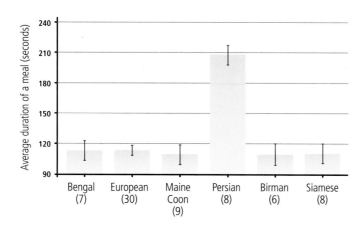

When cats are fed a standard dry food they feed around a dozen times in a 24-hour period. The average duration of each meal is 2 minutes ('), all breeds included. This average is however twice as long among Persians: 3'27", compared with 1'49" among all other breeds (unpublished Royal Canin data, 2005).

Domesticated cats have however retained the principle features of their wild feeding behavior. This feeding behavior continues to be studied frequently to evaluate the impact of commercial food on the oral health of cats as precisely as possible.

2 - Common oral diseases

▶ Prevalence of feline oral diseases in wild and domesticated populations

Whether wild or domesticated, a cat's diet is dictated by its environment. In this respect, commercial food preparation is often considered to be an aggravating factor in the event of oral diseases. The analysis of the oral diseases of a population of wild cats provides an opportunity to study the potential link between a well-defined diet and the various diseases identified.

Four cats were introduced on Marion Island in the Indian Ocean in 1949 and the cat population grew rapidly. The diet of these cats is mostly seabirds (96%) associated with the ingestion of some pebbles. The postmortem analysis of a collection of 300 skulls from this cat population enabled the study of oral health. Despite the average age of the group being estimated at 2-3 years, the prevalence of periodontal disease in a moderate to severe form, was 48%. Taking account of missing teeth (probably due to periodontal disease), periodontal disease was prevalent in 61.8% of cats and 14.8% of the teeth observed. The prevalence of dental trauma and feline odontoclastic resorptive lesions (FORLs) was also high, statistically associated with the prevalence of periodontal disease. On the other hand, only 9% of cats in this study presented calculus, and then typically on the upper carnassials.

The highly specific diet of this wild cat population undoubtedly explains the high frequency of periodontal lesions and the low prevalence of dental calculus observed in such a young colony. When the cat tears apart the carcasses of seabirds, the sharp bone sections are probably responsible for gum trauma, which is assumed to favor the development of more severe periodontal inflammation (*Verstraete et al, 1996*).

In an Australian study, the analysis of oral diseases based on clinical and radiographic criteria in 29 wild cats and 20 domesticated cats (*Clarke & Cameron, 1998*) established that the prevalence of periodontal disease was not significantly different in cats fed with commercial foods and cats whose diet was mainly made up of small prey. A hunting-based diet does not provide natural protection from oral diseases for wild cats.

Veterinarian examination of 15,226 domesticated cats (*Lund et al, 1998*) showed that oral diseases are the most common of all diseases observed. Calculus is present in 24% of cats and 13% of them suffer from some form of gingivitis.

A more detailed analysis conducted by veterinarians specialized in dentistry confirms a strong prevalence of oral diseases. 73% of a population of 753 cats studied presented gingivitis; 67% presented dental calculus; 28% of them had missing teeth; 25% FORLs; 19% severe periodontitis; 12% stomatitis and 11% tooth fractures *(Verhaerte & Van Wetter, 2004)*.

Periodontal disease is found in 32% of individuals presented to veterinarians specialized in dentistry. Out of a population of 152 cats, gingivitis and missing teeth were observed in 59% of cases, FORLs in 57% of cases, teeth fractures in 23% of cases and stomatitis in 2.6% of cases. The prevalence of dental calculus was estimated at 90% *(Crossley, 1991)*.

The postmortem analysis of 81 cats whose death was unrelated to an established oral disease, based on pathological and clinical examination, reported a high prevalence of periodontal disease. 52% of cats older than 4 years of age presented a form of periodontal inflammation. More than 40% of animals aged over 9 years presented a severe form of the disease. Less than 3% of animals aged over 15 years presented any form of lesion due to periodontal disease *(Gengler et al, 1995)*.

To summarize the studies above, the high prevalence of periodontal disease in cats cannot be ignored. There are no major differences between wild and domesticated populations and no apparent influence of commercial food. The presence of oral diseases is therefore not something that characterizes domesticated cats alone and is not necessarily associated with the feeding of commercial foods.

This information is unfortunately always underestimated. It does however shed light on the fact that the high prevalence of oral inflammation in cats is the most common cause of infectious disease in the species. The clinical impact turns out to be much greater than it appeared at first sight. It is especially clear in groups of wildcats whose health is generally related to interspecies competition and conditions the very survival of individuals. In the case of domesticated cats, the pain caused by oral disease is typically underestimated. Once they have been treated, these cats do show major behavioral modifications. Some owners describe this return to health as a "rebirth".

In wild cat populations, oral inflammation could threaten the health and even the survival of individuals.

▶ Periodontal disease

Periodontal disease is the most common disease in cats. It is an inflammatory oral disease associated with the development of dental plaque. Periodontal disease is not a disease as such as much as a collection of periodontal inflammations with varied clinical characteristics chronic or aggressive, local or generalized. All stages are possible: from early-stage periodontal disease to moderate or severe forms. The way periodontal disease develops depends on the mechanical constraints that oppose the development of dental plaque, but also the local immune response of each individual.

The incidence of periodontal disease on the general health of cats is widely underestimated. It is the source of chronic pain that owners are often unaware of and chronic bacterial diseases whose effects on the kidneys, lungs and heart are just starting to be better understood. Periodontal disease is the most common disease reported in cats, with a prevalence estimated at 30-70% of individuals according to studies and the evaluation criteria.

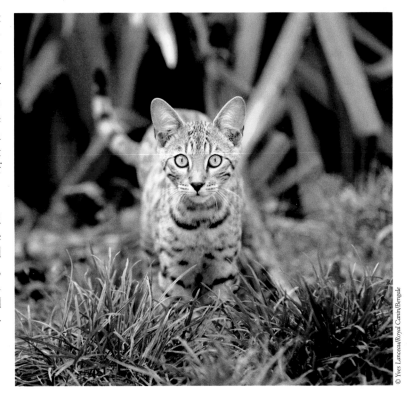

© Yves Lanceau/Royal Canin/Bengale

FIGURE 9 – COMPOSITION OF THE PERIODONTIUM

1. Jaw bone
2. Periodontal ligament
3. Gum
4. Sulcus
5. Cement (covers the root)
6. Dentine
7. Pulp
8. Enamel (covers the crown)

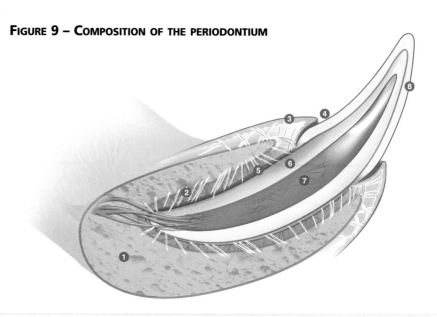

> Description and function of the periodontium

The periodontium is the tissue that supports the teeth in the oral cavity. It connects the teeth, the bone structure of the jaws and the oral mucosa. Its development is associated with the eruption of the tooth and it disappears with its exfoliation. The periodontal tissue guarantees the integrity of dental structures and effectively protects the underlying anatomical structures from aggressions in the oral environment.

The periodontium is composed of the gum, the periodontal ligament, cement and the alveolar bone **(Figure 9)**.

The alveolar bone is a differentiated part of the jawbone. It is responsible for positioning the roots of the teeth in depressions known as dental alveoli.

The periodontal ligament is composed of collagen fibers, which connects the surface of the tooth root (cement) to the alveolar bone. Like a hydraulic shock absorber the periodontal ligament absorbs the pressures placed on the alveolar bone during prehension and the tearing of food. These specialized fibers improve the resistance to pressure of underlying bone tissue and generate a pain signal when the limit of its mechanical resistance is reached.

The cement covers the root of the tooth. It has a similar structure to bone, but without lacunas and channels.

The gum covers the underlying alveolar bone and tightly hugs the base of the crown of the tooth. The gum is composed of a squamous, keratinized epithelium, which is different from the loose, vascularized and non-keratinized alveolar mucosa. It is made up of two parts.

- *The free gum* is located at the level of the crown. It defines a space against the crown known as the gingival crevice, whose physiological depth is less than 0.5 mm in cats. The weak point of the tooth/gum junction is always the gingival crevice. The delimited space is fairly closed and is predisposed to accumulating dental plaque and various food debris. As its histological nature makes it more sensitive to the inflammatory process, the gingival crevice forms a gateway for periodontal disease. As a consequence, all attention must be focused on periodontal disease treatment and prevention programs.

- *The gum attached* to the tooth and the alveolar bone is an essential barrier against bacterial aggression. The seam of the gum is stuck against the bulge of the base of the crown and enhances this protective action.

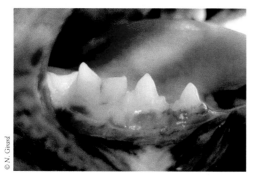

© N. Girard

Healthy gum.

Some 100 billion bacteria are discharged in the saliva every day. The oral cavity is therefore never sterile. There is always a minimal residual inflammation of the mucosa and the oral epithelium. A "healthy" periodontium is therefore defined clinically. The criteria for evaluating a healthy periodontium in cats are the absence of visual evidence of inflammation and the depth of the gingival crevice less than 0.5 mm.

> Pathogenesis of periodontal disease

The development of dental plaque in contact with all the surfaces of the tooth is a natural process resulting from the interaction between tooth and saliva. The anatomical sites predisposed to the deposition of dental plaque are the limit of the crown and the seams of the gum as well as the contacts between the teeth.

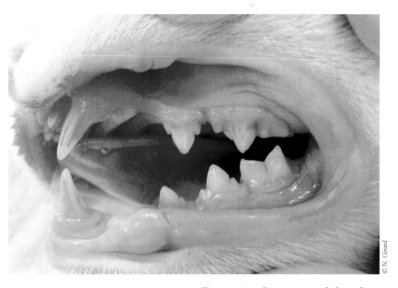

Figure 10 - Supragingival dental plaque on healthy teeth and gums.
The phenomena of bacterial coaggregation and coadhesion facilitate the installation of 90% of the biomass of the dental plaque within 24 hours (the dental plaque is revealed using eosin-type vital staining).

The adhesion and proliferation of bacteria on the surface of the enamel is not possible as such. The gradual colonization of the tooth surfaces by the bacteria is a succession of steps that steadily facilitate the adhesion and multiplication of bacteria:
- physical adhesion of an organic film to the surface of the teeth.
- secondary colonization by specific or pioneer bacteria.
- bacterial proliferation from the colonized organic film.

The adhesion of pioneer bacteria to the tooth surface is possible only after the development of an organic film (acquired pellicle) essentially formed from salivary components (glycoprotein, polypeptides, carbohydrate). Within a few hours of its development, specific bacteria (*Streptococcus sanguis, Actynomyces viscosus*) arrive to colonize the acquired pellicle, gradually saturating the entire surface (>6 million/sq. mm) and forming a biofilm, **dental plaque (Figure 10)**. New bacterial appositions, which stimulate the phenomena of coaggregation and coadhesion, establish 90% of the dental plaque's biomass within 24 hours.

Initially, dental plaque is essentially composed of aerobic Gram+ bacteria but this population develops rapidly. With the increase in the bacterial population comes the fall in oxygen in the air, from 12-14% in the mouth to 1-2% at the base of the gingival crevice. These new environmental conditions, which are associated with various sources of nutrients (diet, bacterial degradation, epithelial degradation), lead to the development of an anaerobic bacterial flora.

As the inflammatory process advances, so the proportion of Gram– bacteria (*Porphyromonas sp, Prevotella sp, Peptostreptococcus sp*), *Fusobacterium* and spirillians increases. The pathogenic role of these aggressive bacteria is much more pronounced and is exercised through various enzymes, toxins and degradation products (*Haake et al, 2002*).

To summarize, the dental plaque is a biofilm that forms on the tooth surface. It is composed of a community of bacterial species embedded inside an extracellular matrix of polymers produced by the hosts and the bacteria themselves (*Marsh, 2004*). Modification of its composition is closely associated with the development of periodontal inflammation. Its interrelation with the cat's immune defense mechanisms conditions to some extent the scale of the periodontal inflammation.

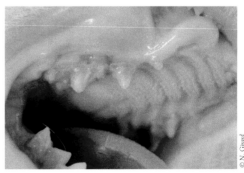

Figure 11 - Deposit of dental calculus in the cat. Accumulation of calculus on 100% of the upper PM4 associated with gum recession and exposure of the furcation.

Calculus is only a mineralized, fossilized form of dental plaque, consequential to the catalytic activity of some bacteria. It is deposited both above and under the gum **(Figure 11)**. While calculus does not contain any pathogenic bacteria, its porous character favors the new accumulation of dental plaque. So while it does not cause the inflammation of the periodontium it is an aggravating factor.

Oral Health

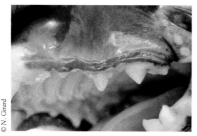

Figure 12 - Generalized gingivitis.
Pronounced gum edema from the canine to the carnassial; spontaneous bleeding around PM3.

The accumulation of dental plaque in the gingival crevice leads to inflammation of the gum seams **(Figure 12)**. At this point, professional care together with the removal of the dental plaque will ensure full remission of the lesions. Without treatment, the dental plaque continues to accumulate and inflammation advances. The environmental conditions in the oral cavity become more favorable to an anaerobic bacterial population containing more and more Gram negative bacteria. **Gingivitis**, the reversible inflammatory stage, may stabilize or develop into periodontitis.

The advancement of the inflammatory process inexorably leads to the collapse of the connecting tissues on the surface of the tooth. Dental plaque then colonizes the tooth root further down. The epithelium of the junction, which constitutes the lower limit of the gingival crevice, migrates to an apical region to heal in the "non-inflammatory" zone, creating a periodontal pocket. **Periodontitis (Figure 13)** is the irreversible stage of periodontal disease. The lesions are final and the main objective of treatment is to halt their advancement. The main cause of the development of periodontal disease is the disruption of the balance between the pathogenic bacterial flora of the dental plaque and the host's immune response.

> Description of periodontal disease in cats

First and foremost, it should be noted that few publications deal with periodontal disease in cats, contrary to a large quantity of publications on the disease in dogs. We would also observe that the expression of periodontal disease in cats is generally described on the model of the dog or human, without taking account of any feline particularities.

- A clinical radiographic and histological study has helped outline the development of periodontal disease in 15 cats *(Reichart et al, 1984)*. A loss of attachment appeared in 25% of premolars and molars, essentially localized to the buccal surface. A pronounced to severe gingivitis was shown in 56% of premolars and molars (buccal surface) and 25% of canines and incisors (buccal surface). After radiographic analysis, alveolar bone loss appeared to be significant in 77% of premolars and molars. Bone loss was also observed on the buccal surface of 82% and on the oral surface of 75% of incisors and canines. The general distribution of observed lesions in cats (gingivitis, alveolar bone loss, inflammatory FORL) was more pronounced in the premolars and molars.

Bearing in mind the high percentage of bone loss shown in the canines and incisors, however, together with the high percentage of missing incisors, it would appear that these teeth are highly susceptible to periodontal disease *(Reichart et al, 1984)*.

A form of periodontitis was shown using dental radiography in 69% of cats presented to the specialist veterinary dentistry department of the University of California, Davis. The results of this

FIGURE 13 - SEVERE LOCAL PERIODONTITIS OF THE UPPER LEFT PM4

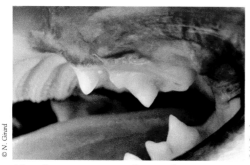

13A - *Severe gingivitis on the mesial and vestibular surface.*

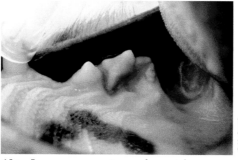

13B - *Severe gum recession on the mesial and palatine surface.*

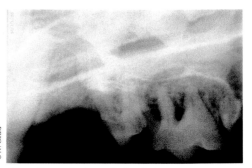

13C - *Severe horizontal alveolysis.*

FIGURE 14 - GENERALIZED HORIZONTAL BONE LOSS DURING PERIODONTAL DISEASE IN THE CAT WITH RESPECT TO THE RIGHT LOWER CARNASSIAL

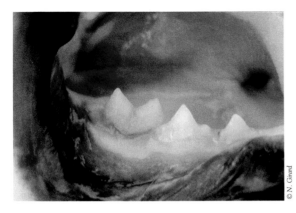

Severe periodontitis.

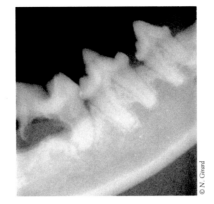

Generalized severe horizontal bone loss.

study confirm that generalized horizontal bone loss **(Figure 14)** is the most common form of bone loss in cats (38%). In total, the height of the alveolar bone was normal in just 28% of cases *(Lommer & Verstraete, 2001)*.

A clinical and radiographic study based on the oral examination of 109 healthy cats fed with dry food confirms these results. The presence of moderate to severe gingivitis associated with the presence of bleeding during periodontal probing was 13%. The average loss of periodontal attachment observed was 0.49 mm (c=1.28) with higher average values in the canines: 1.2 mm in the upper canine and 0.8 mm in the lower canine. Loss of attachment greater or equal to 2 mm was observed in 3.4% of examinations of the vestibular surface, 3% of the distal surface, 2.3% of the mesial surface and 2.2% of the lingual part. Gum recession **(Figure 15)** was observed in 10% of teeth. Absent teeth were most often upper premolars and incisors (21.1% and 11.4% respectively). Furcation **(Figure 16)** was observed in 18% of multi-root teeth and on average in two teeth of every cat examined. The radiographical analysis revealed a high prevalence of bone loss with respect to the dental arches: 21% of upper teeth and 42% of lower teeth. Horizontal and/or vertical bone loss was revealed in 52% and 14% of lower teeth respectively. The simplified analysis of premolars and molars underlines the importance of the inflammatory process: bone loss was observed in 66.5% of teeth *(Girard et al, 2008)*.

Periodontal disease in cats is characterized by a low proportion of periodontal pockets **(Figure 17)**, the strong prevalence of osteolysis in its horizontal form, a high proportion of gum recession and the early appearance of furcation.

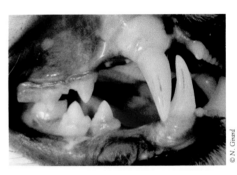

Figure 15 - Severe gum recession around a canine tooth in the cat.
Pronounced gum recession and alveolar bone loss around the upper and lower canines.

Oral Health

FIGURE 16 - FURCATION AROUND THE UPPER PM3 IN THE CAT

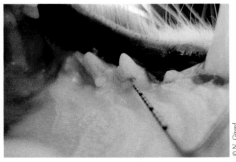

Profuse bleeding following periodontal probing of the furcation.

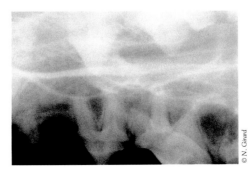

Vertical bone loss.

FIGURE 17 - PERIODONTAL POCKET IN THE CAT

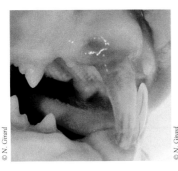
© N. Girard
Pronounced recession and severe gingivitis.

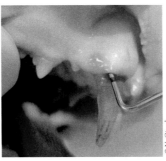
© N. Girard
Insertion of the periodontal probe.

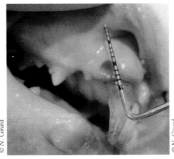
© N. Girard
Evaluation of the depth of the periodontal pocket: 13 mm.

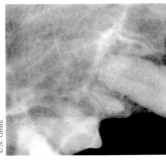
© N. Girard
Severe horizontal alveolar bone loss.

> Predisposing factors

Many factors have an influence on the development of periodontal disease:
- excessive accumulation of dental plaque in the junction between the tooth and gum (absence of oral hygiene, low fiber diet)
- inflammation promoted by a probable insufficiency of the local immune system or in the presence of systemic diseases such as diabetes mellitus, thyroid, liver or kidney insufficiency
- a familial and/or genetic effect is often evoked but never proven
- facial conformation, malocclusion, occlusion trauma.

▶ Tooth resorptions

> Definition

Tooth resorptions are lesions by which the gradual loss of tooth substance is observed **(Figure 18)**. In cats, they are commonly known as feline odontoclastic resorptive lesions (FORLs), as the process of tooth resorption is controlled by multinuclear odontoclastic cells (odontoclasts) *(Gautier et al, 2001)*. These lesions affect the interior and/or exterior of the tooth and their clinical diagnosis is often delicate. Tooth resorptions are also observed in humans and dogs. They are generally due to periodontal inflammation or mechanical constraints with respect to the periodontal ligament (orthodontic treatment, tooth trauma).

FIGURE 18 - FELINE ODONTOCLASTIC RESORPTIVE LESION

Feline odontoclastic resorptive lesions are initiated in the radicular cement and then develop through the dentine and/or the crown. The alveolar bone and the adjacent periodontal ligament are also included locally in the tooth resorption process. The tooth canal is only affected at the end of the process, signaling an internal tooth resorptive lesion.

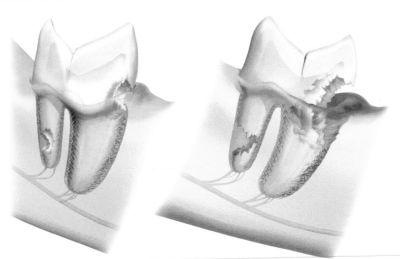

> Prevalence

A high prevalence of FORL has been shown in various cat populations and especially in domestic cats. According to the populations studied and/or the methodology used, the results were between 28% and 67% *(Coles, 1990; Van Messum et al, 1992)*. Such a variation is connected with the choice of population studied (specialist dental department, general dental department, healthy population) or the diagnostic methods used (clinical examination +/- radiological examination). Two studies of healthy cat populations reporting both a clinical and radiological examination revealed an average prevalence of 30% *(Ingham et al, 2002a; Girard et al, 2008)*.

> Pathogenesis

FORLs in cats are mostly external tooth lesions. The resorbed tooth tissue is gradually replaced by newly formed cement or bone tissue. FORLs are initiated in the radicular cement and then develop through the dentine and/or the crown. The alveolar bone and the adjacent periodontal ligament are also included locally in the tooth resorption process.

The tooth canal is only affected at the end of the process, signaling an internal tooth resorptive lesion. Inflammation of the tooth pulp is rare except at the end, when a degenerative state is described. The enamel of the crown may resorb itself in time, but more commonly it fractures due to the absence of underlying support, leading to the clinical appearance of a tooth cavity *(Okuda & Harvey, 1992)*.

FORLs mainly appear in the buccal part of the crown. Sixty-nine percent of the FORLs revealed are associated with an inflammatory phenomenon and 30% display signs of repair *(Reichart et al, 1984)*.

> Etiologies of FORLs

External FORLs may have one or more origins. In human dentistry, the disease may be associated with:
- a chronic inflammatory process adjacent to a cyst, benign or malignant tumor,
or
- be the consequence of dental trauma (mechanical/occlusal) or orthodontic tooth displacement. Lesions are qualified differently depending on whether an inflammatory process is present. Surface FORLs, dentoalveolar ankylosis and replacement lesions are considered to be the consequence of tooth traumas and qualified as non-inflammatory. On the other hand, apical FORLs and periradicular periodontitis are the consequence of lesions of the tooth pulp and are qualified as inflammatory lesions (radicular inflammatory tooth resorptions).

FORLs of the neck of the tooth are often confused with radicular inflammatory tooth resorptions. They are considered to be inflammatory because they are associated with inflammatory damage to the epithelial attachment (in the event of periodontal disease for example) *(Andreasen, 1985; Trope et al, 2002)*.

The precise etiology of FORLs remains unknown and is still the subject of discussion and research. The suspected role of masticatory mechanical constraints and chronic inflammation due to periodontal disease is underlined in various histological *(Gorrel & Larsson, 2002; Roux et al, 2002)* and radiographic *(DuPont & DeBowes, 2002)* studies as well as one clinical study *(Girard et al, 2008)*. Excessive vitamin D intake through the diet *(Reiter et al, 2005)* is proposed as a cofactor, although this continues to be debated. The precise role of specific histological dental structures in cats (vasodentine, osteodentine) has not been fully explained. Any interactions in the calcium regulation process associated with resorptions have been proposed *(Okuda & Harvey, 1992)*.

FIGURE 19 - TYPE 1 FORL OF THE LOWER M1

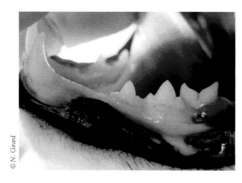 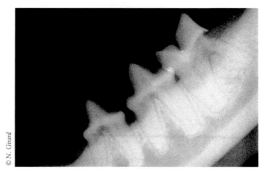

Severe gingivitis in the distal part.   *Inter-oral radiography: type 1 FORL.*

Current veterinary recommendations propose the differentiation of FORLs based on the results of the radiographic evaluation:

- **type 1 FORL:** observation of a physiological periodontal ligament space (*lamina dura*) and radio density of the affected root similar to that of healthy adjacent roots **(Figure 19)**

- **type 2 FORL:** disappearance of the lamina dura in the radiographic examination and radio density of the affected root similar to that of the adjacent alveolar bone (bone remodeling) **(Figure 20)**.

The combined study of the location of FORLs depending on their radiographic type shows significant differences *(Girard et al, 2008)*. Among house cats, the greater prevalence of type 1 lesions is observed in the lower carnassial and type 2 lesions in PM3. Among purebred cats a significant difference is observed for incisors (Type 2 FORL) and the lower carnassial (Type 1 FORL). The distribution of FORLs in the mouth is not uniform according to the type of lesion observed radiographically. This information corroborates the hypothesis that different etiologies cause feline resorptive lesions.

The analysis of FORLs in a population of cats treated at the dentistry department of the University of California, Davis, reveal a significant association between FORL and the presence of severe localized vertical alveolar bone loss *(Lommer & Verstraete, 2001)*.

FIGURE 20 - TYPE 2 FORL OF THE LOWER LEFT PM3

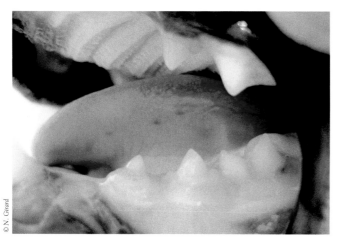 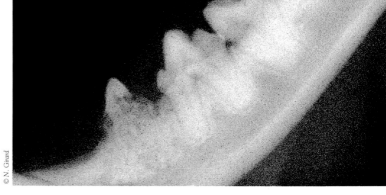

Early gingivitis.   *Type 2 FORL.*

The high prevalence of FORLs in the wild cat population on Marion Island (see above) fed almost exclusively with seabirds reduces the role some authors feel commercial food plays in the appearance of these tooth lesions. The author rather sees a consequence of feline oral inflammatory pathologies like periodontal disease and feline stomatitis (*Verstraete et al, 1996*).

An in-depth statistical analysis of the distribution of FORLs and 14 clinical and radiographic criteria associated with periodontal disease underlines a strong association (*Girard et al, 2008*). The global prevalence of FORLs may be significantly correlated to 6 of these periodontal parameters as well as age. Type 1 and 2 resorptions appear as two different phenomena without any association criteria. Type 1 FORL is significantly associated with 8 of the periodontal variables and so is strongly associated with periodontal disease. Type 2 FORL is correlated with just 2 periodontal parameters so the correlation to periodontal disease is low.

Age appears to be a factor strongly associated with the presence of type 2 FORL and weakly associated with type 1 FORL. All of these observations suggest that type 1 FORL is less sensitive to age with regard to its supposed link to the development of periodontal disease.

► Stomatitis

The term feline stomatitis covers all the oral diseases characterized by a pronounced inflammation of the oral mucosa **(Figure 21)**. Their prevalence appears to be low, although few statistical studies have been published on the subject (2.6% according to *Crossley, 1991*; 12% according to *Verhaert & Van Wetter, 2004*). Studies of large human populations show a prevalence of 5-15% of aggressive forms of periodontal inflammation, supposedly associated with ethnic predisposition (*Wolf et al, 2005*).

The analysis of tooth diseases in a population of 109 cats reveals 5.5% cases of stomatitis (3.7% buccal stomatitis, 1.8% caudal stomatitis) and 12.8% aggressive periodontitis (*Girard et al, 2008*). All these aggressive inflammatory diseases affected purebred cats, none of them housecats. The real impact of breed is still undergoing evaluation with respect to the probable familial effect.

The different types of stomatitis are known and dreaded, because they are generally a real therapeutic challenge. They are so painful that they disrupt the appetite and even the very survival of affected animals. The veterinarians' feeling of helplessness is amplified by the many uncertainties related to the etiology of these diseases.

The clinical management of feline stomatitis demands great diagnostic and therapeutic rigor. Recent studies confirm the role of the Calicivirus in the development of caudal stomatitis (*Addie et al, 2003*). The most descriptive clinical examination is needed to advance the etiological analysis of feline stomatitis. Few published studies use an appropriate terminology to correctly evaluate a given type of medication, complementary examination or viral etiology. More precise information on the therapeutic benefits of selected substances, the role of selected viruses (FCV, HV1, FIV, FeLV) and the best histopathological (especially immunohistological) knowledge in this disease is expected to be found in the years to come.

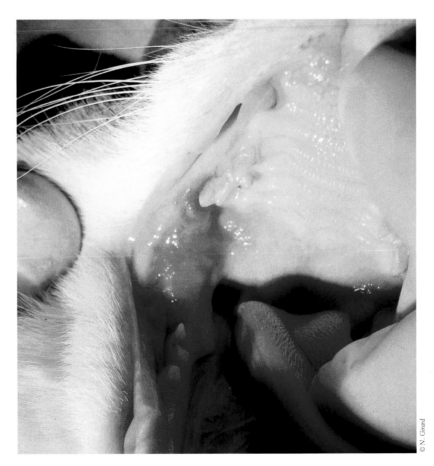

© N. Girard

Figure 21 - Stomatitis lesions in a cat. Jugal buccal stomatitis.

Oral Health

**FIGURE 24 – INFLUENCE OF ERGONOMICS
AND KIBBLE TEXTURE ON MECHANICAL TOOTH BRUSHING**

Indicative value (Newton) measured at the Royal Canin Research Center (2002)

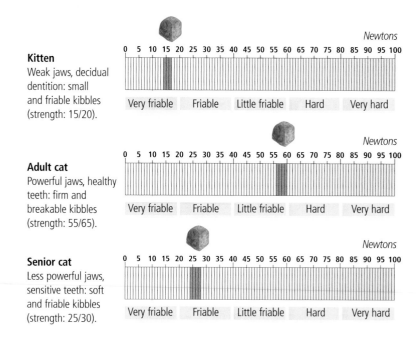

Kitten
Weak jaws, decidual dentition: small and friable kibbles (strength: 15/20).

Newtons

0 5 10 15 20 25 30 35 40 45 50 55 60 65 70 75 80 85 90 95 100

| Very friable | Friable | Little friable | Hard | Very hard |

Adult cat
Powerful jaws, healthy teeth: firm and breakable kibbles (strength: 55/65).

Newtons

0 5 10 15 20 25 30 35 40 45 50 55 60 65 70 75 80 85 90 95 100

| Very friable | Friable | Little friable | Hard | Very hard |

Senior cat
Less powerful jaws, sensitive teeth: soft and friable kibbles (strength: 25/30).

Newtons

0 5 10 15 20 25 30 35 40 45 50 55 60 65 70 75 80 85 90 95 100

| Very friable | Friable | Little friable | Hard | Very hard |

Due to its particular texture, the kibble encourages deeper penetration by the tooth, improving the efficacy of mechanical brushing.

FIGURE 25 - ACTION OF SODIUM POLYPHOSPHATE SALTS WITH CALCIUM IN SALIVA

Without sodium polyphosphate

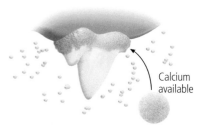

Calcium available

With sodium polyphosphate

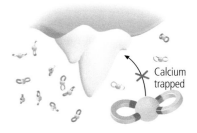

Calcium trapped

The chelated calcium ions are unavailable for the formation of calculus.

with small triangular kibbles **(Figure 24)**. This reduction in dental plaque is explained by the more complete mechanical action of large kibbles. When brushing is encouraged and the kibble texture enables the tooth to penetrate deeper before it fractures, the dental friction time is longer and the efficacy of brushing is improved *(Servet et al, 2003)*.

► Role of the composition of the food

The food may also contain certain ingredients that act against dental plaque and calculus, and so help prevent periodontal disease, when they are released in the oral cavity during mastication.

> Benefit of polyphosphate salts

The efficacy of some polyphosphate salts **(Figure 25)** in curbing the development of calculus is well known and clinically validated. The Ca^{2+} cations in the saliva are responsible for calcifying the dental plaque and transforming it into calculus. If polyphosphates with the capacity to chelate the versatile cations (e.g. Ca^{2+}, Mg^{2+}) are released in the oral cavity they naturally trap the calcium in the saliva in an ionic form, limiting its integration in the dental calculus matrix. The calcium is then released normally in the digestive tract so that it can be absorbed in accordance with the individual's needs. A significant reduction in the accumulation of calculus (-32%) has been observed in cats fed with a food coated with a calcium chelator, compared with a control group fed with the same kibbles without polyphosphate salts *(Servet et al, 2003; 2006)* **(Figure 26)**.

> Benefit of essential oils

The use of essential oils (thymol, eucalyptol, menthol, methyl salicylate) has also undergone long-term clinical evaluation in human dentistry. A reduction of dental plaque (-20-35%) as well as a significant reduction in associated gingivitis (-25-35%) has been obtained by using mouth-rinse solutions containing essential oils *(Perry & Schmidt, 2002)*. The benefit of this type of substance has gradually led to its incorporation in commercial foods. However, no study has yet been published on its specific efficacy.

> Other agents active against dental plaque

Current oral health research focuses on the development of new active components to combat the development of dental plaque.

In cats, an ingredient identified in research for human cosmetics (plaque reduction nutrient or PRN) has been shown to inhibit the development of dental plaque in a standardized comparative study. Its inclusion in a dry reference food (already possessing beneficial mechanical properties due to its special texture) led to a significant reduction in the accumulation of dental plaque (*Servet et al, 2006*). After one month, a 12% reduction in dental plaque **(Figure 27)** was observed on all teeth tested (upper C, P3 and P4; upper P3, P4 and M1). A more detailed analysis of the gum line showed a reduction in plaque of 22% on all teeth tested **(Figure 28)** and 36% when the following teeth were excluded: upper premolars P3-P4 and lower M1. This validates the chemical effect on all the cat's dentition. This study also highlights the greater efficacy with respect to the food's target teeth: upper P4, P3 and lower M1.

New plaque reduction nutrients will probably be developed with the discovery of substances that act not only on bacteria cell integrity but also on the physical interface between dental plaque and the tooth, to facilitate its detachment.

Combining the impact of size/texture and the composition of daily food, it is now possible to promise a significant reduction in the deposition of dental plaque in cats in the region of 30% and of calculus in the region of 50%. Given the cat's very particular chewing mechanism, the action due to the food's physical properties is more pronounced on the carnassials. The addition of PRNs also produces this effect in the rostral part of the oral cavity (canines and incisors).

Conclusion

The prevalence of oral inflammation in cats is widely underestimated. The clinical impact proves to be more important than it appears. In fact it is the number one cause of infectious disease in the species. Contrary to what many people think, periodontal disease is not the same in cats and dogs. It is expressed differently. The most recent studies to evaluate the secondary systemic effects of periodontal inflammations cast new light on the benefit with respect to oral diseases. The aim is not simply to combat bad breath, it is much more ambitious. It is to improve the cat's medical health and life expectancy.

Appropriate treatment reduces the chronic pain and infections associated with oral diseases. Owners are often amazed by the positive effects on their cat when the appropriate care is given. Toothache often produces major behavioral change. After treatment, the cats are generally more active, they eat better and their general condition by and large improves.

Full attention needs to be focused on preventing the development of dental plaque. The potential role of the food as an effective support for oral hygiene is now accepted. It is especially beneficial in cats, bearing in mind the difficulty of daily tooth brushing and their low interest in objects for chewing. The efficacy of this approach will no doubt be improved by working on the physical presentation of the food and searching for new PRNs.

FIGURE 26 - REDUCTION IN CALCULUS ACCUMULATION
(Royal Canin, 2005)

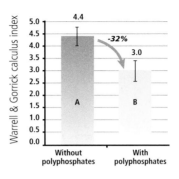

Global calculus deposit index before and after two months of a dry food enriched with polyphosphates.

FIGURE 27 - REDUCTION IN PLAQUE ACCUMULATION
(Royal Canin, 2005)

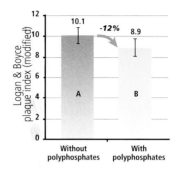

Global dental plaque accumulation index before and after one month of a dry food enriched with PRN.

FIGURE 28 - REDUCTION IN PLAQUE ACCUMULATION
(Royal Canin, 2005)

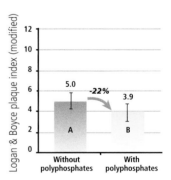

Dental plaque gingival index before and after one month of a dry food enriched with PRN.

Fallacies regarding oral diseases in cats

F	A
"Cats rarely suffer from oral lesions."	Pain is difficult to evaluate in cats by simply observing their day-to-day behavior. Dental care often leads to an improvement in the animal's health a posteriori. Any oral lesion (periodontitis, tooth resorption, stomatitis) must therefore always be considered potentially painful.
"Dental caries is common in cats."	Caries is NEVER observed in cats. The absence of caries is thought to be due to several factors: the conical shape of the teeth, the peculiarities of the diet and the composition of the dental plaque.
"Regular scaling prevents the emergence of periodontal disease in cats."	Calculus as such does not cause inflammation of the periodontium, but rather the daily accumulation of dental plaque and the bacterial populations it is composed of. There are therefore few benefits of removing calculus. Scaling helps suppress the dental plaque in a specialized dental procedure, but it does not unfortunately address the problem of permanent plaque development on the surface of the teeth. To prevent chronic periodontitis, regular scaling must always be combined with other oral hygiene techniques.
"The regular distribution of antibiotics eliminates dental plaque."	Unfortunately not. The bacteria in dental plaque are trapped in a protective complex that strengthens their cooperation. At best, antibiotics will be effective on a very superficial part of the bacterial population. Furthermore, their regular use contributes to the emergence of new strains in the plaque that have developed resistance to antibiotics.
"You have to start looking after a cat's teeth when it gets older."	The prevention of oral disease is always more effective when lesions are diagnosed early. Most cats less than 3 years of age already have tooth lesions that justify specific care. An inspection of the cat's mouth should accordingly be part of every vaccination visit.
"It's not possible to brush a cat's teeth."	While it is clearly difficult to get owners to brush their cat's teeth, the procedure is not impossible. Patience and motivation are often keys to surprising prophylactic results.
"Feeding a cat kibbles helps prevent the development of chronic periodontitis."	Simply giving your cat dry food kibbles will not be enough to reduce dental plaque. Kibble shape, size and texture need to be studied extensively to produce mechanical friction on the tooth surface enough to slow down plaque deposits and calculus formation. It now appears to be very important to combine this mechanical effect with the organic effect produced by nutritional factors that can act by diffusion on the composition of the oral flora.

References

Addie DD, Radford A, Yam PS, et al. Cessation of feline calicivirus shedding coincident with resolution of chronic gingivostomatitis in a cat. J Small Anim Pract 2003; 44: 172-176.

Andreasen JO. External root resorption: its implication in dental traumatology, paedodontics, periodontics, orthodontics and endodontics. Int Endodon J 1985; 18: 109-118.

Barbieri B. Biofilm et maladies parodontales. Inf Dent 2000; 40: 3451-3457.

Boutoille F, Dorizon A, Navarro A, et al. Echocardiographic alterations and periodontal disease in dogs: a clinical study. In Proceedings:15th European Congress of Veterinary Dentistry 2006, Cambridge (UK): 63-65.

Boyce EN. Feline experimental models for control of periodontal disease. Vet Clin North Am Small Anim Pract 1992; 22: 1309-1321.

Brandtzaeg P. The significance of oral hygiene in the prevention of dental diseases. Odont T 1964; 72: 460.

Buckland-Wright JC. Structure and function of cat skull bones in relation to the transmission of biting forces. PhD thesis, university of London, 1975.

Clarke DE, Cameron A. Relationship between diet, dental calculus and periodontal disease in domestic and feral cats in Australia. Aust Vet 1998; 76: 690-693.

Coles S. The prevalence of buccal cervical root resorptions in Australian cats. J Vet Dent 1990; 7: 14-16.

Crossley DA. Survey of feline problems encountered in a small animal practice in New England. Brit Vet Dent Ass J, 1991; 2: 3-6.

DeBowes LJ, Mosier D, Logan E, et al. Association of periodontal disease and histologic lesions in multiple organs from 45 dogs. J Vet Dent 1996; 13: 57-60.

DuPont GA, DeBowes LJ. Comparison of periodontitis and root replacement in cat teeth with resorptive lesions. J Vet Dent 2002; 19: 71-75.

Egelberg J. Local effect of diet on plaque formation and development of gingivitis in dogs. I. Effect of hard and soft diets. Odont Revy 1965; 16:31-41.

Gauthier O, Boudigues S, Pilet P, et al. Scanning electron microscopic description of cellular activity and mineral changes in feline odontoclastic resorptive lesions. J Vet Dent 2001; 18: 171-176.

Gengler W, Dubielzig R, Ramer J. Physical examination and radiographic analysis to detect dental and mandibular bone resorption in cats: a study of 81 cases from necropsy. J Vet Dent. 1995; 12: 97-100.

Girard N, Servet E, Biourge V, et al. Feline Dental Resorptions in a colony of 109 cats. J Vet Dent 2008; in press.

Girard N, et coll. Periodontal status in a colony of 100 cats. J Vet Dent 2008: in press.

Gorrel C, Larsson A. Feline odontoclastic resorptive lesions: unveiling the early lesion. J Small Anim Pract 2002; 43: 482-488.

Gorrel C, Inskeep G, Inskeep T. Benefit of a dental hygiene chew on the periodontal health of cats. J Vet Dent 1998; 15: 135-138.

Haake SA, Newman NG, Nisengard RJ, et al. Periodontal microbiology. In: Caranza's Clinical periodontology. 9th ed. Newman Takei Carranza: Saunders 2002.

Haberstroh LI, Ullrey DE, Sikarski JG, et al. J Zoo Anim Med 1984; 15: 142.

Harvey C, Emily PP. Function, formation, and anatomy of oral structures in carnivores. In: Small animal dentistry. St Louis: Mosby, 1993.

Harvey CE, Orsini P, McLahan C, et al. Mapping of the radiographic central point of feline dental resorptive lesions. J Vet Dent 2004; 21: 15-21.

Harvey C, Shofer FS, Laster L. Correlation of diet, other chewing activities and periodontal disease in North American client owned-dog. J Vet Dent 1996; 13: 101-105.

Houle MA, Grenier D. Maladies parodontales: connaissances actuelles. Current concepts in periodontal diseases. In: Médecine et maladies infectieuses. Elsevier ed, 2003; 33: 331-340.

Ingham KE, Gorrel C, Blackburn JM, et al. Prevalence of odontoclastic resorptive lesions in a population of clinically healthy cats. J Small Anim Pract 2001; 42: 439-443.

Ingham KE, Gorrel C, Bierer BS. Effect of a dental chew on dental substrates and gingivitis in cats. J Vet Dent 2002 (a); 19; 201-204.

Ingham KE, Gorrel C, Blackburn JM, et al. The effect of tooth brushing on periodontal disease in cats. J Nutr 2002 (b); 132:1740S-1741S.

Kays RW, DeWan AA. Ecological impact of inside/outside house cats around a suburban, nature preserve. Animal Conservation 2004; 7: 273-283.

Liberg O. Food habits and prey impact by feral and house-based domestic cats in a rural area in Southern Sweden. J Mamm 1984; 65: 424-432.

Lommer M, Verstraete FJ. Prevalence of resorptive lesions and periapical radiographic lucencies in cats: 265 cases (1995-1998). J Am Vet Med Assoc 2000; 217: 1866-1869.

Lommer MJ, Verstraete FJ. Radiographic pattern of periodontitis in cats: 147 cases (1998-1999). J Am Vet Med Assoc 2001; 218: 230-234.

Lund EM, Bohacek LK, Dahlke JL, et al. Prevalence and risk factors for odontoclastic resorptive lesions in cats. J Am Vet Assoc 1998; 212: 392-395.

Marsh PD. Dental plaque as a microbial biofilm. Caries Res 2004; 38: 204-211.

Orsini P, Hennet P. Anatomy of the mouth and teeth of the cat. Vet Clin North Am Small Anim Pract 1992; 22: 1265-1277.

Okuda A, Harvey C. Ethiopathogenesis of feline dental resorptive lesions. Vet Clin North Am Small Anim Pract 1992; 22: 1385-1404.

Pavlica Z. Periodontal disease and its systemic effects in the risk population for dogs. Clinical and nutritional management of senior dogs and cats. In: Proceedings. 28th World Small Animal Veterinary Association Congress 2002: 19-24.

Pavlica Z, Petelin M. Systemic effects on chronically infected wound in oral cavity of dogs. In: Proceedings. 12th Congress of European Veterinary Dental Society (EVDS) 2003: 29-32.

Perry DA, Schmidt MO. Phase 1 Periodontal therapy. In: Caranza's Clinical periodontology. 9th ed. Newman Takei Carranza: Saunders 2002.

Reichart PA, Durr UM, Triadan H, et al. Periodontal disease in the domestic cat: a histopathologic study. J Periodontal Res 1984; 19: 67-75.

Reiter AM, Lewis JR, Okuda A. Update on the etiology of tooth resorption in domestic cats. Vet Clin Small Anim 2005; 35: 913-942.

Richardson RL. Effect of administering antibiotics, removing the major salivary glands, and tooth brushing on dental calculi formation in the cat. Arch Oral Biol 1965; 10: 245-253.

Roux P, Berger M, Stoffel M, et al. *Observations of the periodontal ligament and cementum in cats with dental resorptive lesions.* J Vet Dent 2005; 22: 74-85.

Servet E, Hendricks W, Clarke D. *Kibbles can be a useful means in the prevention of feline periodontal disease.* Waltham Focus 2003; 13: 32-35.

Servet E, Hendriks W, Clarke D. *Dietary intervention can improve oral health in cats.* J Vet Dent 2008 (in press).

Studer E, Stapley B. *The role of dry food in maintaining healthy teeth and gums in the cat.* Vet Med Small Anim Clin 1973; 68: 1124-1126.

Theyse LFH. *Hill's prescription diet feline t/d: results of a field study, in Proceedings.* Hill's oral symposium (19th-21st March 2003): 60-63.

Tou AP, Adin DB, Castelman WL. *Mitral valve endocarditis after prophylaxis in a dog.* J Vet Intern Med 2005; 19: 268-270.

Tromp JAH, Jansen J, Pilot T. *Gingival health and frequency of the tooth brushing in the beagle dog model.* J Clin Periodontol 1986 (a);13: 164-168.

Tromp JAH, van Rijn LJ, Jansen J. *Experimental gingivitis and frequency of tooth brushing in the beagle dog model.* J Clin Periodontol 1986 (b); 13:190-194.

Trope M, Chivian N, Sigurdsson A. *Traumatic injury.* In: Cohen S, Burns RC, eds. *Pathways of the pulp.* 8th ed. St Louis: Mosby, 2002; 623-632.

Van Messum R, Harvey CE, Hennet P. *Feline dental resorptive lesions, prevalence patterns.* Vet Clin N Amer.1992; 1405-1416.

Verhaert L, Van Wetter C. *Survey of oral disease in cats in Flanders.* Vlaams Diergeneeskundig Tijdschrift 2004; 73: 331-341.

Verstraete FJM, van Aarde RJ, Nieuwoudt BA, et al. *The dental pathology of feral cats on Marion Island, part 2: Periodontitis, external odontoclastic resorption lesions and mandibular thickening.* J Comp Path 1996; 115: 283-297.

Wiggs RB, Lobprise HB. *Oral anatomy and physiology.* In: *Veterinary Dentistry, principles and practice.* Blackwell Publishing, Lippincott-Raven, 1997: 55-86.

Wolf H, Rateitschak EM, Rateitschak KH, et al. *Periodontology.* In: Rateitschak EM, et al. *Color Atlas of Dental Medicine.* 3rd ed: Thieme Medical Publishers, 2005; 95-98.

Oral Health

Focus on:
Nutrients acting on oral health in cats

Servet E., Hendriks W., Clarke D., Biourge V. - Royal Canin Research Center, Aimargues, France - Massey University, New Zealand

Introduction

It has been shown that diets consisting of dry, hard foods result in less accumulation of plaque and tartar compared to canned or other soft foods. This is due to the abrasive nature of the dry food which can scrape or brush the accumulated materials off the tooth surface. In addition, the shape of the kibble has an important role in efficacy of brushing the tooth (when the owner cannot perform tooth brushing of the cat on a regular basis). A previous study *(Servet et al, 2003)* has reported that in cats, a rectangular kibble is more effective in preventing plaque than a triangular kibble.

The purpose of this study was to determine if chelated polyphosphates (sodium polyphosphate- SPP), a unique plaque reducing nutrient (PRN) and a larger kibble size would result in a significant reduction in calculus and plaque formation. SPP is a cation sequestrant that forms soluble complexes with calcium within dental plaque, thereby preventing the accumulation of calculus. A larger kibble of a rectangular shape should require additional prehension, biting and chewing to impact calculus and plaque formation.

Materials and methods

Animals

A total of 30 healthy mixed breed cats were used in the study. To be included in this study, cats had to have normal dentition, scissor-configuration occlusion, dental plaque accumulation and no or mild gingivitis. Cats were housed in groups of 10 and provided their respective diet *ad libitum*. Fresh water was also provided *ad libitum*.

Diets

Cats were exclusively fed dry extruded diets throughout the study. No snacks, calculus or plaque control treats, chews or chew toys were allowed. Three different dietary regimens were compared:

- Diet A: A dry-expanded diet with triangular kibble shape and no oral care purpose, as a negative control diet

- Diet B: A dry-expanded diet with rectangular kibble shape formulated for oral care purpose, including SPP and PRN

- Diet C: A dry-expanded diet with triangular kibble shape and oral care provided by SPP.

All diets were formulated to meet the nutritional levels established by the AAFCO Cat Food Nutrient Profiles for adult maintenance.

Study design

All 30 cats were fed Diet A for 14 days in a pre-study phase **(Table 1)**. At the end of the pre-study phase, all cats were anesthetized and a dental prophylaxis performed to remove all supra and subgingival calculus and plaque. Each cat was deemed to begin the study with a "clean tooth model". All cats remained on Diet A and after a further seven days, plaque indexes were evaluated according to the Logan & Boyce procedure *(Logan & Boyce, 1994)*. Cats were then randomly assigned by gender and plaque forming ability to one of 3 diets. Plaque indexes were evaluated at 7 days. At 28 days, plaque and calculus indexes were evaluated by the *Logan & Boyce* (plaque) and *Warrick & Gorrel* (calculus) procedures *(Warrick & Gorrel, 1995)*. Calculus formation was evaluated a

second time at day 56 **(Table 2)**. One scorer was used to score all cats in a blinded procedure to the different feeding regimens and the scoring order of the cats.

The scored teeth were the canines (C), pre-molar 3 and 4 (PM3 and PM 4) for the upper jaw (maxilla) and C, PM3, PM 4, and molar 1 (M1) for the lower jaw (mandible).

Gingivitis was evaluated according to the method of *Loe & Silness*. Teeth scored were incisor 3 (I3), C, PM3, PM4, M1 for the maxilla and C, PM2, PM3, M4, M1 for the mandible.

TABLE 1 - STUDY DESIGN

Day -28	
Pre-study period	
Day -7	Dental scaling Plaque evaluation Allocation to group
Dietary transition	
Day 0	Dental scaling Plaque evaluation
Day 7	Plaque evaluation
Day 28	Plaque and calculus evaluation
Day 56	Calculus evaluation

Oral Health

ROYAL CANIN

TABLE 2 – CRITERIA FOR CALCULUS DETERMINATION

Coverage
0 - no observable calculus
1 - scattered calculus covering less than 24% of the buccal tooth surface
2 - calculus covering between 25-49% of the buccal tooth surface
3 - calculus covering between 50-74% of the buccal tooth surface
4 - calculus covering more than 75% of the buccal tooth surface

Thickness
L = light = 1 (for calculations)
M = moderate = 2 (for calculations)
H = heavy = 3 (for calculations)

Data Analysis

Dental plaque and calculus scores were expressed as a whole mouth score for each cat and were calculated from the mean value of the scores for each target tooth. Data were expressed as mean ± standard error of the mean (sem). Repeated-measures ANOVA tests were used to derive F-tests for significant differences between treatments. F-values with p-values less than 0.05 were considered significant. Analyses were performed using the General Linear Model procedures in Statgraphics V5 statistical software.

Results

Plaque score at day 7 **(Figure 1)** was significantly lower for Diet B compared to Diet A and Diet B compared with Diet C (28.3% and 28.1%, respectively). In addition, gingival plaque score at Day 7 **(Figure 2)** was significantly lower for Diet B compared with Diet A and Diet C (27.3% and 30.5%, respectively). Diet B was associated with a 30.3% lower plaque score at day 28 compared to Diet A, and 30.1% lower plaque score at day 28 compared to Diet C **(Figure 3)**. Likewise, Diet B was associated with a significant reduction in gingival plaque scores at day 28 **(Figure 4)** compared to both Diet A and Diet C (31.7% and 29.2%, respectively).

Calculus score at day 28 **(Figure 5)** was significantly lower for Diet B compared to Diet A and Diet B compared with Diet C (47.4% and 23.8%, respectively). In addition, there was a significant reduction (30.9%) in calculus score for Diet C compared with Diet A. The calculus score **(Figure 6)** for Diet B was significantly lower than Diet A or Diet C at 56 days (44.6% and 18.9%, respectively). The calculus score for Diet C was significantly lower (31.7%) than Diet A at 56 days.

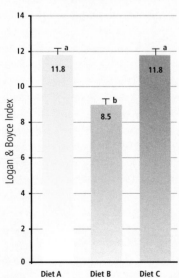

FIGURE 1 - PLAQUE SCORE DAY 7
Logan & Boyce Index
Diet A: 11.8 (a), Diet B: 8.5 (b), Diet C: 11.8 (a)

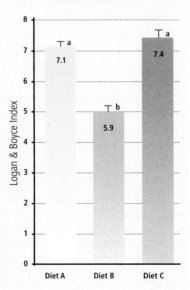

FIGURE 2 - GINGIVAL PLAQUE SCORE DAY 7
Logan & Boyce Index
Diet A: 7.1 (a), Diet B: 5.9 (b), Diet C: 7.4 (a)

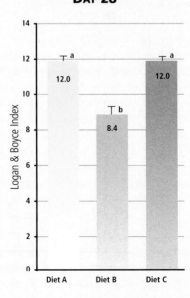

FIGURE 3 - PLAQUE SCORE DAY 28
Logan & Boyce Index
Diet A: 12.0 (a), Diet B: 8.4 (b), Diet C: 12.0 (a)

Oral Health

Discussion

The results of this study demonstrated that plaque and calculus accumulation can be significantly reduced in cats when they are fed a diet that has been specifically formulated with a larger rectangular kibble coated with sodium polyphosphate and a specific plaque reducing nutrient. Plaque was reduced by approximately 30% and calculus was reduced by approximately 45%.

Coating the kibble with sodium polyphosphate alone (Diet C) resulted in significantly less calculus build up compared to the control diet (Diet A), but no significant reduction in plaque was observed. These results confirm that sodium polyphosphate has a significant impact only on calculus, and the results are in agreement with other available feline calculus data *(Stookey, 1995; Johnson & Cox, 2002)*.

Sodium polyphosphate, coated on the external surface of the kibble is released into the oral cavity where it chelates salivary calcium so that it is unavailable for plaque calcification into calculus. When swallowed, the calcium polyphosphate complexes are not stable in the acid environment of the stomach and are rapidly converted to orthophosphates and used as a dietary phosphate source.

The larger, rectangular kibble coated with sodium polyphosphate resulted in significantly less calculus accumulation compared to the smaller triangular kibble coated with sodium polyphosphate (Diet C). Previous studies have shown that diet texture, kibble shape, size and design all impact calculus formation in cats (Servet et al, 2003). Indeed, it has been shown that dry kibble in a rectangular shape as opposed to a triangular shape aids in scraping away plaque when the cat bites and chews the kibble (Servet et al, 2003). This lower plaque deposition rate is attributed to the specially designed kibbles that convey an enhanced mechanical action, attributed to increased friction, induced both a higher crunching rate and by optimized crushing with greater teeth penetration into the kibbles. This process mimics tooth brushing. The significant impact on plaque deposition was attributed to the addition of the unique plaque reducing nutrient, coupled with the size, shape and texture of the kibble, which enhanced the mechanical action and simulated a brushing effect.

Conclusion

A 30% reduction in plaque and 45% reduction in calculus accumulation can be achieved when cats are fed a diet that has been specifically formulated with a larger rectangular kibble coated with sodium polyphosphate and a specific plaque reducing nutrient.

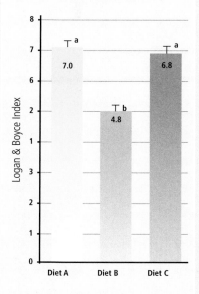

FIGURE 4 - GINGIVAL PLAQUE SCORE DAY 28

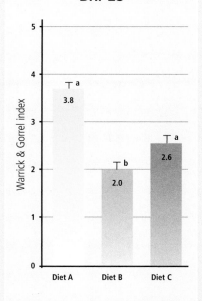

FIGURE 5 - CALCULUS SCORE DAY 28

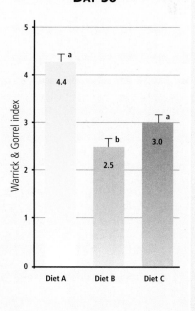

FIGURE 6 - CALCULUS SCORE DAY 56

Oral Health

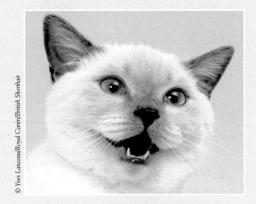

© Yves Lanceau/Royal Canin/British Shorthair

70% of cats aged over 3 years old present oral lesions (Harvey, 2004).

Key points
to remember:

Periodontal disease in cats

Oral Health

Dental health can have repercussions for the cat's general health. It is important that the teeth and oral cavity are regularly examined during a veterinary check-up.

Periodontal disease is the most common disease, affecting 70% of cats aged 20-27 months to various degrees *(Ingham et al, 2002)*. It develops in three phases:

- **phase 1:** deposition of dental plaque, constituting an organic film of salivary polysaccharides and glycoproteins, colonized by aerobic bacteria;

- **phase 2:** development of gingivitis and mineralization of the dental plaque into calculus. The aerobic bacteria are replaced by anaerobic bacteria and bad breath is caused by the formation of volatile sulfur compounds;

- **phase 3:** destruction of the periodontal ligament (periodontitis). The bacteria reach the base of the root and attack the bone in which the tooth is embedded. Gum recession and osteolysis facilitate the tooth's loosening.

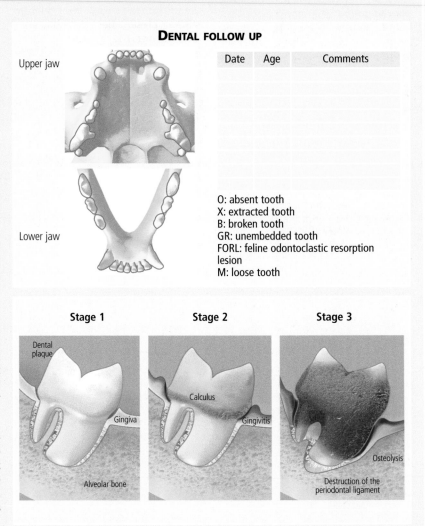

DENTAL FOLLOW UP

Upper jaw

Lower jaw

Date	Age	Comments

O: absent tooth
X: extracted tooth
B: broken tooth
GR: unembedded tooth
FORL: feline odontoclastic resorption lesion
M: loose tooth

Stage 1

Dental plaque

Gingiva

Alveolar bone

Stage 2

Calculus

Gingivitis

Stage 3

Osteolysis

Destruction of the periodontal ligament

ROYAL CANIN

Nutritional responses

Tooth brushing is the best means of preventing the development of periodontal disease. When it is not possible because the owner is not available or the cat is uncooperative, the food can play a beneficial preventive role based on its mechanical and/or chemical effects. The expected benefits are observed only when the cat eats nothing else on a daily basis.

Mechanical effect

Dry foods can have a light abrasive effect on the teeth when they are chewed correctly before swallowing. This permits the destruction of the bacterial mesh that constitutes dental plaque. It is important not to crush or mash the kibbles, as this will negate these benefits.

The mechanical effect is based on matching the appropriate kibble size, shape and texture to the age and size of the individual animal. The aim is maximum penetration of the kibble by the tooth before the kibble crumbles, so as to obtain relative "brushing".

The fact that the cat chews also stimulates the production of saliva, which has a beneficial antibacterial role.

Effect on bacterial flora

Some nutrients can inhibit the deposition of dental plaque by curbing the adhesion of bacteria and/or acting as a bactericide *(Servet et al, 2006)*. The aim is to reduce the proliferation of the anaerobic bacterial population and the production of volatile sulfur compounds responsible for halitosis.

While no specific studies have been published on cats, several studies have demonstrated the efficacy of some nutrients in limiting bad breath. Of the nutrients studied, organic zinc salts (e.g. zinc citrate) and inorganic zinc salts (e.g. zinc sulfate: $ZnSO_4^{2-}$) present beneficial bacteriostatic properties *(Weesner, 2003; Waller, 1997)*.

There are also bacteriostatic and bactericidal oils. Eucalyptus oil for example helps actively reduce the production of sulfur fatty acids *(Pan et al, 2000)*. Lastly, some bacteria are highly sensitive to the action of tea polyphenols *(Isogai et al, 1995)*, the antioxidant properties of which are well known.

Chemical effect

Sodium polyphosphates have a chelator effect on the calcium in saliva and so help limit the calcification of dental plaque.

Conclusion

Adding up the impact of size/texture and composition of daily food, it is now also possible to promise a significant reduction in the deposition of dental plaque in cats.

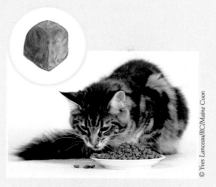

© *Yves Lanceau/RC/Maine Coon*

Oral Health

References

Harvey CE. The oral cavity. In: Chandler EA, Gaskell CJ, Gaskell RM; Feline medicine and therapeutics 2004; Blackwell Publishing & BSAVA: 379-395.

Ingham KE, Gorrel C, Blackburn JM, et al. The effect of tooth brushing on periodontal disease in cats. J Nutr 2002; 132: 1740S-1741S.

Isogai E, Isogai H, Kimura K, et al. Effect of Japanese green tea extract on canine periodontal diseases. Microbial Ecology in Health & Diseases 1995; 8: 57-61.

Pan P, Barnett ML, Coelho J, et al. Determination of the in situ bactericidal activity of an essential oil mouth rinse using a vital stain method. J Clin Periodontol 2000; 27: 256-261.

Servet E, Hendriks W, Clarke D, et al. Dietary intervention can improve oral health in cats. J Vet Dent 2008 (in press).

Waler SM. The effect of some metal ions on volatile sulphur-containing compounds originating from the oral cavity. Acta Ondontol Scand 1997; 55: 261-4.

Weesner BW Jr. Curing Halitosis: the sweet smell of success. J Tenn Dent Assoc 2003; 83: 20.

Kathryn E. MICHEL
DVM, Dipl. ACVN

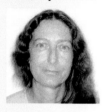

Karin U. SORENMO
DVM, Dipl. ACVIM,
Dipl. ECVIM-CA
(Oncology)

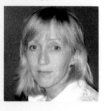

Nutritional status of cats with cancer: nutritional evaluation and recommendations

1 - Characteristics of the feline cancer population 387

2 - Clinical nutritional assessment of cancer patients 388

3 - Cancer cachexia syndrome 392

4 - Nutritional consequences of anti-cancer therapy 393

5 - Dietary intervention 394

6 - Pharmacological intervention 396

Conclusion 399

Frequently asked questions 400

References 401

Cancer

ABBREVIATIONS USED IN THIS CHAPTER

BCS: body condition scoring
CNS: central nervous system
FeLV: feline leukemia virus
MER: maintenance energy requirement
NSAIDs: non-steroidal anti-inflammatory drugs
RER: resting energy requirement
SGA: subjective global assessment

Nutritional status of cats with cancer: nutritional evaluation and recommendations

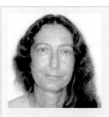

Kathryn E. MICHEL
DVM, Dipl. ACVN

Kathryn Michel graduated from the school of Veterinary Medicine at Tufts University with a doctorate in Veterinary Medicine in 1983. She completed a residency in small animal clinical nutrition and a master's degree at the University of Pennsylvania, followed by a postdoctoral fellowship with the Nutrition Support Service at the School of Medicine. She is a diplomate of the American College of Veterinary Nutrition and currently an associate professor of nutrition and chief of the Section of Medicine at The University of Pennsylvania. Her research interests include nutritional assessment, nutritional requirements of hospitalized companion animals, and nutrient modulation of gastrointestinal and endocrine diseases.

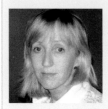

Karin U. SORENMO
DVM, Dipl. ACVIM, Dipl. ECVIM-CA (Oncology)

Karin Sorenmo graduated from the Norwegian School of Veterinary Science. She completed a residency in oncology at the School of Veterinary Medicine of the University of Pennsylvania where she is currently an associate professor of oncology and serves as the chief of the Oncology Section. Her main research interests include mammary gland tumors in dogs and cats, and cancer immunotherapy.

The impact of diet on neoplastic disease is multi-faceted. Both dietary habits and nutritional status have been found to be risk factors for the development of certain types of cancer. Nutrition, including special diets and specific nutrients, has also been investigated for its therapeutic role in cancer patients. In addition, the response to chemotherapy and tolerance of treatment has been found to be associated with nutritional status.

With the current lack of nutritional investigation specific to feline cancer patients, the focus of this chapter will be on what we know about the clinical presentation of this population, the process of assessing nutritional status in cats, the significance of poor nutritional status in cats affected with neoplasia, and what strategies we currently have at our disposal to intervene in cancer patients who are experiencing anorexia, weight loss, and a decline in body condition.

Cancer

The interactions of diet and neoplasia have been much more extensively investigated in human patients, and what preliminary studies exist in veterinary medicine almost all focus on canine cancer patients. Cats, however, do make up a substantial portion of the oncological caseload and one might be tempted to apply findings in other species to the feline patient. This, however, should be done with caution given the many unique aspects of feline physiology, metabolism, and disease. For example, one report found that the minority of canine cancer patients (5%) had an underweight body condition (*Michel et al, 2004*). Conversely, the clinical impression has been that feline cancer patients are often in poor body condition. A recent investigation at the University of Pennsylvania found this to be the case with 44% of patients assessed as having an underweight body condition and > 90% as having evidence of muscle wasting (*Baez et al, 2007*) (**Figure 1**).

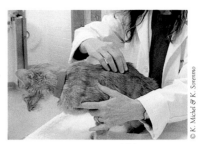

Figure 1 - *Over 90% of feline cancer patients examined in an investigation at the University of Pennsylvania were found to have experienced muscle wasting (Baez et al, 2007).*

1 - Characteristics of the feline cancer population

Cats comprise approximately 26% of all cancer patients seen by the oncology service of the University of Pennsylvania and the fraction of cats versus dogs has remained constant over the past decade. Despite the fact that cats represent a significant portion of patients that undergo treatment through the oncology section, there is limited information regarding the feline cancer population on how nutritional factors might influence treatment and outcome. In order to characterize the feline cancer population better in terms of age, breed, sex, body weight, and what types of malignancies they were treated for, information on all cats with malignancies that were seen by all sections of the Veterinary Hospital of the University of Pennsylvania over the past three years was collected. This population may be representative of the feline cancer population in many other larger urban referral centers.

► Epidemiologic data

A total of 712 cats with a diagnosis of various types of cancer were evaluated. Eighty percent were domestic short hair cats, with a slight over-representation of males versus females (52.7 versus 47.3%) of which all but one cat was neutered. The majority of cats were middle-aged to older, with a mean age of 11 years and a mean body weight of 4.58 kg. Sixty percent of the cats had different types of solid tumors and 40% had lymphoma or leukemia. When comparing cats with solid tumors to cats with lymphoma or leukemia, we found that these two groups differed significantly in age and body weight; cats with solid tumors were significantly older and heavier than cats with lymphoma/leukemia with a mean age of 12.0 years versus 10.5 years (p< 0.0001) and a mean body weight of 4.7 kg versus 4.4 kg (p= 0.049). This difference is not surprising since most cats with lymphoma present with signs of systemic disease and multi-organ involvement at the time of diagnosis.

► Feline lymphoma

Cats with lymphoma represent a significant portion (40%) of the total hospital feline cancer population and an even higher proportion of the oncology section's cat population, since many of these are treated with systemic chemotherapy. The original World Health Organization Classification system listed the various anatomic forms as generalized, alimentary, thymic, skin, leukemia (true, i.e. only blood and bone marrow involved) and others (*Owen, 1980*). A more simplified and practical classification system includes only 4 groups and feline lymphoma is typically classified according to anatomic site: the thoracic form, the alimentary form, the multicentric form, and an unclassified form (skin, leukemia, CNS, nasal etc) (*Moore et al, 2001*).

Alimentary lymphoma is the most common anatomic form of lymphoma currently seen in our hospital. This is probably also representative of the situation in most other oncology practices since most cats with lymphoma that are diagnosed today are FeLV negative with primary alimentary involvement. Cranial mediastinal lymphoma typically found in FeLV positive younger outdoor cats is not as common anymore (*Gabor et al, 1998; Vail et al, 1998; Richter, 2003;*

Louwerens et al, 2005; Milner et al, 2005). The alimentary forms of lymphoma often pose a challenge to the clinician both from a therapeutic and a nutritional point of view.

The list of which signs qualify as B-signs has not been completely defined, and leave some room for subjectivity, but in general include any signs of systemic disease at diagnosis, regardless whether these signs are directly associated with the lymphoma, are paraneoplastic, or are from other concurrent illness. Many of these B-signs are typical presenting complaints when cats with lymphoma present for initial evaluation and diagnostics. The typical clinical signs associated with alimentary lymphoma include: decreased appetite, anorexia, vomiting, diarrhea, weight loss and fatigue *(Richter, 2003).* The clinical signs might have lasted for weeks to months, and many of these cats present in poor nutritional condition. Successful management of these patients requires effective treatment of the underlying malignancy, i.e. chemotherapy, while at the same time controlling nausea, vomiting, diarrhea, anorexia and instituting adequate nutritional support.

Unlike many dogs, cats with lymphoma are typically diagnosed when they have clinical signs from their lymphoma. Systemic signs secondary to lymphoma will constitute a sub-stage B category, which according to many studies is associated with a worse prognosis. In fact, sub-stage B is a more consistent negative prognostic factor in the canine lymphoma literature than stage of disease *(Valerius et al, 1997; Baskin et al, 2000; Garrett et al, 2002; Simon et al 2006).*

2 - Clinical nutritional assessment of cancer patients

The process of nutritional assessment involves evaluation of not only the patient's nutritional status but also the diet it is receiving and how that diet is being fed. Furthermore, this process should not be an initial one time exercise but an on-going practice throughout the patient's course of treatment so that adjustments can be made in diet and feeding recommendations based on the patient's response to therapy. The actual task of nutritional assessment involves several steps **(Figure 2)**. First determine the patient's nutritional status which is a subjective evaluation based on the medical history and physical examination. Next the patient's voluntary food intake should be assessed. Once the patient's nutritional status and food intake have been evaluated, other aspects of the patient's clinical presentation should be considered, including the specific type and stage of cancer, the intended course of therapy, and whether or not there are any pre-existing or concur-

FIGURE 2 - A STEP-BY-STEP APPROACH FOR THE NUTRITIONAL ASSESSMENT OF FELINE CANCER PATIENTS

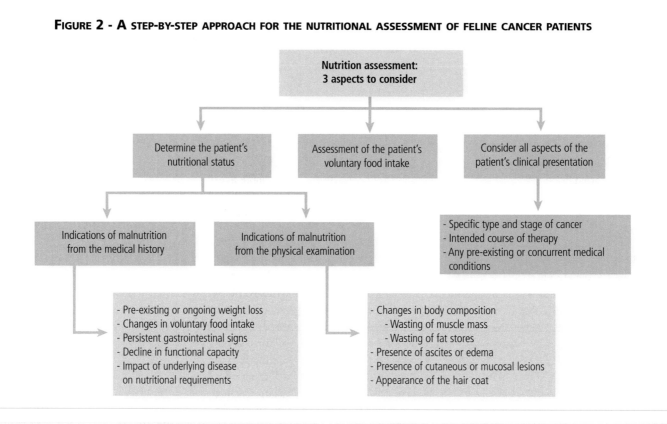

rent medical conditions. Formulating a suitable nutritional plan for each patient needs to encompass all of this information.

The nutritional assessment will help determine whether the patient is experiencing malnutrition or at risk of becoming malnourished, whether the diet and the intake of that diet are adequate to the patient's nutritional needs, whether any specific dietary management, including assisted feeding, is indicated and, in the case of assisted feeding, which route of feeding will be the safest, most effective and best tolerated by the patient. The process of nutritional assessment can also identify potential problems that might arise as a consequence of the dietary management, and allow for planning to prevent them or anticipate them through appropriate monitoring.

► Determining nutritional status

A technique referred to as subjective global assessment (SGA) was developed for the nutritional assessment of human patients approximately 20 years ago (Detskey et al, 1987). The technique was designed to utilize readily available historical and physical parameters in order to identify malnourished patients who are at increased risk for complications and who will presumably benefit from nutritional intervention. The assessment involves determining:
- whether nutrient assimilation has been restricted because of decreased food intake, maldigestion or malabsorption;
- whether any effects of malnutrition on organ function and body composition are evident;
- and whether the patient's disease process influences its nutrient requirements.

To adapt the SGA to cancer patients, the medical history should be assessed in five areas:
- pre-existing or ongoing weight loss
- extent of voluntary dietary intake
- the presence of persistent gastrointestinal signs either from the primary disease or treatment the patient is receiving
- the patient's functional capacity (e.g., weakness, presence of exercise intolerance)
- and the impact of the patient's underlying disease state.

When dealing with cancer patients one must consider the ways in which the tumor could directly or indirectly affect food intake, the impact that cancer therapy may have on food intake and metabolism, and the recognition that the tumor itself may exert effects on metabolism that negatively influence nutritional status.

It is often difficult to document a history of weight lost since most animals are only weighed when they come in to a veterinary clinic and not always then. It is critical that cats being treated for cancer are weighed consistently on the same scale and that the scale is sensitive and accurate for animals in the feline weight range. It is also important to know the time course over which the weight loss has occurred. Rapid weight loss is generally of greater concern because it is more likely to involve a greater percentage of lean tissue catabolism than a more gradual weight loss. Having said that, cancer cachexia syndrome, as documented in human cancer patients is characterized by loss of both lean body mass and adipose tissue and can take a chronic course.

The physical examination focuses on changes in body composition, specifically wasting of fat stores and muscle mass, the presence of edema or ascites, the presence of mucosal or cutaneous lesions, and the appearance of the patient's hair coat. Several excellent body condition scoring systems (BCS) have been developed for cats (Laflamme, 1997; German et al, 2006). However, these systems do not apply well to cats with cancer because they depict patients that deviate from optimal based on under- or overconsumption of protein and calories. It has been reported in a study from the University of Pennsylvania that over 90% of cats diagnosed with cancer have evidence of muscle wasting even in cases where the patient had adequate or even excessive fat stores (Baez et al, 2007). Without careful examination, which involves palpation of skeletal muscle mass over bony prominences (such as the scapulae or vertebral column), some of these patients might be misclassified as overweight

Regardless of the reason a cat is presented at the clinic, the body weight must be recorded.

Cancer

Figure 3 - Evaluation of the cat's body composition.

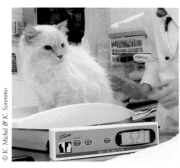

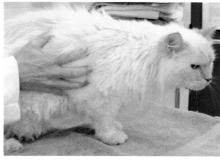

Feline cancer patients can present with a relatively normal body silhouette and weight.

Hence, body condition scoring requires manual palpation to assess both fat and lean body mass.

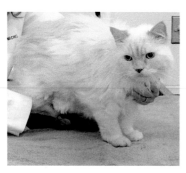

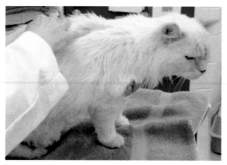

Assessment of body fat in cats should always involve palpation of the abdominal fat pad, in addition to palpation over the rib cage.

In addition to the standard techniques used for body condition scoring, feline cancer patients should always be assessed for evidence of muscle wasting by palpation for muscle mass over boney prominences such as the vertebral spinous processes.

TABLE 1 - MUSCLE MASS SCORING SYSTEM	
Score	**Muscle Mass**
0	Severe muscle wasting as evidenced by pronounced decreased muscle mass palpable over the scapulae, skull, or wings of the ilia.
1	Moderate muscle wasting as evidenced by clearly discernable decreased muscle mass palpable over the scapulae, skull, or wings of the ilia.
2	Mild muscle wasting as evidenced by slight but discernible decreased muscle mass palpable over the scapulae, skull, or wings of the ilia.
3	Normal muscle mass palpable over the scapulae, skull, or wings of the ilia.

or even obese (**Figure 3**). Thus we recommend subjectively evaluating muscle mass (**Table 1**) in addition to using one of the standard body condition scoring systems available.

The findings of the historical and physical assessment are used to categorize the patient as:
A: well nourished
B: borderline or at risk of becoming malnourished
C: significantly malnourished.

Coupling this assessment with the patient's cancer diagnosis, stage, treatment protocol, and prognosis will aid in making decisions about nutritional therapy.

► Assessment of voluntary food intake

In order to be able to assess whether that patient's food intake is adequate, you must have a caloric goal, select an appropriate food, and formulate a feeding recommendation for the patient. By doing so, you will have an accurate account of how much food is offered to the patient, and will be able to evaluate the patient's intake based on how much of the food is consumed.

> Hospitalized patients

For hospitalized patients, we recommend using an estimate of resting energy requirement (RER) as your initial caloric goal (**Table 2**) as most hospitalized patients are not expending much more energy than RER while they are caged. Under such conditions most patients eating at least RER will

Cancer

lose little if any weight. Clearly if a patient is willing to consume calories in excess of RER it should be permitted to do so. However, starting out with this amount of food will provide a goal to aim for with patients who have a decreased appetite. It is critical to monitor both the patient's food intake and body weight to establish whether the patient is in energy balance or not and to permit timely adjustment of the dietary plan if the patient is not responding as anticipated (see chapter 13)

> Out-patients

The majority of cancer patients are treated as out-patients and therefore will require additional caloric intake to compensate for energy expended on voluntary physical activity. Under these circumstances, the daily maintenance energy requirement (MER) should be estimated (Table 3) and used to calculate the initial caloric goal.

This information should be converted into clear feeding directions for the cat's caregiver using specific portions of whichever foods are being offered to the patient in a manner analogous to how a drug dosage would be calculated and prescribed. There should be a plan for reporting back to the clinician about daily food intake and for accurately monitoring body weight on a regular basis to assess the patient's response and allow for modification of the feeding plan as appropriate.

TABLE 2 - ESTIMATION OF RESTING ENERGY REQUIREMENT (RER)

$RER = 70\ BW(kg)^{0.73}$
or $RER = 30\ BW(kg) + 70$*

BW (kg)	$RER = 70\ BW(kg)^{0.73}$
1	70
1.5	94
2	116
2.5	137
3	156
3.5	175
4	193
4.5	210
5	227
5.5	243
6	259
6.5	274
7	290
7.5	305
8	319

*patients weighing >2 kg
[For patients with excessive adipose tissue use a conservative estimate of the individual's lean body weight for the calculation.]
BW: body weight

TABLE 3 - ESTIMATION OF DAILY MAINTENANCE ENERGY REQUIREMENT (MER)
$MER = 1.1\ to\ 1.2 \times RER$

BW (kg)	1.1 x RER (kcal)	1.2 x RER (kcal)
1	77	84
1.5	103	113
2	128	139
2.5	151	164
3	172	187
3.5	193	210
4	212	232
4.5	231	252
5	250	272
5.5	267	292
6	285	311
6.5	301	329
7	319	348
7.5	336	366
8	351	383

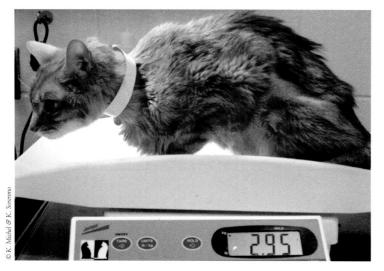

Figure 4 - Assessment of weight loss. *Many feline cancer patients have already experienced weight loss at the time of diagnosis and are at risk of further deterioration in body condition during the induction phase of chemotherapy.*

► Determining the need for assisted feeding

Patients who are unable to eat or whose voluntary food intake is insufficient to maintain energy balance will require some form of intervention whether it is as simple as coax feeding or a more aggressive approach using some form of assisted feeding **(see chapter 13)**. Clearly the feeding management of those patients who are already significantly malnourished at the time of presentation should receive immediate attention.

It is often the case that reduced food intake as a consequence of cancer therapy can be anticipated. Therefore a plan should be in place for nutritional intervention should the need arise, particularly in the case of patients whose nutritional status is considered borderline at the commencement of therapy.

3 - Cancer cachexia syndrome

► Distinction between weight loss due to starvation and cachexia

It is well recognized that weight loss is a common finding in human cancer patients and one which has been shown to have associations with clinical outcome *(Tisdale, 1997)*. As already stated, weight loss in association with neoplasia can occur for a number of reasons including the effects of the tumor and the cancer therapy. However, the weight loss seen in many human cancer patients does not appear to be attributable to decreased food intake alone. In simple starvation, individuals lose principally adipose tissue, whereas patients with neoplasia can experience loss of both lean and adipose tissues *(Moley et al, 1987)*. Furthermore, the magnitude of the weight lost often does not correspond to the amount of food consumed, and this weight loss cannot be reversed by a concomitant increase in caloric intake *(Costa et al, 1980)*.

This paraneoplastic syndrome of cancer cachexia is hypothesized to result from metabolic alterations that exist as a consequence of the underlying tumor. Derangements in carbohydrate, lipid, and protein metabolism have been found in both human and canine cancer patients that may contribute to weight loss *(Shapot & Blinov, 1974; Nixon et al, 1980; Nolop et al, 1987; Shaw & Wolfe, 1987; Vail et al, 1990; Tayek, 1992; McMillan et al, 1994; Ogilvie et al, 1994;1997; Vail et al, 1994; Dworzak et al 1998)*. There is also evidence that cytokines, including TNFα, IL-1, and IL-6, could play a role in these metabolic alterations *(Gelin et al, 1991; Moldawer and Copeland, 1997)*.

What remains unknown is to what extent the weight loss seen in feline cancer patients is attributable to decreased appetite or the direct effects of the tumor or therapy on nutrient assimilation or metabolism and to what extent cancer cachexia syndrome **(Figure 4)** may be responsible. This is important because in the former situation careful attention to feeding management should be able to avert or ameliorate loss of weight and body condition, whereas in the latter situation, effective means of counteracting the progression of cachexia remain elusive.

► Body condition as a prognostic factor

Cancer cachexia syndrome has been implicated as a negative prognostic factor for survival, surgical risk, response to chemotherapy, and tolerance of treatment in human cancer medicine *(Daly et al, 1979; DeWys et al, 1980; McCaw, 1989)*. There have been some preliminary studies in companion animal cancer patients looking at body condition and weight loss. When body condition was evaluated in dogs seen at the oncology service at the University of Pennsylvania only 5% of the dogs were considered significantly underweight with a BCS <2.5/5 (1= cachectic, 3=optimal; 5=obese) while 29% were classified as significantly overweight (>4/5) *(Michel et al, 2004)*.

Conversely, an investigation of feline cancer patients at the same institution documented that up to 44% of cats with cancer treated through the oncology service had a BCS <3/5 (*Baez et al, 2007*).

This study also found that both a low BCS as well as a low body weight had a negative impact on prognosis. Both cats with solid tumors and cats with lymphoma have significantly shorter survival times if their BCS or their body weight were low. Furthermore, a positive correlation between remission status and BCS was found.

The presence of weight loss or cachexia was not found to be an independent negative prognostic indicator as it has been in similar studies in human oncology (*Vigano et al, 2000*). Nevertheless, the results suggest that weight loss and deterioration of body condition are significant problems in feline cancer medicine and may have consequences for response to treatment, remission duration and quality of life.

> Cats in remission are more likely to weigh more and have a higher body condition score.

4 - Nutritional consequences of anti-cancer therapy

Debilitated cats with advanced alimentary lymphoma represent some of the most challenging cases in medical oncology. The poor nutritional status in these patients is typically a result of a combination of factors resulting in prolonged inadequate nutrition. These signs may be direct effects of gastrointestinal involvement, stage of disease or may also, in part, be due to a deranged metabolic state secondary to cancer cachexia syndrome.

▶ Secondary effects of chemotherapeutic protocols

Regardless of the pathogenesis, in order to reverse these signs, treatment of the underlying malignancy is necessary. This requires the use of chemotherapy. The choice of chemotherapeutic protocol is influenced by cell type or lymphoma grade. Most oncologists use a combination of chemotherapeutic drugs including, prednisone, asparaginase, vincristine, cyclophosphamide, methotrexate, and doxorubicin to treat cats with intermediate to high grade lymphoma (intermediate to large cell type) (*Moore et al, 1996; Valerius et al, 1997; Vail et al, 1998; Zwahlen et al, 1998; Krystal et al, 2001; Teske et al, 2002; Richter, 2003; Milner et al, 2005*). Many of these drugs are associated with gastrointestinal signs such as nausea, vomiting, anorexia, diarrhea, and fatigue; clinical signs which many of these cats already exhibit. Debilitated patients may be more likely to experience adverse reactions to treatment, require dose reductions, have a decreased response to treatment and have a worse outcome. The induction phase can be particularly difficult and requires careful monitoring of tumor response, addressing toxicity from treatment as needed and constant assessment of the general status of the cat.

A cat with alimentary lymphoma and severe weight loss.

▶ Variability of individual responses

Lymphoma is a chemotherapy-responsive malignancy and some cats with high grade lymphoma may go into remission quickly, tolerate the chemotherapy and improve without specific nutritional intervention. However, others may take longer to respond and/or become increasingly intolerant to chemotherapy and suffer progressive weight loss through the induction phase. Some of these cats may never attain remission and fail early, and others may be taken off chemotherapy prematurely due to unacceptable toxicity and poor quality of life. These cats require intervention.

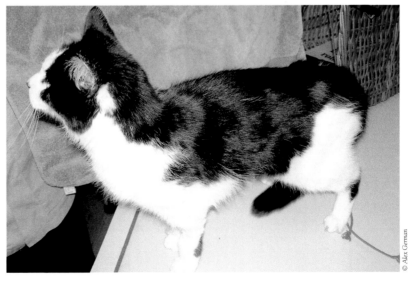
© Alex German

DIETARY AVERSION

If a food is associated with distress, an unpleasant experience (hospitalization) or digestive problem (poisoning), the food is likely to be avoided in the future. This phenomenon is known as aversion. Aversion is a form of negative conditioning used by animals to avoid foods that are unsuitable for them.

In cats, aversion sets in very quickly. A single meal associated with unpleasantness leads to a refusal to eat. Such aversion can persist for at least 40 days (Bradshaw et al, 1996). The smell alone of a food associated with digestive disorders is enough to elicit aversion. Cats even go so far as to show aversion for their usual food if it is served in the presence of an air current bearing the odor of a food to which they have developed an aversion.

TABLE 4 - SIGNS OF LEARNED FOOD AVERSION

The patient initially shows interest in food when it is offered but backs away after smelling or tasting the food.

The patient salivates, swallows repeatedly or turns its head away when food is offered.

A caged patient positions itself as far away as possible from the feeding bowl.

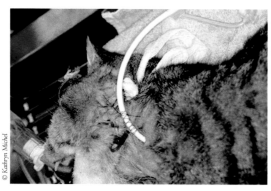

© Kathryn Michel

Figure 5 - Assisted feeding by esophagostomy tube.
Esophagostomy tubes are relatively non-invasive and simple to place and provide well-tolerated access for assisted feeding in feline patients.

A prospective study on the incidence of toxicity and overall quality of life in dogs and cats treated with chemotherapy at the University of Pennsylvania confirmed that weight loss, vomiting, and anorexia were more common in cats than dogs (Bachman et al, 2000). Sixty percent of the cats lost weight in the induction phase, this is in sharp contrast to the situation in dogs, where close to 70% gained weight (p = 0.0077). Doxorubicin was the drug most often associated with weight loss and vomiting in both cats and dogs. These results reflect the complexity of the situation. Chemotherapy is necessary to treat the underlying malignancy, yet it may also exacerbate the clinical signs and contribute to further weight loss, vomiting, diarrhea and reduced quality of life. The overall median survival of cats with lymphoma is less than one year; poor nutritional status and low body weight are associated with worse outcome in cats (Baez et al, 2007). It is unknown whether early intervention to reverse the loss of weight and body condition improve outcome in these cats, but these results clearly show that more attention should be paid to ensuring adequate nutritional support, both to improve quality of life as well as to potentially prolong survival.

5 - Dietary intervention

► Coax feeding

When a cat exhibits a decreased appetite it is natural to try to tempt it to eat by offering a variety of palatable foods. Very often the caregiver will further attempt to coax the patient to eat by putting the food close to the cat's face or actually placing food in its mouth. Sometimes these techniques can be successful and lead to adequate food intake by the patient. However, such efforts are labor intensive and time consuming. A feeding plan with specific caloric goals should be formulated in advance so the caregiver can assess the adequacy of the patient's food intake. Furthermore, it is very important to recognize that cats sometimes associate nausea, general indisposition, or pain with the act of eating or even the sight or scent of food. This is called learned food aversion and can further complicate achieving adequate food intake in a patient.

Therefore, whenever attempting to coax feed a cat, one must remain alert to the signs of food aversion **(Table 4)** and recognize that there will be circumstances when it will be necessary to resort to assisted feeding for a time because of the risk of causing or exacerbating this condition. **Table 5** lists some general guidelines on how to approach these patients. However, every patient will be different and it is necessary to observe each individual's behavior in order to decide how best to proceed.

► Assisted feeding

Much of the information gleaned in your nutritional assessment will aid in making the choice of the best route for assisted feeding access. Other information to evaluate in the decision making process should include:

- assessment of gastrointestinal tract function
- assessment of other organ systems that may have an impact on the patient's ability to tolerate specific nutrients
- assessment of the patient's ability to tolerate a feeding tube and tube placement
- assessment of the patient's risk for pulmonary aspiration.

If parenteral nutrition is contemplated, it is also necessary to include assessment of the ability to obtain vascular access and the patient's fluid tolerance.

There are some additional considerations to take into account when assessing cancer patients for assisted feeding. Certain chemotherapeutic agents can impair wound healing with the consequence of a greater risk of septic complications with tubes that are placed into the peritoneal cavity (e.g. gastrostomy and enterostomy tubes). This risk can be magnified if the patient is receiving immunosuppressive drugs. Radiation therapy can have similar consequences if the tube placement is within the field of treatment. The esophagostomy tube has many of the advantages of a gastrostomy tube but carries a lower risk of serious septic complications (**Figure 5**). These tubes are simple and inexpensive to place and usually well-tolerated by feline patients.

One final consideration is the fact that assisted feeding is a form of life-support. Used properly it could have the benefit of both prolonging life and ensuring a better quality of life for the patient. However, there may be circumstances, in terminal patients, where humane euthanasia is in the better interest of the patient then prolonging life. It is often more difficult for involved pet owners to terminate life supporting therapies than to initiate them and therefore the decision to use assisted feeding in a patient should bear in mind these ethical issues.

Figure 6 is a decision tree that illustrates how these various factors should be taken into account to choose the safest and most effective route of assisted feeding. Assisted feeding in feline patients is covered in more detail in chapter 13.

▶ Diet selection

In general, diet selection is based on which of patient's problems can and should be addressed with nutrition and the nutritional requirements of the patient. While there have been many investigations of ways in

TABLE 5 - GUIDELINES FOR COAX FEEDING
Resist the temptation to coax a cat to eat when it is showing overt signs of nausea and discomfort. Cats that gulp or salivate at the sight or scent of food, who turn their heads away from the food or spit it out when it is placed in their mouths should not have food forced on them.
Consider the possibility of using anti-emetic drugs if vomiting and nausea are a problem.
Consider the use of assisted feeding as an alternative.
Consider appetite stimulant drugs; however, these should only be used in patients that either have no signs of food aversion or who have begun to feel better and may now be able to overcome a food aversion.
For cats that are showing some interest in food: - try novel food items. Remember that table foods will not provide all of the nutrients that a cat requires and if a cat eats an exclusively home cooked diet for more than a few days, that diet should be evaluated by a veterinary nutritionist for nutritional adequacy; - make mealtimes as comfortable and unstressful as possible. Try not to schedule them at the same time as other treatments such as the administration of medications; - divide the day's food into as many small meals as possible. Offering small meals of fresh food is more likely to meet with success than a few large meals no matter how tempting the food is; - the food ingredients that increase palatability for most cats include moisture, fat, and protein. Switching from a dry pet food to a canned food or the other way around may improve food acceptance; - remember that "mouth feel" (the texture and consistency of food) is an important aspect of palatability for cats (so switching to canned foods will not always meet with success).
Trying foods with increased fat or protein content should be done with consideration of the patient's tolerance for these nutrients.
The standard advice for getting anorexic cats to eat has been to warm the food to just below body temperature. This is believed to increase the aroma of the food, which in turn will enhance the taste. However, this might be counterproductive in patients that are showing food aversion.

FIGURE 6 - DECISION TREE TO DETERMINE THE ROUTE OF ASSISTED FEEDING

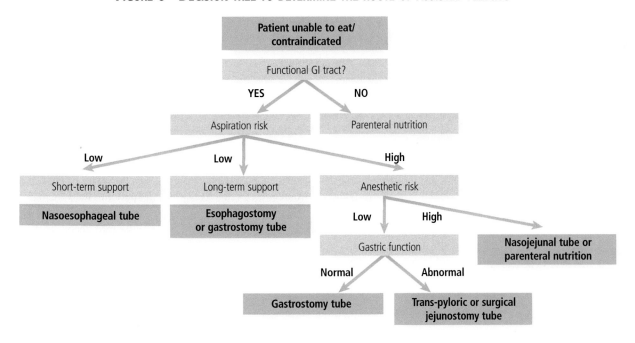

which diet and specific nutrients may be used to slow or antagonize tumor growth, modulate immune function, or counteract the cancer cachexia syndrome, most of this research has been done in rodent models or human patients. There have been preliminary clinical investigations involving canine cancer patients, but none to date that have involved cats. A canned low carbohydrate diet that was fortified with fish oil and arginine was found to increase survival time and disease free interval in dogs with stage III lymphoma *(Ogilvie et al, 2000)*. With the exception of the additional fish oil, many conventional canned cat foods have a similar formulation to the diet that was used in this investigation.

The major consideration for diet selection for cats with cancer should be acceptance by the patient. The diet should meet feline nutritional requirements and if it does not, it should be supplemented to address any deficiencies. Ideally, the diet should be of high caloric density, as this will aid in ensuring sufficient energy intake by the patient, especially in cases when appetite is decreased. In addition, if the patient has clinical signs or disease secondary to or in addition to cancer that would benefit from dietary management, efforts should be made to select and feed a diet formulated to address those conditions.

Lastly, in patients with alimentary neoplasia, in particular lymphoma, nutrient malabsorption can occur. While this can lead to generalized protein-calorie malnutrition, it can also lead to specific micronutrient deficiencies. One nutrient deficiency which has been reported in cats with gastrointestinal disease, including lymphoma, is cobalamin deficiency *(Simpson et al, 2001)*. Cats with inflammatory bowel disease complicated by cobalamin deficiency have shown improved weight gain and response to therapy with parenteral supplementation of this vitamin (cobalamin, 250 µg SC once weekly, for 4 weeks) *(Ruaux et al, 2005)*. It is our clinical impression that cats with alimentary lymphoma also can benefit from parenteral cobalamin supplementation.

6 - Pharmacological intervention

In addition to treating the underlying malignancy with surgery, radiation therapy, chemotherapy or a combination of these modalities, additional medications may be indicated and necessary to reverse weight loss and improve quality of life. In order to choose the most effective drugs and provide the optimal care for the individual patient it is important to determine the cause for the inadequate food intake and weight loss.

► Causes of dysorexia and anorexia

Anorexia is the failure of the usual appetite signals and can be a direct or indirect effect of the cancer itself or the cancer treatment, specifically chemotherapy. Decreased or loss of appetite may be a direct result of abdominal pain or discomfort, and early satiety due to restricted gastric accommodation or delayed emptying secondary to tumor infiltrate. Primary intestinal tumors may lead to complete or incomplete obstruction, ileus, malabsorption, diarrhea or constipation which again can lead to discomfort, bloating, anorexia or nausea *(Uomo et al, 2006)*.

Chemotherapy may contribute to further decreasing appetite by its effects on the vomiting center as well as the effect on the gastrointestinal tract. Certain chemotherapeutic drugs such as vincristine can cause ileus and constipation, which again may feed into the cycle of anorexia and depression *(Ogilvie et al, 2001)*. The direct cytotoxic effects on the intestinal epithelial lining may lead to sloughing and make possible bacterial translocation and secondary intestinal bacterial overgrowth.

Chemotherapy induced gastroenteritis can induce nausea, vomiting and diarrhea. The risk for sepsis is especially important if the patient experiences concurrent myelosuppression. If there is a potential for sepsis, broad-spectrum antibiotics with good gram positive and gram negative coverage are indicated in these patients.

► Analgesia

Pain and discomfort may contribute to anorexia and weight loss. It is often difficult to determine whether veterinary patients are in pain, especially visceral pain. Visceral pain is commonly reported in human cancer patients with abdominal organ cancer, especially pancreatic cancer. Cancer cachexia is more common in pancreatic cancer than in any other cancer type and up to 80% of the patients are reported to be cachetic *(Splinter, 1992; Ryan et al, 1998)*. Pain medications are routinely provided to palliate these patients *(Li et al, 2004)*.

It is feasible that cats with alimentary lymphoma experience some degree of discomfort or pain, however, the effectiveness of pain medications in improving appetite and reversing the cycle of weight loss in these patients has not been evaluated, and pain medications may not be routinely prescribed. Pain is easier to recognize and therefore more likely to be treated in cats with visible non-resectable solid tumors that invade or destroy bone or that compress nerves. Palliative care with the focus of treating the cancer pain with oral or parenteral pain medication and/or palliative radiation therapy is routinely offered to cats with oral squamous cell carcinoma or osteosarcomas. It is the authors' subjective impression that some of these cats improve and increase their voluntary food intake with such measures. However, there are no studies to confirm these observations.

► Anti-inflammatory drugs

The systemic effects of cancer and metabolic changes associated with cancer cachexia syndrome are mediated by a complex network of pro-inflammatory cytokines *(Jatoi et al, 2001; Walker, 2001)*. Anti-inflammatory drugs may therefore have a role in reversing some of these effects. Nonsteroidal anti-inflammatory drugs (NSAIDs) include several different drugs with anti-cycloxogenase activity. These drugs have both analgesic and well as anti-inflammatory effects, and may therefore provide dual benefits to patients suffering from a painful non-resectable tumor and/or the systemic inflammatory effects of the tumor and cancer cachexia syndrome. In addition, the effects against cycloxogenase-2 may have direct anti-cancer effects, especially in tumors overexpressing this enzyme. The direct anti-cancer affects of NSAIDs have been reported only in dogs at this point *(Schmidt et al, 2001; Knapp et al, 2002; Mustaers et al, 2003; Mohammed et al, 2004; Mustaers et al, 2005)*. NSAIDs have been reported to improve some of the symptoms associated with cancer cachexia syndrome and improve quality of life in human pancreatic and other gastrointestinal cancer patients *(Wigmore et al, 1995; McMillian et al, 1997; McMillian et al, 1999)*.

► Appetite stimulating drugs

The use of appetite stimulating drugs and anti-depressants may also be indicated in some patients. It can be very difficult and often impossible to distinguish between anorexia resulting from nausea and anorexia as part of the cancer cachexia syndrome.

Therefore anti-emetics should always be considered first or in conjunction with drugs to stimulate appetite. Administering appetite stimulating drugs without providing effective anti-emetics may worsen nausea and cause more vomiting with the potential of creating a learned food aversion. It is also important to rule out and treat any physical causes of nausea, vomiting and subsequent anorexia such as gastrointestinal tumors, intestinal obstruction or chemotherapy-induced gastroenteritis prior to prescribing appetite stimulating drugs.

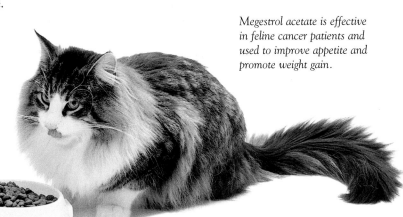

Megestrol acetate is effective in feline cancer patients and used to improve appetite and promote weight gain.

© Yves Lanceau/RC/Norwegian Forest Cat

Megestrol acetate is the most effective and commonly prescribed drug to combat weight loss and cachexia in human oncology. A large meta-analysis found that cancer patients receiving megestrol acetate were significantly more likely to gain or maintain weight than those who did not receive the drug *(Berenstein et al, 2005)*. The exact mechanism of action of megestrol acetate is complex and thought to involve stimulation of appetite by both direct and indirect pathways as well as antagonism of the metabolic effects on the principal catabolic cytokines *(Uomo et al, 2006)*. Megestrol acetate is also effective in feline cancer patients and used to improve appetite and promote weight gain.

However, **corticosteroids** are used more commonly in the USA, especially in feline lymphoma. Corticosteroids are part of the chemotherapy protocol for lymphoma and used for their cytotoxic effects, however, corticosteroids have additional benefits including appetite stimulation and anti-inflammatory effects which might be beneficial in combating the cancer cachexia syndrome.

Cyproheptadine, an anti-serotonergic, is another appetite stimulant used relatively frequently in cats and still favored by many veterinarians despite the fact that prospective trials in human cancer patients found no improvement in nutritional status in patients receiving cyproheptadine versus placebo *(Kardinal et al, 1990)*.

Appetite stimulating drugs are often used in conjunction with other palliative measures in cats. Some seem to benefit from these measures, but it may be impossible to determine which of the palliative drugs is indeed effective in patients where many different strategies to improve appetite are instituted simultaneously; the improvement may in fact be a result of synergistic or complimentary additive effects of a combination of drugs. A combination of drugs or a multimodality approach may indeed be necessary to maintain weight or reverse weight loss.

Nevertheless, it is important to assess all of the above potential contributing factors, i.e. tumor stage and direct gastrointestinal involvement, presence of nausea, pain or discomfort, chemotherapy induced gastroenteritis, or the presence of the cancer cachexia syndrome, so that the most appropriate drugs or drug combinations are administered. There may be a practical limitation to how many different oral medications a cat will tolerate, and forceful administration of excessive unnecessary medications may make the situation worse. **Tables 6** and **7** include drugs with recommended dosages used to decrease nausea, stimulate appetite, improve nutritional status and combat weight loss in cats with cancer.

TABLE 6 - ANTI-EMETIC DRUGS		
Drug	**Dosage**	**Comments**
Metoclopramide	0.2-0.4 mg/kg [0.1-0.2 mg/lb], SC or PO q6-8 1-2 mg/kg/day [0.5-1 mg/lb], IV CRI	Promotes gastric emptying and acts centrally on the chemoreceptor trigger zone (central effects are less potent in the cat than in other species)
Prochlorperazine	0.1-0.5 mg/kg [0.05-0.2 mg/lb], SC or IM q6-8	Sedative and hypotensive effects (adrenergic antagonist) acts centrally on the vomiting center and chemoreceptor trigger zone
Dolasetron Mesylate Ondansetron	0.5-1.0 mg/kg [0.2-0.5 mg/lb], IV or PO q24 0.3-1.0 mg/kg [0.1-0.5 mg/lb], PO q 24 hr	Acts centrally on the chemoreceptor trigger zone
Dexamethazone	1-3 mg/cat (given as a single dose in conjunction with other anti-emetics)	Unknown mechanism of action; potentates the effect of other anti-emetics

The licensing arrangements for therapeutic agents varies worldwide. Some of these agents may not be licensed or approved for use in cats.

TABLE 7 - APPETITE STIMULANT DRUGS

Drug	Dosage	Comments
Benzodiazepine Derivatives* Diazepam Oxazepam	0.2 mg/kg [0.1 mg/lb], IV 0.5 mg/kg [0.2 mg/lb], PO q12-24	Causes sedation Contraindicated in cats with hepatic failure Effects wane with time when used in sick animals
Cyproheptadine*	0.2-0.5 mg/kg [0.1-0.2 mg/lb], PO q12	Anti-serotonergic Can cause excitability, aggression and vomiting
Megestrol Acetate	0.25-0.5 mg/kg [0.1-0.2 mg/lb], q 24 hr for 3-5 days, then q 48-72 hr	Stimulates appetite by direct and indirect pathways Antagonistic effects on the principal catabolic cytokines Diabetogenic
Prednisone	0.5-1.0 mg/kg [0.2-0.5 mg/lb], q 24	Direct central effects Inhibition of tumor and host-induced substances Direct cytotoxic effects in lymphoma

Both the benzodiazepine derivatives and cyproheptadine cause only a momentary increase in appetite and are unreliable for ensuring adequate caloric intake.

The licensing arrangements for therapeutic agents varies worldwide. Some of these agents may not be licensed or approved for use in cats.

Conclusion

The primary goals of cancer therapy are to prolong life and maintain a good quality of life. Ensuring adequate nutrition is a requirement for both goals to be fulfilled. Human cancer studies have found that cachectic patients have a worse outcome, more complications and a lower response to therapy. The situation is likely similar in cats, as illustrated by one recently published investigation, where:
- remission was positively correlated with a higher BCS
- cats with solid tumors and lymphoma that had an underweight body condition had significantly shorter survival times than cats with a higher BCS (*Baez et al, 2007*).

Weight loss and the associated reduced quality of life may not only have a negative impact on treatment, but may also have direct consequences for survival, because it may lead to a decision to euthanize. The ability, interest, and willingness to eat voluntarily are major components of having a good quality of life. Most owners and veterinarians will likely agree that a cat that does not eat voluntarily or adequately over long periods of time may not feel well and may be suffering.

Therefore, providing effective nutritional support and offering the appropriate palliative medications to decrease nausea, improve appetite and facilitate voluntary food intake become crucial for prolonging survival. On our service we have found that the majority of cats with lymphoma lose weight in the induction phase of chemotherapy (*Bachman et al, 2000*). A significant proportion of cats with lymphoma die or are euthanized within the first months of starting chemotherapy. These facts suggest that more focus should be directed towards ensuring adequate nutrition and preventing weight loss in these patients. Early nutritional intervention may not only improve quality of life in cats with cancer but may also have positive impact on survival.

Cancer

Frequently asked questions

Q	**A**
How do we know whether it is the treatment or the cancer itself that makes the cat appear nauseated and have a reduced appetite?	This is probably one of the most frequently asked questions by both veterinarians and owners. In order to answer this it is necessary to re-assess the remission status of the cat and to perform a thorough review of the previous treatment history in order to determine whether there is a pattern to the weight loss or whether the nausea might be associated with certain chemotherapeutic drugs. This may require performing an abdominal ultrasound in cats with gastro-intestinal lymphoma and comparing the findings to the pre-treatment staging ultrasound. If the results suggest improvement or even clinical remission, the suspicion is that it is the chemotherapy that is the culprit. If this is the case, giving the cat a short break from treatment may result in a resolution of the problem. Continued chemotherapy should be initiated carefully with prophylactic anti-emetics and dose-reductions should also be considered. If the ultrasound shows persistent lymphoma or even worsening status, other chemotherapeutic drugs with concomitant anti-emetics may be needed.
Is my cat suffering because it is not eating?	It is reasonable to assume that a cat that does not eat does not feel well. There is a gradual scale from not "feeling well" to suffering. A temporary decrease in appetite or even anorexia may be acceptable in most owners' and veterinarians' opinion as long as it is assumed that it does not significantly impact on or interfere with other aspects of the cat's life. However, severe prolonged anorexia and weight loss secondary to any terminal disease for which there is no treatment or palliation is a clear sign of an unacceptable quality of life.
What can I do to improve my cat's food intake?	Appetite is affected by many internal and external signals. Many cancer patients may experience a reduction in appetite due to direct or indirect effects of the tumor and the treatment they are undergoing. Every effort should be made to optimize the patient's wellbeing including addressing conditions such as dehydration, fever, pain, and nausea. Make feeding times as unstressful as possible. Try offering small amounts of a variety of tempting foods but be alert for signs of learned food aversion. Offering many small meals through out the day may meet with more success than fewer larger meals. Sometimes warming the food to body temperature will increase its appeal.
My cat's appetite is very poor and he is losing weight despite a good response to chemotherapy. I have been told a feeding tube could help him through this period but I am concerned about the impact this would have on his quality of life.	Tube feeding is well-tolerated by many feline patients. Esophagostomy tubes, in particular, seem to cause little discomfort to the patient and provide access that permits the feeding of canned cat foods. Tube feeding is not possible in patients that have uncontrolled vomiting. However, when these conditions are not present or are properly managed, tube feeding will improve the patient's nutritional status, energy level, and overall sense of well-being. Since the cat is in remission but still losing weight, the weight loss may be due to chemotherapy induced nausea and fatigue, minor dose reductions and effective anti-emetics should also be considered in addition to feeding tube placement.

Cancer

Bachman R, Shofer F, Sorenmo K. A study of the quality of life in dogs and cats receiving chemotherapy. In Proceedings. 20th Annu Conf Vet Can Soc 2000; 15-18.

Baez JL, Michel KE, Sorenmo K, et al. A prospective investigation of the prevalence and prognostic significance of weight loss and changes in body condition in feline cancer patients. J Fel Surg 2007; 9: 411-417.

Baskin CR, Couto CG, Wittum TE. Factors influencing first remission and survival in 145 dogs with lymphoma: a retrospective study. J Am Anim Hosp Assoc 2000; 36: 404-409.

Berenstein EG, Ortiz Z. Megestrol acetate for the treatment of anorexia-cachexia syndrome. Cochrane Database Syst Rev 2005; 2: CD004310.

Bradshaw JWS, Goodwin D, Legrand-Defretin V, et al. Food selection by the domestic cat, an obligate carnivore. Comp Biochem Physiol 1996; 114A: 205-209.

Costa G, Lane WW, Vincent RG, et al. Weight loss and cachexia in lung cancer. Nutr Cancer 1980; 2: 98-103.

Daly JM, Dudrick SJ, Copeland EM. Evaluation of nutritional indices as prognostic indicators in the cancer patient. Cancer 1979; 43: 925-931.

Detsky AS, Mclaughlin JR, Baker JP, et al. What is subjective global assessment of nutritional status? J Parenter Enteral Nutr 1987; 11: 8-13.

DeWys WD, Begg C, Lavin PT, et al. Prognostic effect of weight loss prior to chemotherapy in cancer patients. Am J Med 1980; 69: 491-497.

Dworzak F, Ferrari P, Gavazzi C, et al. Effects of cachexia due to cancer on whole body and skeletal muscle protein turnover. Cancer 1998; 82: 42-48.

Gabor LJ, Malik R, Canfield PJ. Clinical and anatomical features of lymphosarcoma in 118 cats. Aust Vet J 1998; 76: 725-732.

Garrett LD, Thamm DH, Chun R, et al. Evaluation of a 6-month chemotherapy protocol with no maintenance therapy for dogs with lymphoma. J Vet Intern Med 2002; 16: 704-709.

Gelin J, Moldawer LL, Lonnroth. Role of endogenous tumor necrosis factor α and interleukin 1 for experimental tumor growth and the development of cancer cachexia. Cancer Res 1991; 51: 415-421.

German AJ, Holden SL, Moxham G, et al. A simple, reliable tool for owners to assess the body condition of their dog or cat. J Nutr 2006; 136: 2031S-2033S.

Jatoi A, Loprinzi CL. Current management of cancer associated anorexia and weight loss. Oncology (Williston Park) 2001; 15: 497-502.

Kardinal CG, Loprinzi CL, Schaid DJ, et al. A controlled trial of cyproheptadine in cancer patients with anorexia and/or cachexia. Cancer 1990; 65: 2657-2662.

Knapp DW, Glickman NW, Mohammed SI, et al. Antitumor effects of piroxicam in spontaneous canine invasive urinary bladder cancer, a relevant model of human invasive bladder cancer. Adv Exp Med Biol 2002; 507: 377-380.

Kristal O, Lana SE, Ogilvie GK, et al. Single agent chemotherapy with doxorubicin for feline lymphoma: a retrospective study of 19 cases (1994-1997). J Vet Intern Med 2001; 15: 125-30.

Laflamme, DP. Development and validation of a body condition score system for cats: A clinical tool. Feline Practice 1997; 25: 13-18.

Li D, Xie K, Wolff R, et al. Pancreatic Cancer. Lancet 2004; 363: 1049-1057.

Louwerens M, London CA, Pedersen NC, et al. Feline lymphoma in the post-feline leukemia virus era. J Vet Intern Med 2005; 19: 329-335.

McCaw DL. The effects of cancer and cancer therapies on wound healing. Semin Vet Med Surg 1989; 4: 281-286.

McMillan DC, Preston T, Watson WS, et al. Relationship between weight loss, reduction of body cell mass and inflammatory response in patients with cancer. Br J Surg 1994; 81: 1011-1014.

McMillian DC, O'Gorman P, Fearon KC, et al. A pilot study of megestrol acetate and ibuprofen in the treatment of cachexia in gastrointestinal cancer patients. Br J Cancer 1997; 76: 788-790.

McMillian DC, Wigmore SJ, Fearon KC, et al. A prospective randomized study of megestrol acetate and ibuprofen in gastrointestinal cancer patients with weight loss. Br J Cancer 1999; 79: 495-500.

Michel KE, Sorenmo K, Shofer FS. Evaluation of body condition and weight loss in dogs presenting to a veterinary oncology service. J Vet Intern Med 2004; 18: 692-695.

Milner RJ, Peyton J, Cooke K, et al. Response rates and survival times for cats with lymphoma treated with the University of Wisconsin-Madison chemotherapy protocol: 38 cases (1996-2003). J Am Vet Med Assoc 2005; 227: 1118-1122.

Mohammed SI, Khan KN, Sellers RS, et al. Expression of cyclooxygenase-1 and 2 in naturally-occurring canine cancer. Prostaglandins Leukot Essent Fatty Acids 2004; 70: 479-483.

Moldawer LL, Copeland EM. Proinflammatory cytokines, nutritional support, and the cachexia syndrome. Cancer 1997; 79: 1828-1839.

Moley JF, Aamodt R, Rumble K, et al. Body cell mass in cancer bearing and anorexic patients. J Parenter Enteral Nutr 1987; 11: 219-222.

Moore AS, Cotter SM, Frimberger AE, et al. A comparison of doxorubicin and COP for maintenance of remission in cats with lymphoma. J Vet Intern Med 1996; 10: 372-375.

Moore A, Ogilvie GK. Lymphoma, Section VI: Management of Specific diseases. In: Yvonne Stecher, ed. Textbook: Feline Oncology a comprehensive guide to compassionate care. Trenton: Veterinary Learning Systems, 2001; 191-219.

Mustaers AJ, Mohammed SI, DeNicola DB, et al. Pretreatment tumor prostaglandin E2 concentration and cyclooxygenase-2 expression are not associated with the response of canine naturally occurring invasive urinary bladder cancer to cyclooxygenase inhibitor therapy. Prostaglandins Leukot Essent Fatty Acids 2005; 72: 181-186.

Mustaers AJ, Widmer WR, Knapp DW. Canine transitional cell carcinoma. J Vet Intern Med 2003; 17: 136-144.

Nixon DW, Heymsfield SB, Cohen AB, et al. Protein-calorie undernutrition in hospitalized cancer patients. Am J Med 1980; 68: 683-690.

Nolop KB, Rhodes CG, Brudin LH, et al. Glucose utilization in vivo by human pulmonary neoplasms. Cancer 1987; 60: 2682-2689.

Ogilvie GK, Ford RB, Vail DM. Alterations in lipoprotein profiles in dogs with lymphoma. J Vet Intern Med 1994; 8: 62-66.

Ogilvie GK, Walters L, Salman MD, et al. Alterations in carbohydrate metabolism in dogs with nonhematopoietic malignancies. Am J Vet Res 1997; 58: 277-281.

Ogilvie GK, Fettman MJ, Mallinckrodt CH et al. Effect of fish oil, arginine, and doxorubicin chemotherapy on remission and survival time for dogs with lymphoma: a double-blind, randomized placebo-controlled study. Cancer 2000; 88: 1916-1928.

Cancer

Ogilvie GK, Moore A. Chemotherapy - Properties, uses, and patient management. Section III: Common therapeutic and supportive procedures. In: Yvonne Stecher, ed. Textbook: Feline Oncology a comprehensive guide to compassionate care. Trenton: Veterinary Learning Systems, 2001; 62-75.

Owen LN. World Health Organization TNM Classification of Tumors in Domestic Animals. 1st ed. Geneva, 1980.

Richter KP. Feline gastrointestinal lymphoma. Vet Clin North Am Small Anim Pract 2003; 33: 1083-1098.

Ruaux C, Steiner JM, Williams DA. Early biochemical and clinical responses to cobalamin supplementation in cats with signs of gastrointestinal disease and severe hypocobalaminemia. J Vet Intern Med 2005; 19: 155-160.

Ryan DP, Grossbard MI. Pancreatic cancer: local success and distant failure. Oncologist 1998; 3: 178-188.

Schmidt BR, Glickman NW, DeNicola DB, et al. Evaluation of piroxicam for the treatment of oral squamous cell carcinoma in dogs. J Am Vet Med Assoc 2001; 218: 1783-1786.

Shapot VS, Blinov VA. Blood glucose levels and gluconeogenesis in animals bearing transplantable tumors. Cancer Res 1974; 34: 1827-1832.

Shaw JH, Wolfe RR. Fatty acid and glycerol kinetics in septic patients and in patients with gastrointestinal cancer. Ann Surg 1987; 205: 368-376.

Simon D, Nolte I, Eberle N, et al. Treatment of dogs with lymphoma using a 12-week, maintenance-free combination chemotherapy protocol. J Vet Intern Med 2006; 20: 948-954.

Simpson KW, Fyfe J, Cornetta A, et al. Subnormal concentrations of serum cobalamin (vitamin B12) in cats with gastrointestinal disease. J Vet Intern Med 2001; 15: 26-32.

Splinter TA. Cachexia and cancer: a clinician's view. Ann Oncol 1992; 3(Suppl): 25-27.

Tayek JA. A review of cancer cachexia and abnormal glucose metabolism in humans with cancer. J Am Coll Nutr 1992; 11: 445-456.

Teske E, van Straten G, van Noort R, et al. Chemotherapy with cyclophosphamide, vincristine, and prednisolone (COP) in cats with malignant lymphoma: new results with an old protocol. J Vet Intern Med 2002; 16: 179-186.

Tisdale MJ. Biology of cachexia. J Natl Cancer Inst 1997; 89: 1767-1773.

Uomo G, Gallucci F, Rabitti PG. Anorexia-cachexia syndrome in pancreatic cancer: recent development in research and management. J Pancreas 2006; 7: 157-162.

Vail DM, Ogilvie GK, Wheeler SL, et al. Alterations in carbohydrate metabolism in canine lymphoma. J Vet Intern Med 1990; 4: 8-11.

Vail DM, Panciera DL, Ogilvie GK. Thyroid hormone concentrations in dogs with chronic weight loss, with special reference to cancer cachexia. J Vet Intern Med 1994; 8: 122-127.

Vail D, Moore AS, Ogilvie GK, Volk LM. Feline lymphoma (145 cases): proliferation indices, cluster of differentiation 3 immunoreactivity, and their association with prognosis in 90 cats. J Vet Intern Med 1998; 12: 349-354.

Valerius KD, Ogilvie GK, Mallinckrodt CH, et al. Doxorubicin alone or in combination with asparaginase, followed by cyclophosphamide, vincristine, and prednisone for treatment of multicentric lymphoma in dogs: 121 cases (1987-1995). J Am Vet Med Assoc 1997; 214: 512-516.

Viganò A, Bruera E, Jhangri GS, et al. Clinical survival predictors in patients with advanced cancer. Arch Intern Med 2000; 160: 861-868.

Walker PK. The anorexia/cachexia syndrome. Primary Care Cancer 2001; 21: 13-17.

Wigmore SJ, Falconer JS, Plester CE, et al. Ibuprofen reduces energy expenditures and acute phase protein production compared with placebo in pancreatic cancer patients. Br J Cancer 1995; 72: 185-188.

Zwahlen CH, Lucroy MD, Kraegel SA, et al. Results of chemotherapy for cats with alimentary malignant lymphoma: 21 cases (1993-1997) J Am Vet Med Assoc 1998; 213: 1144-1149.

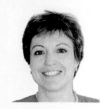

**Isabelle
GOY-THOLLOT**
DVM, MSc, PhD

Denise A. ELLIOTT
BVSc (Hons), PhD,
Dipl. ACVIM,
Dipl. ACVN

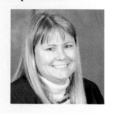

Nutrition and critical care in cats

Introduction 407

1. Nutritional requirements and starvation in healthy cats 407

2. Consequences of starvation in critically ill cats 409

3. Nutritional assessment 412

4. Calculating nutritional requirements 416

5. Enteral nutrition 418

6. Parenteral nutrition 426

Conclusion 431

Fallacies regarding feeding during intensive care 432

References 433

Royal Canin nutritional information 435

ABBREVIATIONS USED IN THIS CHAPTER

ATP: adenosine triphosphate	**EPA**: eicosapentaenoic acid	**PEG**: percutaneous endoscopic gastrostomy
BCAA: branch-chain amino acid	**FFA**: free fatty acid	**PN**: parenteral nutrition
BER: basal energy requirement	**FHL**: feline hepatic lipidosis	**PPN**: partial parenteral nutrition
CK: creatine kinase	**GI**: gastrointestinal	**PUFA**: polyunsaturated fatty acid
CPN: central parenteral nutrition	**GLN**: glutamine	**RER**: resting energy requirement
DPG: diphosphoglycerate	**IGF1**: insulin growth factor 1	**SGA**: subjective global assessment
DHA: docosahexaenoic acid	**IV**: intravenous	**TNF-α**: tumor necrosis factor
EFA: essential fatty acid	**MER**: maintenance energy requirement	

Critical care

Nutrition and critical care in cats

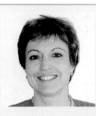

Isabelle GOY-THOLLOT
DVM, MSc, PhD

Isabelle Goy-Thollot graduated from Maisons-Alfort's École Nationale Vétérinaire in 1989. She was a medical intern at Maisons-Alfort between 1989 and 1991, specializing in companion animals. She co-founded the SIAMU, the critical care, anaesthesia and emergency medicine unit at Lyon's École Nationale Vétérinaire in 2000. She currently leads the SIAMU as well as being in charge of instruction in emergencies and critical care for companion animals. Isabelle has been President of the European Veterinary Emergency and Critical Care Society (EVECCS) since 2005. She is a member of the scientific committees of various journals and veterinary associations in France. Isabelle has developed her expertise in various placements in Utrecht (Netherlands) and Davis (USA) as well as participating in many activities for journals and conferences.

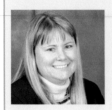

Denise A. ELLIOTT
BVSc (Hons) PhD Dipl. ACVIM, Dipl. ACVN

Denise Elliott graduated from the University of Melbourne with a Bachelor in Veterinary Science with Honors in 1991. After completing an internship in Small Animal Medicine and Surgery at the University of Pennsylvania, Denise moved to the University of California-Davis where she completed a residency in Small Animal Internal Medicine, a fellowship in Renal Medicine and Hemodialysis, and a residency in Small Animal Clinical Nutrition. Denise received board certification with the American College of Veterinary Internal Medicine in 1996 and with the American College of Veterinary Nutrition in 2001. The University of California-Davis awarded a PhD in Nutrition in 2001 for her work on Multifrequency Bioelectrical Impedance Analysis in Healthy Cats and Dogs. Denise is currently the Director of Scientific Affairs for Royal Canin USA.

*T*he cat is not a small dog especially with respect to critical care medicine. The physiologic response to shock, the procedures required for resuscitation, and the parameters that require careful monitoring present specific challenges that are unique for the critically ill cat. Although some feline disorders cause an increased appetite (diabetes mellitus or hyperthyroidism), the majority of feline illnesses result in partial or total anorexia.

Critical care

Introduction

With the emphasis in first diagnosing the underlying disease process, nutrition is often relegated as a late therapeutic process, typically considered when the patient has already been hospitalized for 4-5 days and has received little to no nutritional support. Moreover, a common practice is to wait just one more day, whereby there is some unreasonable expectation that anorexia that persisted for days will simply reverse itself because intravenous (IV) fluids have been administered. In reality, loss of appetite is one of the most powerful and long lasting features of severe disease. Therefore, the correct assumption should be that appetite will not resolve with supportive care and timely nutritional intervention should be implemented.

As more and more research uncovers the benefits of enteral nutrition and the complications that are derived from gut atrophy, critical care human specialists now feed patients much earlier than before in the disease process. This practice has resulted in improved outcomes and fewer complications. In veterinary medicine a similar transition has begun over the last few years, and is gaining momementum.

The two approaches to feeding critically ill cats are:
- enteral feeding, in which some portion of the gastrointestinal tract is utilized
- and parenteral feeding, in which nutrients are administered in a manner other than using the gastrointestinal tract, most commonly via central or peripheral venous access.

In the past several years, transitioning from ineffective strategies such as force- or syringe-feeding, warming foods, and adding flavor enhancers, to more recent recommendations for early tube feeding, novel methods of administrating nutrition to critically ill cats have resulted in increased survival rates.

1 - Nutritional requirements and starvation in healthy cats

▶ Specific requirements

> Cats are carnivores

Carnivorous by nature, cats require few carbohydrates but need high levels of protein. Adult cats require two to three times more dietary protein than omnivorous species, and have a high requirement for essential amino acids as energy sources (Zoran, 2002). Unable to adapt their urea cycle enzymes or aminotransferases to reduced protein intake, cats possess limited ability to adjust protein metabolic pathways for conserving nitrogen. Feline metabolism mandates cats to use protein for maintenance of blood glucose concentrations even when sources of protein in the diet are limited. These peculiarities help to explain the rapid onset of protein malnutrition in anorectic cats (Zoran, 2002; Center 2005) (Figure 1).

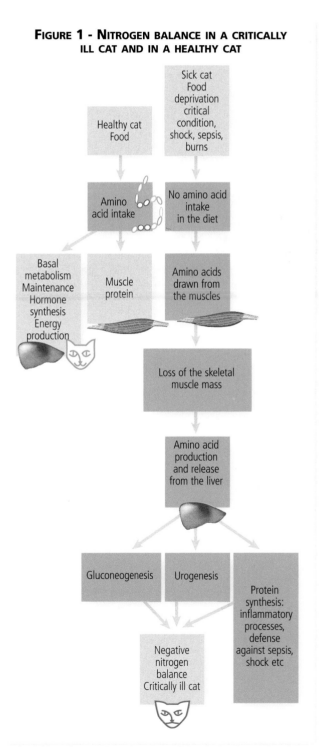

FIGURE 1 - NITROGEN BALANCE IN A CRITICALLY ILL CAT AND IN A HEALTHY CAT

Hastened use coupled with an inability to conserve or synthesize certain amino acids, necessitates a higher dietary amino acid intake for cats compared with most other species (*Kerl & Johnson, 2004; Kirby, 2004; Center, 2005*).

- **Taurine** deficiency has been proven to cause dilated cardiomyopathy, reproductive disorders and retinal degeneration.
- **Arginine** has important roles in nitrogen elimination and the urea cycle in addition to stimulating endocrine secretagogue activity, improving nitrogen retention, reducing nitrogen loss in post-operative patients, enhancing collagen deposition in wounds, enhancing T-cell function, and growth of lymphocytes (*Morris & Rogers, 1978; Barbul & Hurson, 1994; Zoran, 2002; Center, 2005; Saker, 2006*). Arginine is also a precursor of nitric oxide (NO) (*Barbul & Hurson 1994*).
- **Methionine and cysteine** are key methyl group donors important for the production of many metabolites such as glutathione, which is an important antioxidant and scavenger of free radicals (*Zoran, 2002; Center, 2005*).
- **The amino acid glutamine** (GLN) has been described as a "conditionally essential amino acid". Increased demand coupled with poor supply in critical patients may result in compromise of the gut mucosal barrier, with subsequent bacterial translocation and systemic infection. Impairment of reticuloendothelial function, in conjunction with a reduction in antibody production increases the risk of sepsis and multiple organ failure (*Elliott & Biourge, 2006*). Glutamine also has an important role in acid-base balance. Plasma glutamine levels have been reported to decrease by 58% after critical illness or injury, to remain decreased for up to 3 weeks and was associated with increased mortality in critically ill patients (*Wischmeyer, 2003*).

> Cats need minimal amounts of carbohydrates

Cats have several physiologic adaptations that reflect their low carbohydrate intake. Cats lack salivary amylase, the enzyme responsible for initiating starch digestion. Cats also have low activities of intestinal and pancreatic amylase and reduced activities of intestinal disaccharidases that digest carbohydrates in the small intestine. These species specific differences however, do not mean that cats cannot use starch. In fact, cats are extremely efficient in their use of digestible carbohydrates. Cats also have minimal activity of hepatic glucokinase and glycogen synthetase probably as a result of a metabolism designed to use gluconeogenic amino acids and fat, rather than starch. As a result, cats have limited ability to rapidly minimize hyperglycemia from a large dietary glucose load (*Zoran, 2002*).

High levels of dietary carbohydrates may also decrease protein digestibility in cats. This is due to a combination of factors, including increased passage rate. Increased amounts of carbohydrates in diets also results in increased microbial fermentation in the colon and increased production of organic acids (*Kienzle, 1994*).

> Cats have a specific requirement for polyunsaturated fatty acids

Fat typically provides most of the fuel for energy. Essential fatty acids (EFAs) for cats include linoleic, linolenic, arachidonic, eicosapentaenoic and docosahexaenoic acid. Most species can convert linoleic acid to arachidonic acid, the primary precursor for the 2-series prostaglandins, leukotrienes and thromboxanes. Arachidonic acid is required for maintenance of cell wall and tissue integrity and can be found in diets containing animal sources of fats. Cats however, do not have the enzymatic machinery (lack adequate hepatic Δ-6-desaturase activity and other hepatic desaturases) to synthesize derivatives of arachidonic acid (Zoran, 2002). Therefore arachidonic acid is an essential nutrient needed in the feline diet (*Kirby, 2004*).

> Vitamin needs of cats are unique

Cats require higher amounts of several water soluble B-vitamins including niacin, thiamine and pyridoxine compared with other species, and are predisposed to depletion during prolonged starvation. In addition, in some disease states, cats also require additional supplementation with cobalamin (B_{12}) (*Zoran, 2002; Kirby, 2004*).

Cats do not have the ability to convert beta-carotene to active vitamin A (retinol). Cats lack dioxygenase enzymes in the intestinal mucosa that split the beta-carotene molecule to vitamin A aldehyde (retinal). Therefore, preformed vitamin A must be supplied in the diet. Vitamins E and K are also important and may become deficient in cats that have prolonged anorexia (*Zoran, 2002*).

► Effect of fasting and starvation in healthy cats

TABLE 1 - HORMONAL CONTROL AND EFFECTS ON NUTRITION
Adapted from Atkinson & Worthley, 2003

Hormone	Secretion stimulated by	Stimulates	Inhibits
Insulin	Hyperglycemia Amino acids (e.g., arginine, leucine)	Glycogenesis Lipogenesis Protein synthesis	Gluconeogenesis Ketogenesis Proteolysis Lipolysis
Glucagon	Hypoglycemia Sympathetic stimulation Alanine	Gluconeogenesis Ketogenesis Glycogenolysis	Glycogenesis Lipogenesis
Catecholamines	Sympathetic stimulation Hypoglycemia	Gluconeogenesis Glucagon release Lipolysis	Insulin release Insulin effect

The normal nutrient-metabolism cycle in healthy animals involves an alternating system of feeding and fasting. In the fed state, the hormonal response to the nutrients glucose and amino acids, is stimulation of insulin secretion coupled with a reduction of glucagon secretion (substrate control) **(Table 1).** This results in stimulation of glycogenesis and repletion of the glycogen reserves, an increase in protein synthesis and the storage of fats. During the fasted state, plasma levels of glucose and amino acids fall, insulin secretion is reduced and glucagon secretion is increased which stimulates gluconeogenesis and glycogenolysis.

Periods of fasting longer than three to five days induces a state of starvation. In this situation, there is a further reduction in insulin levels and an increase in glucagon secretion. In addition, mild sympathic activation stimulates hormone-sensitive lipoprotein lipase which increases the release of free fatty acids (FFAs) from adipose tissue. Excess FFAs are converted by the liver to ketone bodies, which substitute for glucose as energy substrates in the brain and other organs. Ketones help to decrease skeletal muscle breakdown and amino acid release by reducing the obligatory demand for glucose, and gluconeogenesis. With chronic starvation, glucagon levels return to their post absorptive levels and catecholamine levels decrease. The basal metabolic rate decreases due to a reduction in the peripheral conversion of thyroxine (T4) to triiodothyronine (T3) (*Atkinson & Worthley, 2003*).

In carnivores such as cats, glycogen stores are quickly depleted and this leads to the initial mobilization of amino acids from muscle stores. Within days, a metabolic shift occurs toward the preferential use of fat deposits, which spares the catabolic effects on lean muscle tissue (*Chan, 2006; Chan & Freeman, 2006*) **(Figure 1)**.

2 - Consequences of starvation in critically ill cats

► General consequences of "stressed starvation"

Critical illness induces unique metabolic changes in cats that predispose them to malnutrition and its deleterious effects. An important distinction in the body's response to inadequate nutritional intake occurs in disease or stressed starvation compared with healthy starvation (*Michel, 2004; 2006; Chan & Freeman 2006*) **(Table 2)**.

TABLE 2 - UNSTRESSED STARVATION VERSUS STRESSED STARVATION
Adapted from Michel (2004; 2006)

Unstressed starvation	Stressed starvation
- Mediators secreted in response to the lack of food - Conservation of endogenous proteins - Resolves with feeding	- Mediators secreted in response to tissue injury or inflammation - Catabolism of endogenous proteins - Resolves with healing or treatment of the underlying disease

Critical care

FIGURE 2 - GENERAL CONSEQUENCES OF STARVATION IN CRITICALLY ILL CATS

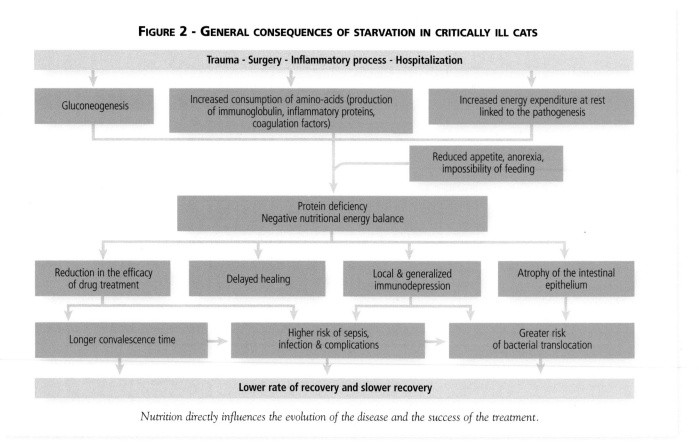

Nutrition directly influences the evolution of the disease and the success of the treatment.

During a critical pathological process, the nutritional hormones are no longer substrate controlled. To maintain hemodynamic homeostasis during acute injury, an increase in sympathetic tone and catecholamine (e.g., epinephrine and norepinephrine) secretion occurs. The catecholamines stimulate glycogenolysis and sensitive hormone protein lipase to increase the plasma levels of FFAs, glucose and insulin. Insulin inhibits ketogenesis. The increase in sympathetic tone increases the resistance of the peripheral tissues to insulin. In septic patients the stress response is exacerbated by the release of polypeptide mediators including tumor necrosis factor (TNF-α) and interleukin-1 that cause functional hepatic abnormalities, increase glucose intolerance and increase skeletal muscle protein catabolism (via the ubiquitin-conjugation proteasome pathway) (*Atkinson & Worthley, 2003*). The inflammatory response also triggers alterations in cytokines and hormone concentrations and shifts metabolism toward a catabolic state with accelerated proteolysis that typically results in significant negative nitrogen balance (**Figure 1**). Paradoxically, these patients may preserve fat deposits in the face of lean muscle tissue loss (*Chan & Freeman, 2006*). The consequences of lean body mass loss include delayed wound healing, immunosuppression, reduced muscle strength (both skeletal and respiratory), and ultimately increased morbidity and mortality (*Marik & Zaloga, 2001; Atkinson & Worthley, 2003*) (**Figure 2**).

► Specific topics in critically ill cats

> Alterations in carbohydrate metabolism in critically ill cats

Similar to critically ill humans, alterations in carbohydrate metabolism are present in critically ill cats and likely contribute to the hyperglycemia commonly observed in this population. Alterations in carbohydrate metabolism in critical illness include increased glucose production (gluconeogenesis), depressed glycogenesis, glucose intolerance, and peripheral insulin resistance. Concentrations of counter-regulatory hormones, such as glucagon, cortisol, and epinephrine are increased and these hormones play a role in up-regulating gluconeogenesis. In addition, hepatic gluconeogenesis appears to become resistant to the regulatory effects of insulin and blood glucose, further contributing to hyperglycemia.

Activation of inflammatory cytokines and neuroendocrine pathways are believed to play a key role in lipid, protein and carbohydrate metabolism. Interactions between the various metabolic pathways are also believed to contribute to hyperglycemia. Glucose intolerance has also been found to parallel the severity of illness. Hyperglycemia has been associated with poorer outcome in critical human patients (*Van den Berghe, 2004*), and studies have demonstrated the benefits of insulin administration in the critically ill population (*Van den Bergh, 2004*).

The impact of hyperglycemia on outcome in critically ill cats has not been as well characterized. In a retrospective study, *Chan et al* (2006) reported that cats presented to the emergency service with hyperglycemia were significantly more likely to die or be euthanized than those without hyperglycemia. However, in this study, the degree of hyperglycemia did not appear to impact outcome. Critically ill cats have also been reported to be at risk for developing hyperglycemia associated with parenteral nutrition (PN). Hyperglycemia was documented to occur in 75% (*Lippert et al, 1993; Syring et al, 2001*) and 20% (*Crabb et al, 2006*), respectively of cats receiving PN. More importantly, the development of hyperglycemia in cats receiving PN was shown to negatively impact survival (*Pyle et al, 2004*). *Chan et al* (2006) reported that critically ill cats had higher circulating concentrations of glucose, lactate, glucagon, non-esterified fatty acids, and cortisol compared with healthy controls. Critically ill cats also had lower insulin and insulin:glucagon ratios compared with healthy controls. The phenomenon of hyperglycemia in critically ill cats is complex, remains incompletely understood and likely involves multiple pathophysiological mechanisms.

> Gastro-intestinal motility and mucosal integrity

Cats that are post-anesthetic, postoperative (especially abdominal surgery), hypokalemic, suffering from gastrointestinal, reticuloendothelial, or neuromuscular diseases, or on narcotic analgesics have a strong likelihood of gastrointestinal paresis. Several aspects of digestive physiologic and intestinal microbiologic characteristics of cats suggest a possible role of bacteria in these abnormalities. It has been suggested that increased numbers of bacteria in the feline intestine serve to enhance digestion of protein and fat (*Zoran, 2002*). Ileus predisposes the patient to bacterial and endotoxin translocation, poor intestinal nutrient digestion and absorption, gastrointestinal ulceration and vomiting. The patient should be auscultated at least three times daily for bowel sounds (*Kirby, 2004*). In addition, critically ill cats receive numerous medications that can cause anorexia, nausea and vomiting (**Table 3**). These clinical symptoms contribute to the inappetance characteristic of critically ill cats.

> Feline hepatic lipidosis

Feline hepatic lipidosis (FHL) is the most common metabolic hepatic disease for cats; especially cats that are obese or stressed (*Zoran, 2002; Center, 2005*). Although the etiopathogenesis of FHL is still incompletely understood, it is now clear that most cats (over 95%) have an illness or circumstance directly causing a catabolic state (*Center, 2005*). Nutrients including taurine, arginine, non esterified FFAs and B-vitamins have been suggested, but not proven, to be involved in the pathogenesis of FHL (*Zoran, 2002*).

Successful treatment of FHL is based on early intervention and adequate nutritional support. In cats that receive early aggressive nutritional support, the prognosis for survival approaches 90%, but in cats not receiving such treatment, the chance of survival is only 10 to 15%. The best diet for treatment of cats with FHL is unknown, but evidence clearly suggests that dietary protein reduces hepatic lipid accumulation and maintains nitrogen and energy balance in cats with FHL (*Biourge et al, 1994; Center, 2005*) (see chapter 4).

TABLE 3 - LIST OF SELECT MEDICATIONS WHICH MAY CAUSE ANOREXIA, NAUSEA AND VOMITING IN CATS
Adapted from Michel, 2006

Amoxicillin
Cephalexin
Chloramphenicol
Amoxicillin/clavulanate
Erythromycin
Tetracyclines
Trimethoprim/sulphadiazine
Cardiac glycosides
Non-steroidal anti-inflammatory drugs
Chemotherapeutic agents
Narcotic agents

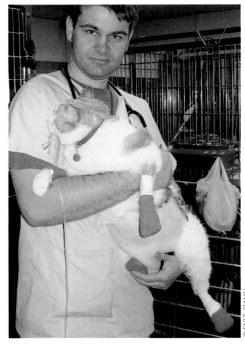

Obesity is a form of malnutrition often responsible for complications in the event of intensive care.

Critical care

411

► Goal of nutritional support in critically ill cats

The immediate goal of providing nutritional support to hospitalized cats is not to achieve weight gain, which mostly likely reflects a shift in water balance, but rather to minimize further loss of lean body mass. Nutritional support will not reverse the factors causing proteolysis, gluconeogenesis or lipolysis associated with sepsis or stress. Therapy should therefore focus upon decreasing catecholamine secretion by correcting hypotension, hypoxia and pain, and decreasing the levels of catabolic polypeptide mediators by treating sepsis (e.g., antibiotics, fluid therapy). Nevertheless, while nutrition may not reverse the catabolic response, it enhances protein synthesis and may retard protein catabolism, and therefore may reduce the total burden of body protein loss if introduced early in the management of the acutely ill patient (*Atkinson & Worthley, 2003; Kirby, 2004; Chan & Freeman, 2006*).

3 - Nutritional assessment

Nutritional assessment identifies malnourished patients that require immediate nutritional support and also identifies patients at risk for developing malnutrition in which nutritional support will help to prevent malnutrition. Moreover, nutritional assessment aims not simply to diagnose whether a patient is malnourished but whether the malnutrition will have an impact on clinical outcome. Currently used indications for nutritional support include a history of illness or weight loss, current poor body condition or acute loss of 5% body weight, or a history of anorexia or inappetence over 3 days (real or anticipated).

Nutritional assessment first determines the patient's nutritional status. This is a subjective evaluation based on the medical history and physical examination. Next the patient's caloric intake should be assessed. The patient's nutritional status and food intake are considered in conjunction with the severity of the patient's current illness, factors such as cardiovascular instability, electrolyte abnormalities, hyperglycemia, and hypertriglyceridemia and concurrent conditions such as renal or hepatic disease that will impact the nutritional plan.

Considering all this information will allow the clinician to determine what method of feeding is necessary, how aggressive they should be in initiating assisted feeding, and which route of feeding will be the safest, most effective and best tolerated by the patient (*Michel, 2006*). An important fact to remember is that many critically ill cats present to the veterinarian after several days if not weeks of inadequate nutritional support. Therefore, provision of nutrition to critically ill patients should occur as soon as it is safe to provide nutrition. This will vary from patient to patient, but the tendency has been to wait too long (*Chan, 2006; Chan & Freeman 2006*).

► Determining nutritional status

In humans, a technique referred to as Subjective global assessment (SGA) was developed approximately 20 years ago as a standardized tool to assess the nutritional assessment of patients (*Detsky et al, 1987*). Although no standardized scoring system currently exists in veterinary medicine, the principles of SGA can be applied to ensure the appropriate history, physical examination, laboratory data and diagnostic techniques are applied for the assessment of critically ill patients (*Michel, 2006; Elliott, 2008*).

> History

The dietary history should record if the patient is or is not consuming food. It is important to record the total duration of inappetence, which is the number of days the cat was inappetant in both in the home prior to hospitalization, and the hospitalized environment. It is also important to differentiate between how much food the pet is offered, versus how much of the food the cat consumed at home and in the hospital. This could be particularly difficult if the cat is both an

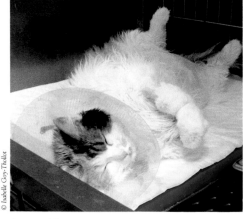

© Isabelle Goy-Thollot

Successful treatment of feline hepatic lipidosis is based on early intervention and adequate nutritional support.

indoor/outdoor cat, or is in a multi-cat free-feeding environment. The frequency and amount of vomiting and/or diarrhea should also be noted.

> Physical examination

The physical examination focuses on changes in body composition, specifically wasting of fat stores and muscle mass, the presence of edema or ascites, the presence of mucosal or cutaneous lesions, and the appearance of the patient's hair. Indications for nutritional support include the presence of injuries which prevent adequate oral intake (facial injuries, prolonged or unmanaged pain, injuries requiring surgical correction), and conditions of excessive protein loss (peritoneal drainage; open discharging skin wounds; hepatic or renal failure; protein-losing nephropathy or enteropathy).

> Body weight

Body weight provides a rough measure of total body energy stores and changes in weight typically parallel energy and protein balance. In the healthy animal, body weight varies little from day to day. However, additional challenges may arise in the critically ill patient. Edema and ascites cause a relative increase in extracellular fluid and mask losses in muscles or fat mass. Conversely, massive tumor growth or organomegaly can mask loss in fat or lean tissues. In addition, body weight can be falsely altered by dehydration or fluid accumulation. There can also be wide variation between scales, so it is important to use the same scale for an animal to avoid inter-scale variation. Finally, body weights are relatively small in cats and variations could be subtle and the scale must be precise (*Chan, 2006; Elliott, 2008*).

Finally, a single body weight measurement by itself has little meaning. It is important to know if and how it changes.

> Body condition score

Several excellent body condition scoring systems have been developed for cats. The most common is a 5-point system **(Figure 3)** where a body condition score of 3 is ideal, 5 is obese, and 1 is cachetic (see chapter 1). The body condition scoring systems are designed to evaluate fat stores on the body. In critically ill cats, there is often a disproportional loss of lean body tissue, while the fat stores appear to be adequate. Therefore, careful examination of the muscle stores by palpation of the skeletal muscle mass over bony prominences, such as the scapula or vertebral column is also necessary. Indeed, *Freeman et al* (2006) have recommended the use of a cachexia scoring system to evaluate lean body mass, where a score of 0 is normal and 4 represents severe cachexia.

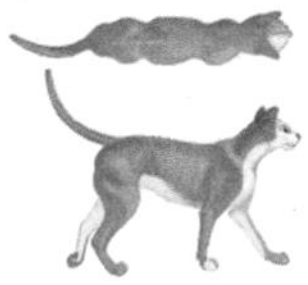

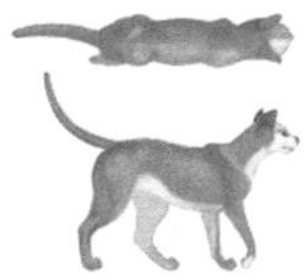

> Laboratory indicators of malnutrition

There are no biochemical analyses that will reliably identify malnourished cats or enable monitoring them during supportive alimentation. Currently used laboratory indicators of malnutrition include hypoalbuminemia, decreased blood urea nitrogen, hypocholesterolemia, anemia and lymphopenia. However alterations of these common indicators are often indistinguishable from those that can occur with concurrent disease. Albumin loss, for example, rather than undernutrition, may decrease plasma albumin levels (*Atkinson & Worthley, 2003*). *Fascetti et al* (1997) reported that anorectic cats have significantly higher serum creatine kinase concentrations compared to healthy cats. Furthermore, the creatine kinase concentration significantly decreased within 48 hours of implementation of nutritional support. The availability and ease of quantification of creatine kinase (CK) activity make it a promising method of nutritional assessment and monitoring in cats.

FIGURE 3 - BODY CONDITION SCORING IN CATS

Grades	Criteria
1 Emaciated:	- Ribcage, spine, shoulder blades and pelvis easily visible (short hair) - Obvious loss of muscle mass - No palpable fat on rib cage
2 Thin:	- Ribcage, spine shoulder blades and pelvis visible - Obvious abdominal tuck (waist) - Minimal abdominal fat
3 Ideal:	- Ribcage, spine not visible but easily palpable - Obvious abdominal tuck (waist) - Little abdominal fat
4 Overweight:	- Ribcage, spine not easily palpable - Abdominal tuck (waist) absent - Obvious abdominal distension
5 Obese:	- Massive thoracic, spinal and abdominal fat deposits - Massive abdominal distension

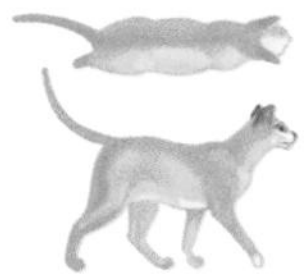

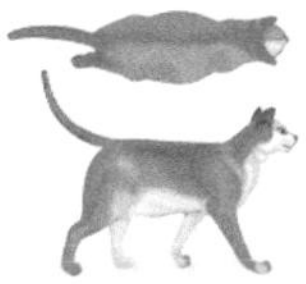

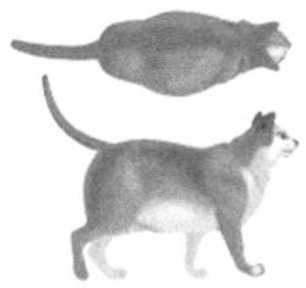

Other markers of nutritional status including prealbumin, transferrin, total iron binding capacity, fibronectin, IGF1, retinal binding protein, ceruloplastin, α-1-antitrypsin, α-1-acid glycoprotein and C-reactive protein have not been evaluated in feline patients (*Elliott, 2008*).

> Integrating the data

All steps in nutritional management should be documented completely and clearly in the medical record. The importance of clear documentation is exemplified by the study of 276 dogs in which a negative energy balance occurred in 73% of the hospitalization days. The negative energy balance was attributed to poorly written orders in 22% of cases (*Remillard et al, 2001*). Accurate documentation facilitates communication between the various members of the veterinary care team and strengthens the importance of nutrition in the overall care of the patient.

▶ Assessment of voluntary food intake

In order to assess whether that patient's food intake is adequate, it is necessary to determine the caloric goal, to select an appropriate food and to write precise feeding orders for the patient. Precise documentation allows an accurate accounting of how much food is offered to the patient and an easier evaluation of intake based on how much of the food is consumed (*Michel, 2006*).

▶ Determining the route of feeding

Nutritional support of critically ill patients can be administered via enteral or parenteral routes. Considerable debate and controversy has existed for several decades as to which method may be superior. The answer, or at least the current consensus, is that both methods are valuable and have important roles in managing critically ill patients. The goal of nutritional support should remain to utilize all tools that are available to prevent malnutrition in critically ill patients, while maximizing the benefits and minimizing the risks of the modality that is chosen.

The choice of the best route for assisted feeding is based principally upon evaluation of the patient and to a lesser extent upon logistical factors such as the availability of special diets and nutrient solution or access to 24 hour nursing care (*Michel, 2006*) **(Table 4)**. Whenever possible, the enteral route should be the first choice (*Chan, 2006*). Enteral nutrition is preferable as it is the most physiological, easy and safe method to institute; it is also the least expansive (*Yam & Cave 1998*). While the enteral route is commonly held as the method of choice, in practice gastrointestinal dysmotility or diarrhea may cause suboptimal results with failure to deliver the desired daily requirements (*Atkinson & Worthley, 2003*). However, even if patients can only tolerate small amounts of enteral nutrition, this route of feeding should be pursued and supplemented with PN as necessary to meet nutritional needs. Critically ill cats that are completely intolerant to enteral feeding, should receive parenteral nutrition **(Figure 4)**.

The assessment of gastro-intestinal (GI) tract function should include evaluation of the patient for nausea and vomiting and indications of GI dysfunction such as ileus or malabsorption. It is important to consider if the patient is receiving any medications that might cause nausea or GI ileus and whether the patient has had any recent gastrointestinal surgery or injury that will require bypass.

The patient is further assessed for indications of other organ systems that may impact the patient's ability to tolerate specific nutrients. Renal or hepatic failure may affect protein tolerance. Infiltrative mucosal disease may affect the patient's ability to assimilate dietary fat. With the exception of nasoesophageal tubes, placement of enteral feeding tubes requires general sedation or anesthesia. Therefore veterinarians should anticipate the need to place an enteral feeding tube when the patient is undergoing diagnostic procedures or surgery. If an enteral feeding tube is to be surgically placed, the patient should be assessed for a coagulopathy. Patients should also be evaluated for underlying conditions or the use of medications that might impair wound healing. Even the placement of a nasoesophageal tube will require physical restraint and some patients with respiratory compromise may not be able to tolerate this simple procedure.

TABLE 4 - PERTINENT INFORMATION TO EVALUATE IN THE NUTRITIONAL ASSESSMENT
Adapted from Michel, 2006

1. Assessment of gastrointestinal (GI) tract function
2. Assessment of the other organ systems that have an impact on the patient's ability to tolerate specific nutrients
3. Assessment of the patient's ability to tolerate placement of a feeding tube
4. Assessment of the patient's risk for pulmonary aspiration
5. Assessment of the ability to obtain vascular access
6. Assessment of the patient's fluid tolerance

FIGURE 4 - INTEGRATING NUTRITIONAL SUPPORT: DECISION TREE
(Adapted from Delaney et al, 2006)

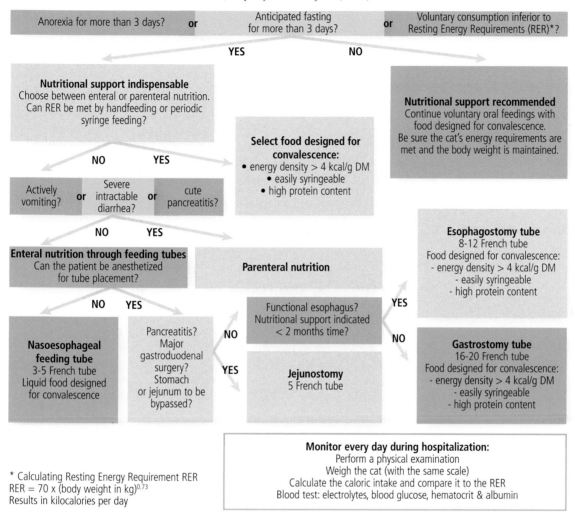

* Calculating Resting Energy Requirement RER
RER = 70 x (body weight in kg)$^{0.73}$
Results in kilocalories per day

If PN is considered, it is necessary to determine whether venous access can be obtained and whether that access will be central or peripheral. In addition, the patient's fluid tolerance must be assessed (Michel, 2004; Michel, 2006). The optimal delivery of PN is via a central venous catheter which requires close monitoring of the patient for metabolic complications. Therefore the patient receiving PN should be cared for in a facility that has 24 hour nursing care and the ability to perform serum chemistry tests.

The type of nursing care that the patient will receive should influence the choice of tube and feeding route. For example, if a cat is expected to go home with a feeding tube then it must be a type through which bolus feeding is possible unless the owner is capable of caging and monitoring their pet at home for continuous feeding.

The type of diet will influence the choice of tube type and site. If the only available food is blenderized then the choice is limited to using large bore tubes placed in the esophagus or stomach (Michel, 2004; Michel, 2006).

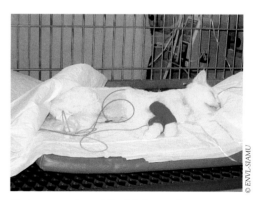

Patients must be stabilized before undergoing anesthesia, regardless of the urgency to implement nutritional support (Chan & Freeman, 2006a).

4 - Calculating nutritional requirements

Once the decision to implement nutritional support has been achieved, a stepwise process to calculate the energy requirements and to select the appropriate nutrient profile with respect to protein, carbohydrate, and fat is necessary. In addition to nutrients, the water requirement of the cat also needs to be evaluated.

► Energy

The calculation of the energy requirement of critically ill patients has been the subject of some controversy. Direct measurement of patient's energy consumption is not readily available. Consequently, several equations have been recommended to estimate the requirement. These equations utilize the resting energy requirement (RER), the basal energy requirement (BER), or the maintenance energy requirement (MER). The RER accounts for the energy required by the animal in a resting state and it includes physiologic influences and the assimilation of nutrients (*Elliott & Biourge, 2006; Michel 2006*). The interspecies formula (1) is most commonly used by the authors. Formula (2) is an alternative equation that can be used for to estimate RER in cats.

Formula 1 $RER = 70 \times (\text{current body weight in kg})^{0.73} \text{ kcal/day}$

Formula 2 $RER = 40 \times (\text{current body weight in kg}) \text{ kcal/day}$

To avoid complications associated with refeeding critically ill patients (see below), the cat's current body weight should be used for the initial RER calculation, regardless of whether the cat is underweight or overweight. The caloric intake can then be adjusted on a day-to-day basis to ensure the appropriate amounts of calories are administered to maintain current body weight. With resolution of the critical illness, caloric intake is further adjusted to either achieve weight gain in underweight cats, or for obese cats, a healthy weight loss program can be implemented (see chapter 1).

Some authors have recommended multiplying the RER with an illness factor (0.5 to 2.0) to account for hypermetabolism (*Bartges et al, 2004*). Other authors suggest that the RER of critically ill dogs, determined with indirect calorimetry, indicates that their energy expenditure is only slightly increased from normal (*O'Toole et al, 2004*). In addition, feeding excess calories can be associated with gastrointestinal complications, electrolyte imbalances, hepatic dysfunction, or cardiac abnormalities, complications commonly referred to as the refeeding syndrome (*Solomon & Kirby, 1989; Miller & Bartges, 2000; Armitage-Chan et al, 2006*). Furthermore, overfeeding energy can result in increased carbon dioxide production which can challenge patients with respiratory compromise (*Lippert et al, 1993*). Finally, a study showed an association between the use of illness factors and the development of hyperglycemia in cats administered parenteral nutrition (*Crabb et al, 2006*). Therefore, these studies support the recent trend of formulating nutritional support in critically ill patients to meet the RER rather than the more generous illness energy requirements (*O'Tool et al, 2004*).

► Protein

To abolish negative nitrogen balance in a severely hypermetabolic and hypercatabolic patient it may be necessary to supply protein in amounts in excess of normal minimum requirements (*Elliott & Biourge, 2006*) **(Table 5)**. Although nitrogen balance is often used to determine the protein requirements of critically ill people, this is not commonly measured in critically ill animals. In critically ill cats, protein should reach 30 to 50% of the calories (*Chan & Freeman, 2006*). Protein requirements are usually estimated based on clinical judgment and the recognition that protein requirements are markedly increased during certain diseases (e.g., peritonitis, draining wounds, severe burns) or require adjustement with other diseases (e.g., uremia, hepatic encephalopathy). The dietary source of protein should be highly digestible and contain all the essential amino acids. Human liquid formulas should be used cautiously, if at all in cats. Human formulations typically do not meet the high protein requirements of the cat, and are deficient in essential nutrients such as arginine, taurine and arachidonic acid.

TABLE 5 - PROTEIN REQUIREMENT IS USUALLY HIGHER IN CRITICALLY ILL CATS COMPARED TO HEALTHY CATS

Protein to calorie ratio is 110g/1,000 kcal versus 80 g/1,000 kcal in normal cats.

Proteins represent 40% RER versus 28% in normal cats.

Specificities of cats:
- Higher protein requirements
- Higher taurine and arginine requirements

Critical care

The branch-chain amino acids (BCAAs) leucine, isoleucine and valine (or their metabolites) may have a regulatory and anabolic role in protein metabolism by either increasing the rate of muscle protein synthesis or by decreasing the rate of protein degradation. Some, but not all, human studies have reported that BCAAs have a positive effect on nitrogen balance in the stressed patient (*Skeie et al, 1990*). To date, studies to evaluate the benefits of BCCA in critically ill cats have not been reported. However, the metabolism of these amino acids in this species, suggest that BCAA's could have positive benefits (*Elliott & Biourge, 2006*).

There are limited studies in critically ill or diseased companion animals supplemented with GLN. *Marks et al* (1999) were unable to preserve intestinal function in cats with methotrexate-induced enteritis that were fed a glutamine-supplemented amino acid-based purified diet. However, there are numerous studies evaluating the effects of enteral or parenteral glutamine in critically ill humans. Some studies report positive effects of glutamine supplementation on the gastrointestinal barrier and outcome, whereas other studies report no differences. Summarizing the numerous human studies certainly suggests that glutamine could have positive benefits on gastrointestinal health in critically ill cats.

► Carbohydrates

Cats do not have an absolute requirement for carbohydrates other than as an alternative source of energy. However, supplementation with carbohydrates may help to preserve lean body mass by down regulating gluconeogenesis. Excess simple carbohydrates should be avoided in critically ill cats as they can predispose to hyperglycemia (*Lippert et al, 1993; Chan et al 2002; Pyle et al, 2004*) **(Table 6)**. The subsequent release of insulin may lead to or exacerbate hypophosphatemia, hypokalemia, and other metabolic derangements (*Elliott & Biourge 2006*). In addition, cats have difficulty metabolizing large loads of highly digestible carbohydrate. Therefore, carbohydrates as source of energy are not recommended for critically ill cats.

Conversely, the inclusion of fermentable fibers or prebiotics such as beet pulp or fructo-oligosaccharides may have several beneficial effects in critical illness. Fermentable fibers have a positive effective on the mucosal barrier by stimulating the growth of intestinal bacteria such as Lactobacilii and Bifidobacteria. These bacterial species are considered to be beneficial to gastrointestinal health as they decrease the growth of pathogens such as *Clostridia* and *E. coli*. In addition, they produce the short chain fatty acids butyrate, acetate and propionate, which provide fuel for colonocytes. Short chain fatty acids enhance sodium and water absorption, increase mucosal blood flow and increase gastrointestinal hormone release. These mechanisms contribute to the trophic role that short chain fatty acids have on the intestinal mucosa, stimulating enterocyte and colonocyte proliferation (*Elliott & Biourge, 2006*).

► Fat

High fat diets (over 40% of calories) have been recommended for critically ill patients because free fatty acids rather than glucose provide the principal fuel in the catabolic patient. The preferential use of fat as a fuel may also help spare protein from catabolic processes for energy generation so that the protein can be used for anabolic processes. In addition, fat provides more than twice the energy density per unit weight than protein or carbohydrates, which helps to make the diet more concentrated **(Table 7)**.

Polyunsaturated fatty acids (PUFA's) are essential for the maintenance of membrane integrity as constituents of membrane phospholipids and the provision of substrates for eicosanoids synthesis (protaglandins, thromboxanes, and leukotrienes). The eicosanoids regulate the production of several cytokines such as interleukin-1 and TNF-α and are involved in critical inflammatory and immune responses. The long chain omega-3 fatty acids such as EPA (eicosapentanoic acid) and DHA (docosahexaenoic acid) decrease the synthesis of inflammatory mediators (COX-2 inhibitor-like action, PGE$_2$ production inhibition, NF-ÎB nuclear translocation decrease, and cytokines production inhibition), and they have been shown to have clinical benefits in a variety of disea-

TABLE 6 - THE CARBOHYDRATE INTAKE SHOULD BE LOWER IN CRITICALLY ILL CATS COMPARED TO HEALTHY CATS

Carbohydrate to calorie ratio is 40-60 g/1,000 kcal in normal cats.
Carbohydrates represent 15-20% RER versus 20-30% in normal cats.

TABLE 7 - THE FAT REQUIREMENT IS USUALLY HIGHER IN CRITICALLY ILL CATS COMPARED TO HEALTHY CATS

Fat to calorie ratio is 60-80 g/1,000 kcal versus 60 g/1,000 kcal in normal cats.
Fat represents 50-70% RER versus 50% in normal cats.

Critical care

se states, including sepsis. Conversely, omega-6 fatty acids have a significant role in immunosuppression, tumorinogenesis, and inflammation (*Kerl & Johnson, 2004; Saker, 2006*).

► Vitamins and minerals

Vitamins and minerals facilitate complex metabolic reactions and are key components of antioxidant activities (*Saker 2006*). Electrolytes (phosphorus, sodium, potassium and magnesium) should be closely evaluated in diets formulated for the critically ill patient to prevent the refeeding syndrome (*Solomon & Kirby, 1989; Justin & Hohenhaus, 1995; Miller & Bartges, 2000; Armitage-Chan et al, 2006*). Zinc supplementation may be beneficial in the critical patient to support the immune system and help promote wound healing. Critically ill cats may also have increased requirements for the water-soluble B vitamins. Vitamin B_{12} is particularly important for cats with pancreatitis or chronic intestinal disease.

► Special nutrients

The association of malnutrition with reduced resistance to infections has been observed for centuries. Numerous studies have evaluated the clinical effectiveness of specific nutrient supplementation in modulating the immune system (*Heyland & Dhaliwal, 2005*). Immunomodulating nutrients that have been evaluated include glutamine, arginine, long chain omega-3 fatty acids, antioxidants (such as vitamin C, vitamin E, taurine, caroteinoids), and nucleotides (*Chan & Freeman, 2006a*). However, the optimal combination and level of immune modulating nutrients to support the immune system of the critically ill cat is not yet known (see chapter 14).

Free radicals are unstable molecules generated by numerous exogenous and endogenous mechanisms. Hypovolemia, ischemia and reperfusion injury, common components of critical illness, can increase the production of free radicals. Free radicals cause oxidative damage to cellular components, which may ultimately contribute to organ dysfunction. The body counteracts oxidative damage by using free radical scavenging systems such as superoxide dismutase, glutathione peroxidase, catalase, vitamin E, vitamin C, taurine, and carotenoids. However, in critical illness, an imbalance between oxidant production and antioxidant protection can arise. Therefore it is prudent to supplement the diet of the critically ill patient with antioxidants.

In summary, the beneficial effects derived from adequate nutrititional support include: enhanced immune fonction, wound repair, response to therapy, recovery time and survival time (**Figure 5**).

► Water

The water needs of cats reflect their evolutionary status as desert-dwelling carnivorous animals who evolved to obtain most of their water requirements from the consumption of prey. Cats also have a less sensitive response to thirst and dehydration than dogs.

Nevertheless, critically ill cats are generally dehydrated or hypovolemic and restoration of fluid and electrolyte balance, and circulating blood volume typically requires intravenous support. However, consideration should also be given to critically ill cats to ensure adequate intake of free water, which can be administered enterally or parentally.

5 - Enteral nutrition

A study investigated the percentage of prescribed enteral nutrition delivered to 23 cats and 2 dogs (*Michel & Higgins, 2006*). This investigation reported a good rate of success for delivery of clearly prescribed enteral nutrition. In addition, consultation with the Nutritional Support Service improved the likelihood that prescribed nutrition would meet the patient's estimated RER.

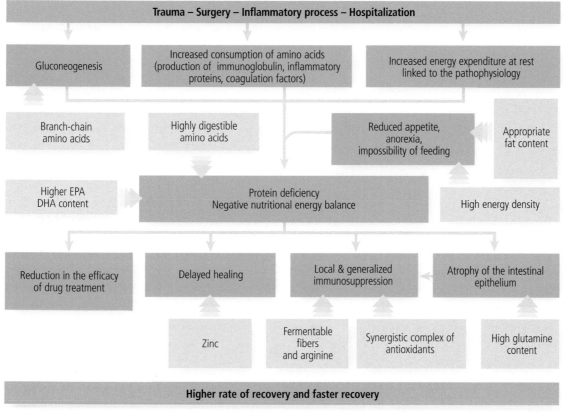

FIGURE 5 - NUTRITIONAL KEYPOINTS TO IMPROVE THE SPEED OF RECUPERATION AND TO IMPROVE CLINICAL SUCCESS

▶ "Assisted" feeding

Cats are known for a tendency to have fixed food preferences and therefore may refuse a new food. When smell or food is associated with positive consequences, the food will be eaten again. Conversely, if the smell or food is associated with distress, such as an unpleasant experience or hospitalization, the food will be avoided in the future. This phenomenon is known as aversion and in cats, aversion sets in very quickly. It is recommended to resist the temptation to coax a cat to eat. Forcing food on a cat who clearly does not want it may risk inducing aspiration pneumonia and a learned food aversion.

The smell alone of a food associated with digestive disorders is enough to elicit aversion. Cats even go so far as to show aversion for their usual food if it is served in the presence of an air current bearing the odor of a food to which they have developed an aversion. Therefore, it is important to be careful when preparing foods for cats at the hospital. Odors may travel and could trigger an aversion reaction even in cats being fed their usual diet. It is best to prepare the cats' food in a place where food odors cannot reach the cats.

For cats that show some interest in food, several methods can be tried to increase the inclination to eat. One can offer food in a novel setting or have someone different to do the feeding. Stroking and talking to a cat with the food nearby may stimulate interest to eat (**Figure 6**).

Cats need to feel safe and secure within their environment. To this end veterinarians and owners need to provide facilities for the main behavioral functions of eating, sleeping and playing and also ensure that the cat has the ability to control its own stress through the natural mechanisms of hiding and retreating. One of the problems with hospitalization is that the cat finds itself

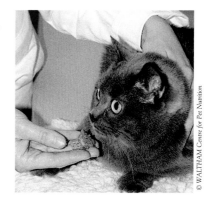

© WALTHAM Centre for Pet Nutrition

Figure 6 - *Sometimes a cat will be stimulated to eat if a small amount of food is placed in the mouth or on the lips or paws.*

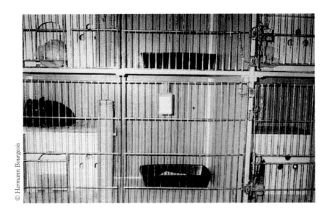

Figure 7 - *Moving the cats to larger dog cages which permits the separation of food, lodging and litter may restore the appetite of some cats.*

constantly on display and correspondingly vulnerable. Taking steps to provide the cat with a constant and predictable environment, both in terms of physical structure and scent profiles, will help to increase the cat's security. Hospitalized cats may be uncomfortable eating because the lack of space causes the spatial requirements of cats to be disrespected **(Figure 7)**.

Early satiety is common in anorectic patients, so it is recommended to divide the day's food up into as many small fresh meals as possible. This is particularly important in cats as their natural behavior is to eat a large number of small meals each day. They also eat day and night. Therefore, mimicking natural behavior in the hospitalized environment by providing multiple small fresh meals during the day and night may facilitate food intake.

It is important to keep in mind that "mouth feel" is very important to cats. Nutrients that increase palatability for most cats are moisture, fat and protein, and cats prefer foods with an acidic flavor and strong aromas. Adding water to a dry cat food or switching to a canned food may improve food acceptance. Most cats prefer their food at body temperature. Therefore warming the food prior to serving may encourage anorectic cats to eat. For cats showing interest in food but an unwillingness to eat warm food, it is suggested to try offering chilled food *(Michel, 2001)*. For cats that do not achieve adequate caloric intake using the above mention methods, enteral or parenteral feeding is indicated to achieve effective dietary management *(Michel, 2001; Elliott, 2008)*.

► Pharmacological appetite stimulation

Only a few drugs have been used as appetite stimulants in feline patients **(Table 8)**. There are a number of adverse effects associated with these medications. In numerous authors'opinion they have no place in the nutritional management of hospitalized critically ill patients. The only means of ensuring adequate caloric intake is through nutritional support (i.e. tube feeding or PN). Appetite stimulants could be used once the patient is recovering from its disease in the home environment *(Chan, 2006)*.

► Enteral feeding tubes

Enteral feeding can be achieved via nasoesophageal, esophagostomy, gastrostomy or jejunostomy devices *(Marks, 1998)*. Enteral feeding tubes are available in several sizes and designs, and are constructed of latex or silicone. Latex tubes are less expensive but generally require replacement within 8-12 weeks due to tube wear and tear. Silicone tubes typically survive 6-12 months and are less irritant at the stoma site. An array of feeding adapters can be attached to the enteral tube.

The use of these agents in cats can be restricted according to the licence applicable in each country.

TABLE 8 - APPETITE STIMULANTS Adapted from Chan, 2006		
Drug	**Dosage**	**Comments**
Benzodiazepine derivatives: - Diazepam - Oxazepam	- 0.2 mg/kg IV - 0.5 mg/kg PO SID to BID	Sedation, contraindicated in cats with hepatic failure, effects wane with time when used in sick animals
Cyproheptadine	0.2-0.5 mg/kg PO BID	Antiserotoninergic, can cause excitability, aggression and vomiting
Mianserine chlorhydrate	2-4 mg/kg PO SID	Excitability, aggression and vomiting

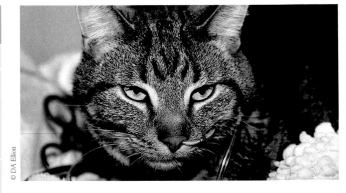

Figure 8 - Nasoesophageal tube placed in a cat.
Most critically ill patients will tolerate nasoesophageal tube placement, but some individuals may require sedation.

Critical care

> Nasoesophageal tubes

Nasoesophageal tubes are an excellent option for short-term feeding (< 5 days) of hospitalized cats **(Figure 8)**. Placement is described in **Table 9**. The tip of the nasoesophageal tube should not enter the stomach, but rather, sit in the distal esophagus. If the tube traverses the esophageal-gastric junction, acid reflux is likely, causing esophagitis and contributing to vomiting and irritation.

TABLE 9 - NASOESOPHAGEAL TUBES
Verset et coll, 2008; adapted from Bosworth & Snow 2004; Chan 2006

Indications	Contraindications
• Anorexic animals with a functional lower digestive system • Short-term tube feeding (< 5 days) • Spontaneous feeding contraindicated or impossible: mandible fractures, post oral surgery	• Uncontrollable vomiting • Surgery on the mouth, pharynx, esophagus • Trauma or esophageal stenosis • Deglutition/esophagus transit disorder • Altered state of consciousness • Delayed gastric emptying • Hepatic duct surgery • Fractures of nasal cavities or rhinitis • Severe thrombocytopenia/pathy • Brain trauma or intracranial hypertension (increased intra cranial pressure due to sneezing)

Pros	Cons
• Inexpensive • Easy to place • No anesthesia required • Animals can drink and swallow around the tube • No wait time before use or withdrawal	• Short-term nutrition • Uncomfortable tube of small diameter • Liquid food and large volumes due to small diameter • Elizabethan collar interferes with resumption of spontaneous feeding

Preparation	
Equipment	**Cat**
• 3-5 Fr Pediatric feeding tube (PVC, silicon, Teflon) • Lidocaine spray • Lidocaine gel • Non-resorbant monofilament thread and needle and/or cyanoacrylate • Elizabethan collar	• Spray lidocaine in the nose • Animal sitting or in sternal decubitus position • Flexed neck

Insertion
• Measure the placement length of the tube (from nasal meatus to 9th intercostal space) and mark the tube with indelible ink • Apply lidocaine gel around the tube • Insert the tube ventromedially and feed to the position of the insertion guide • Secured the tube with glue spot, suture or surgical staple at the nares laterally to the face and head • Verify the tube's position by radiograph • Place an Elizabethan collar

Post insertion	
Supportive care	**Complications/withdrawal**
• Progressive refeeding • Prior to each and every use: Confirm placement by aspiration and check for gastric contents • Following each and every use: Rise with lukewarm water (5-10mL) to prevent obstruction	• Overfeeding (nausea, reflux, vomiting, diarrhea) • Aspiration pneumonia • Epistaxis, rhinitis, dacryocystitis • Gastro-esophageal reflux and esophagitis • Obstruction of the tube • Withdrawal: resumption of spontaneous feeding

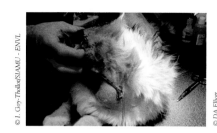 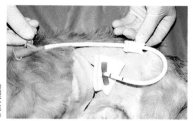 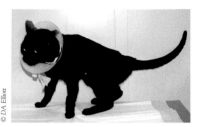

Figure 9 - Esophagostomy tube in a cat.
Esophagostomy tubes can easily be placed under a light anesthetic with minimal equipment.

Figure 10 - Gastrotomy tube in an anesthetized cat.
A gastrotomy tube must remain in place for a minimum of 7-10 days to allow a seal to form with the abdominal wall.

Figure 11 - Gastrotomy tube in a conscious cat.
Most patients tolerate the tubes quite well.

FIGURE 12 - PERCUTANEOUS ENDOSCOPIC GASTROSTOMY (PEG)

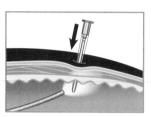

The endoscope is introduced into the stomach, which is dilated, then the skin and stomach are punctured using the trocar.

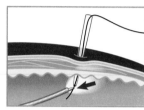

A guide is passed through the trocar and gripped with the endoscope forceps in the direction of the muzzle until it re-emerges.

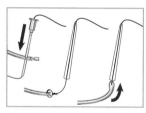

The tube is fixed to the guide using attachment.

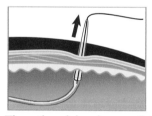

The guide and the tube are pulled towards the stomach until the end of the tube reaches the stomach wall.

Contraindications for nasoesophageal tubes include patients that have severe facial trauma involving the nares, protracted vomiting and/or regurgitation, semiconsciousness, or those patients that have laryngeal, pharyngeal, or esophageal physical or functional abnormalities *(Marks, 1998)*. Nasoesophageal tubes, are small, typically 3 to 5 Fr. Therefore, the selection of diet to feed via a nasoesophageal tube is limited to liquid or reconstituted powder diets. Some critically ill cats may not tolerate the large volumes required of such mixtures. *(Marks, 1998; Yam & Cave, 2003; Chan, 2006)*.

> Esophagostomy tubes

Esophagostomy tubes can easily be placed under a light anesthetic with minimal equipment **(Table 10)**. The only major associated complication is the potential for infection at the entry site and meticulous care of the surgical wound is essential to maintain the tube. In a study of 67 cats, esophagostomy feeding tubes were placed in 46 cats and percutaneous endoscopic gastrostomy (PEG) feeding tubes were placed in 21 cats. The authors reported that esophagostomy tubes were an excellent and less invasive alternative to the PEG tube *(Ireland et al, 2003)*. Critical care nutritionists believe that mastering the placement of esophagostomy feeding tubes is essential in the management of critically ill cats and this technique should be adopted in almost all practices *(Chan, 2006)* **(Figure 9)**.

> Gastrostomy tubes

Gastrostomy tubes are invaluable for the long-term nutritional support of critically ill patients **(Figure 10)**. Gastrostomy tubes may be placed surgically, or by percutaneous technique assisted with an endoscopic or blind placement apparatus. 16-20 Fr tubes are appropriate for cats. They must remain in place for a minimum of 7-10 days to allow a seal to form with the abdominal wall. These tubes can be easily maintained for many weeks to months in the chronically ill or anorexic patient *(Elliott et al, 2001; Luhn et al, 2004, Mesich & Snow 2004, Thompson et al 2004)* **(Figure 11)**. Peritonitis is a potential complication if the gastrostomy tube leaks or is removed early. The PEG technique is presented in **Figure 12**.

> Jejunostomy tubes

The jejunostomy tube by-passes the stomach and pancreas and can be used in case of severe pancreatitis, diffuse gastric mucosal disease, protracted vomiting or delayed gastric emptying. The jeju-

TABLE 10 - ESOPHAGOSTOMY TUBES

Verset et coll, 2008; adapted from Von Werthern & Wess 2001; Bosworth et al, 2004; Vannatta & Snow 2004; Chan, 2006

Indications	Contraindications
• Enteral nutrition > 7 days • Prolonged anorexia • Post-op mouth and head surgery • Oral cavity disorders • Contraindications of nasoesophageal tubes	• Uncontrollable vomiting • Primary or secondary esophageal disorders (esophagitis, megaesophagus, trauma, stenosis) • Foreign body, surgery or esophageal tumor • Delayed gastric emptying • Hepatic duct surgery

Pros	Cons
• Well tolerated • Inexpensive • Easy to place • Large diameter tubes • Can use calorically-dense diets • Long-term nutrition (1-12 weeks)	• General anesthesia needed for placement • Surgical procedure

Preparation

Equipment	Animal
• Endotracheal tube • Curved Rochester carmalt • 8-12 Fr 40 cm Pediatric feeding tube (PVC or silicon) • Non-resorbant monofilament thread and suture equipment • Elizabethan collar	• General anesthesia with placement of endotracheal tube • Right lateral decubitus • Clip and surgically prepare the left lateral cervical zone

Insertion

- Measure the placement length of the tube (from 1/3 proximal of the esophagus to 8th or 9th rib), and mark with indelible ink
- Elongate the side exit side hole on the tube with a small blade
- Identify the position of the jugular, retromandibular and oral-facial veins
- Introduce the carmalt in the mouth and direct it down the proximal esophagus with outward pressure, caudally to the hyoid and the entrance to the larynx
- Rotate the tip of the carmalt dorsally, pushing the esophagus towards the skin
- Palpate the tip of the carmalt over the skin
- Incise through the skin into the esophagus over the tip of the instrument (the mucosa of the esophagus is more difficult to incise than the skin)
- Gently force the tip of the instrument through the incision when the mucosa
- Enlarge the incision slightly to allow the tip of the carmalt to open
- Place the esophagostomy tube within the tips of the carmalt
- Close the carmalt and remove it from from the oral cavity, with the attached tube
- Disengagement of the tip of the carmalt
- Curl the tip of the tube back into the mouth and feed it into the esophagus
- As the curled tube is pushed into the esophagus, the proximal end is gently pulled outwards simultaneously
- Redirect the tube within the esophagus and creat a subtle "flip"
- Visually inspect the oropharynx to confirm that the tube is no longer present within the oropharynx
- Re-scrub the incision site, place a pursestring suture followed by a "Chinese finger trap"
- Apply a light trap around the neck
- Confirm correct placement with radiography

Post insertion

Supportive care	Complications/withdrawal
• Monitor the wound and change the dressings for 3-5 days then every 2-3 days • Wait 24 h before use • Progressively refeed • Prior to each and every use: Confirm placement by aspiration and check for gastric contents • Following each and every use: Rise with lukewarm water (5-10mL) to prevent obstruction	• Overfeeding (nausea, reflux, vomiting, diarrhea) • Perforation of the jugular at placement • Aspiration pneumonia • Esophageal reflux, vomiting/regurgitation • Local infection at stoma site • Obstruction • Cellulitis if tube is prematurely removed

TABLE 11 - DETERMINATION OF A REFEEDING PROGRAM

Case A anorexic for <3 days: plan to meet Resting Energy Requirement (RER) in 3 days

Day 1: 1/3 of RER
Day 2: 2/3 of RER
Day 3: Full RER

Case B anorexic for >3 days: plan to meet RER in 5 days

Day 1: 1/4 of RER
Day 2: 1/2 of RER
Day 3: 2/3 RER
Day 4: 3/4 of RER
Day 5: Full RER

nostomy tube requires surgical placement with general anesthesia and laparotomy. New placement techniques have been described whereby the jejunostomy tube is introduced via a gastrostomy tube and directed down through the pylorus with an endoscope (*Heuter 2004; Jergens et al 2007*). Due to the narrow diameter of the tube, and placement in the jejunum, feeding must be by a continuous infusion pump with a liquid diet. Therefore jejunostomy tubes are limited to in-hospital use. Peritonitis can occur if the tube is prematurely removed. Contraindications include ascites, peritonitis, immunosuppression and distal small bowel obstructions (*Heather et al, 2004*).

> Feeding protocols

Nutritional support should be introduced gradually. Generally one-third to one-quarter of the daily caloric intake is administered on the first day. If no complications occur, the amount fed is successively increased to reach total caloric requirements by the third or fourth day (*Bartges et al, 2004; Elliott & Biourge, 2006*) **(Table 11)**. If necessary, the diet can be modified by blenderizing with water to ensure passage through the feeding tube. The total daily volume is divided into 4-6 feedings depending on duration of anorexia and patient tolerance.

Gastric dysmotility is a common abnormality in critically ill patients. Prokinetic agents appear to have a beneficial effect on gastrointestinal motility and feeding tolerance in critically ill patients (*Corke, 1999; Booth et al, 2002*). The use of anti-emetic drugs should be considered in cats where vomiting and nausea are a problem **(Table 12)**. Metoclopramide, in addition to having some anti-emetic effects, may be beneficial in patients where delayed gastric emptying is a problem (*Michel, 2001; Mohr et al, 2003*). *Chan & Freeman* (2006) recommend continuous infusions of metoclopramide at 1-2 mg/kg/day. More recently, potent anti-emetics belonging to the HT3-antagonist family of drugs (ondasetron, dolansteron) have been recommended, however efficacy trials are lacking. A new type of anti-emetic (maropitant, an NK-1 antagonist), has been introduced. However, clinical experience in cats is not yet available.

A common misconception is that animals fed via enteral tubes will not eat voluntarily, and therefore ad-libitum feedings are withheld. Anorexia typically resolves once the primary disease is addressed. Therefore, food can be offered to cats to assess their appetite, and to help to determine when to wean them from enteral tube feeding.

> Complications

• *Aspiration pneumonia*

The most serious complication of enteral feeding is aspiration pneumonia. This can be a fatal complication in critically ill cats. Patients at risk of pulmonary aspiration include patients who have had a prior episode of aspiration pneumonia, patients with impaired mental status including those receiving sedatives and certain analgesics, patients with neurological injuries, patients with reduced or absent cough or gag reflexes, and patients receiving mechanical ventilation (*Michel, 2004; 2006*). Nasoesophageal tube displacement from the esophagus into the trachea will cause aspira-

TABLE 12 - SELECT ANTI-EMETIC AGENTS
Adapted from Michel 2001

Drug	Dosage	Comments
Metoclopramide	0.2-0.4 mg/kg IV, SC or PO TID 1-2 mg/kg/day IV CRI	Promotes gastric emptying and acts centrally on the chemoreceptor trigger zone (central effects are less potent in the cat than in other species)
Ondansetron	0.1-0.15 mg/kg slow IV push BID	Acts centrally on the chemoreceptor trigger zone ($5HT_3$ antagonists)

The use of these agents in cats can be restricted according to the licence applicable in each country.

tion pneumonia. The risk of aspiration pneumonia can be minimized by ensuring correct positioning of the feeding tube prior to each and every feeding.

• Mechanical complications

Mechanical complications such as tube obstruction, premature removal or dislodgement are the common complications seen with enteral nutrition. Tube obstruction can be minimized by adequate dilution and blending of the diet prior to administration. The enteral formula should never be allowed to sit in the feeding tube and the tube should be flushed with warm water after every feeding or whenever GI contents are aspirated via the tube. Obstruction of esophagostomy tubes can be dramatically reduced, by enlarging the distal exit hole prior to placement. Techniques to facilitate removal of the obstruction include massaging the outside of the tube while simultaneously flushing and aspirating with water; instilling carbonated drinks, meat tenderizers or pancreatic enzyme solutions for 15 to 20 minutes; or gently using a polyurethane catheter to dislodge the obstruction. The final resort is tube removal and replacement.

While it is tempting to employ a feeding tube for medicating a patient, this practice should be used with caution. If possible, only liquid medications should be given through feeding tubes. Viscous medications should be diluted with water and tablets crushed to a fine powder before mixing with water. Only one medication should be administered at a time and with the exception of phosphate binders for renal disease, separately from enteral feedings to avoid drug-drug and drug-nutrients interactions.

Premature tube removal or dislodgement is best prevented by choosing a tube that the patient will be comfortable with and by using Elizabethan collars or body wraps as appropriate. Marking the tube where it exits the body at the time of tube placement with indelible ink will aid in monitoring whether a tube has migrated from its original position. Whenever the location of a tube is in doubt it should be verified radiographically. Iodinated contrast media can be infused through a gastrostomy or enterostomy tube to check for leaks into the peritoneal cavity *(Michel, 2004)*.

• Feeding intolerance

Feeding intolerance is a common complication, especially in critically ill animals. Animals that vomit persistently and frequently (more than 3 times a day) probably should not be fed via the enteral route. Altering the feeding strategy is recommended for cats that vomit small amounts and infrequently (less than 2 times a day). For example, smaller volumes administered over a longer duration, more frequently can improve feeding tolerance. If bolus feeding is still not tolerated, feeding via continuous infusion could improve feeding tolerance. It is recommended to start at a very low rate, e.g. 2 mL/hour and slowly increase the rate based on patient response, until the daily caloric intake is achieved. In such cases, reaching caloric target may be delayed by a few days *(Marks, 1998; Michel, 2004; Chan, 2006; Chan & Freeman, 2006)*.

• Metabolic complications

Different types of metabolic disturbances can occur with nutritional support.

- Patient's inability to assimilate nutrients
For example, a cat with impaired renal function might become azotemic on a high protein diet. This disturbance can be anticipated by a thorough nutritional assessment of the patient before formulating the nutritional regiment.

- Refeeding syndrome
The refeeding syndrome can develop in patients who have experienced severe muscle wasting as a result of prolonged starvation or catabolic disease *(Michel, 2004; Armitage-Chan et al, 2006)*. This is perhaps the more severe complication associated with nutritional support of critically ill patients and may develop after oral, enteral or parenteral nutrition although this remains a rare

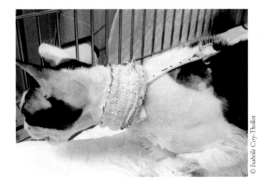

While it is tempting to employ a feeding tube for medicating a patient, this practice should be used with caution.

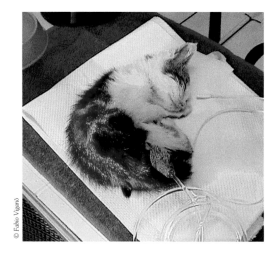
© Fabio Viganò

Prevention of the refeeding syndrome requires stabilization of the fluid, electrolyte and acid-base status of the patient before starting nutritional support (Armitage-Chan et al, 2006).

occurrence. In people, this syndrome results in widespread systemic effects including depression of myocardial function, cardiac arrhythmias, hypoventilation, seizures and mental dysfunction, poor neutrophil function, muscle weakness, and hemolytic anemia.

Most of these effects occur secondary to hypophosphatemia however deficiencies of magnesium and potassium may also contribute. Hypophosphatemia develops due to the rapid increase in insulin release upon reintroduction of nutrition. Increased insulin activity stimulates anabolic processes, which require incorporation of phosphate into high-energy substrates such as adenosine triphosphate (ATP) and 2,3-diphosphoglycerate (2,3-DPG). There is a transcellular shift of phosphate, which in the face of whole-body phosphate depletion results in hypophosphatemia. The reduction in ATP synthesis and consequent energy deficit, contributes to many of the clinical signs associated with the refeeding syndrome (*Solomon & Kirby, 1990; Miller, 2000; Armitage-Chan et al, 2006*). Hemolytic anemia secondary to hypophosphatemia associated with the refeeding syndrome has been reported in cats (*Justin & Hohenhaus, 1995*). Patients identified with severe hypophosphatemia usually respond to phosphate supplementation at a rate of 0.01-0.06 mmol/kg/hour (*Justin & Hohenhaus, 1995*).

- Hyperglycemia

Hyperglycemia is another common metabolic complication that has only recently received attention in veterinary medicine. Possible consequences of hyperglycemia in critically ill animals include higher infection rates and increased mortality, however, it is not yet clear if insulin administration is indicated or influences outcome (see § 2,b,1) (*Chan et al, 2006; Crabb et al, 2006*). The risk of hyperglycemia associated with nutritional support is more common with parenteral nutrition (*Crabb et al, 2006*).

- Fluid overload

Diets used for enteral tube feeding are > 80% water, and water is used to flush the enteral tube upon conclusion of feeding. Therefore, fluid overload can occur in cats receiving nutritional support. Patients with pre-existing cardiac disease on high volumes of enteral tube feeding and receiving intravenous fluids are most at risk of fluid overload. Clinical signs consistent with fluid overloaded include dyspnea, pulmonary edema, and pleural effusion. Prevention requires thorough clinical evaluation to identify those patients most at risk, and to formulate an appropriate nutrition and fluid therapy plan to maintain hydration and yet avoid fluid overload (*Chan & Freeman, 2006*).

> Monitoring and reassessment

Monitoring parameters for patients receiving enteral nutrition include body weight, serum electrolytes, the patency of the enteral feeding tube, the appearance of the stoma site, and clinical signs consistent with gastrointestinal intolerance, volume overload or pulmonary aspiration (*Chan & Freeman, 2006*). The number of calories, and indeed the macronutrient composition of the diet selected may need to be adjusted according to the patient's changing needs and tolerance. In patients unable to tolerate the prescribed amounts, the clinician should consider reducing the amounts of enteral feedings and supplementing the enteral feeding with parenteral nutrition. With continual reassessment, the clinician can determine when to transition the patient from assisted feeding to voluntary consumption of food. The discontinuation of nutritional support should only begin when the patient can consume at least 75% RER, without coaxing (*Chan, 2006*).

6 - Parenteral nutrition

Principal indications for parenteral nutrition include uncontrollable vomiting, regurgitation, acute pancreatitis, intestinal obstruction, severe malabsorption, prolonged ileus, and inability to guard the airway. Parenteral nutrition can be delivered through a central vein (central PN or CPN) or a peripheral vein (partial PN or PPN). CPN is the provision of all of the animal's calorie and protein requirements. PPN only supplies part of the animal's energy and nutrient requirements (*Chan & Freeman, 2006; Delaney et al, 2006*).

CPN is often the preferred modality for a cat requiring parenteral nutrition. A disadvantage of CPN includes the requirement for central venous access (jugular or femoral venous catheter), it is slightly more expensive, and it may be associated with more metabolic complications. CPN requires central venous access as the solution is hyperosmolar. The higher the osmolality of the solution, the higher the incidence of thrombophlebitis (*Chandler et al, 2000*). Relatively few reports are available regarding the use of parenteral nutrition in cats (*Lippert et al, 1993; Chan et al, 2002; Pyle et al, 2004; Crabb et al, 2006*). The major indication of parenteral nutrition in cats appears to be pancreatitis (*Chan et al, 2002; Pyle et al, 2004; Crabb et al, 2006*).

▶ Components

Both CPN and PPN are a combination of a dextrose solution, an amino acid solution, and a lipid solution. The most commonly used amino acid solutions contain most essential amino acids for cats, except taurine. However, because parenteral nutrition is typically not used beyond 10 days, taurine deficiency is not a clinical complication in most circumstances. Amino acids solutions are available with and without electrolytes. Cats that have normal serum electrolytes typically receive amino acid solutions with electrolytes, whereas patients who have electrolytes disturbances may benefit from amino acid solutions without electrolytes so that the electrolyte disturbances can be individually corrected (*Chan & Freeman, 2006; Freeman & Chan, 2006*). The osmolality of the amino acid solutions with and without electrolytes is also significantly different. Consequently, PPN, which requires the osmolality of the final solution to be less than 600 mmOsm/L, is typically formulated using an amino acid solution without electrolytes.

Lipid emulsions are the calorically dense component of parenteral nutrition and a source of essential fatty acids. The ratio of dextrose to lipid should be selected to reflect the hormonal milieu and metabolic condition of the liver. Lipid emulsions are isotonic. Typical lipid emulsions consist of soybean and safflower oil and provide predominantly long-chain polyunsaturated fatty acids, including linoleic, oleic, palmitic, and stearic acids. These solutions are emulsified with egg yolk phospholipids and their tonicity is adjusted with glycerol. The emulsified fat particles are comparable in size to chylomicrons and are removed from the circulation through the action of peripheral lipoprotein lipase. Infusions of lipid have not been shown to increase pancreatic secretion or worsen pancreatitis, excepted in cases where serum triglycerides are elevated, indicating a failure of triglyceride clearance. Although specific data on the maximal safe level of lipid administration in veterinary patients are not available, maintaining normal serum triglycerides levels in cats receiving parenteral nutrition seems prudent. (*Chan & Freeman, 2006; Freeman & Chan, 2006*).

The parenteral solution should be formulated to contain 40 mEq/L of potassium to compensate for the insulin mediated transcellular potassium shift associated with refeeding. Similarly, the parenteral solution should be formulated to contain a minimum 5-10 mM/L of phosphorus. Water soluble vitamins can be provided by the addition of a multivitamin B complex preparation. These preparations typically do not include folic acid due to incompatibility with riboflavin in solution. Fat soluble vitamins, trace elements, and calcium are not generally included in the parenteral nutrition solution if the duration of treatment is expected to be less than 1-2 weeks. The addition of calcium is not routine because of the risk of precipitation of the parenteral solution, and calcium deficiency appears to be well tolerated in the short term. The dose of trace minerals to include in the parenteral nutrition is uncertain. Vitamin K should not be added to the parenteral nutrient solution, but should be administered subcutaneously once weekly.

Critical care

427

TABLE 13 - WORKSHEET FOR CALCULATING PARTIAL PARENTERAL NUTRITION FOR CATS

Adapted from Freeman et Chan, 2006

1. Caculate the resting energy requirement (RER)
70 x (current body weight in kilograms)$^{0.73}$ = ☐ kcal/day

2. Calculate the partial energy requirement (PER)
PER = RER x 0.70 = ☐ kcal/day

3. Determine the nutrient composition
For animals under 3 kg, the formulation will provide a fluid rate higher than maintenance fluid requirements. Be sure that the animal can tolerate this volume of fluids
a. Cats weighing 3 - 5 kg
   PER x 0.20 = ☐ kcal/day from dextrose
   PER x 0.20 = ☐ kcal/day from protein
   PER x 0.60 = ☐ kcal/day from lipid
b. Cats weighing 6 - 10 kg
   PER x 0.25 = ☐ kcal/day from dextrose
   PER x 0.25 = ☐ kcal/day from protein
   PER x 0.50 = ☐ kcal/day from lipid

4. Calculate the volume of nutrient solutions required each day
a. 5% dextrose solution = 0.17 kcal/mL and 253 mOsm/L
   ☐ kcal from dextrose ÷ 0.17 kcal/mL = ☐ mL dextrose/day
b. 8.5% amino acid solution without electrolytes= 0.085 g protein/mL
   = 0.34 kcal/mL and 890 mOsm/L
   ☐ kcal from protein ÷ 0.34 kcal/mL = ☐ mL amino acids/day
c. 20% lipid solution = 2 kcal/mL and 260 mOsm/L
   ☐ kcal from lipid ÷ 2 kcal/mL = ☐ mL lipid/day

5. Calculate the total daily volume of parenteral solution
☐ mL total volume of PPN solution = ☐ mL 5% dextrose solution + ☐ mL 8.5% amino acid solution + ☐ mL 20% lipid solution

6. Calculate the osmolality
mOsm/L should be less than 600 mOsm/L for peripheral administration
☐ mL 5% dextrose solution * 0.253 mOsm/mL = ☐ mOsm
☐ mL 8.5% amino acid solution * 0.890 mOsm/mL = ☐ mOsm
☐ mL 20% lipid solution * 0.26 mOsm/mL = ☐ mOsm
☐ mL total volume of PPN solution
☐ mOsm of PPN solution
☐ mOsm/L of PPN solution = 1000*(☐ mOsm of PPN solution ÷ ☐ mL total volume of PPN solution)

7. Calculate the administration rate
This formulation provides approximately a maintenance fluid rate.
☐ mL/hour PPN solution = ☐ mL total volume of PPN solution/24 hrs

Foot notes
Calories supplied by proteins: 4 kcal/g
Calories supplied by carbohydrates: 4 kcal/g
Calories supplied by lipids: 9 kcal/g

► Compounding and prescription

Parenteral nutrition requires specific compounding practices to maintain sterility and to prevent precipitation of the components. The macronutrients should be combined in the following order: glucose then amino acids then lipids. For logistical and economical reasons, more than one day's supply of PN usually is typically compounded at one time, however, no more than a 3-day supply of parenteral nutrition should be compounded and stored (refrigerated) at a time. Parenteral admixtures should never be frozen or heated, and any unused portions should be discarded (*Campbell et al, 2006; Freeman & Chan, 2006*).

The worksheets presented in **Table 13** and **Table 14** are designed to provide an admixture that is intended to last 24 hours when administered at a constant-rate infusion. Bags of parenteral nutrition should not be at room temperature for more than 24 hours.

► Administration

Parenteral nutrition requires a dedicated catheter (central or peripheral) placed aseptically **(Table 15)**. Strict asepsis and regular catheter care should minimize the risk of bacterial colonization and a catheter-related infection. The choice of catheter type may vary depending on the desired formulation (osmolarity and composition), the bleeding propensity of the cat and the available venous access. Triple lumen central IV catheters are often used for CPN. These catheters allow the first port to be used for blood sampling and intermittent drug administration, the second port to be used for continuous medications and fluid adminstration and the third port to be soley dedicated to CPN (*Campbell et al, 2006; Delaney et al, 2006*). CPN solutions should be administered through a 1.2 μm in-line filter, and as continuous rate infusions utilizing infusion pumps (*Chan & Freeman, 2006*).

Hydration status, electrolyte abnormalities and acid-base disturbances should be corrected prior starting parenteral nutrition administration, as provision of nutritional support can cause alterations that may initially worsen these changes. CPN should be instituted gradually over 24 to 48 hours. If there are no complications, the rate of administration can be increased every 4 hours, until the goal rate is achieved (*Campbell et al, 2006*). Most cats tolerate receiving 50% of total requirements on the first day and 100% on the second day. Cats that have been without food for long periods may require slower introduction (33% on the first day, 66% on the second day, and 100% on the third day). PPN does not require gradual introduction and can be initiated at 100% on the first day. It is important to adjust the cat's intravenous fluids when initiating parenteral nutrition to avoid fluid volume overload (*Campbell et al 2006, Delaney et al 2006; Freeman & Chan 2006*).

TABLE 14 - WORKSHEET FOR CALCULATING CENTRAL TOTAL PARENTAL NUTRITION FOR CATS

Adapted from Freeman & Chan, 2006

1. Calculate the resting energy requirement (RER)

70 x (current body weight in kilograms)$^{0.73}$ = ☐ kcal/day

2. Calculate the protein requirements

Standard   6 g/100 kcal

Decreased requirements (hepatic, renal failure)   3-4 g/100 kcal

RER ÷ 100 x ☐ g/100 kcal = ☐ g protein/day

3. Calculate the volumes of nutrient solutions required each day

8.5% amino acid solution with electrolytes = 0.085 g protein/mL = 0.34 kcal/mL

☐ g protein required/day ÷ 0.085 g/mL = ☐ mL of amino acids/day

Non-protein calories

The calories supplied by proteins are subtracted from the RER to get total non-protein calories needed

☐ g protein required/day x 4 kcal/g = ☐ kcal provided by protein

RER - kcal provided by protein = ☐ nonprotein kcal needed/day

Non-protein calories are usually provided as a 50/50 mixture of lipid and dextrose. However, if the patient has been preexisting condition (diabetes, hypertriglyceridemia), this ratio may need to be adjusted.

To supply 50% of nonprotein kcal with lipid

Volume of lipid required = (☐ nonprotein kcal needed/day * 0.5) ÷ 2 kcal/mL = ☐ mL of 20% lipid

To supply 50% of nonprotein kcal with dextrose

Volume of dextrose required (☐ nonprotein kcal needed/day * 0.5) ÷ 1.7 kcal = ☐ mL of 50% dextrose

4. Total volume of the solution

Total volume of TPN solution = ☐ mL 8.5% amino acid solution with electrolytes + ☐ mL 20% lipid solution + ☐ mL 50% dextrose solution = ☐ mL

5. Calculate the amount of potassium and phosphorus to add to the solution

The desired potassium concentration = ☐ mEq/L.

8.5% amino acid solution with electrolytes contains 60 mEq/L potassium.

Calculate the amount of potassium provided by the amino acid solution: = (☐ mL of amino acids *60 mEq/L) ÷ 1000 = ☐ mEq in ☐ mL Total volume of TPN solution = ☐ mEq/L.

The volume of potassium to add to the parenteral solution to achieve the desired potassium concentration = (desired potassium concentration ☐ mEq/L – actual potassium concentration ☐ mEq/L) * ☐ mL Total volume of TPN solution = ☐ mEq K to add.

The desired phosphorus concentration = ☐ mM/L.

8.5% amino acid solution with electrolytes contains 30 mM/L phosphorus.

Calculate the amount of phosphorus provided by the amino acid solution: = (☐ mL of amino acids *30 mM/L) ÷ 1000 = ☐ mM.

Calculate the amount of phosphorus provided by the lipid solution: = (☐ mL of amino acids *15 mM/L) ÷ 1000 = ☐ mM.

The amount of phosphorus provided by the parenteral solution = ☐ mM/L from amino acid solution + ☐ mM/L from lipid solution in ☐ mL Total volume of TPN solution = ☐ mM/L.

The volume of phosphorus to add to the parenteral solution to achieve the desired phosphorus concentration = (desired phosphorus concentration ☐ mM/L – actual phosphorus concentration ☐ mM/L) * ☐ mL Total volume of TPN solution = ☐ mM phosphorus to add.

6. Consider vitamin B supplementation

7. Administration rate

Day 1: ☐ mL/hour

Day 2: ☐ mL/hour

Day 3: ☐ mL/hour

TABLE 15 - CENTRAL AND PERIPHERAL INTRAVENOUS CATHETERS RECOMMENDED FOR PARENTERAL ADMINISTRATION IN CATS

Adapted from Campbell et al, 2006

Catheter use	Material	Lumens	Size	Length
Central jugular for CPN	Polyurethane	2-3	4-5.5 Fr.	8-13 cm
Peripheral lateral saphenous for CPN	Polyurethane	3	5.5-7 Fr	30 cm
Peripheral for PPN	Any	1	-	Any

CPN: central parenteral nutrition - PPN: partial parenteral nutrition

TABLE 16 - POTENTIAL COMPLICATIONS OF PARENTAL NUTRITION

Adapted from Freeman & Chan, 2006

	Type of complication	Methods to reduce the risk
Mechanical	Line breakage Chewed line Disconnected line Perivascular infiltration Catheter occlusion Phlebitis Thrombosis	Aseptic placement of catheter Aseptic handling of catheter and lines Use Elizabethan collars Change bandage and check catheter site daily for swelling, erythema, malpositioning of catheter
Metabolic	Hyperglycemia Hypoglycemia (when discontinuing parenteral nutrition) Hyper/hyopkalemia Hyper/hypochloremia Hyper/hyponatremia Hyper/hypophosphatemia Hyper/hypomagnesemia Hyperbilirubinemia Hypertriglyceridemia Hypercholesterolemia Refeeding syndrome	Use a conservative approach (RER) for the calculation of caloric requirements Initiate and discontinue parenteral nutrition gradually Monitor glucose and electrolytes daily
Septique	Clinical signs of sepsis in conjunction with a positive catheter tip or blood culture	Maintain a dedicated catheter Catheter composed of materials of low thrombogenicity Place and handle catheters and lines with aseptic technique Changing catheters at prescribed time Monitor body temperature, catheter site, general attitude If sepsis is suspected, parenteral solution and catheter tip should be cultured

Routine physical examinations including body temperature, heart rate, respiratory rate, twice daily weight measurements, assessment of hydration status, and attitude should be performed on all critically ill patients receiving parenteral nutritional support. To monitor for complications associated with the parenteral nutrition therapy, the packed cell volume, total protein, blood urea nitrogen, serum electrolytes (sodium, potassium, chloride, ionized calcium), venous blood gas and blood glucose concentrations should be monitored every 4 to 6 hours **(Table 16)**. Urine can be checked daily for glucosuria. Serum triglycerides and ammonia concentrations should be determined daily.

▶ Complications

Metabolic, mechanical and septic complications can occur in cats receiving parenteral nutrition.

Studies report the rates of metabolic complications in critically ill cats receiving parenteral nutrition to range from 28-320% **(Table 16)**. The rates of metabolic complications appear lower when less than full calculated energy requirements are provided *(Crabb et al, 2006)*. The most common metabolic complications described in cats are hyperglycemia, glucosuria, lipemia, hypernatremia, hypokalemia, azotemia, hypocalcemia, hyperchloremia, hypertriglyceridemia, hypophosphatemia, refeeding syndrome and throbocytopenia *(Lippert et al, 1993; Chan et al, 2002; Pyle et al, 2004; Campbell et al, 2006; Crab et al, 2006)*. These may necessitate adjusting the nutrient ratios, slowing the rate of infusion, or administering insulin, potassium or phosphate supplements. Hyperglycemia appears to be the most common metabolic complication *(Crab et al, 2006)*. Congestive heart failure can occur secondary to fluid shifts *(Freeman & Chan, 2006)*.

The rate of mechanical complications in critically ill cats receiving parenteral nutrition have been reported to be between 9-56% *(Lippert et al, 1993; Chan et al, 2002; Pyle et al, 2004; Crab et al, 2006)*. Reported mechanical complications include catheter dysfunction or dislodgements, thrombophlebitis, damaged or leaking administration lines, accidental breaking or occlusion of the administration line, and equipment failure. These mechanical complications were rapidly rectified when recognized and usually had little effect on the cat's outcome *(Campbell et al, 2006)*.

The rate of septic complications has been reported between 3 and 16% *(Lippert et al, 1993; Chan et al, 2002; Pyle et al, 2004)*. Intestinal atrophy that occurs with long-term parenteral nutrition may explain the increased occurrence of bacterial translocation from the gut and sepsis in animals receiving only parenteral nutrition *(Campbell et al, 2006)*. Bacterial infections of the administration line and sepsis can be minimized with sterile placements techniques, sterile parenteral nutrition compounding and regular line care by staff trained specifically in these tasks *(Campbell et al, 2006)*. Rapid removal of any catheter believed to be contributing to localized or systemic infection is advised. The range of potential septic complications includes positive blood cultures, infected catheter sites in febrile animals, positive culture of the catheter tip or the parenteral solution in febrile animals and/or an abnormally high neutrophil concentration (*Campbell et al, 2006*).

Overall mortality rates in feline patients receiving parenteral nutrition have been reported to be between 19-52%, but this is likely influenced by the animal's underlying medical condition(s) (*Lippert et al, 1993; Chan et al, 2002; Pyle et al, 2004; Campbell et al, 2006*). *Chan et al* (2002) found no differences in metabolic, mechanical or septic complications in cats administered parenteral nutrition centrally versus peripherally. In parallel, this study showed that concurrent enteral nutrition during PN administration was associated with improved survival.

▶ Discontinuing parenteral nutrition

Transitioning to oral intake or enteral nutrition should occur as soon as possible to avoid the problem of gut atrophy. In veterinary medicine, parenteral nutrition is typically administered for less than one week. It is important to ensure that the patient is tolerating oral intake or enteral nutrition and is ingesting sufficient amounts (at least 75% of RER) before discontinuing parenteral nutrition. Once the patient is able to eat, it should be offered food regularly to assess its appetite, or a feeding tube should be placed if the animal is anorectic. It is suggested to gradually reduce the rate of administration of CPN over a period of 12 to 24 hours, to allow time for appropriate endocrine equilibration in order to prevent hypoglycemia. PPN can be discontinued abruptly without this gradual decrease (*Campbell et al, 2006; Freeman & Chan, 2006*).

The use of parenteral nutrition as part of the supportive care plan can be an invaluable addition in select animals. Given cats' unique nutritional requirements and metabolic particularities, future additional studies aimed at more closely examining PN formulations may lead to the development of a formulation more suitable for cats with a lower overall rate of complications.

Conclusion

Critical care nutrition is a rapidly evolving field. It is clear, and fortunate that the paradigm has changed from waiting until a cat decides to eat on it's own (and suffers severe body mass loss in the process) to proactively implementing nutritional support as soon as the patient's life threatening conditions are stabilized.

The consequences of critical illness culminate in significant changes that clearly alter not only nutrient metabolism, but also increase the risk of morbidity and mortality to the patient. Critical steps in management include early recognition of the need to feed the patient, adapting the caloric and nutrient intake to match the metabolic environment and continual monitoring to optimize the prescription and minimize the risk of complications. Aggressive nutritional management will not only increase the survival chances of the critically ill patient, but also aid rapid recovery and return to the home environment.

Fallacies regarding feeding during intensive care

F	A
"Nutrition is not a great problem. It is neither a priority nor an emergency compared with the other treatments and care protocols."	Nutritional support is not a substitute for emergency treatment to support the main vital functions. On the other hand, it must not be neglected. Status and nutritional requirements must be evaluated every day as part of a full examination of the cat during intensive care. Nutritional support must be part of the care protocol.
"The cat will be able to eat on its own in one or two days."	Time passes quickly in intensive care and the period the cat does not eat properly is always underestimated. Nutritional support takes time and may demand invasive procedures (e.g. esophagostomy or gastrostomy), which clinicians delay in the hopes that the cat will start eating again on its own. Anorexia is one of the most commonly observed clinical signs in intensive care units: treatment, anesthesia, surgery and the stress of hospitalization are all anorexigenic factors.
"Perfusion feeds the cat."	Although it does provide glucose, maintenance fluid therapy cannot be considered to be a form of nutritional support. While the aim is to correct blood volume, dehydration, and acid-base and electrolyte imbalances, its role is not to feed the cat. Only total or partial parenteral nutrition solutions administered in accordance with precise protocols can do this.
"If the cat does not want to eat, you can just initiate a parenteral nutrition protocol."	Parenteral nutrition is always tempting because it makes it possible to calculate precise intake with total certainty. Parenteral nutrition is not risk free, however, and it demands monitoring by qualified staff. Septic complications are especially common and the numerous required biological analyses are expensive.
"Hyperglycemia induced by parenteral nutrition is not a real problem. At least the cat receives the energy."	In humans, hyperglycemia is correlated with a negative prognostic outcome. In cats, it is correlated with the seriousness of the disease. There is a dearth of studies in this species for determining the influence of hyperglycemia on the prognosis and the necessity of controlling it with insulin therapy. The current recommendation is to avoid treatments that are likely to induce hyperglycemia.
"Cats fed through feeding tubes are not hungry. It's not worth giving them anything else to eat."	On the contrary, it is important to offer food to cats fed through feeding tubes. It helps assess how interested they are in foods and whether they have their appetite back. It helps clinicians determine the best time to withdraw the feeding tube.
"Feeding tubes are very practical for administering drugs."	While tempting, it is inadvisable to administer drugs through a feeding tube. Turning drugs into powder can change their absorption and digestive tolerance. Also, the absorption of some drugs is changed by the composition of foods (depending on their fat content). Lastly, drugs may interact when administered at the same time.
"Parenteral solutions can correct electrolyte imbalances."	The aim of parenteral nutrition is to provide an intake of nutrients bypassing the digestive system, not to correct electrolyte imbalances, which should be done independently using traditional fluid therapy solutions. It is however advisable to check the electrolyte content of common parenteral nutrition solutions. If they contain electrolytes, they can only be administered to animals with a normal electrolyte balance. Furthermore, the electrolyte balance must be monitored in these cats, to identify the appearance of any disruptions caused by the parenteral nutrition. If the cat's electrolyte balance is disturbed, it is advisable to use parenteral nutrition solutions containing no electrolytes and to correct the patient's electrolytes independently at the same time.

References

Armitage-Chan EA, O'Toole T, Chan DL. Management of prolonged food deprivation hypothermia, and refeeding syndrome in a cat. J Vet Emerg Crit Care 2006; 16: S34-35.

Atkinson M, Worthley LIG. Nutrition in the critically ill patient: Part I. Essential physiology and pathophysiology. Critical Care and Resuscitation 2003; 5: 109-120.

Barbul A, Hurson M. Arginine. In: Gay S eds. Nutrition and Critical Care. Missouri, Year Booh Inc., 1994; 107.

Bartges J, Kirk C, Lauten S. Calculating a patient's nutritional requirements. Vet Med 2004; 99(7): 632.

Biourge V, Massat B, Groff JM, et al. Effects of protein, lipid, or carbohydrate supplementation on hepatic lipid accumulation during rapid weight loss in obese cats. Am J Vet Res 1994; 55: 1406-1415.

Booth CM, Heyland DK, Paterson WG. Gastro-intestinal promotility drugs in the critical care setting: A systematic review of the evidence. Crit Care Med 2002; 30: 1429-1435.

Bosworth C, Bartges J, Snow P. Nasoesophageal and nasogastric feeding tubes. Vet Med 2004; 99: 590-594.

Campbell SJ, Karriker MJ, Fascetti AJ. Central and peripheral parenteral nutrition. Waltham Focus 2006; 16(3): 21-29.

Center SA. Feline hepatic lipidosis. Vet Clin Small Animal 2005; 35: 225-269.

Chan DL, Freeman LM, Labato MA, et al. Retrospective evaluation of partial parenteral nutrition in dogs and cats. J Vet Intern Med 2002; 16: 440-445.

Chan DL. Nutritional support of critically ill patients. Waltham Focus 2006; 16(3): 9-15.

Chan DL, Freeman LM. Nutrition in critical illness. Vet Clin of North America: Small Animal Practice 2006; 36: 1225-1241.

Chan DL, Freeman LM, Rozanski EA, et al. Alterations in carbohydrate metabolism in critically ill cats. J Vet Emerg Crit Care 2006; 16: S7-S13.

Chandler ML, Guilford WG, Payne-James J. Use of peripheral parenteral nutritional support in dogs and cats. J Am Vet Med Assoc 2000; 216: 669-673.

Corke C. Gastric emptying in the critically ill patient. Crit Care Resusc 1999; 1: 39-44.

Crabb SE, Freeman LM, Chan DL, et al. Retrospective evaluation of total parenteral nutrition in cats: 40 cases (1991 – 2003). J Vet Emerg Crit Care 2006; 16: S21-26.

Delaney SJ, Fascetti AJ, Elliott DA. Nutrition and critical care in dogs. In: Encyclopedia of Canine Clinical Nutrition. Paris: Aniwa SAS, 2006; 426-447.

Detsky AS, Mclaughlin JR, Baker JP, et al. What is subjective global assessment of nutritional status? J Parenter Enteral Nutr 1987; 11: 8-13.

Elliott DA. Nutritional assessment. In: Silverstein D, Hopper K (eds). Critical Care Medicine, St Louis, Elsevier, 2008.

Elliott DA, Biourge V. Critical care nutrition. Waltham Focus 2006; 16(3): 30-34.

Elliott DA, Riel DL, Rogers QR. Complications and outcomes of gastrotomy tubes used for the nutritional management of renal failure in dogs: 56 cases (1994-1999). J Am Vet Med Assoc 2000; 217: 1337-1342.

Fascetti AJ, Maudlin GE, Maudlin GN. Correlation between serum creatine kinase activities and anorexia in cats. J Vet Intern Med 1997; 11: 9-13.

Freeman LM, Chan DL. Total parenteral nutrition. In: DiBartola SP, editor. Fluid, Electrolyte, and acid-base disorders in small animal practice. 3rd ed. St Louis (MO): Saunders Elsevier 2006; 584-601.

Heather F, Bartges J, Snow P. Enterostomy feeding tubes. Vet Med 2004; 99: 627-630.

Heuter K. Placement of jejunal feeding tubes for post-gastric feeding. Clin Tech Small Anim Pract 2004; 19: 32-42.

Heyland DK, Dhaliwal. Immunonutrition in the critically ill patients: from old approaches to new paradigms. Intensive Care Med 2005; 31: 501-503.

Ireland LM, Hohenhaus AE, Broussard JD, et al. A comparison of owner management and complications in 67 cats with esophagostomy and percutaneous endoscopic gastrostomy feeding tubes. J Am Anim Hosp Assoc 2003; 39: 241-246.

Jergens AE, Morrison JA, Miles KG, et al. Percutaneous endoscopic gastrojejunostomy tube placementin healthy dogs and cats. J Vet Intern Med 2007; 21:18-24.

Justin RB, Hohenhaus AE. Hypophosphatemia associated with enteral alimentation in cats. J Vet Intern Med 1995; 9: 228-233.

Kerl ME, Johnson PA. Nutritional plan: matching diet to disease. Clin Tech Small Anim Pract 2004; 19: 9-21.

Kienzle E. Effect of carbohydrate on digestion in the cat. J Nutr 1994; 69: 102-114.

Kirby R. The cat is not a small dog in ICU: Part I and II. In: WSAVA eds. World Small Animal Veterinary Association congress proceeding. 2004.

Lippert AC, Fulton RB, Parr AM. A retrospective study of the use of total parenteral nutrition in dogs and cats. J Vet Intern Med 1993; 7: 52-64.

Luhn A, Bartges J, Snow P. Gastrostomy feeding tubes: percutaneous endoscopic placement. Vet Med 2004; 99: 612-617.

Marik PE, Zaloga GP. Early enteral nutrition in acutely ill patients: A systematic review. Crit Care Med 2001; 29: 2264-2270.

Marik PE, Zaloga GP. Meta-analysis of parenteral nutrition versus enteral nutrition in patients with acute pancreatitis. BMJ 2004; 328: 1407.

Marks SL. The principles and practical application of enteral nutrition. Vet Clin of North America: Small Animal Practice 1998; 28: 677-709.

Marks SL, Cook AK, Reader R, et al. Effects of glutamine supplementation of an amino acid-based purified diet on intestinal mucosal integrity in cats with methotrexate-induced enteritis. Am J Vet Res 1999; 60: 755-763.

Mesich ML, Bartges J, Tobias K, et al. Gastrostomy feeding tubes: surgical placement. Vet Med 2004; 99: 604-610.

Michel KE. Deciding who needs nutritional support. Waltham Focus 2006; 16(3): 16-20.

Michel KE. Management of anorexia in the cat. J Feline Med Surg. 2001; 3: 3-8.

Michel KE. Preventing and managing complications of enteral nutritional support. Clin Tech Small Anim Pract 2004; 19: 49-53.

Michel KE, Higgins C. Investigation of the percentage of prescribed enteral nutrition actually delivered to hospitalized companion animals. J Vet Emerg Crit Care 2006; 16: S2-S6.

Miller CC, Bartges JW. Refeeding syndrome. In: Bonagura JD. Ed. Kirk's Current Veterinary Therapy XIII, Small Animal Practice. Philadelphia: WB Saunders Co; 2000: 87-89.

Mohr AJ, Leisewitz AL, Jacobson LS, et al. Effect of early enteral nutrition on intestinal permeability, intestinal protein loss, and outcome in dogs with severe parvoviral enteritis. J Vet Inter Med 2003; 17: 791-798.

Morris JG, Rogers QR. Ammonia intoxication in the near adult cat as a result of dietary deficiency of arginine. Science 1978; 199: 431.

O'Toole E, Miller CW, Wilson BA, et al. Comparison of the standard predictive equation for calculation of resting energy expenditure with indirect calorimetry in hospitalized and healthy dogs. J Am Vet Med Assoc. 2004; 225: 58-64.

Pyle SC, Marks SL, Kass PH. Evaluation of complications and prognosis factors associated with administration of total parenteral nutrition in cats: 75 cases (1994-2001). J Am Vet Med Assoc 2004; 225: 242-250.

Remillard RL, Darden DE, Michel KE, et al. An investigation of the relationship between caloric intake and outcome in hospitalized dogs. Vet Therapeutics 2001; 2: 301-310.

Saker KE. Nutrition and immune function. Vet Clin North Am Small Anim Pract 2006; 36: 1199-1224.

Skeie B, Kvetan V, Gil KM, et al. Branch-chain amino acids: Their metabolism and clinical utility. Crit Care Med 1990; 18: 549-571.

Solomon SM, Kirby DF. The refeeding syndrome. A review. J Parenter Enteral Nutr 1990; 14: 90-97.

Syring RS, Otto CM, Drobatz KJ. Hyperglycemia on dogs and cats with head trauma: 122 cases (1997-1999). J Am Vet Med Assoc 2001; 218: 1124-1129.

Thompson K, Bartges J, Snow P. Gastrostomy feeding tubes: percutaneous, nonsurgical, nonendoscopic placement. Vet Med 2004; 99: 619-626.

Vanatta M, Bartges J, Snow P. Esophagostomy feeding tubes. Vet Med 2004; 99: 596-660.

Van den Berghe G. How does blood glucose control with insulin save lives in intensive care? J Clin Invest 2004; 114: 1187-1195.

Verset M, Viguier E, Goy-Thollot I. In: Gestes techniques en urgences, réanimation et soins intensifs. Les Éditions du Point Vétérinaire, Wolters-Kluwer France, 2008 (sous presse).

Von Werthern CJ, Wess G. A new technique for insertion of esophagostomy tubes in cats. J Am Anim Hosp Assoc 2001; 37: 140-144.

Wischmeyer PE. Clinical application of L-glutamine: past, present and future. Nutr Clin Pract 2003; 18: 377-385.

Yam P, Cave C. Enteral nutrition: options and feeding protocols. In Practice 2003: 118-129.

Zoran DL. The carnivore connection to nutrition in cats. J Am Vet Med Assoc 2002; 221: 1559-1567.

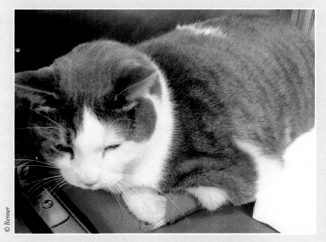

*Nutritional support is an integral part of treating
hospitalized animals in a critical situation.*

Key points to remember

The benefits of nutritional support
in critically ill cats

Factors predisposing to malnutrition

Four risk factors are cited, although there may be more.

- Spontaneous consumption of the cat tends to fall or be interrupted during pathological episodes.

- Some traumas or lesions of the oral cavity may disrupt ingestion.

- Additional examinations or surgical interventions sometimes entail protracted fasting.

- Nutritional requirements increase in the event of acute and/or febrile diseases.

Expected benefits of nutritional support

There is medical consensus on the importance of early nutritional support whatever the cause of the reduced appetite. Whenever possible, oral feeding is preferred ("If the gut is working, use it"). This per os feeding helps preserve the intestinal barrier. In the absence of spontaneous consumption, nutritional support may be provided by nasophageal tube.

Generally speaking, when instigated early nutritional support can:

- achieve clinical improvement and accelerate rehabilitation

- reduce hospitalization time

- reduce complications in the event of surgery

- improve the survival rate in critically ill cats

INDICATIONS OF CONVALESCENCE DIETS FOR DOGS AND CATS IN VETERINARY CLINICS
*Source: Royal Canin survey
(June-September 2006)*

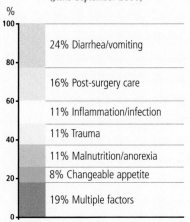

24% Diarrhea/vomiting

16% Post-surgery care

11% Inflammation/infection

11% Trauma

11% Malnutrition/anorexia

8% Changeable appetite

19% Multiple factors

The convenience of the diet given to hospitalized cats is a major selection criteria that may gain time in critical care situations.

Critical care

Select practical criteria for choosing food for critically ill cats

The use of food specially formulated to nourish animals in intensive care facilitates the work of clinicians and care teams.

Maximum palatability

Sick cats generally display a reduced appetite and weight loss. The food must help overcome this by being as palatable as possible.

Formulation adapted to increased nutritional requirements

High-energy concentration

High energy density is important for providing the highest quantity of calories in a low volume. This compensates for a reduced appetite in cats that feed themselves and facilitates administration in the event of enteral-feeding.

To increase the energy density, food for critically ill patients must be high in fat (> 40% of total calories). High-fat diets may present contraindications only in the event of acute pancreatitis and hyperlipidemia.

High protein content

Pathological conditions activate metabolism: tissue catabolism increases and must be compensated for by more intense tissue synthesis. Intake of 30-50% of total energy in the form of protein helps combat loss of lean body mass. This protein must have the following characteristics:

- high biological value to cover the requirement of essential amino acids

- high digestibility to minimize nitrogenous waste and so avoid overloading the liver and kidney functions.

High-protein diets may not be tolerated in hepatic encephalopathy or stage III/IV chronic kidney disease.

Rich in antioxidants

Hypovolemia and reperfusion injury increases the production of free radicals. A complex synergy of antioxidants (vitamins E and C, taurine, carotenoid pigments etc) help combat oxidative stress and facilitate optimal immune defenses.

Convenience

Wet foods are generally more acceptable to cats in the intensive care setting or convalescent cats with a reduced appetite. They can also be warmed to body temperature before feeding.

Wet foods are also better suited to different types of distribution: in a bowl, from the hand or through enteral feeding tubes. The texture must enable administration by syringe, in diluted or undiluted form. The food must be both easy to manipulate, regardless of how it is administered, and easy to split into precise rations.

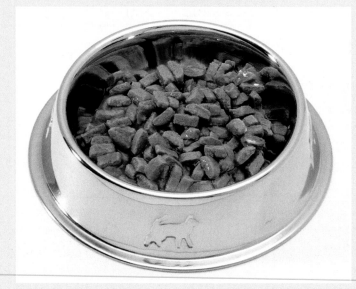

Wet foods are suited to different types of distribution: in a bowl, from the hand or through enteral feeding tubes.

Critical care

Convalescence
rationing sheet

Step 1 • Calculate patient's resting energy requirement (RER)
RER = 70 x (body weight in kg)$^{0.73}$ kcal/day = = ☐ kcal/day

Step 2 • Characteristics of the convalescence diet
Name of the selected food:
Food energy density:
in kcal/g: ☐ [or in kcal/mL]: ☐
    • In case of diluted food*: determine energy density
    Food: kcal/mL ☐ x food volume mixed: mL ☐ = ☐ kcal for total mix
    Water: mL ☐ + food volume mixed: mL ☐ = ☐ mL for total mix
    Total mix: kcal ☐ ÷ total volume: mL ☐ = ☐ kcal/mL for total mix
    *to assist the passage through a syringe or feeding tube

Step 3 • Calculate the total amount to give daily
(In gram [g] or in milliliter [mL])
    If measuring by weight (g)
    RER: kcal/day ☐ ÷ Food: kcal/g ☐ = ☐ g of food/day
    For a liquid diet, if measuring by volume (mL)
    RER: kcal/day ☐ ÷ Food: kcal/mL ☐ = ☐ mL of food/day
    For a liquid mix, if measuring by volume (mL)
    RER: kcal/day ☐ mix: kcal/mL ☐ = ☐ mL of mix/day

Step 4 • Determine the refeeding program
    Case A: if anorexic < 3 days ==> plan to meet RER in 3 days:
    D1: 1/3 of RER = food/day: g (or mL) ☐ x 0.33 = ☐ g (or mL)
    D2: 2/3 of RER = food/day: g (or mL) ☐ x 0.66 = ☐ g (or mL)
    D3: 100% of RER = food/day: g (or mL) ☐ x 1 = ☐ g (or mL)
    Case B: if anorexic > 3 days ==> plan to meet RER in 5 days
    D1: 1/4 of RER = food/day: g (or mL) ☐ x 0.25 = ☐ g (or mL)
    D2: 1/2 of RER = food/day: g (or mL) ☐ x 0.5 = ☐ g (or mL)
    D3: 2/3 of RER = food/day: g (or mL) ☐ x 0.66 = ☐ g (or mL)
    D4: 3/4 of RER = food/day: g (or mL) ☐ x 0.75 = ☐ g (or mL)
    D5: 100% of RER = food/day: g (or mL) ☐ x 1 = ☐ g (or mL)

Step 5 • Select the desired number of meals per day
Typically 4-6 meals evenly distributed throughout the day (as patient volume tolerance and staffing permits)
Number of meals per day: ☐

Step 6 • Calculate the amount to feed at each meal
    Case A: If anorexic for < 3 days (plan to meet RER in 3 days)
    D 1: [g (or mL) for day 1 ÷ number of meals per day] = ☐ g (or mL) per meal
    D 2: [g (or mL) for day 2 ÷ number of meals per day] = ☐ g (or mL) per meal
    D 3: [g (or mL) for day 3 ÷ number of meals per day] = ☐ g (or mL) per meal
    Case B: If anorexic for > 3 days (plan to meet RER in 5 days)
    D 1: [g (or mL) for day 1 ÷ number of meals per day] = ☐ g (or mL) per meal
    D 2: [g (or mL) for day 2 ÷ number of meals per day] = ☐ g (or mL) per meal
    D 3: [g (or mL) for day 3 ÷ number of meals per day] = ☐ g (or mL) per meal
    D 4: [g (or mL) for day 4 ÷ number of meals per day] = ☐ g (or mL) per meal
    D 5: [g (or mL) for day 5 ÷ number of meals per day] = ☐ g (or mL) per meal
Be sure to adjust the patient's intravenous fluids according to the amount of water being added through the diet.

Critical care

Debra HORWITZ
DMV, Dipl. ACVB

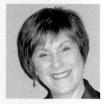

Yannick SOULARD
Eng

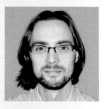

Ariane JUNIEN-CASTAGNA
Eng

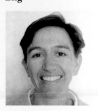

The feeding behavior of the cat

1. Factors affecting the feeding behavior of the cat 441

2. Description of the feeding behavior of the cat 447

3. Determinism and regulation of feeding consumption 454

4. Disorders of ingestion behavior 458

5. Water drinking in cats 466

Conclusion 469

Frequently asked questions 470

References 472

Royal Canin nutritional information 474

Behavior

The feeding behavior of the cat

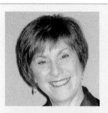

Debra HORWITZ
DVM, Dipl. ACVB
Dr. Horwitz graduated from Michigan State University College of Veterinary Medicine. After several years in general practice, she began to limit her practice to behavioral problems in companion animals. She received board certification from the American College of Veterinary Behaviorists in 1996. She has a private referral practice for behavior problems in dogs and cats and also consults for the Veterinary Information Network and lectures frequently in North America and abroad and is the editor and author of several books on behavior. She is president of the American College of Veterinary Behaviorists 2006-2008.

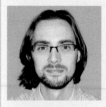

Yannick SOULARD
An agricultural engineer with a Master's degree in managing innovation in biotechnology and the agro-food industry, Yannick Soulard joined Royal Canin's Canadian subsidiary in 1999 as a support technician for the sales team. He was given responsibility for formulating foods for North America until 2001. Back at the Royal Canin Research Center in Aimargues, France, he spent six years in palatability development. Today, he leads the Nutrition research unit.

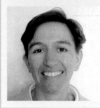

Ariane JUNIEN - CASTAGNA
After graduating from Université de Technologie de Compiègne in 1996 (agro-food process engineering), Ariane joined Royal Canin in 1997, initially in production. She moved to the Research Center that same year, working on an industrial pilot. Since 2001, she has been in charge of palatability development projects.

*F*eeding behavior corresponds to all the motor sequences from the search for food, its recognition, acceptance and intake. It thus begins with exploration and ends with swallowing.

Although feeding behavior is well studied in domestication and production, only empirical data or anthropomorphic analysis is available for cats. Some recent scientific experiments, essentially performed by petfood manufacturers, are completing the scope of data available in pets.

The feeding and social behavior of cats differs greatly from dogs. Not only do their nutritional requirements differ, but the social structure of cats also results in different communication and feeding patterns both between cats and with their human caregivers. Meeting the nutritional needs of cats requires an understanding of their feeding ecology, nutritional needs and social communication and structure.

1 - Factors affecting the feeding behavior of the cat

► Hereditary determinants

> Sensorial aspects

Taste

The sensation of taste in a cat is present 5 days before birth *(Beaver, 1980)* and improves during life. The sensitivity differs between the 4 main types of taste perception, with the following hierarchy from the most to least stimulating (as demonstrated by the simple application of vinegar, salt, quinine, and sugar, on the tongue):

acid > bitter > salty > sweet

(Domestic cats are neither attracted to, nor show avoidance of the taste of sweet carbohydrates and high intensity sweeteners).

Our knowledge of taste has indeed evolved through the study of neurological signals in cranial nerves following the stimulation of the taste buds by different substances. Three cranial nerves are involved in taste. The facial nerves, in particular the chorda tympani, have undergone the most observations. This research has given rise to many theories. For example, *Boudreau (1973,1977)* presented a theory suggesting acid, amino acid and nucleotide taste systems specific to cats. This theory has not been confirmed by other authors.

The number of taste buds is estimated at around 475 **(Figures 1 and 2)**. It is much less than dogs (1700) and man (9000). In dogs, gustatory cell turnover is around 4 days. No data is available in cats, but we may expect that it is similar. This data is interesting to evaluate appetite recovery after insult to the oral epithelium.

FIGURE 1 - LOCALIZATION OF THE TASTE RECEPTORS ON THE TONGUE OF THE CAT

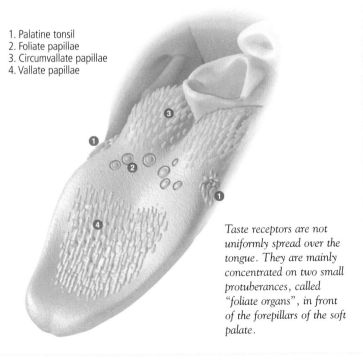

1. Palatine tonsil
2. Foliate papillae
3. Circumvallate papillae
4. Vallate papillae

Taste receptors are not uniformly spread over the tongue. They are mainly concentrated on two small protuberances, called "foliate organs", in front of the forepillars of the soft palate.

FIGURE 2 - DIFFERENT TYPES OF GUSTATIVE RECEPTORS

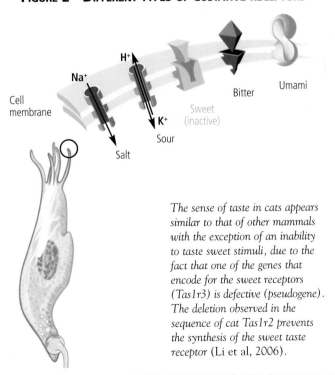

The sense of taste in cats appears similar to that of other mammals with the exception of an inability to taste sweet stimuli, due to the fact that one of the genes that encode for the sweet receptors (Tas1r3) is defective (pseudogene). The deletion observed in the sequence of cat Tas1r2 prevents the synthesis of the sweet taste receptor (Li et al, 2006).

Behavior

Bitter taste

Bitter compounds easily trigger aversions. Bitter taste is due to a wide variety of components (tannins, alkaloids, malic acid, quinine, phytic acid, aminoacids such as tryptophan, isoleucine, leucine, arginine, phenylalanine, etc.).

Cats are very sensitive to bitter tastes (*Houpt, 2005*). Cats are more sensitive than dogs to bitterness and detect it at lower concentrations. They can detect concentrations of bitter taste four hundred times smaller than levels detected by hamsters (*Carpenter, 1956; Houpt, 1991*). This perception enables them to avoid many toxic substances (for example strychnine), which are often very bitter.

Sweet taste

Cats do not appear to care for sweet tastes: receptors have been deactivated. The corresponding gene exists but it has been switched off to a pseudogene (*Brandt, 2006*) through phylogenic adaptation (*Li et al, 2006*). Cats tend to reject synthetic sweeteners like saccharine or cyclamate, since they are perceived as bitter (*Bartoshuk et al, 1975*). The sweet taste of antifreeze appeals to dogs but not to cats. Rather, cats are typically poisoned by cleaning their paws after walking through the antifreeze.

Acid taste

This perceptiveness is widely used by petfood companies. Many commercially available cat food flavors indeed contain phosphoric acid. Excessive acid and phosphorus intakes must be avoided in cats with impaired renal function.

Salty taste

The perception is rather positive in cats and can enhance food or water consumption. Some water taste was hypothesized in early experiments, as taste receptors were thought to be reacting to distillated water. However, these electrophysiological responses were in fact the result of the adaptative neutrality of the cat's taste receptors to saline saliva.

Amino-acids

The taste buds connected to the facial nerve are highly sensitive to amino-acids: a single amino acid is able to stimulate the taste nerve fibers. These changes appear to be a specialization for feeding on prey, which is rich in protein (*Bradshaw et al, 1996*).

Oral sensitivity is not only gustatory, but somesthesia is important for granulometry and temperature detection through the lingual nerve. The ligaments of the teeth also participate. Any paradental disease or the effect of age, through modification of the resistance of the gums and teeth can strongly modify food perception and palatability.

It has been shown that the perception of food flavor is not simply the superposition of the various taste varieties but sensory messages are creating a brain image that is compared to innate or learned schemes (*Gallouin, 1987*). However, no specific data exist for cats.

Olfaction

Olfaction is present at birth and matures by three weeks of age. The cat is less sensitive than the dog to smell. This difference in sensitivity is due to the num-

FIGURE 3 - AIR CIRCULATION IN THE NASAL CAVITIES OF THE CAT

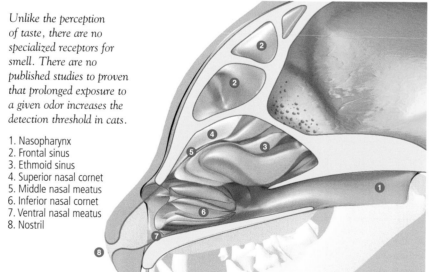

Unlike the perception of taste, there are no specialized receptors for smell. There are no published studies to proven that prolonged exposure to a given odor increases the detection threshold in cats.

1. Nasopharynx
2. Frontal sinus
3. Ethmoid sinus
4. Superior nasal cornet
5. Middle nasal meatus
6. Inferior nasal cornet
7. Ventral nasal meatus
8. Nostril

ber of olfactory cells, rather than their density in the mucosa. Cats have between 60 and 70 million olfactory cells (compared to 80-220 in dogs). In some animal studies, it has been estimated that only 1% of volatile compounds enter the nasal mucosa (**Figure 3**) however, no direct data exist in cats.

The cat is very selective and cautious. Olfaction is THE key factor to trigger food acceptance. Any anosmia will prevent food intake, and this anorexia will last as long as the cat cannot smell (*May, 1987*). Renewal of the olfactory mucosa and appetite recovery requires four to five days.

The range of smells perceived by cats is large but some specific odors are particularly attracting for them:
- mineral origin: bleach
- plant origin: catnip, olive wood, valerian, asparagus, mint, papyrus, cloves, mimosa
- animal origin: pheromones (although they do not have any direct food related meaning, but only territorial or sexual), livers, meats, viscera, etc.

However, detection ability does not mean food preference and no clear data exist on individual variability.
Some unusual odors or pheromones often trigger a specific reaction, called the Flehmen reaction, during which the cat lifts its upper lip and breathes some air through the vomero-nasal organ (Jacobson organ) located in the hard palate.

Petfood manufacturers are of course working on volatile compounds that are able to attract both the cat (when approaching its bowl) and the owner (when opening the can or the bag of kibble). However, as can be expected, this area of research remains very confidential and unpublished.

Vision

Lott-Brown et al (1973) have shown that cats are not able to discriminate between 520 and 570 nm lengthwaves. They thus would be unable to discriminate white from yellow or green. It would be for the cat the same "tonality". Red and blue are conversely clearly differentiated.
As a result, we may assume that colors of food are more important for owners than for cats.

The cat's vision is panoramic and adapted to discriminate movements more so than tonal differences. This ability has clearly evolved to facilitate predation.

> Behavioral aspects

Pre-natal experience

The acquisition of certain preferences may occur very early in life, as early as during gestation. Fetuses are surrounded by amniotic fluid, which contains compounds they assimilate in utero (*Thorne, 1994*). A cat's gustatory system is functional in the final days of gestation (*Tichy, 1994*).

Suckling behavior

Thanks to a burrowing reflex which lasts until the 8th day after birth, the new born kitten chooses a nipple during the first two days of its life. This reduces competition between littermates and decreases the time to initiate suckling (*Foucault, 1992*). Temperature (of the skin) and olfactory stimuli (from Montgomery glands secretion around the nipples) are the most important after birth

The suckling reflex appears from the 50th day of gestation and is gone by the 23rd day of life.

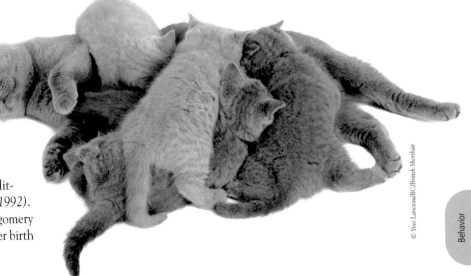

Behavior

443

There is nevertheless a maturation process during which regulatory factors transition from oral stimulation by milk up to the 10th day, to peri-oral stimulation (whatever the food is). The effect of digestive filling appears from 3 weeks of age.

The time allocated to suckling changes during the first month according to a relatively constant scheme. Kittens spend 10% of their time suckling and get milk for the first 2 weeks. Suckling time increases quickly up to 60% at 3 weeks and then decreases to 10% at the end of the first month (*Foucault, 1992*). They also spend time to suckle without drinking any liquid.

The evolution of the kitten – mother bond around food evolves quite significantly during this time. During the first two weeks, 75% of the suckling periods are initiated by the queen. During the two following weeks, the proportion falls from 50 to 5%. The mother then begins to avoid her kittens and allocates them only 20% of her time. Weaning is in fact beginning, with major behavioral and digestive changes.

During lactation, the composition of milk varies with the mother's diet. Kittens may develop certain preferences at this time in their lives (*Thorne, 1994*). Few articles describe this for cats. Weaning has in fact been more throughly studied.

Weaning experience

When eating their first solid food, kittens choose what their mothers eat, even if this food is unusual for cats (*Wyrwicka & Chase, 2001*). Dietary preferences are thus not all innate; they are acquired through social influences after birth.

Kittens whose mothers have been conditioned to eat bananas (usually unpalatable for cats) will eat bananas during weaning even if they have access to more conventional food for cats such as kibbles (*Wyrwicka & Long, 1980*). Kittens imitate their mother's eating behavior down to the smallest detail. They begin by eating from the same plate, at precisely the same spot, as their mother takes its food. There is a correlation between the mother's dietary consumption and that of the kittens. In the above experiment, the kittens that ate the least amount of banana were those whose mothers ate the least. The influence of the queen can last after weaning and separation between kittens and their mother. Food preferences acquired during weaning in their mother's presence persisted in kittens until the age of 4 to 5 months (*Wyrwicka & Long, 1980*).

Weaning is an important time in an animal's dietary history. The moment a cat eats its first solid food is probably crucial in terms of influence, especially if it happens in their mother's presence.

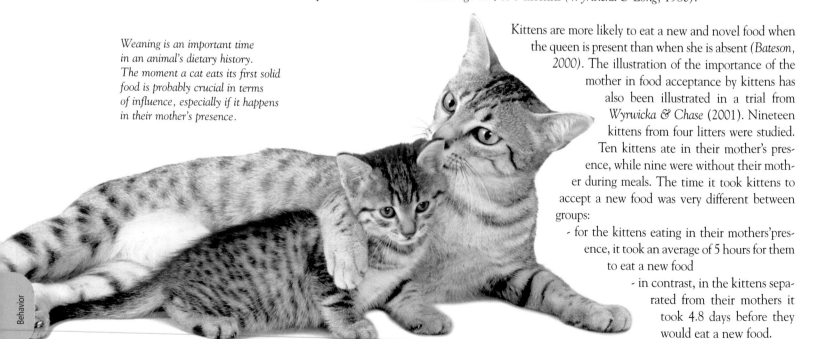

Kittens are more likely to eat a new and novel food when the queen is present than when she is absent (*Bateson, 2000*). The illustration of the importance of the mother in food acceptance by kittens has also been illustrated in a trial from *Wyrwicka & Chase* (2001). Nineteen kittens from four litters were studied. Ten kittens ate in their mother's presence, while nine were without their mother during meals. The time it took kittens to accept a new food was very different between groups:
- for the kittens eating in their mothers' presence, it took an average of 5 hours for them to eat a new food
- in contrast, in the kittens separated from their mothers it took 4.8 days before they would eat a new food.

© Yves Lanceau/RC/Egyptian Mau

Therefore many dietary habits are determined before 6 to 8 weeks of age. The practical consequence is that food education must be done at this stage. A good idea is to select, at least for the first weeks after adoption, the food used by the breeder.

Individual and breed differences

Kittens fed by stomach tube have very limited gustatory experience compared to kittens fed normally. During conditioning tests in which success is rewarded with food, the kittens fed by stomach tube took longer to succeed and even refused to eat the reward (*Stasiak & Zernicki, 2000*). Being deprived of dietary experience then influences future feeding behavior. All the early sensorial or digestive experiences create the individual variability. Learning leads to avoiding harmful or unpleasant foods and to preferably seek for nutritionally or sensorially gratifying ones.

Sex has no recognized effect on food perception in this species, even if feeding behavior can be indirectly affected by acute territorial competition in female cats, and by breeding season in male cats.

Breed may have some influence, although it is difficult to prove it unequivocally. It may be an area of future research.

Age affects ingestion behavior but less than in dogs (*Peachey & Harper, 2002*).The increase of dietary experience and the decline of olfactory and gustatory capabilities may enhance fussiness or even provoke preference inversion.

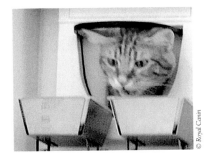

One peculiar feature in cat palatability testing that offers the choice between two bowls, is that some tasters always choose one side, regardless of the diet inside the bowl. Some cats are thus left handed, other are right handed!

▶ Environmental factors

> Social environment

The cat is a solitary hunter, but tends to gather in feeding and breeding spots in wild urban groups. The territory is transient and variable throughout time and space, i.e. it is possible that the territory overlaps between two cats but at different moments. Hierarchy in cats depends on the place and time during the day: it is a relative dominance. Territory may easily trigger aggressiveness and fights.

Unlike dogs **(Table 1)**, household cats do not appear to show social facilitation of eating: they usually eat alone and do not seem to be affected by the presence of another cat (*Houpt, 2005*). Some cats will even share the bowl with another cat, while others may sit calmly and wait for their turn. A female in estrus can have the right to get food first. However, other researchers feel that cats show hierarchical issues regarding the food bowl with higher ranking cats displacing lower ranking cats from the food source in a multi-cat home (*Knowles et al, 2004*). In ad libitum experimental situations, social feeding (as defined by time overlap of at least one minute between meals), occurs in duo with only 20% of meals (*Mugford, 1977*).

For owners of cats living outdoor, feeding is a privileged moment for contacts. Quite often, the feeder has better or, at least, the easier

In collective housing, it appears that some competition may occur. Fights are somewhat rare if food is available in large quantities.

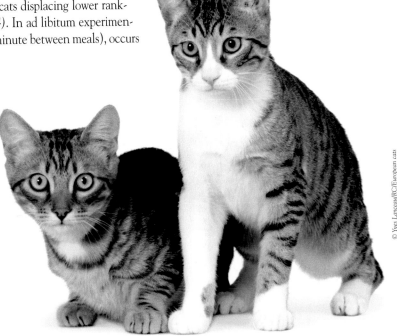

TABLE 1 - THE MAIN DIFFERENCES BETWEEN FELINE AND CANINE FEEDING BEHAVIOR	
Cat	**Dog**
Strict carnivore	Omnivore
12 to 20 meals/day	1 to 3 meals/day
Feed during day and night	Feed during daylight
Regular eaters	Glutton feeders
No social value of the meal	Social value of the meal

Behavior

445

relationship with the cat. *Geering* (1989) has shown that the act of feeding is necessary to reinforce the bond, but is not sufficient to keep it. Other interactions, like petting, grooming, playing, talking, are required to maintain a newly established link *(Bateson & Turner, 1989)*.

In the household environment, the rhythm of the supply of food often reflects the owner's lifestyle. Two or three meals are often fed during the day: in the morning before going to work, at the evening when returning, or even just before going to bed to keep the cat quiet!

Diet acceptance is largely influenced by the psychological, affective and material environment **(Figure 4)**. *Wolter* (1982) mentions various factors likely to influence the feeding behavior of the cat: tension between family members, change of light, sudden noise from stereo systems, different odors of cleaning product for the bowl, arrival of strangers, etc. This has nothing to do with food quality but an involuntary cat disturbance. Checking the feeding behavior during a recovery phase can lead to food refusal or lower acceptance. This situation is also observed when the owner has just bought a new food (new brand or new claim) and wants to check whether or not the animal accepts it. A very first analysis of perceived anorexia should review these unexpected but simple reasons! This disorder will be reviewed in the final section.

> Physical environment

Cats need to feel safe and secure within their home environment. To this end owners need to provide facilities for the main behavioral functions of eating, sleeping and playing and also ensure that the cat has the ability to control its own stress through the natural mechanisms of hiding and retreating. In tidy homes or those with built in furniture, places for cats to hide may be in short supply. This may create a situation where a cat might feel insecure and vulnerable without any escape routes or hiding places. Taking steps to provide the cat with a constant and predictable environment, both in terms of physical structure and scent profiles, will help to increase the cat's security; while the provision of access to high up resting platforms, secure bolt holes and hideaways may decrease the use of oral appeasing behaviors, such as over grooming and over eating. If all of the furniture in the house is built in it may be necessary to put up shelves for the cat to rest on, or clear out part of a cupboard or wardrobe to offer a safe hideout *(Dehasse et al, 1993)*.

FIGURE 4 - FACTORS CONTRIBUTING TO DIET ACCEPTANCE

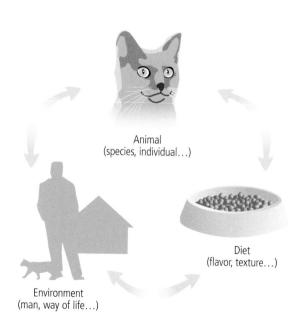

Animal
(species, individual...)

Diet
(flavor, texture...)

Environment
(man, way of life...)

▶ Influence of the food itself on feeding behavior

In the testing done on food choices and taste reactivity in cats *(Van den Bos et al, 2000)* two response sequences were noted and correlated to possible palatability reactions. A preference to consume an offered food was often preceded by a lick or a sniff of the feeding bowl, lip lick and face groom. Cats presented with food that was less desirable would lick or sniff the food and lick their nose. Whether the food was eaten was also partially dependent on the degree of hunger. In general cats will eat more of a desirable food regardless of hunger, but consumption of a less desirable food is often dependent on the hunger status of the cat.

Once a meal is consumed most cats will groom themselves regardless of perceived palatability. As direct gastric canulation leads to the same post-prandial behavior (without soiling lips and cheek), it is considered as an innate neurophysiologic reflex.

One of the most important features to consider is that cats will often eat and prefer a novel diet over a familiar one. The intensity of **neophilic behavior** depends on the foods' relative palatability and on the duration of exposure to the usual food. If the new food is less palatable than the usual food, the effect is shortlived. Twenty four kittens received the same food for 16 weeks, and then underwent a comparative test [two bowl test] for several days with the usual food and a new food of equivalent palatability. The first day, the kittens systematically chose the new food. After the second day, the difference was no longer significant between the two foods (*Mugford, 1977*). The novelty effect lasted only a few days (rarely more than 5 or 6 days), after which dietary preference stabilized.

> **Neophilia** is preference for a food never encountered by the animal or food that has not been recently encountered by the animal. This behavior is quite common in carnivores and has been identified in both dogs and cats. Neophilia enables animals to diversify their diet and achieve a better nutritional balance.

In the home, the preference for frequently changing the diet, a ritual that many owners participate in, is called **metaphilia** (from the greek, meta: "transformation"). This corresponds to an increase in consumption due to the renewal and alternation of known diets (*Rabot, 1994*). This is clearly observable in the cafeteria regimen in practice. This behavioral trait has led some manufacturers to create packaging of multi-single portions containing various varieties.

When changing a pet's diet, one must be prepared for the possibility of neophilia and the associated increase in energy consumption during the first month after the new diet is introduced. The novelty effect is accompanied by temporary caloric overfeeding. In the first month, cats may eat up to100 kcal/kg. The effect then wanes and consumption stabilizes around 60 kcal/kg after two months (*Nguyen et al, 1999*). Whenever a change is made to a pet's diet, owners should take care to measure out the food to ensure proper caloric delivery.

Breaking this natural neophilic trend, an owner can choose to always give the same diet. There is a risk of boredom with a perceived decrease in palatability (even it the food is complete and well balanced). One may relate that phenomenon to the human concept of "oral satiation" (always eating chocolate or eating oysters too often may decrease their palatability). On the other hand, choosing to frequently vary the diets beyond the carnivorous status of cats and to consider them as omnivorous by humanization, may lead to **neophobia** and again food refusal.

Some specific events can trigger fixation to one food and acquired **food aversion**. These disorders will be discussed below.

2 - Description of the feeding behavior of the cat

▶ Predation and hunting

Unlike the domestic dog, the body type of the domestic cat is not far from its wild ancestors. However, differences in prey sizes have led to significant differences, e.g: domestic cats use their incisors less, meals are more frequent and their way of consuming prey is also different: domestic cats begin with the head, large felids begin with the viscera.

> Hunting instinct or learned behavior?

Predatory behavior is innate: all cats probably know how to hunt, but certain aspects seem to be learned. Approach and pursuit are stimulated by littermates. Hunting behavior is more likely seen in kittens from a queen that hunts. Kittens learn to catch and to kill the same prey that their mother hunts (*Bateson & Bateson, 2002*).

Behavior

During weaning, there is an amazing training program for hunting displayed by the queen:

- 4th week: the queen brings meat pieces to the kittens
- 5th week: she eats dead prey in front of her kittens
- 6th or 7th week: she lets them eat the prey
- 8th week: she brings a live prey in order for the young hunters to learn to kill.

The first hunting sessions occur at 3 months. At 4 months of age, the young hunters are confirmed. The absence of predatory experience does not seem to interfere with motor abilities but often reveals prey selectivity issues. A kitten must indeed be taught that a mouse can be eaten. If it is not done before the age of 3 months old, the cat can starve even in the presence of the unknown prey! However, even cats that did not have access to prey when they were kittens can learn to become proficient hunters.

It has been speculated that feeding a cat may reduce its desire to hunt, but evidence to support this is lacking or controversial. Cats that are provisioned with food at home spend less time hunting than cats that are not provisioned with food, but both still hunt even if the number of actual prey caught and consumed is hard to quantify *(Fitzgerald & Turner, 2000)*.

Hunting session

Unlike dogs who hunt in packs, cats in the wild are solitary and opportunistic hunters. They catch small prey and eat alone. Observations show that they often fail in their attempts to catch prey: only 13% of tracked prey is actually caught *(Kays & DeWan, 2004)*, every success representing 3-5 attempts *(Fitzgerald & Turner, 2000)*. A cat brings home an average 0.7 prey a week *(Woods et al, 2003)*.

Hunting sessions can last 30 minutes, on distances between 600 and 1800 m in their territory. An obvious variability exists between individuals: for example, male cats hunt longer and further than female cats.

Cats spend two-thirds of their awake time to hunt in natural conditions. Hunting behavior is composed of several sequences:
- stalking the prey
- approaching and pursuing
- catching the prey by a central leap (their body will be low to the ground and they move slowly toward the prey, pausing prior to leaping to attack)
- killing by biting the neck, following an eventual fight
- consumption rarely occurs at the location of the catch (for the reason of quietness).

As the process progresses, the sequences are less and less modifiable by the cat's experience or it's'environment. The first steps (seeking, stalking and approach) are indeed flexible as a result of adaptation to different situations, while the last ones (e.g. attack and bite) are more stereotyped to secure efficient catch and kill, and thus individual survival.

Cats rarely bury their catch for postponed consumption. Cats eat rather quickly and then regurgitate furs and bones. Prey cleaning is rather poor, unless it is voluminous (such as pigeons or young rabbits). The cat breaks the bones and masticates with its large premolars. It can eat an entire mouse in less than one minute. When consuming a mouse, it starts at the head and eats

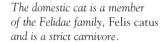

The domestic cat is a member of the Felidae family, Felis catus and is a strict carnivore.

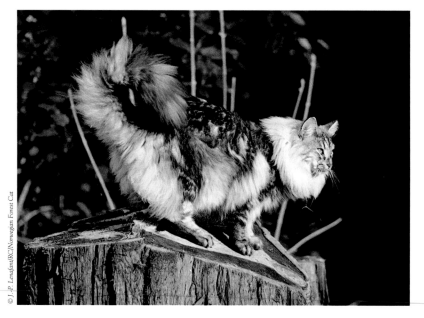

in the direction of the tail (*Case, 2003*). It is often the logical consequence of the killing method, during which the neck is broken. It might also be related to an adaptive behavior, securing prey catch and intake.

Leyhausen (1979) (quoted by *Rabot*, 1994) has shown that the complete hunting sequence is in fact controlled by a system of progressive and different motivation phases:
- interest is awaken by auditory stimuli (scratching, grating), which enables the cat to locate precisely the prey. In veterinary practice, scratching the consultation table is indeed often the best way to draw attention from the cat;
- visualization of rapid movement triggers approach. Experience nevertheless allows the cat to recognize a motionless prey and to attack it;
- catch answers to more precise visual and olfactory clues and is triggered by tactile stimuli.

© C. Chataignier

Feral cats hunt every 2 or 3 days, whereas domestic cats can hunt everyday.

Leyhausen's studies seemed to indicate that prey capture, killing and consumption were indeed independent actions. Capture and killing appeared to be also independent of hunger but if hunger pre-exists, predatory sequence is complete as hunger is the only reason that explains consumption.

Each stage induces in turn the following one, which permits the succession of all sequences by different stimuli. Hunger is not compulsory to trigger prey seeking but increases kill probability. Satiety does not inhibit sacrifice.

The domestic cat hunts quite often but rarely eats the prey. The system of independent phases proposed by Leyhausen would indeed explain that cats just fed can display all sequences without food intake. Some steps can be repeated and the owner can attend a cruel predatory play, during which prey is still alive while being handled in all ways. The fact of bringing back the prey to the owner can be falsely interpreted as a proof of the maternal like type of bond.

> The most common types of prey

Each catch represents only a small percentage of the cat's daily energy requirements (the caloric content of a mouse can be estimated at 30 kcal). It is possible to find up to 12 small preys in a feral cat's stomach. This represents an adaptive behavior to scarcity periods. Continental cats essentially hunt young lagomorphs and rodents. Birds come after in the list and reptiles even lower. Cats living on islands depend mainly on rats, mice and sea birds.

Cats are versatile and generalist hunters. They can easily move from one prey type to another depending upon ecological evolutions. They can even go to some domestic feeding during scarcity periods. On some islands, feline predation has been put as the cause of some species extinction, according to *Bateson and Turner* (1989). Studies focused on the effect of predation on wildlife are however limited and it is unclear whether the extrapolation of these data to the global feline population is accurate.

> Techniques to limit predatory behavior in domestic cats

Attempting to decrease predation by house hold cats is probably a worthy goal. Predatory behavior is a normal behavioral pattern in cats but often distressing to their owners. Although

Behavior

449

6 of 10 cats (in the United States) and most pure breed cats are kept indoors and therefore cannot hunt, in Europe many cats (7 of 10) have an outdoor access so they can hunt and kill small rodents and birds. Owners often find this behavior objectionable especially when cats direct the behavior toward song birds and/or bring prey home.

Predatory behavior is best prevented by keeping cats indoors and obtaining kittens from queens that do not hunt (so as to get inexperienced individuals). In addition, keeping a quick release cat collar with a large bell on the cat may diminish their proficiency. *Nelson et al* (2005) compared collar mounted warning devices on reducing predation in cats in the UK and found that there was no significant difference in the prey return rate between cats wearing collars with one bell, two bells or a sonic device.

The cat has been domesticated for nearly 6000 years but has not lost his exceptional hunting skills thanks to the independency of predatory sequences. Cats can easily return to the wild and survive without human intervention.

► Domestic feeding

Cats spend from 1 to 2% of their awake time eating. When feeding a household cat, the food can be provided either in a controlled manner i.e. as meal feeding or as free choice feeding. Regardless of the type of feeding regime chosen, it is useful to establish regular feeding and eating patterns for house hold cats **(Table 2)**.

> The place of the feeding bowl

The territorial organization of the cat's life must be taken into consideration. Each spot has a defined dedication for the cat: feeding, resting, playing, eliminating. And these functions are not mixed. You would not eat in the middle of the train entrance or in your toilets. It is the same for a cat! **(Figure 5)**.

Bowls have to be small, to control intake and to encourage frequent refilling. Regular cleaning of the bowl is necessary, to avoid off smells and safety issues. In homes with multiple cats, each cat should be offered their own food bowl. Antagonistic interactions between cats may restrict some individuals from access to food and water bowls leading to weight loss and perhaps medical complications. In addition, because cats may not share space equally, food bowls should be allocated through out the environment, not all in one location. Care should be exercised to note where individual cats spend most of their time and place food and water bowls in those locations. Litter boxes should be placed at a significant distance from the feeding location.

> Meal feeding

When pet owners use a meal feeding method to feed their cats they either control the time the food is provided or the portion size provided. It is the best method for canned food so as to secure freshness and safety. Leaving leftovers for hours in the bowl indeed leads to bacteriological risks and palatability decrease due to organoleptic deterioration. Manufacturers have understood this problem and now propose single portions diets. Because cats eat multiple small meals when hunting, most household cats find

TABLE 2 - FEEDING REGIMES IN HOUSE HOLD CATS		
Method	**Advantages**	**Disadvantages**
Meal feeding The owner controls either the time the food is provided and/or the amount of food provided daily. Usually the cat is provided with 2-3 small meals daily at set times.	- Allows the owner to monitor food intake - Helps assess health - Allows all cats access to food - Increases bonding time	- Some cats may solicit food at other times - May not meet the cats internal schedule for eating
Free choice feeding The cat is provided with food at all times.	- Allows the cat to control consumption - The cat can eat multiple small meals daily	- Unable to monitor intake - May lead to over consumption and obesity - Allows no time for human-animal bonding
Combination feeding Free choice dry food, meal feeding wet food once or twice daily.	- Allows multiple small meals daily - Allows for bonding time	- Unless closely regulated over consumption can occur - Some individuals may not get enough to eat

single meal feeding unsatisfactory if it is the only method chosen. If an owner chooses to feed its cat in a time controlled manner, at least two meals per day should be provided. However, an increased frequency of meals may help control hunger and decrease excessive food soliciting behavior. It is indeed amazing to see cats learning to detect when they can get extra food. They associate some events to a high probability to get reward e.g. during the advertising break of the evening TV movie or when the owner puts the kitchen in order (they can be warned by the noise of plates in the dishwashing machine!).

Meal feeding methods

- With **time controlled feeding**, the food is left available for a set amount of time and then picked up and not provided again until the next feeding time. For most cats, 30-60 minutes should be allotted for eating when fed in a time controlled manner (*Case, 2003*).

- With **portion controlled feeding**, the amount of food provided is measured and placed in the bowl and once it is consumed, no more food is provided until the next meal. For a single household cat, portion control can help control weight while potentially allowing the cat to eat several meals through out the day, something that cannot occur with timed feeding.

FIGURE 5 - THE MINIMAL DISTANCE BETWEEN THE FEEDING PLACE AND THE ELIMINATION AND RESTING PLACES

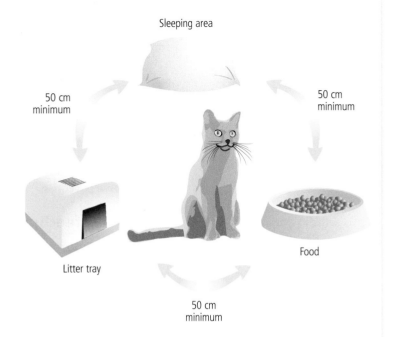

Sleeping area

50 cm minimum

50 cm minimum

50 cm minimum

Litter tray

Food

The feeding station must be in a quiet place (not close to the washing machine), at the right distance from the litter box.

Meal feeding in either manner has several advantages. It allows owners to determine how much food the cat consumes in a 24 hour period. Food consumption is often a good marker of health and knowing how much the cat eats can help an owner determine how the cat feels. If multiple cats reside in the home it may allow the caregivers to assess each cats eating pattern and access to food and may help the owner to recognize health or social problems in the cats. Meal feeding also allows the pet and the owner to interact several times a day strengthening the human-animal bond.

Free choice feeding

In free choice feeding food is provided to the cat at all times so that the cat can eat multiple small meals in a 24 hour period. Domestic cats often eat multiple small meals through out the day. Depending upon observations, this number varies from 8 to 16. This is linked to the evolution of the cat to an opportunistic feeding pattern, nibbling small amounts of food on numerous occasions. This method relies on the cat ability to self regulate intake. This is the best option when the cat is fed with dry food. However, due to the increased palatability of commercial cat foods coupled with reduced exercise, cats may over eat and become obese. In addition, self feeding does not necessarily allow the human caregiver to determine daily intake especially in homes with multiple cats. With self feeding, a change in food consumption and resultant weight loss may not be noticed for some time perhaps imperiling pet health. Self feeding also limits the pet-owner interaction around feeding time.

Some pet owners may combine meal feeding and free choice feeding by providing set meals of small amounts of wet food and provide dry food in free choice. It creates a social re-enforcement of food intake, although this effect is much less important than in dogs. The cat is invited to eat wet food as a "plus" and the calorie content is added to the normal dry food ration spread over the day. In some cases the energy balance can be excessive. The practitioner must keep in mind that some cats may have difficulties to regulate their energy consumption when fed two different

Behavior

types of food: a strict control of the quantities fed to the cat and of the nutritional balance of both types of foods is highly recommended.

> The role of the human in feline feeding

Because most household cats do not hunt to meet their nutritional needs, when they are hungry they target their pre-meal behaviors and food soliciting behaviors towards the humans within the home. These behaviors include vocalization, rubbing on nearby objects and on the humans. Often if the person moves in the direction of where the food is provided or stored, the cat may run in that direction or continue to wind between the legs actually impeding progress. It has been suggested that people who feed the cat have a better relationship with the cat perhaps because of these opportunities to interact (Geering, 1989).

Owners often inadvertently assume all vocalization and attention is in fact a food soliciting behavior. They then respond by feeding the cat, resulting in a potent learning process. The owner's response is acting as a reward for vocalization and attention seeking behaviors which usually will increase in frequency and intensity. Not only can these behaviors be distressing to the owner, excessive food intake will also lead to obesity and related medical problems. Owners should learn to recognize when enough food has been provided and consumed, and not reward these behaviors with food. They then should find an alternate activity such as play or grooming once the nutritional needs have been met.

> Observations of feeding behavior: how the cat eats

Many nutritional studies are based on the study of the factors affecting the amount of food that cats ingest. The regulation of ingestion is a complex and still poorly understood phenomenon. The frequency and size of meals represent two key parameters of feeding behavior.

Number of meals per day

Each cat has its own way to dispatch its meals throughout the day. A cat generally needs 3 weeks to get a stable life pattern. In an ad libitum situation, it ranges from 3 to 20 meals per day (Kane et al, 1981; Houpt, 2005), like water intake (Mac Donald et al, 1984). In cattery conditions, when cats are fed ad libitum with dry food, the dietary consumption is influenced by the night and day alternance: the dietary consumption at night is often inferior to consumption during the day, but during the night, the meals are larger and longer (Kanes et al, 1981; Royal Canin Research Center: internal data, 2004).

Meal size, meal duration and speed of eating

Meal size increases with palatability (especially the first meal) or when the feeder goes from meal feeding to ad libitum feeding. The average duration of a meal is almost 2 minutes (**Figure 6**). The speed of eating is an important criterion for the owner's perception. It is in fact much more influenced by food structure than palatability. For dry kibbles, the eating rate increases from 2 to 4 grams per minute. For canned product, it lies between 4 and 8 grams per minute.

Studies done at the Royal Canin Research Center illustrate how the number of meals, quantity of ingested food

FIGURE 6 - THE FEEDING PATTERN OF THE CAT OVER 24 HOUR
(*Source: Royal Canin Research Center; internal data, 2004*)

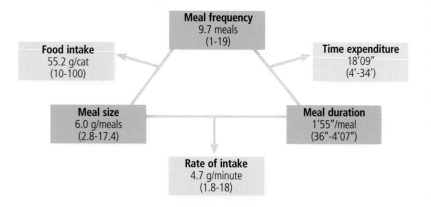

The feeding behavior of cats living together in groups was followed using an electronic scale with access controlled by an electronic chip. This system makes it possible to follow in real time each cat's consumption profile in terms of the number of meals, the meal size and the duration of the meal (between brackets: mean-extremes).
Data were collected with 8 adult domestic cats (2 to 3 years old), fed ad libitum with the same dry food over 17 days.

452

- it is easier to store, to keep for a longer period of time
- it can easily be fed free choice without concerns of spoilage
- it may offer dental hygiene properties. The chewing and grinding may help prevent plaque and calculus development (see chapter 10) and dry diets have been specifically formulated to increase their dental cleaning properties.

Some cats show a preference for certain shaped kibble morsels and have preferences for mouth feel and surface to volume ratio of the food (*Crane et al, 2000*). Cats reject broken kibbles.

Canned cat food can either be a complete and balanced diet or just a supplement that is primarily meat. Canned foods are blended and contain additional water; in some cases the moisture of the product reaches 85%. It can result in a low caloric density and thus promote higher intake on a long term basis Many cats find canned foods extremely palatable due to the high water, fat and protein content (*Case, 2003*). Product texture is very important to determine eating patterns:

Minced products are continuously swallowed, the cat staying crouched and never lifting its head. The speed of eating is high and owners may perceive that this is a reflection of palatability, whereas the reason is more mechanical than sensorial!

Jelly products lead cats to take large gulps of meat. They have to chew a bit and lift their head simply to swallow. Some owners may have the perception that their cat is more reluctant to eat. Others may feel that the cat is appreciating the food, tasting it quietly, thanking them by looking at them and licking their lips!

Semi moist foods: most of these products are marketed as treats for cats and are not meant to be used as the sole dietary source of nutrition. They are softer in texture than dry food, but they are not as moist as canned food. They do not require refrigeration and have long shelf lives. Some ingredients, used as preservatives of the water level, may even negatively affect palatability.

Homemade diets are not usually recommended since cats have specific dietary requirements that may be hard to meet.

> Taste and the composition of the food

Food palatability is the very first key factor of success for petfood acceptance, for both cats and owners. Despite a lot of publications concerning feline food preferences or aversions, cat's preferences are more nutrient-orientated than ingredient-orientated. Quality and freshness of raw materials are nevertheless important.

An important technological know how (enzymatic hydrolysis, fermentation, etc.) has been developed, leading to the commercialization of very efficient natural flavors, homogeneously coated onto the kibbles in order to drastically increase their acceptance **(Figure 8)**. However, there is little information that the authors can provide in this text as the data remains strictly confidential among palatability experts in petfood companies.

Proteins (especially hydrolysed proteins from meats, and sometimes plants such as soyabean) as well as fat are both palatable for cats. Some ingredients like yeasts and specific acids are also appreciated by cats.

The selection of fat is important, and above all their protection against oxidation. Fat can also interfere with palatability through some texture effects. Short and medium chain fatty acids (caprylic acid, coconut oil, etc.) are sometimes associated with altering the palatability of the food

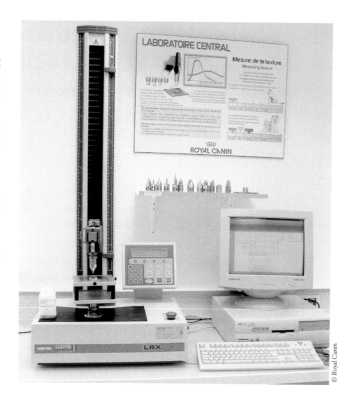

The texturometer is used to measure the kibble's resistance to the force of the cat's teeth and jaws. Interchangeable modules imitate the shape and size of teeth according to the size and age of the cat.

Behavior

FIGURE 8 - MAIN TECHNOLOGIES USED IN THE DEVELOPMENT OF AROMAS

1. Hydrolysates are often obtained from heated, acidified poultry proteins. Enzymes are used to breakdown protein into palatable compounds.

2. Maillard reactions are used to aromatize various products (coffee, biscuits, roasted meats, etc).

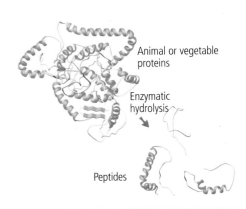

Animal or vegetable proteins

Enzymatic hydrolysis

Peptides

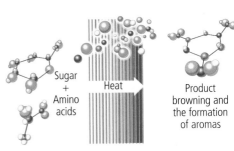

Sugar + Amino acids

Heat

Product browning and the formation of aromas

(Mac Donald et al, 1985) but this effect can be hidden when the ingredients and the surrounding formula are appealing for the cat.

Palatability has too often been blamed for feline obesity. However, the food's energy concentration is more important than palatability. An inactive, neutered cat that has access to food with a high-energy concentration will inexorably gain weight. Prevention is about maximizing activity and optimizing the composition of the food.

A cat has more difficulty limiting its food consumption if the kibbles are very rich in fat. Cats fed ad libitum with a food containing 20% fat develop greater adipose reserves than when the fat level is halved, regardless of the animal's sex: male or female, intact or neutered *(Nguyen et al, 1999)*.

► Elements of the regulation of hunger

Global palatability of the food is crucial, but hunger is a sine qua non condition for the cat to eat.

> General principles

Energy supply is controlled by homeostatic regulatory processes for food intake and body expenditure or both. Nutrient supply to the body must be constant. However, food intake is a discontinued and periodic behavior. A medium and long term regulation system thus exists; with the involvement of body storages (essentially fat). Everything is done homeostatically to prevent loss of tissues and weight loss.

Controls of food intake can be classified by several pathways:
- **behavioral pathways**: habits and learning such as sensorial or metabolic conditioning
- **nervous pathways**: mastication effecting oral satiation, stomach filling effecting physical satiation
- **metabolic pathways**: short term glucostatic theory, long term lipostatic theory

Glucostatic theory in cats

A low level of glucose in the hypothalamic cells triggers hunger *(Rowland, 1985)*.

Lipostatic theory

The endocrine role of adipose cells has been studied during the past few years. Many cytokines have been identified that act on insulin metabolism, inflammation, etc. Among these, leptin, the satiety hormone discovered in 1994, has been clearly involved in appetite regulation *(Bouret et al, 2004)* however, there are few studies in cats.

One satiation signal cannot act alone to control body balance which is the result of a series of separated control points, acting on a different time scale. Animals control their food consumption through 3 major food compounds:
- water
- sodium (all other mineral are consumed in relation to caloric density)
- energetic nutrients

If formulation is correctly done and if the feeding distribution well adapted to behavior requirements, energetic regulation is then efficient.

It has been suggested that the sensorial properties of a food become more important than metabolic ones for deprived cats. This could be an adaptative protective behavior during which cats seeking desperately for food become more discriminating to avoid poisoning risks in excessive hunger states. For well-fed cats, both palatability and nutritional values are acting in the regulation process.

From a practical standpoint, the only valid clue of efficient regulation is the stability of body weight. Significant inter-individual variability does exist. When analyzing publications and the possibly contradictory conclusions, it is important to perform a critical evaluation of what kind of regulatory processes are explored in relation to the beginning (animal reaction), the duration (constant modification) and termination (new equilibrium status).

> Energy regulation

Many experiments on caloric dilution of food content have been performed. Some contradictory conclusions have been drawn, that are often linked to the methodology employed (e.g. the addition of cellulose, water, clay etc).

Under very stable conditions, the cat seems able to control its food intake in relation to caloric density (more precisely in relation to dry matter caloric density). This process starts within 2 to 3 days and requires at least 3 or 4 weeks (*Rowland, 1981*). Meal size is most affected, secondarily meal frequency. However cafeteria feeding (i.e. changing and varying daily dry matter content and palatability) disturbs this natural ability. This is typically what happens in the home when the owner frequently alternates canned and dry foods, brands, varieties, etc.

> Protein regulation

In cats, contrary to humans or dogs, protein has been shown to increase food intake (*Servet et al, 2008*). Therefore, limiting the amount of protein (with a fiber substitution) is an original strate-

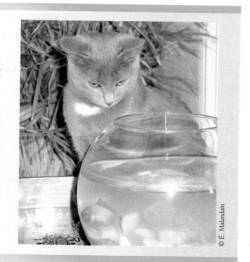

WHY DO SOME CATS LIKE FISH SO MUCH?

In its original environment – the cat is adapted to deserts – where there is limited availability of fish. So where does this attraction for fish flesh come from - even to the extent that certain cats take great delight in raiding garden ponds, and feasting on gold fish and young koi?

Fish is a source of protein. Historically, cats have always been very opportunistic and quickly realized that there was obvious benefit in hanging around the quays when fishing boats returned to port because they could eat the remains from cleaning and gutting of the fish. In the time of sailing boats, voyages took a long time and boats took on board provisions of cereals - unfortunately accompanied by mice and rats that fed on them. Cats were therefore taken on board as well in order to control the population of these undesirable rodents and, once their mission was accomplished, the sailors would therefore show their gratitude by giving them fish.

In Asia, similar to human food, ocean-products are very commonly used in catfood.

© E. Malandain

gy to limit spontaneous food/energy intake. These observations might be useful in the design of a diet to manage feline obesity (see chapter 1).

It has been suggested that some specific amino acids, such as tryptophan can affect general behavior (agression, excitability or territoriality modulation) in dogs *(Bosch et al, 2007)*. There may be a relationship between tryptophan intake by the brain and the level of carbohydrate in the diet. However, changes of the level of carbohydrate in the diet are often linked to concommittant change in the protein level, which can also affect behavior. The mechanism how the intake of nutrients that act as precursors of neurotransmittors (choline for acetylcholine, tyrosine for catecholamines, and tryptophan for serotonin) effect food composition is unclear and obviously needs more scientific work.

> Physical satiety

It has been proposed that the receptors for physical satiety in cats may be more efficient in regulating food intake than the energy pathways. In the single meal feeding situation, the cat is able to achieve its daily needs, even within 5 days following a transition from ad libitum to one hour distribution *(Thorne, 1982; Finco et al, 1986)*.

Ranking of control pathways is logically linked to the action level: physical satiation in the short term and caloric satiation in the medium term. The link is the fact that dry matter is both responsible for filling the stomach and for providing energy.

From a developmental standpoint, experiments on new born kittens *(Hinde, 1975)* would suggest that oral satiation is acting first before the development of gastric satiation: in other words, milk intake is less important than suckling movements.

Sleep is increased after meals. The effect is noticeable 3 hours after intake. Latency is variable: the quicker it appears, the longer it lasts. It is medidated by endocrine pathways and depends upon nutrients, duodenum pH, and gastric emptying.

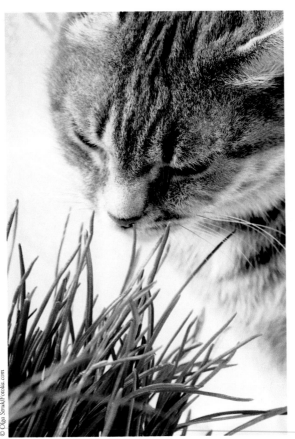

Nepeta cataria (catnip plant)
The catnip plant is usually well appreciated by cats. It is a generic name that applies to various plants sold for cats.

4 - Disorders of ingestion behavior

In the owner's mind, feeding behavior is associated with health, well being and pleasure, especially in mature markets where anthropomorphism is strongly present. This is probably why so many clients regularly question veterinarians about the relationship of food intake to some disturbances.

We will distinguish qualitative troubles (plant eating, pica and wool sucking, fixation on one food, learned aversion) from quantitative troubles (hyperorexia and anorexia).

► Qualitative disorders

> Grass and plant eating and catnip

Cats frequently eat grass if they have access to it and/or they may ingest house plants. Plant ingestion may be considered as a natural phenomenon which makes vomiting easier and thus the expulsion of hairballs. It becomes a behavioral issue when addiction occurs, i.e. if a cat systematically seeks a specific plant.

The **catnip plant** *(Nepeta cataria)* often induces a reaction in cats. Not all cats respond to catnip: 30-50% of cats do not respond at all and the response appears to be inherited and modified by both age and experience *(Beaver, 2003)*. When exposed to catnip a cat who responds will usually smell it, lick it, chew or eat it. The cat may hold the catnip in their paws if it is fresh. Cats will often roll in the plant. Some cats become quite animated and leap and play. The sequence is accompanied by head shaking, rubbing of the cheek and chin against the plant and profusely salivating. This may be perceived by an unexperienced owner as an estrus-like behavior. The response lasts 5-15 minutes and cats may be refractory to catnip exposure for about an hour. This is a sort of satiation phase following the excitement. The active component, or at least the most powerful one, is a nepetalactone, a terpenoid with a special attraction effect to female cats *(Sakurai, 1988)*.

Valerian *(Valeriana officinalis)* produces similar effects to catnip. Cats roll on roots, urinate over it and exhibit signs of great excitement. After chewing the plant, the cat will roll for 10-15 minutes on the floor, rub against objects and exhibit estrus-like behavior.

Actinidia (including chinese gooseberry): when presented with this plant, the cat stops eating and even stops sexual activity. On detection of the smell, they will seek its origin and roll on their backs in a state of total ecstasy.

Olive wood

Most cats chew and lick olive wood objects and rub at them. Olive flesh is not attractive to cats, it is more the nut.

This attraction to plants may become annoying and more importantly, as many house plants are poisonous, can have serious consequences when ingested. In addition, most owners find the consumption of houseplants objectionable and punish the cat for doing so if they catch the cat in the act. This can often result in a cat that is frightened of the owners. Treatment aims at providing acceptable plant material for ingestion by creating a cat garden of grasses (sold in many petshops) and plants that are acceptable and safe for consumption by the cat. Other plants should be placed out of reach either high off the ground, secured in another room or outdoors. In some cases making the plants aversive using hot-pepper solutions sprayed on the leaves or a water sprayer if the cat gets too close diminishes the behavior.

> Pica and wool sucking/chewing behavior

Pica

Pica refers to the voluntary ingestion of non dietary, non nutritional items and can include clothing, electric cords, wool, fabric, cardboard, plastic and many other items. Some cats may actually ingest the items and intestinal blockage is possible.

It represents between 5 to 10% of behavioral problems in cats. Often pica occurs in young, active animals and in some cases a genetic predisposition is suspected but has not been proven *(Beaver, 2003)*. It is important to keep in mind that kittens actively explore orally their environment up to 6 weeks of age and voluntary intake of unedible items can occur without being pica. Beyond that, special attention is due.

The origin of pica is in fact not very well known. Some mineral or vitamins deficiencies had been incriminated in the past, but the tremendous formulation improvement of cat food has eliminated this possible theory. Massive parasitism may be a similar contributing factor in farm cats.

Medical conditions such as feline leukemia and feline immunodeficiency should be investigated since they may contribute to abnormal behaviors. In dogs, exocrine pancreatic insufficiency has been associated with pica, but that has not been noted in the cat *(De Braekeleer et al, 2000)*. In other situations a lack of an enriched environment, dental problems, teething, attractive odors on objects and attention seeking have all been considered as contributory factors for pica.

Pica is thought to first be exhibited in situations of conflict and/or anxiety for the pet. In cats the initial situations may be social situations between cats, changes in social interactions with family members, moving house, etc. Over time the problem behavior occurs in other situations and more frequently until it interferes with function. Diagnosis of a compulsive disorder is based on exclusion of other causes for the behavior.

Wool sucking

Wool sucking has to be distinguished from true pica. This behavior is considered to be a compulsive disorder (*Luescher, 2002*). Wool sucking occurs when a cat takes clothing items, usually woolens (but other fabrics may be chosen) and sucks or chews. Some kittens are naturally sucking their littermates or their own skin: later, this habit can extend to other species, cushions, or the owner's clothes. Under natural conditions, kittens can suckle their mother up to 6 months of age. In domestic conditions, weaning is earlier (6 to 8 weeks). *Houpt* (1982) hypothesized that it was the result of a suckling deprivation as a consequence of early detachment, however, nothing has yet been definitively proven. The strong or excessive affective link with the mother and with the owner (in oriental breeds) may also be part of the explanation.

Treatment

Treatment of pica and wool sucking includes a mix of the following strategies:
- in some cases merely keeping the pet away from items is useful.
- making items aversive with unpleasant smelling or tasting detergents: garlic or red pepper mashes, aloes, quinine, strong perfumes (avoid chlorinated agents which attract cats)
- redirect the cat to other items: increasing feeding opportunities through the use of feeder type toys may help.
- keeping the materials out of reach (*Houpt, 2005*), when possible
- offer derivations to the cat, such as toys, possibilities to go out for a walk or a hunt
- behavior modification, creating a predictable and reliable environment avoiding anxiety sources
- restructuring the interactions with the owner, by discouraging over-attachment syndrome (regular and increasing separation phases from the owner, compensated by physical contacts initiated only by this latter while ignoring cat solicitations: it is hard to get observance but it is efficient)
- in some cases use psychotropic medication e.g. a Selective Serotonin Reuptake Inhibitor (SSRI) such as fluoxetine or a tricyclic antidepressant (TCA) such as clomipramine (*Luescher, 2002*).

Because Siamese and Burmese cats are over-represented up to 8 months of age; a genetic predisposition toward wool sucking is suspected but not yet proven.

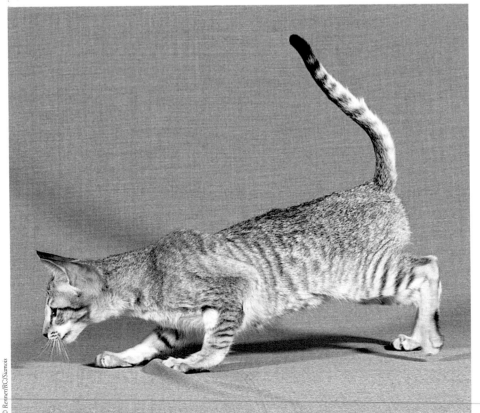

© Renner/RC/Siamois

> Fixation on one type of food and neophobia

Neophobia is the opposite of neophilia and corresponds to avoidance of a new food compared to the usual food. Also called "fixation of food habits", neophobia has been identified in cats. This behavior is part of a food selection strategy.

Omnivorous animals consume foods that provide a balanced diet and avoid taking the risk of eating new unknown foods. However, carnivores in the wild display more neophilic than neophobic behavior (*Thorne, 1982*). Neophobia is more common when meals are served in unusual conditions (*Thorne, 1982*) or if the animal is under stress (*Bradshaw, 1991*).

It is not uncommon for a cat to become fixated on a particular type or flavor of food and reject all others. Often this can be prevented by offering a diversity of flavors and textures of appropriate complete and balanced diets when the cat is young. Willingness to try new foods and food preferences may be influenced by the queen and the weaning conditions: kittens fed since weaning with the same cereal-based food preferred this type of food to more palatable canned food with tuna (*Wyrwicka & Long, 1980*). Neophobia, the lack of recognition of food as being edible (*Bradshaw et al, 2000*), exists in varying degrees. The more regular the diet, the more persistent is the neophobia.

In some cases it may be medically necessary to switch a cat to a new diet. If the diet texture and shape are the same as the previous one, the cat may accept it readily by adding it step by step in the new food while decreasing the proportion of the old food over a week of time. For some cats, offering the new food and old food side by side will also help the transition. In other situations, a cat may need to be transitioned from a canned food to a dry food or vice versa. This is often difficult since many cats seem to have preferences for certain shapes and/or textures of food. Increasing the smell may enhance eating for some cats and this often can be accomplished by warming the food.

A few days are required to overcome neophobia and for an animal to experiment with the new food (*Cheney & Miller, 1997*). To overcome neophobia towards a new flavor, cats should not be exposed to the smell alone; they must also taste it. In a study on cats, *Bradshaw (1986)* showed that neophobia disappeared after the third day of presentation of food flavored with lamb. Neophobia reappeared three months later if the cat was not regularly exposed to the new flavour. One solution devised to overcome neophobia towards a flavor involves using drinking water as a support. Although neophobia toward new foods is common in many species, neophobia toward flavored drinking water is indeed rare.

Introducing a new diet under unusual circumstances or when a cat is stressed (by pain or illness, by being away from its owner, in a veterinary clinic etc) is more likely to result in neophobia (through an aversion learning process) than if the new food is introduced under familiar, positive circumstances. It is recommended to always introduce a new diet under the least stressful conditions for the pet and use a food transition program.

> Learned taste aversions

Aversion is a strategy used by animals to avoid foods that are unsuitable for them. It is a form of negative conditioning. If the smell of food is associated with distress, with an unpleasant experience (hospitalization, forced or hidden drug administration) or with a digestive problem (poisoning, allergies), the food will be avoided in the future. This phenomenon is known as aversion (*Cheney & Miller, 1997*).

In cats, aversion sets in very quickly. A single meal associated with unpleasantness leads to a refusal to eat. Such aversion can persist for 40 days (*Bradshaw et al, 1996*) or more (*Mugford, 1977*). The smell alone of a food associated with digestive disorders is enough to elicit aversion. Cats even go so far as to show aversion for their usual food if it is served in the presence of an air current bearing the odor of a food to which they have developed an aversion (*Mugford, 1977*). Be careful when preparing foods for cats being boarded at the hospital. Odors may travel and could trigger an aversion reaction even in cats being fed their usual diet. It is best to prepare the food in a place where food odors cannot reach the cats.

▶ Quantitative disorders

> Polyphagia

It is crucial to remember that feeding is an affective and rewarding act for the owner. It is the moment of the day during which the owner can get attention from the cat. However owners have to understand that the dietary behavior of cats is different from humans. For humans, the kitchen is often a social place. Cats like contact and will therefore go to the kitchen just to share social interactions. These requests for interaction are misinterpreted by the owner as begging for food. Owners do not recognize food soliciting behavior as an attention seeking behavior, not hunger and provide the cat with too much food which it willingly consumes. Most cats

> **THREE APPROACHES WHICH MAY HELP OVERCOME NEOPHOBIA**
>
> 1 - Offer the new diet each day for at least three days (offering fresh food each time). Persistent exposure, even if the cat initially refuses the new food, may help overcome neophobia.
> 2 - Try putting a small piece of the new food in the cat's mouth, so that the cat can taste the new food.
> 3 - If the diet is a wet food (can or pouch), try smearing a little of the food onto the cat's front legs. Most cats will lick off the food and this can habituate the cat to a new food.

TABLE 5 - CREATING GOOD FEEDING AND EATING HABITS IN CATS

1. Pick a diet appropriate for the life stage (kittens, adult cats, elderly cats), physical activity and environment
2. Provide food in an appropriate bowl in a safe, secure, quiet location
   a. When multiple cats reside in the home each cat should have their own bowl
   b. If social conflicts between cats are evident then some cats may need to be fed in separate locations
3. Calculate the appropriate amount needed to meet the nutritional needs of each cat in the home
4. Feed close to the same time each day
5. Avoid excessive solicitations for food if nutritional needs have been met
   a. Substitute play time, exercise, grooming or attention rather than supplementing dietary intake

TABLE 6 - CAUSES OF POLYPHAGIA
From: Masson, 2004

Transient			Persistant	
Reactional		Induced	Weight gain	Weight loss
Physiological	Psychological	Orexigen drugs	Dysregulation	Metabolic
Gestation Lactation Cold temperature Sustained exercise	High palatability	Megestrol Acetate	Hypothalamic lesions (unusual)	Diabetes mellitus Hyperthyroidism Malassimilation Chronic kidney disease
	Owner solicitation	Glucocorticoids		
		Anticonvulsivants		

are obese because they are provided with a highly palatable, energy rich diet in excessive of their metabolic needs. Starting out with a good feeding routine and pattern may help prevent obesity (**Table 5**).

It is important to remember that neutering is responsible for decreasing energy expenditure. The balance between energy intake and energy requirements is usually disturbed after neutering.

Pathological and medical reasons

If the cat consumes excessive amounts of food without gaining weight then a metabolic problem (such as hyperthyroidism, pancreatic insufficiency, diabetes mellitus), massive parasitism or sometimes brain tumors, should be considered and a full medical evaluation obtained.

Some drugs such as diazepam, megestrol acetate and corticosteroids may also induce polyphagia (**Table 6**).

"Hypersensitivity/Hyperactivity syndrome"

Some European behaviorists recognize a syndrome of excess food intake which may be due to lack of self control. Kittens scratch, bite, run everywhere and play constantly. Owners are impressed by the amount of food eaten without becoming fat. Some cats gulp their food, eat it quickly and then regurgitate it. This syndrome is due to a lack of mother regulation between the 5th and 6th week. This often happens when adopting young kittens from an outdoor life, that are not handled and not well fed during this crucial period of their life (Beata, 2007).

Social problems

A cat may consume large quantities of food if it is anxious due to overcrowding, tense social relationships between cats in the home and lack of privacy while eating. Some kittens coming from large litters can maintain the habit to overeat to compensate for competition to the access of food, even when they are later in a single cat household, without competition.

If the problem of excessive food consumption is due to social problems between cats within the home, some simple environmental manipulations can be useful. Food and water bowls should be provided in all areas of the home, after paying special attention to which cats frequent what areas and where they spend their time. Some cats may be more agile than others and the provision of food bowls on elevated locations may allow them to eat with privacy. If one cat consistently eats more than its share of food, then set feeding times and separating cats for feeding may allow all cats to eat their required allotment.

Anxiety

The cat that is permanently looking for food may meet the European criteria for bulimia which can be a symptom of permanent anxiety. The excessive eating and food seeking are a substitution activity for frustration or conflict. If anxiety is the source of overeating then the individual conditions causing anxiety must be addressed (changes in schedules or territory organization, etc.).

These treatments are beyond the scope of this article but are detailed in other sources (*Horwitz, et al, 2002*).

Excessive food solicitation behaviors and overfeeding

When cats become hungry they may engage in bothersome food solicitation behaviors. These can be especially problematic if the cat does not have access to the outdoors to hunt, or if food is provided in a meal format or set amount daily to prevent obesity. In an attempt to get noticed, food solicitation behaviors include vocalization, climbing, jumping, running, even destruction or agressivity (especially when meal feeding is chosen vs ad libitum distribution, creating some food frustration). Often these behaviors occur during night time hours, waking their owners. In an attempt to placate the cat many owners will get up and feed the cat. Unfortunately, although the cat will stop bothering the owner after being fed that time, the act of feeding the cat when they are noisy will result in the behavior continuing since the cat has been successful, i.e. they received food. The reward (food gift) is indeed reinforcing the undesirable behavior.

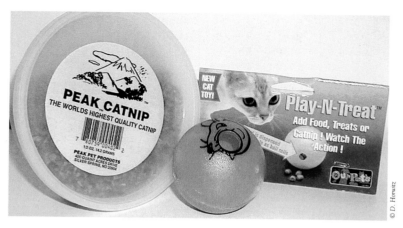

Figure 9 - *Examples of food dispensing toys.*

Owners need to be counseled on how to avoid giving into demands for additional food. First, they must realize that not all vocalization (even that which occurs in the food preparation area) is a request for food. In some cases, it is just a request for interaction such as petting, grooming or play. A lot of owners wrongly interpret some marking behaviors (such as rubbing against the legs) like begging and they fill the bowl! They will effectively think they were right because they see the cat grabbing some kibbles in a very short meal. This will install a nibbling feeding habit in the cat that can eventually facilitate the development of obesity. If the owner responds to these solicitations with food, then food solicitation behavior can become a ritual, helped by the same reinforcement process explained in the previous paragraph.

Feeding the cat on a set feeding schedule allows owners to control food intake. The daily amount provided should be calculated so that the proper amount is fed daily. In some cases providing the food in a food dispensing toy **(Figure 9)** will slow down the rate of consumption and perhaps increase satiety thereby helping to decrease food solicitation behavior.

Figure 10 - *Cats need to be stimulated by new toys to encourage play behavior.*

Daily play sessions limit the risk of obesity. Research has indicated that cats may quickly tire of a toy and the intensity of play diminishes within a few minutes. However, the presentation of a new toy stimulates the return of play (*Hall et al, 2002*) **(Figure 10)**. Exercise can also be increased by placing food bowls at distant locations requiring the cat to walk longer distances to obtain food.

Globally, two methods are employed to stop excessive food solicitation behaviors:
1. to ignore the cat and stop feeding the cat on demand, a process called **extinction**. When the owners attempt to do so, the cat will usually escalate their attempts for a few days, before it decreases. This intensification phase is hard to manage for owners. They

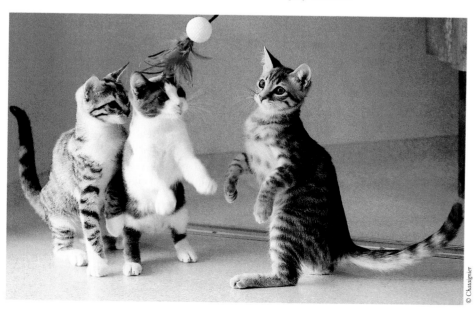

must be aware of such process and must hold out. With time, they will finally see a decrease in the demands. To facilitate success in this intensification phase, the owners can also either confine the cat to an area where they cannot hear it, or interrupt the behavior with a noise stimulus that discourages the cat from continuing.

2. to provide food in a way that is not connected to the owners using **a timed feeding system.** Electronic feeders that operate on a timer can be programmed to provide food at a set time each day and the cat may learn to wait until that time to be fed. In other cases, the feeding time must be slowly manipulated to teach the cat to eat at a later time each day.

Habits have to change to stop the reinforcement process. The owner may change the meaning of some daily situations or clues to play, petting, walking etc.

> Finicky eating patterns

Many pet owners complain that their cat is finicky and eats poorly. While many medical problems can influence hunger and subsequent food intake, these will not be considered here. Only the behavioral issues will be discussed, although all cats with suspected diminished appetite should undergo a complete medical and dental evaluation.

In certain cases a cat may refuse food from time to time simply because they are overfed, not hungry and/or exercising self-regulation of intake. Many new owners are unaware of the nibbling pattern of cat feeding behavior. Other cats may show finicky behavior due to excessive rotation of dietary choices. In other cases the cat has learned that waiting and not eating will result in a different, perhaps more desirable food choice being offered. It is important to take time to explain that too many changes in food varieties or giving treats can be harmful for cats.

Body weight of a finicky cat should be assessed. If the cat is obese and if no disease is suspected, you can hypothesize that the cat may obtain food from additional sources (perhaps from a neighbor, another pets food etc).

The first step is to evaluate the actual amount of food provided daily and the actual amount consumed by the pet. This must also include all treats and human foods provided to the pet. The pet must be weighed: cats that are of normal weight and maintaining their weight over time are usually consuming adequate nutrition to maintain body weight. Body condition score should also be assessed. If the cat is obese then finicky behavior is not a nutritional problem, rather an emotional and behavioral one.

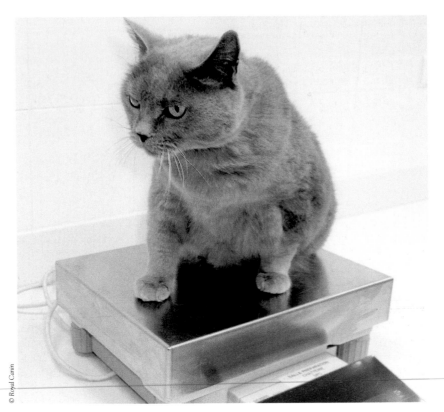

© Royal Canin

Once any underlying medical and dental problems have been identified and treated, behavioral treatment strategies can be employed. Daily caloric needs should be evaluated so that they can be met. The appropriate amount of food that should be provided daily to meet the animal's nutritional needs should be calculated for the owner. Often this is less than the owner has been feeding and this simple reassessment can help the owner understand that the cat is consuming adequate amounts of food. For many animals, setting a feeding routine is useful. The food should be provided at the same time daily in a quiet location and with each cat having its own bowl. Limiting treats can also help increase the desire to eat the provided commercial preparation.

Feeding diets that have increased levels of fat will allow for more nutrition with each mouthful. Excessive attention at meal times should be avoided since this can increase finicky behavior if it becomes an attention seeking tactic. Regular follow up both to weigh the pet and discuss progress with the owner should be scheduled to assess improvement and keep the treatment program on track.

> Anorexia

Anorexia is defined as a diminished appetite. It is associated with many disease processes, trauma and psychological disturbances. In complete anorexia the animal does not eat at all. In partial anorexia the animal may eat some food but not enough to meet its metabolic requirements. Although it is often the reason for consulting the veterinarian, anorexia can result from either an organic or behavioral pathology. It can be due to:
- illness such as fever syndromes or cancer (anorexia may appear before tissue destruction and is the result of tumor metabolites).
- any parodontel disease (creating pain), face or jaw trauma (leading to an inability to eat)
- loss of olfaction: anorexia will last as long as the olfactory mucosa is not restored (renewal needs 4 to 5 days after the destructive agent has been removed)
- psychological stress (depression in reaction to the absence of the owner, even loss of close companions) or physical stress (e.g. excessive handling) (Beaver, 2003): anorexia is accompanied by behavioral escape and withdrawal, house soiling, inhibition of play and exploration.
- anxiety triggered by social stress (antagonistic relationships between household cats, schedule changes, new household members (human or animal)
- anxiety that occurs with transportation, boarding or hospitalization (which can lead to specific learned aversion associated with the diet given during the event).

Cats that are anxious may hide and refuse to come out to eat. In this situation, the anorexia may simply be due to a lack of access to the food bowl. In some individuals anorexia may last only a few days, resolving when the stressful event ends or within a short period of time (2 to 3 days after boarding, house move, or transportation). Often these individuals do not need intervention other than providing easily accessible food and water bowls, possibly located where the cat is hiding. They then compensate by a huge meal. Forcing the cat to come out of hiding to eat is counter productive and may increase rather than decrease anxiety and the resultant loss of appetite.

In multiple cat homes partial anorexia may be ongoing especially if the social situation creates anxiety, stress and aggressive encounters between cats. If food and water bowls are not placed through out the environment, some cats may be unable to access them except at odd times. Even then, they may risk being attacked by other cats within the home for entering their territory. Understanding how the cats use the space provided to them and where various cats spend their time within the space provided can indicate where food, water bowls and litter boxes should be placed. Owners may need to be educated on aggressive interactions between cats. Not all aggressive interactions are overt (hissing, growling, chasing and fighting) but in many cases the actions are covert such as staring, blocking access or displacing the cat from resources (Table 7).

In cats that are anorexic for more than 4 to 5 days, early intervention is suggested. Meal feeding in quiet, dark locations may help some individuals. The use of pheromone diffusers may calm some cats and increase food consumption both in the home and in the kennel or hospital situation, by their appeasing effects. Griffith et al (2000) found that both well and ill cats exposed to the pheromone showed increased interest in food and eating and increased grooming. In the second phase of the same

TABLE 7 - SOCIAL STRESS IN THE DOMESTIC CAT AND ITS EFFECT ON BEHAVIOR

Problem	Effect	Solution
Too many cats in the home	Social stress leads to problems with eating or access to the feeding bowl	One food bowl per cat in various locations
To little space for so many cats	Aggressive interactions and/or hiding possible	Create additional vertical space
Aggression between cats	Chasing, injury, hiding, weight loss due to lack of access to food or anxiety	Create separate territories for cats, perhaps with barriers. Have adequate resources through out the environment
House soiling	Owner distress, relinquishment of cats	More litter boxes in multiple locations (hygiene?)

study, cats exposed to the pheromone and a cat carrier showed significant increase in food intake over 24 hours compared to cats exposed to pheromone alone. Providing secure quiet locations, hiding spots within the cage or kennel and pheromones may therefore help increase eating in some hospitalized and kenneled cats.

When anorexia becomes profound, medical intervention is required. In the early stages some individuals may respond to benzodiazepines which may stimulate appetite. Diazepam however has only a transient effect (3 to 4 days) and acute hepatoxicity is often a serious risk. Mianserine has a quick orexigenic effect, but leads to some desinhibition to be controlled (*Coupry, 2007*). Food should be nearby after administration in case the cat shows interest in eating. Cyproheptadine has also been used in some cases to stimulate appetite. Progestins and anabolic steroids have been tried in the past but, due to potential adverse side effects, they are not recommended and rarely used. Should anorexia persist, enteral feeding tubes need to be employed to allow for supplemental nutrition until the cat recovers and begins to eat on its own. Forced feeding presents however a disadvantage: digestion and absorption are indeed incomplete compared to voluntary eating (food intake stimulates the cephalic phase of digestion which can account for up to half of the gastric acid production).

To summarize, the following simple actions can help solve the problem (*Rabot, 1994*):
- pay attention to any causes of uncomfort (dirty bowl, noisy place, strong smell of litter box, feeding spots with frequent passage, air flows)
- warm the food to 38-40°C (instead of receiving the canned portion directly out of the refrigerator)
- move the bowl to a quieter place (by looking at the cat activity program and locating preferred spots) or separate each cat (to avoid rivalry), at set times
- introduce a novel and very palatable food (the effect only lasts 2 to 3 days), in a sudden way, or spread over several days by increasing proportions into the daily ration
- attend meals for strongly dependent cats or put some food on the fingers to make them linked (especially in the case of reactional depression, but beware of the risk of ritualization)
- ensure renewal of canned food (to avoid oxidative and bacteriological damage).

One must remember that the efficacy of these recommendations may vary between cats and situations. Felines are rarely deceived and often stubborn.

5 - Water drinking in cats

Perhaps because of their evolutionary history, cats tend to have a relatively low intake of water. *Felis lybica*, the European cat ancestor, lived in the desert and was able to concentrate its urine to avoid water losses. Today's cat has kept this ability, but with the risk of forming bladder calculi. Although a cat can be food deprived for several weeks, a few days of water deprivation are enough to put its life in serious danger.

In a multiple cat home food and water bowls must be spread through out the environment so that all cats may access them easily without encountering cats that they have a conflict with. In many cases this will resolve the anorexia and the cat will begin to eat normal amounts of food.

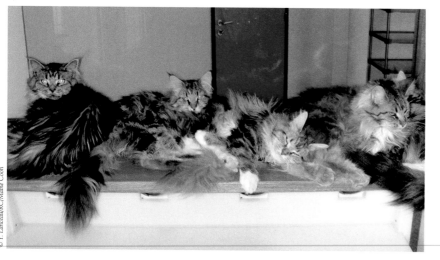

© Y. Lanceau/RC/Maine Coon

Animals have three sources available to meet their water needs:
- water offered for drinking
- water in the food
- water created by the metabolism of nutrients (*Beaver, 2003*). Water is produced by substrate oxidation (fat providing the greatest quantity but carbohydrates providing the best output).

▶ Some pathophysiological considerations

Water needs for cats vary from 55 to 70 mL/kg BW/day. The requirement is in fact related to the dry matter intake: 2mL per gram of dry matter eaten.

Behavior

> Intrinsic regulation of drinking behavior

Thirst is the sensation which triggers water intake. The signal comes from the lateral hypothalamus, close to the hunger center. Regulation is complex and closely linked to variation of plasma osmolarity, controlled by vasopressin.

Drinking satiation is first triggered by oral stimulation on a short term basis (one hour). Gastric distension interferes later, acting mainly on the frequency of intake. Finally, cellular hydration controls water satiation through complex interactions.

Cats are not as sensitive to water loss as the dog and may not drink additional water until they have lost as much as 8% of their body water (*Case, 2003*).

Water intake varies depending upon water losses:
- physiological losses: urination (40mL/kg/day), feces and respiration, lactation
- pathological losses: diarrhea, vomiting, edema, skin injuries, diabetes mellitus, renal failure, etc...

A reduction of blood pressure and blood volume also provoking thirst, through the renin-angiotensin-aldosterone system.

> External factors that influence drinking behavior

The composition of the food

Water intake is affected by food type and moisture content. Cats fed a canned food drink virtually no water since they meet most of their water requirement with their food intake. It is the same with fish or meat fed animals.

Dry food contains only 7-8% water, requiring the animal to consume more water to meet their daily needs. It has been shown that dry food increases fecal water loss but decreases urinary loss (*Jackson & Tovey, 1977*). However, it is important to mention that, while intake is strongly modified, the general water balance is not modified by the moisture content of the food. Urinary calculi are more strongly linked to the urinary mineral composition and urinary pH than to the moisture content of the diet. The only risky situation occurs when there is a transition from canned to dry diet.

Caloric density does not affect water intake. Increasing the dietary protein level results in increased water intake (due to the increased diuresis required to eliminate urea). Carbohydrates decrease water intake, due the higher output of metabolic water from carbohydrate metabolism. Sodium chloride increases water intake. Hypernatremia (> 160 mEq/L) triggers thirst and water consumption in cats.

Temperature

The drinking behavior of the cat is much less influenced by temperature and effort compared to the dog. This can be readily explained as salivary and perspiration losses are not significant in the cat. To facilitate water intake the temperature of the water must not be too cold (not less than 10°C).

Food supply

This factor has been better studied in dogs than in cats. In a restricted regimen, the rate of water intake increases to 2.5 mL per gram of dry matter eaten. A one hour per day feeding pattern leads to a decrease of food and water consumption, compared to the ad libitum situation. In this latter context, water intake is linked to the meals. This is a learned process.

► Practical considerations to encourage a cat to drink

Like food intake, cats drink throughout the entire twenty-four hour period. They drink 12 to 16 times a day but water intake each time is small: 10 to 12 mL. Tremendous variation exists between individuals: this is linked to the sum of physiological effects described above.

To help promote optimal water intake, cats should be provide with fresh, clean water daily from easily accessible water bowls. Owners must pay attention that their cat can have access to water at any time. It is dangerous to provide only one bowl in one room, which could remain closed for a period of time, thus preventing the animal to drink enough. A second bowl elsewhere in the house is recommended, particularly when leaving the cats unsupervised e.g. for a weekend.

Spoiled water is rejected by cats. Glass, metal or porcelain bowls are preferred to plastic ones. The location of the water bowl is important: it has to be put at least 50 cm away from the food bowl and the litter. This distance is sometimes critical when the cat is hospitalized. Water must be palatable: cats are extremely sensitive to odors and some can display preferences for water taken from toilets, sink, etc. Some cats prefer electronic water fountains that aerate the water on a regular basis. One way to increase water palatability is to add meat juice, some milk or some salt. Feeding either a canned food or a liquid food is another alternative.

► Drinking disorders

> Adipsia or hypodipsia

Any cause of hyponatremia (such as severe hepatic disease, congestive heart failure, acute kidney failure, nephrotic syndrome) can stop water intake. These causes of adipsia are in fact compensatory mechanisms.

Conditions of the oral cavity (gingivitis, abscess, tumors, ulcers, fractured jaws, foreign bodies, etc.) may reduce drinking, due to either mechanical or painful reasons.

Adipsia may be simply the result of poor water quality (e.g. water left too long in a dirty bowl). It is nevertheless important to remember that water intake will be still nil as far as all water needed will have been supplied by the food!

> Polydipsia

The average water consumption of a cat depends on the dry matter ingested: around 2mL of water is required for each gram of dry matter consumed.

Any change of drinking behavior must be carefully evaluated. Water intake becomes pathologic beyond 100 mL/kg/day. Any cause of polyuria (> 50 mL/kg) will logically lead to polydipsia (**Table 8**).

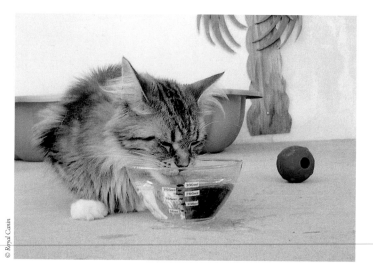

Plasma osmolarity facilitates the identification of what is primary polydipsia and what is compensatory *(Remy, 1986)*:
- if plasma osmolarity is greater than 310 mOsm/L, polyuria is primary and urinary loss creates polydipsia
- when plasma osmolarity is below 290 mOsm/L, polydipsia is primary and the low osmotic pressure leads to polyuria.

Intake of salty foods (fish scraps…) leads to polydipsia, and then to polyuria.

Polydipsia may be a reaction to stress or a substitution activity of a permanent anxiety. Hypercortisolemia triggers excessive water intake *(Landsberg, 2003)*. Situations of conflict situations must be identified and corrected.

Hypercalcemia linked to secondary hyperparathyroidism can stimulate thirst.

TABLE 8 - DIFFERENTIAL DIAGNOSIS POLYDIPSIA *From: Masson, 2004*					
Cause and intensity	**Urinalysis**		**Blood analysis**		
	Osmolarity	Abnormal elements	BUN	Glucose	Other
Chronic kidney disease +	⇩	Protein	⇧	N	
Pyometra +	N	Protein	⇧	N	
Diabetes mellitus ++	⇧	Glucose	N	⇧	
Diabetes insipidus +++	⇩		N	N	
Hyperadrenocorticism ++	N		N	Slight ⇧	Hypercortisolemia ⇧
Hyperthyroidism ++	N		N	N	
Liver failure ++	N	Bilirubin	N or ⇧	N or ⇩	SGPT ⇧
Gastro-enteritis +	⇧		N or ⇧	N	
Hypercalcemia +	N		N	N	Calcium ⇧

N = no change

Hepatic failure can lead to polydipsia through decreased renin degradation and increased angiotensin activity.

Conclusion

The data presented provides an understanding of the normal eating patterns of domestic cats. Some of the information is empirical. Others come from research, in both the natural condition and in the laboratory. Extrapolation from other species and large felids should be avoided.

The data can help veterinarians and pet owners make relevant choices for feeding routines and food types. The domesticated way of life, with increased social relationships and and evolutionary predator behavior must be considered when designing feeding protocols.

Medical problems can often contribute to changes in the selectivity and regulation of food ingestive behavior. Obesity is a major feline health problem. Proper client education and feeding regimes can help prevent and control excessive weight gain. The opposite problem of the fussy or finicky cat is only a problem if the cat is loosing weight. The real issue is in the owner's mind and belief.

Behavioral problems related to feeding and drinking can be due to anxiety, inappropriate provisioning of the cats within the home, learned eating patterns or compulsive disorders. A complete medical and behavioral evaluation should enable the clinician to determine the cause of the problem and therefore prescribe appropriate intervention.

Although the integration of the cat into the family can bring well being and happiness to everyone, the veterinarian will also have to explain to owners to avoid "thinking too human" when taking care of the cat, especially when feeding.

Frequently asked questions about the feeding behavior of the cat

Q	A
Do cats need to have several different flavors?	No, as long as they have a well-balanced diet, cats do not need flavor variety from day to day.
Why are cats fussier than dogs?	In fact, cats are not fussier than dogs. This commonly held belief is untrue. A poorly reared dog may be very hard to please. For some dogs, refusing food is a way of asserting their position in the family. Cats on the other hand, attribute no "social" value to food. If they refuse to eat, it's either because they're sick or because they have a genuine dislike of the food. The competition that exists in a pack always lead dogs to gulp down a maximum amount of food in the shortest possible time, i.e. dogs display "gluttonous" behavior. Cats, as solitary hunters, can take their time to dissect and savor their prey. Their behavior can be described as "tasting".
Are cats sensitive to sweet and salty taste?	Cats are different from dogs and humans. Cats have no preference for sweet tasting foods. This is due to their strictly carnivorous nature. Cats are also less sensitive to salt and have a higher NaCl or KCl detection threshold. Since salt is found naturally in their prey, cats have not been selected for this gustatory capacity present in other mammals, especially herbivores.
Every time I go to the kitchen my cat follows me and cries, what does he want?	Often the most frequent location and time for the cat to interact with the owner is around feeding so they may also choose that location or time to solicit attention. If the cat has been fed and consumed the proper amount to meet their nutritional needs, then they should not be fed when they vocalize. Feeding the cat every time it vocalizes will be seen by the cat as a reward for their behavior and therefore vocalization will increase. Try substituting play, grooming or social interaction rather than feeding the cat when it is not feeding time.
I have two cats and one is overweight and one is not. How can I provide an appropriate diet for each cat?	Each cat may need a different diet to meet their nutritional needs. One solution is to use timed meal feeding. Several times a day each cat is provided their diet and given a certain amount of time to consume their food. To facilitate each cat eating the appropriate food, the cats should be separated during feeding time. Once feeding time is over, the bowls should be put away until the next feeding session. In other situations, the thinner cat may be more agile than the larger cat and can have their food bowl in an elevated location that the heavier cat cannot access.

Q	A
How should I react when my cat refuses to eat the prescription diet?	Transitions to a new diet are best done slowly. The new diet can be offered next to the old diet to help the cat become familiar with the new food. In some cases it might help to mix the food together. If the texture of the two foods (old and new) are very different, this may be a problem for some cats. Using a similar texture food if possible may help the transition.
How can I prevent my cat from hunting birds?	Although unwanted by humans, predatory behavior is a normal cat behavior. Keeping the cat indoors will prevent predation. If that is not possible, some cats will be deterred by wearing a quick release cat collar that is equipped with large bells to warn the birds of their impending approach. Naturally, removing temptation in the form of bird feeders and bird houses is prudent.
I need to increase the amount of liquid (water) that my cat ingests every day. How can I do that?	Water consumption will vary according to the food type provided. Cats on dry kibble diets will drink more water than cats on moist, canned food. Water consumption can be increased by adding water to the canned food or providing water that has been enhanced with fish flavoring. Some cats prefer water that is fresh and aerated and will drink more water if provided water from a running faucet or a pet drinking fountain.

Behavior

References

Bartoshuk LM, Jacobs HL, Nichols TL, et al. Taste rejection of non nutritive sweeteners in cats. J Comp Physiol Psychol 1975; 89: 971-975.

Bateson P. Behavioural development in the cat. In: Turner DC, Bateson P eds. The Domestic Cat; the biology of its behaviour. 2nd ed. Cambridge UK, 2000: 9-22.

Bateson P, Bateson M. Post-weaning feeding problems in young domestic cats - a new hypothesis. Vet J 2002; 163: 113-114.

Beata CA. Feline behavior: can nutrition really make a difference? In: Proceedings, Royal Canin Feline Symposium, 2007: 30-33.

Beaver BV. Feline Behavior. In: A Guide for Veterinarians. 2nd ed. Elsevier Science, USA, 2003: 212-246.

Beaver BV. Sensory development of Felis catus. Lab Anim 1980; 14: 199-201.

Bosch OJ, Sartori SB, Singewald N, et al. Extracellular amino acid levels in the paraventricular nucleus and the central amygdala in high- and low-anxiety dams rats during maternal aggression: regulation by oxytocin. Stress 2007; 10: 261-270.

Boudreau JC. Chemical stimulus determinants of cat neural taste responses to meats. J Am Oil Chem Soc 1977; 54: 464-466.

Boudreau JC, Alev N. Classification of chemoresponsive tongue units of the cat geniculate ganglion. Brain Res 1973; 17: 157-75.

Bouret SG, Draper SJ, Simerly RB. Trophic action of leptin on hypothalamic neurons that regulate feeding. Science 2004; 304: 108-110.

Bradshaw JW. Sensory and experiential factors in the design of foods for domestic dogs and cats. Proc Nutr Soc 1991; 50: 99-106.

Bradshaw JW, Goodwin D, Legrand-Defretin V, et al. Food selection by the domestic cat, an obligate carnivore. Comp Biochem Physiol 1996; 114A: 205-209.

Bradshaw JW, Healey LM, Thorne CJ, et al. Differences in food preferences between individuals and populations of domestic cats Felis sylvestris catus. Appl Anim Behav Sci 2000; 68: 257-268.

Brandt J. Taste receptor genes in carnivore and their relationship to food choice. In: Proceedings, Monell Chemical Senses Center PA USA; Symposium Panelis, Arzon, France, 2006.

Carpenter JA. Species differences in taste preferences. J Comp Physiol Psychol 1956; 49: 139-144.

Case L. The cat: Its behavior, nutrition and health. Iowa State University Press, 2003: 289-341.

Cheney CD, Miller ER. Effects of forced flavor exposure on food neophobia. Appl Anim Behav Sci 1997; 53: 213-217.

Crane SW, Griffin RW, Messent PR. Introduction to commercial pet foods cats. In: Hand MS, Thatcher CD, Remillard RL, Roudebush P eds. Small Animal Clinical Nutrition. 4th ed. Kansas: Mark Morris Institute, 2000: 111-126.

De Braekeleer J, Gross KL, Zicker SC. Normal Dogs. In: Hand MS, Thatcher CD, Remillard RL, Roudebush P eds. Small Animal Clinical Nutrition. 4th ed. Kansas: Mark Morris Institute, 2000: 227.

Dehasse J, De Buyser C. Socio-écologie du chat. Prat Med Chir Anim Comp 1993; 28: 469-478.

Finco DR, Adams DD, Crowell WA, et al. Food and water intake and urine composition in cats: influence of continuous versus periodic feeding. Am J Vet Res 1986; 47: 1638-1642.

Fitzgerald BM, Turner DC. Hunting behaviour of domestic cats and their impact on prey populations. In: Turner DC, Bateson P eds. The Domestic Cat: the biology of its behaviour. 2nd ed. Cambridge University Press, 2000: 152-175.

Foucault V. Contribution à l'étude du comportement alimentaire du chat domestique, Thèse de Doctorat Vétérinaire (Lyon), 1992.

Geering KB. The effect of feeding in the human-cat relationship. In: Proceedings 5th International Conference on the relationship between human and animal, Monaco, 15-18 Nov 1989.

Griffith CA, Steigerwald ES, Buffington CA. Effects of a synthetic facial pheromone on behavior of cats. J Am Vet Med Assoc 2000; 217: 1154-1156.

Hall SL, Bradshaw JWS, Robinson IH. Object play in adult domestic cats; the roles of habituation and disinhibition. Appl Anim Behav Sci 2002; 79: 263-271.

Hinde RA. Animal behavior: a synthesis of ethology and comparative ethology. Mac GrawHill book company, 2nd ed, 1975: 551-555.

Horwitz DF, Mills DS, Heath S. In: BSAVA Manual of Canine and Feline Behavioural Medicine; Gloucester UK, 2002.

Houpt, KA. In: Domestic Animal Behavior. Blackwell Publishing, Ames, Iowa, 2005: 329-334.

Houpt KA. Gastrointestinal factors in hunger and satiety. Neurosci Biobehav Rev 1982; 6: 145-164.

Houpt KA. Feeding and drinking behavior problems. Vet Clin North Am Small Anim Pract 1991; 21: 281-298.

Jackson OF. Urinary pH effects of diet additives. Vet Rec 1977; 101: 31-33.

Kane E, Morris JG, Rogers QR. Acceptability and digestibility by adult cats of diets made with various sources and levels of fat. J Anim Sci 1981; 53: 1516-1523.

Kays RW, DeWan AA. Ecological impact of inside/outside house cats around a suburban nature preserve. Animal Conservation 2004; 7: 273-283.

Knowles RJ, Curtis TM, Crowell-Davis SL. Correlation of dominance as determined by agonistic interactions with feeding order in cats. Am J Vet Res 2004; 65: 1548-1556.

Landsberg G, Hunthausen W, Ackerman L. Handbook of behavior problems of the dog and cat. Elsevier Saunders, Toronto, 2003.

Leyhausen P. Cat Behaviour: the predatory and social behavior of domestic and wild cats. Garland Press, New York 1979.

Li X, Li W, Wang H, et al. Cats lack a sweet taste receptor. J Nutr 2006; 136: 1932S-1934S.

Lott Brown J, Shively DF, Lamotte HR, et al. Color discrimination in the cat. J Comp Physiol Psychol 1973; 81: 534 – 544.

Luesher AU. Compulsive Behaviour In: Horwitz DF, Mills DS, Heath eds. BSAVA Manual of Canine and Feline Behavioural Medicine. Gloucester (UK): BSAVA ed, 2002: 229-236.

Mac Donald LM, Quinton RR, Morris GJ. Aversion of the cat to dietary medium chain triglycerides and caprylic acid. Physiol Behav 1985, 35: 534-544.

May K. Association between anosmia and anorexia in cats, Sciences (New York) 1987; 510: 480-482.

Mugford AR. *External influences on the feeding of carnivores*. The chemical senses and Nutrition, Academic Press, NY 1977: 25-50.

Nelson SH, Evans AD, Bradbury RB. *The efficacy of collar-mounted devices in reducing the rate of predation of wildlife by domestic cats* Appl Anim Behav Sci 2005; 94: 273-285.

Nguyen P, Dumon H, Martin L, et al. *Effects of dietary fat and energy on bodyweight and body composition following gonadectomy in cats.* In: Proceedings 17ᵗʰ ACVIM Congress 1999; Chicago (IL): 139.

Peachey S.E. et Harper E.J. *Ageing does not influence feeding behaviour in cats.* In: J Nutr 2002 (139): 1735-1739.

Remy S. *Étude du comportement alimentaire et de l'élimination fécale et urinaire de l'eau chez des chats nourris avec différents types d'aliments riches en eau.* Thèse de Doctorat Vétérinaire (Toulouse), 1986.

Rabot R. *Le comportement alimentaire et dipsique du chat et ses troubles.* In: Proceedings Séminaire Société Féline Française, 1994: 42-47.

Rowland N. *Glucoregulatory feeding in cats.* Physiol Behav 1981; 26: 901-903.

Rowland NE, Bellush LL, Carlton J. *Metabolic and neurochemical correlates of glucoprivic feeding.* Brain Res Bull 1985; 14: 617-624.

Servet E, Soulard Y, Venet C, et al. *Evaluation of diets for their ability to generate "satiety" in cats.* J Vet Intern Med 2008; 22: in press.

Stasiak M, Zernicki B. *Food conditioning is impaired in cats deprived of the taste of food in early life.* Neurosci Lett 2000; 279: 190-192.

Thorne CJ. *Cat feeding behavior*, Waltham Symposium n° 4, Vet Clin North Am Small Anim Pract 1982: 555-562.

Thorne CJ. *Feline and canine fads.* Vet Rec 1994; 135: 48.

Van den Bos R, Meijer MK, Spruijt BM. *Taste reactivity patterns in domestic cats (felis silvestris catus).* Appl Anim Behav Sci 2000; 69: 149-168.

Woods M, McDonald Ra, Harris S. *Predation of wildlife by domestic cats Felis catus in Great Britain.* Mammal Review 2003; 33: 174-188.

Wyrwicka W, Chase MH. *Importance of the environment in conditioned behavior.* Physiol Behav 2001; 73: 493-497.

Wyrwicka W, Long AM. *Observations on the initiation of eating of new food by weanling kittens.* Pavlov J Biol Sci 1980; 15: 115-22.

Behavior

Palatability and nutritional precision are interconnected

Palatability is essential if the cat is to take in what it needs. The best-balanced food in theory is useless if the cat turns its nose up at it. Even more so when its health demands a special diet that is theoretically not favorable to palatability: limited sodium, fats and proteins. There are various solutions for overcoming this obstacle and retaining an adequate palatability level.

Palatability is not a luxury: it's a vital obligation

The fundamental aim of nutrition is to provide all essential nutrients every single day in a sufficient quantity to cover all needs. The first of these needs is energy, in whatever form the calories are provided.

The formulation of feline diets is above all based on energy density: the ration volume offered to the cat must be compatible with its capacity of digestion:

- too low a volume does not give the cat a feeling of satiety

- too high a volume may not be consumed properly or may cause digestive problems.

Palatability helps the cat overcome certain kinds of stress

For many cats, a loss of appetite is one of the first signs of stress. If the food is not sufficiently palatable and if the period of stress is prolonged, there will be a risk of chronic underconsumption and the appearance of nutritional deficiencies. The cat will lose weight, the quality of its hair will deteriorate and its immune defences will be weakened.

Examples of situations in which the cat's appetite is disturbed

- Changes of environment: when a kitten or an adopted cat arrives in a new home, moves house or is put in a cattery during the holidays.

- Changes to diet: some cats tend to reject a new food (neophobia). This phenomenon is especially observed when the food is offered in unfavorable environmental conditions or when cats have been given the same food for a very long time. Conquering neophobia entails realizing the most gradual dietary transition possible **(Figure 1)** in conditions that are ideal for the cat's well-being, thus preventing the development of an aversion that would be even more difficult to overcome.

FIGURE 1 - TECHNIQUE TO ENSURE GOOD DIETARY TRANSITION

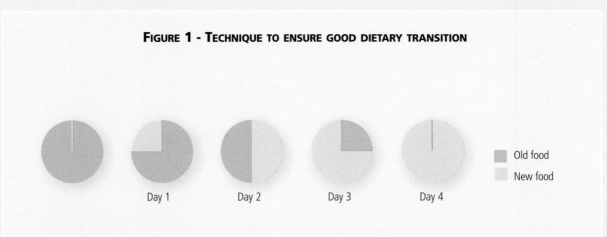

Day 1 Day 2 Day 3 Day 4

Old food
New food

It is advizable to change a diet gradually. For example, mix 25% of the new food with 75% of the old food on day 1. The next day mix together equal quantities and on day 3 mix 75% of the new food with 25% of the old food. On day 4 you can give the cat only the new food.

Behavior

ROYAL CANIN

How is palatability evaluated?

Palatability is measured through objective studies to assess the cat's behavior in the presence of one or several foods. It is mostly interesting to try to estimate the cat's preferences and the way the food is ingested.

The cat's preference for a given food

This can be realized by measuring the respective consumption of two different foods freely available to the cat **(Figure 2)**. The cat's selection criteria are subsequently analysed.

The reliability of the result depends on the number of cats used and the duration of the study among other things. The selection of the most discriminating cats helps increase the sensitivity of the tests.

The way the food is ingested

This reflects the attractiveness of the food for the cat. The quantity of food spontaneously ingested within a given time or the time needed to ingest a given quantity are important data. Videos showing the prehension method and any consumption difficulties provide some useful additional data.

The information obtained at the cattery is confirmed by studying cats owned by private individuals when evaluating palatability in diverse environmental conditions and taking into account such notions as the owner's appreciation of the look of a product and his or her attitude when serving the food, the variable conditions of serving a meal, etc.

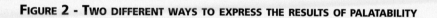

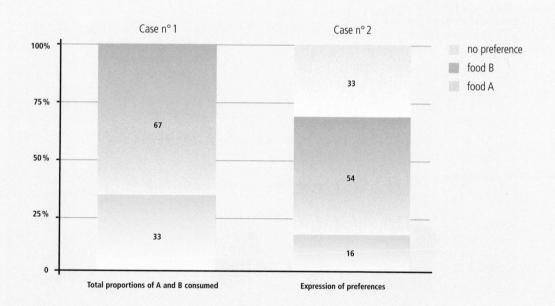

FIGURE 2 - TWO DIFFERENT WAYS TO EXPRESS THE RESULTS OF PALATABILITY

The results can be expressed in two ways:
- Case n°1: the graph only indicates the proportions of foods A and B consumed by all cats.
- Case n°2: 16% of cats preferred food A (i.e. they consumed at least twice as much of food A as they did of food B),
* 54% preferred food B and 33% showed no preference.*
The second method best reflects the differences, because it takes into account the number of cats that show a clear preference.

Does palatability diminish with time?

All food products tend to deteriorate with time. Guaranteeing good palatability during the whole shelf life of a product entails slowing down the aging of the product.

Quality of fats

The conservation of the fats in a food demands close monitoring, particularly those in the kibble coating. In contact with the oxygen in the air, the fat molecules generate the production of unstable molecules – free radicals – that cause oxidation. Liquid fats at ambient temperature (poultry fats, vegetable oils) are the most sensitive to oxidation, because they are unsaturated. Keeping food in the light at a warm temperature accelerates the process.

The role of antioxidants is to block the free radicals before they provoke chain reactions that lead to the appearance of peroxides, then secondary oxidation compounds, aldehydes and ketones. All of these compounds are potentially toxic. It is rare for the cat to consume a food that contains deteriorated fats however, as it is very sensitive to the rancid smell emitted by oxidation. The use of truly effective antioxidants is indispensable to conserve palatability and protect the health of the animal.

Development of the aromatic profile

Expertise on palatability is not restricted to the development of aromas that are particularly attractive to the cat. These aromas are essentially volatile, so they can be easily picked out by the cat's sense of smell. That means they risk evaporating in the ambient air. As a result, the kibbles internal odors come to the fore. The cat does not necessarily find this different aroma profile as pleasant.

Another risk is the deterioration of aromas with time. What starts out being a pleasing flavor may ultimately turn into a negative palatability factor.

The research carried out on palatability entails following the development of these substances to verify their behavior as the product ages. Palatability must remain satisfactory throughout the life of the product, right up to the best before date on the pack.

To limit the risk of the loss of palatability after the pack has been opened, it is important to select the right size of pack for a particular cat's daily consumption. A 4 kg cat that eats an average 50 g of kibbles per day, consumes the equivalent of

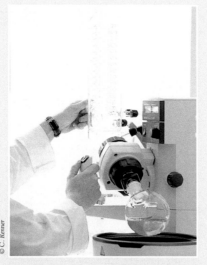

The quality of fats is monitored in the ingredients and in the final product. The freshness and the resistance to oxidation of oils and fats are major criteria for good palatability.

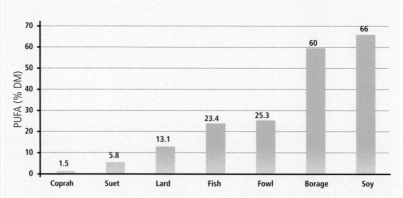

FIGURE 3 - COMPARISON OF THE QUANTITY OF POLYUNSATURATED FATTY ACIDS (PUFA) IN DIFFERENT OILS AND FATS

The higher the PUFA content and the longer the fatty acid chains, the greater the fat's sensitivity to oxidation if not adequately protected.

ROYAL CANIN

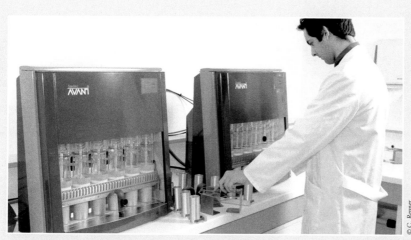

The role of all the antioxidants is to stabilize the fat in the product and the kibble coating to preserve palatability and the health of the cat.

a 1.5 kg (3 lb) bag in a month. The aromas will be conserved well during that period as long as the bag is stored in a dark place in a hermetically sealed container at a stable temperature. It's better not to select a larger bag as this would require a longer period of storage.

Working on conserving the nutritional qualities of the product

The preservation of a product's organoleptic qualities entails vigilance at various levels.

The choice of ingredients

Palatability must be a key factor to take into account from the moment of formulation. The thermal treatment used to separate proteins and fats from a meat has an impact on palatability for example. Likewise, a given source of fat will be favored depending on its resistance to oxidation **(Figure 3)**.

The process

All the technology involved in kibble grinding, cooking, drying and coating is oriented to preserving the original qualities of the ingredients. The time between manufacture and packing is minimized.

Antioxidation

To prevent the oxidative reactions from beginning, it is preferable to use chelated trace minerals (especially iron and copper). Once chelated, their bioavailability is increased and they are unable to catalyze oxidation reactions in the food.

All fats in the food must be fresh and protected before they are transported and used: substances used in cat food are the same as those used in food for human consumption. They are selected on the basis of their safety and efficacy.

Packaging

To rule out the loss of aromas and oxidation the food is kept in an airtight pack totally devoid of oxygen, a technique called modified atmosphere packaging (Figure 4). The air is replaced by a neutral gas (nitrogen) during packaging. The food conserved in this way is protected as the bag is closed. After opening, the aromas are preserved properly by keeping the bag away from light and humidity at a constant, low temperature.

FIGURE 4 - PRINCIPLE OF THE CONTROLLED ATMOSPHERE

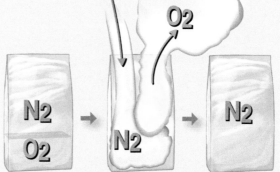

Sealed airtight bag modified
atmosphere = NITROGEN

The air is made up of around 20% oxygen and 80% nitrogen.
The modified atmosphere in the bag is 100% nitrogen, which prevents oxidation phenomena from taking place.

Behavior

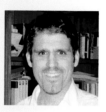

Nicholas J CAVE
BVSc, MVSc,
MACVSc,
Dipl. ACVN

Nutrition and immunity

1 - Nutrition and immunity – Complex interactions 481

2 - The immune system 481

3 - Nutritional requirements for immunity 485

4 - Effects of malnutrition on immunity 488

5 - Effects of immune responses on nutritional status 489

6 - Immune response to dietary antigens (oral tolerance) 493

7 - Nutritional modulation of immunity 497

8 - Effect of route of nutrition 503

Conclusion 504

Frequently asked questions 505

References 507

ABBREVIATIONS USED IN THIS CHAPTER

α LA: alpha linolenic acid
APC: antigen presenting cell
APR: acute phase response
ARA: arachidonic acid
CAM: cell adhesion molecule
CD80/CD86: costimulatory molecules
COX: cycloxogenase
DGLA: dihomo-γ-linolenic acid
EPA: eicosapentaenoic acid
FHV: feline herpes virus

HETE: hydroxyeicosatetraenoic acid
HPETE: hydroperoxy-eicosate-traenoic acid
IFN: interferon
Ig: immunoglobulin
IL: interleukin
iNOS: nitric oxide synthetase
LOX: lipoxogenase
LPS: lipopolysaccharide
LT: leukotriene

MHC: major histocompatibility complex
NF-κB: nuclear transcription factor
NK: natural killer cell
NO: nitric oxide
NOS: nitric oxide synthase
PAMPS: pathogen associated molecular patterns
PG: prostaglandin
PPAR: peroxisome proliferator-activated receptor

PUFA: polyunsaturated fatty acids
SIRS: systemic inflammatory response syndrome
TGF β: transforming growth factor
Th₁: lymphocyte Th_1
TLR: toll-like receptors
Th₂: lymphocyte Th_2
TNF-α: tumor necrosis factor
TX: thromboxane

Nutrition and immunity

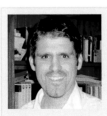

Nicholas J CAVE
BVSc, MVSc, MACVSc, Dipl. ACVN

Nick Cave graduated from Massey University (New Zealand) in 1990 and worked in private practice for 7 years before completing a residency in internal medicine and Masters in Veterinary Science at Massey University. He then completed a residency in clinical nutrition and studied for a PhD in nutrition and immunology at the University of California, Davis, and became a diplomate of the American College of Veterinary Nutrition in 2004. He is now senior lecturer in small animal medicine and nutrition at Massey University.

There are few, perhaps no, diseases in which the pathogenesis does not in any way involve the immune system. The involvement may be primary as in hypersensitivities, secondary as in infectious diseases, or in more obscure and surprising ways such as in the effect of obesity on immunity. Immune function ranges from simple, innate, barrier defenses, through to complex, highly adaptive, antigen-specific multi-cellular responses.

From basic to complex, the immune system is, like any other body system, dependant on the appropriate supply of nutrients and sensitive to nutritional deficiencies and imbalances. But unlike other body systems, the rapid changes in nutrient requirements associated with cellular replication, cellular synthesis, and highly energetic activities makes the immune system very responsive to both long term and short term nutrition. Given the vital role that the immune system has both for the benefit, and in certain diseases the detriment of the animal, it is important to understand how nutrition affects immunity in health and disease. This chapter aims to explore some of the most important aspects of how nutrition affects immunity in cats.

1 - Nutrition and immunity – Complex interactions

As indicated in **Figures 1 and 2**, nutrition directly affects the immune response. This can be in three general ways:
1. enhancement or exaggeration of the response
2. suppression or limitation of the response
3. changing the nature of the response

Whether a change is good or bad depends upon the specific disease state, and the individual patient. Attenuation of an immune response may be beneficial in hypersensitivity diseases (e.g. atopic dermatitis) or in overwhelming systemic immune activation (i.e. systemic inflammatory response syndrome or SIRS). Likewise, enhancement of an immune response may be desirable for prevention or elimination of infection, or immunity to tumor development.

In contrast, modulation of immunity can be detrimental or even fatal to the host. Immunosuppression in the face of infection can lead to prolonged morbidity or even overwhelming sepsis. Enhancement of immunity may lead to increased self-damage in states already characterized by excessive or poorly regulated immune activation (e.g. SIRS, hypersensitivity diseases). Clearly then, one diet cannot fit the needs of all.

To understand how nutrition can affect immunity, once must first understand the nature of immunity.

2 - The immune system

► Function

The immune system, in all its complexity, has evolved for the defense against infectious organisms from viruses, bacteria, and fungi, to large multicellular parasites. Immune responses range from non-specific barrier-type functions, to phylogenetically advanced, complex, adaptive responses that may involve destruction or elimination of the pathogen (**Figure 3**). A perfect response to infection would result in elimination without self damage. Immune responses are never perfect however, and damage to the host always occurs, ranging from undetectable to disproportionate, and at its most extreme, fatal.

Remembering this basic concept is essential in interpreting the effect of nutrition on immunity.

FIGURE 1 - NUTRITION AND IMMUNITY

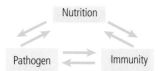

The interaction between nutrition and immunity is complex and incompletely understood.
An important basic concept is that the interaction is bi-directional.

FIGURE 2 - NUTRITION, PATHOGEN AND IMMUNITY

Nutrition

Pathogen ⇄ Immunity

If one takes into account the specific pathogen or tumor cell that is initiating the immune response, the interaction becomes even more complex.

FIGURE 3 - FEATURES AND FUNCTIONS OF INNATE AND ADAPTIVE IMMUNITY
Key points of nutritional modulation

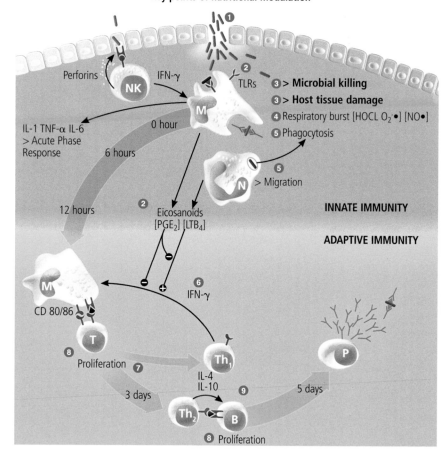

Site of effect: nutritional modification
1. Vitamin A, protein-energy malnutrition
2. Polyunsaturated fatty acids (PUFA)
3. Antioxidants, protein-energy malnutrition
4. Antioxidants, arginine, glutamine, genistein, carotenoids
5. Glutamine, genistein, iron
6. Lutein, genistein
7. Leptin, vitamin E, PUFA
8. Nutrients presented in **Table 2**, lutein, genistein (in cats?), copper, zinc
9. Lutein, vitamin A, iron

TABLE 1 - KEY COMPONENTS OF INNATE IMMUNITY

Component	Examples	Functions
Epithelial secretions		Exclusion of infection, transport of antimicrobial molecules
Epithelial barriers		Exclusion of infection
Antimicrobial molecules	Defensins, lysozyme	Microbial killing
Natural antibodies	IgM	Opsonization, complement fixation
Phagocytes	Neutrophils, macrophages	Phagocytosis and killing of microbes
Killing cells	NK cells	Lysis of infected or neoplastic cells, activation of macrophages
Coagulation proteins	Thrombin	Physical confinement of microbes
Complement		Microbial killing, opsonization, chemotaxis, leukocyte activation
C-reactive protein		Opsonization

FIGURE 4 - LIGANDS AND EFFECTS OF TOLL LIKE RECEPTORS (TLR) SIGNALING

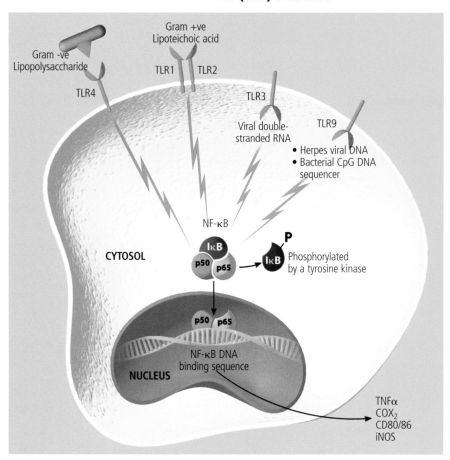

One common signaling pathway after engagement of TLRs is the activation of the nuclear transcription factor NF-κB. The activated NF-κB dimer then diffuses into the nucleus where it promotes the transcription of a variety of pro-inflammtory genes.

► General aspects of immune responses

> Innate

Anatomical and physiological mechanisms that contribute to immunity and that are in place regardless of previous exposure, are referred to as "innate". Many of these mechanisms are phylogenetically ancient (e.g. lysozyme, phagocytes), whilst others are complex and have only evolved in vertebrates, becoming refined in mammalian species (e.g. natural killer cells) (Table 1).

In mammals, the initial role of innate immunity is to exclude micro-organisms where possible. When infection occurs, the innate responses to the pathogen result in any, or a combination of:

1. elimination of infection
2. limiting the initial progression of infection (the "speed-bump" for initial infectious agents)
3. stimulation of adaptive immunity through the production of the early inflammatory response to infection. Thus innate immunity provides the "danger signals" that alert and activate adaptive immune responses.

Recognition of microbes

Cells of innate immunity have evolved receptors that recognize phylogenetically conserved molecules. These molecular patterns have been termed **pathogen associated molecular patterns** or "PAMPS". Examples of PAMPS are lipopolysaccharide (LPS) from gram negative bacterial cell walls, lipoteichoic acid from gram positive bacterial cell walls, and double-stranded RNA from viruses. The PAMP receptors include scavenger receptors, mannose receptors, and the family of Toll-like receptors (TLR) (Akira, 2003). To date there are 10 known mammalian TLRs, although the expression of all 10 types has not yet been described in cats. Most TLRs are membrane proteins, although the TLR 9 binds to its ligand intracellularly (bacterial DNA). Binding of a TLR with its ligand results in the generation of the nuclear transcription factor NF-κB, which diffuses into the nucleus and binds to specific sites on the DNA of the host cell, leading to the transcription of a variety of pro-inflammatory genes. In macrophages and neutrophils these genes include cytokines (TNF-α, IL-1, and IL-12), adhesion molecules (E-selectin), cycloxogenase (COX), nitric oxide synthase (iNOS), and on macrophages the co-stimulatory molecules CD80 and CD86.

The net effect of TLR signaling in leukocytes is migration into inflamed tissues, enhanced killing of microbes or infected cells, and the production of inflammatory cytokines and chemokines to signal and activate the cells of the adaptive immune response **(Figure 4)**.

Killing of phagocytosed microbes

Phagocytosed microbes remain within the membrane bound phagosome in the cytoplasm. Once internalized, these phagosomes then fuse with preformed lysosomes, which contain several proteases (e.g. elastase). In addition, activation of the phagocyte (e.g. by signaling through TLRs) results in assembly of the multi-subunit machinery of the NADPH-oxidase in the phagosome membrane, and within the plasma membrane. This enzyme complex catalyses the reduction of diatomic oxygen (O_2) to the superoxide radical ($O_2^{\bullet -}$). The $O_2^{\bullet -}$ is then enzymatically dismutated to produce hydrogen peroxide, a potent oxidant that may be partially responsible for microbial killing. However, the presence of myeloperoxidase within the phagosome utilizes the peroxide to produce a more potent antibacterial, **hypochlorous acid** (HOCl). This process of producing powerful oxidants following activation and phagocytosis by neutrophils and macrophages rapidly utilizes large amounts of available oxygen and is termed the **respiratory burst (Figure 5)** (*DeLeo et al, 1999*).

Following activation of the phagocyte, the inducible form of **nitric oxide synthetase** (iNOS) is also expressed, resulting in the production of the free radical **nitric oxide** (•NO), which reacts with superoxide to form the toxic metabolite peroxynitrite (*Eiserich et al, 1998*). These various oxidants are not only confined to the phagosome, but are also released extracellularly to contribute to microbial killing in the immediate vicinity. Inevitably, this results in collateral oxidative damage to surrounding tissues.

FIGURE 5 - RESPIRATORY BURST AND HOCL PRODUCTION

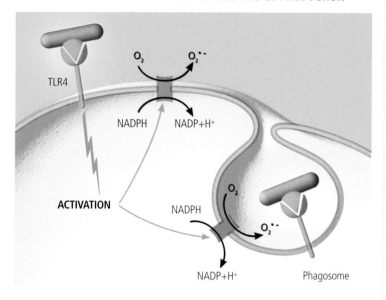

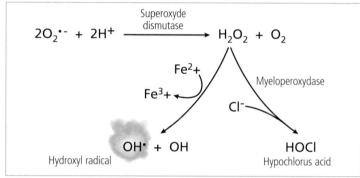

A: *NADPH oxidase is assembled at the outer and phagosome membranes to produce extra and intracellular superoxide (O_2^-).*

B: *Superoxide will then be dismutated to H_2O_2 which will react with a transition metal (Fenton reaction) to form the highly reactive hydroxyl radical (OH $^-$), or to be converted into hypochlorus acid ("bleach").*

To protect themselves from massive autogenously derived oxidative damage, phagocytes require greater concentrations of cytosolic (aqueous) and membrane (lipophilic) antioxidants, which are degraded and rapidly replenished during the respiratory burst. The most important antioxidants in this regard appear to be glutathione, ascorbate, tocopherol, and taurine. Feline neutrophils contain high intracellular concentrations of taurine. In fact, taurine constitutes 76% of the free amino acid cytosolic pool, compared with 44% in lymphocytes (*Fukuda et al, 1982*). Elimination of HOCl by the conversion of taurine to taurine chloramine protects cells against endogenously created oxidants. It has been also suggested that the taurine chloramine may also act as an intracellular signaling molecule that limits further $O_2^{\bullet -}$ and •NO production.

However, in cats maintained on taurine deficient diets, suppression of both phagocytosis and respiratory burst activity by neutrophils occurs, consistent with its role primarily as an antioxidant (*Schuller-Levis et al, 1990*).

Natural killer cells

Natural killer cells (NK cells) are large granular lymphocytes, distinct from T and B lymphocytes. NK cells are responsible for the identification and killing of virally infected and neoplastic cells, without prior exposure (sensitization). NK cells lyse target cells by releasing granules of the enzymes perforin, which creates pores in cell membranes, and granzyme, which enters the perforated cell and induces programmed cell death (apoptosis). Activated NK cells are also important secretors of IFN-γ, and are thus important activators of macrophages in the vicinity, increasing their phagocytic and respiratory burst capabilities.

> Adaptive immunity

Adaptive immunity is stimulated by infection, and by signaling from the innate immune system. With subsequent re-exposure to the infectious organism, the magnitude, specificity, and speed of the response increases, hence the term **adaptive immunity**. Adaptive immunity is the domain of the T and B lymphocytes, whereby humoral (antibody) responses or cellular responses are generated against specific molecules termed **antigens (Figure 3).**

> Eicosanoids

Eicosanoids are a group of lipid messengers synthesized from the 20-carbon polyunsaturated fatty acids (PUFA) dihomo-γ-linolenic acid (DGLA; 20:3n-6), arachidonic acid (ARA; 20:4n-6) and eicosapentaenoic acid (EPA; 20:5n-3). Eicosanoids include prostaglandins (PGs), thromboxanes (TXs), leukotrienes (LTs), lipoxins, hydroperoxy-eicosatetraenoic acids (HPETE) and hydroxyeicosatetraenoic acids (HETE).

FIGURE 6 - THE PRODUCTION OF EICOSANOIDS FROM FATTY ACID PRECURSORS RELEASED FROM CELL MEMBRANE PHOSPHOLIPIDS BY THE ACTION OF PHOSPHOLIPASE A2

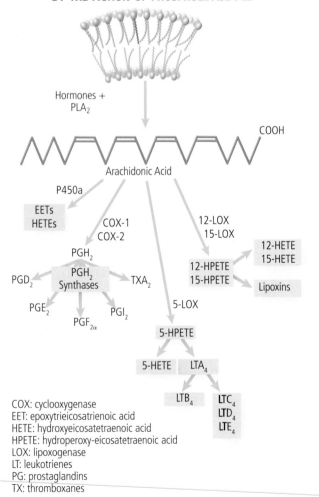

COX: cyclooxygenase
EET: epoxytrieicosatrienoic acid
HETE: hydroxyeicosatetraenoic acid
HPETE: hydroperoxy-eicosatetraenoic acid
LOX: lipoxogenase
LT: leukotrienes
PG: prostaglandins
TX: thromboxanes

The fatty acid precursor for eicosanoid synthesis is released from cell membrane phospholipids, usually by the action of phospholipase A2, which is activated in response to a noxious cellular stimulus **(Figure 6)**. Generally, the membranes of cells in cats on most commercial diets contain 5 to 10 times more ARA than EPA; thus ARA is usually the principal precursor for eicosanoid synthesis, giving rise to the 2-series PGs and TXs, and the 4-series LTs *(Plantinga et al, 2005)*. However, the exact proportion of other 20 carbon PUFA in cell membranes is determined by the relative proportions of them, and their shorter 18 carbon precursors in the diet of the animal.

PGE_2 has a number of pro-inflammatory effects including inducing fever, increasing vascular permeability and vasodilation and enhancing pain and edema caused by other agents such as histamine *(Harris et al, 2002)*. PGE_2 suppresses lymphocyte proliferation and natural killer cell activity and inhibits production of tumor necrosis factor (TNF)-α, interleukin (IL)-1, IL-6, IL-2 and interferon (IFN)-γ In these respects then, PGE_2 is also immunosuppressive and anti-inflammatory. PGE_2 does not affect the production of the Th2-type cytokines IL-4 and IL 10, but promotes immunoglobulin E (IgE) production by B lymphocytes. Therefore PGE_2 supports a Th2-biased adaptive response, and inhibits Th1 responses.

LTB_4 increases vascular permeability, enhances local blood flow, is a potent chemotactic agent for leukocytes, induces release of lysosomal enzymes, enhances the respiratory burst, inhibits lymphocyte proliferation and promotes natural killer cell activity. LTB_4 enhances production of TNFα, IL-1 and IL-6 by monocytes and macrophages, and enhances Th1 cytokine production.

To add to the complexity, PGE_2 inhibits 5-lipoxogenase, thereby interfering with production of LTB_4, and ARA also gives rise to anti-inflammatory lipoxins. Thus, eicosanoids are pro- as well as anti-inflammatory, and together they regulate inflammation. The overall effect will depend upon the timing of production of the different eicosanoids, the sensitivity of target cells, and the concentrations of the different eicosanoids produced.

3 - Nutritional requirements for immunity

▶ During the development period

The first and perhaps most significant effect of nutrition on immunity occurs during the development of the immune system (*Cunningham-Rundles et al, 2005*). Cells of the immune system develop in utero, but this is followed by an important period of maturation soon after birth, continuing to develop throughout life. Deficiencies of zinc, protein, essential amino acids, vitamin A, and copper are only some of the many nutritional variables that can impair development of the immune system in young, growing animals. Micronutrient deficiencies affect the adaptive immune responses, and innate responses **(Table 2)**. Thymic and splenic lymphocyte numbers can be greatly reduced by maternal deficiencies, most notably zinc. Serum antibody responses in young animals to vaccination can be affected by maternal deficiencies of nutrients such as of zinc, iron, copper, selenium, and magnesium.

The net effects of malnutrition during development are altered microbial colonization of mucosal surfaces, impaired responses to commensals and pathogens, increased susceptibility to infection, and decreased ability to resolve infection once established. Such defects may last well beyond the initial period of malnutrition and alter an animal's immunophenotype for life.

TABLE 2 - THE EFFECTS OF SPECIFIC NUTRIENT DEFICIENCIES ON IMMUNITY

Primary nutrient deficiency	Immunological defects	Clinical manifestation
Zinc	Thymic atrophy, lymphopenia, altered T-lymphocyte differentiation, reduced Th1 cytokine production, decreased antibody production	Diarrhea, increased susceptibility to infection from skin commensals
Copper	Lymphopenia, reduced lymphocyte proliferation	Neutropenia, anemia
Selenium	Decreased, increased viral virulence??	Increased susceptibility to infection, increased organ oxidative damage
Iron	Decreased humoral responses, decreased phagocytosis and respiratory burst, reduced T-lymphocyte proliferation	Anemia, increased susceptibility to infection
Vitamin E	Increased IgE, increased PGE_2 production	Increased atopic disease signs? Increased organ oxidative damage
Vitamin A	Mucosal barrier defects (squamous metaplasia), Lymphopenia, depressed antibody production, decreased Th2 responses, depressed neutrophil and macrophage maturation	General increased susceptibility to infection - especially respiratory infections, diarrhea
Protein	Impaired cell mediated responses, decreased cytokine production	General increased susceptibility to infection
Protein – energy malnutrition	Thymic atrophy, reduced lymphoid tissue mass (lymph nodes), decreased circulating T-lymphocytes and B-lymphocytes, Impaired cell mediated responses, decreased cytokine production, reduced neutrophil migration	General increased susceptibility to infection from exogenous and endogenous sources, increased morbidity and mortality, diarrhea (villous blunting, chronic enteritis)

Figure 7 - Anerobic glycolytic pathway

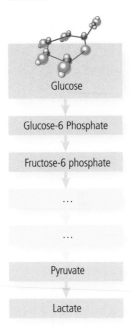

Glucose

↓

Glucose-6 Phosphate

↓

Fructose-6 phosphate

↓

…

↓

…

↓

Pyruvate

↓

Lactate

► Essential nutrients for fuel

> Glucose

Glucose is essential for monocytes, neutrophils, and lymphocytes. Following activation of macrophages and neutrophils, or stimulation of lymphocyte proliferation, glucose oxidation increases dramatically, although it is only partially oxidized, with lactate being the predominant end product **(Figure 7)**. Glutamine is another vital fuel for both cell types, and at rest, may account for more than 50% of ATP production by these cells. Like glucose, glutamine is only partially oxidized, with glutamate, aspartate, and lactate as the end products, and only a small amount being oxidized completely to CO_2, H_2O, and NH_3. Although fatty acids and ketones can be oxidized for ATP production, cellular activation and proliferation of leukocytes does not increase the rate of usage of either substrate *(Newsholme et al, 1987; Newsholme & Newsholme, 1989)*.

Incomplete oxidation of glucose and glutamine occurs despite the presence of mitochondria and functioning citric acid cycles. This is consistent with the need for these cells to operate in areas of low oxygen availability (e.g. ischemic tissue, or unvascularized spaces). The high rates of glucose and glutamine utilization is partly to provide intermediates for the biosynthesis of purine and pyrimidine nucleotides which are required for the synthesis of DNA and mRNA by these cells, and partly to maintain high rates of metabolic flux through the pathways to allow for rapid large changes in utilization that follows activation.

> Glutamine

Plasma glutamine concentrations affect the susceptibility of cells to different apoptosis triggers: where glutamine-starving cells are more sensitive to apoptosis *(Oehler and Roth, 2003)*. In contrast, glutamine may protect activated T cells from apoptosis. A similar protective effect against apoptosis has been demonstrated in neutrophils, in which glutamine also appears to positively regulate the expression of the NADPH oxidase. The immunosuppressive effect of asparaginase has been shown to be due to its ability to hydrolyse glutamine, rather than to the reduction of asparagines *(Kitoh et al, 1992)*. In addition, states associated with low plasma glutamine concentrations are also associated with suppression of both innate and adaptive immunity.

Plasma glutamine is almost entirely derived from skeletal muscle, since dietary glutamine is either utilized by the intestine or the liver, and plasma glutamine only rises very slightly following a meal. During inflammatory responses, muscle catabolism increases in response to low plasma insulin, or muscle insulin resistance induced by cortisol and catabolic cytokines *(Kotler, 2000)*. This provides a source of glutamine both for hepatic gluconeogenesis, but also directly to leukocytes. Thus feeding in systemic inflammatory disease states with glutamine free amino acid sources would be expected to inhibit muscle glutamine release, suppress plasma glutamine concentrations, and thus lead to relative immunosuppression. Conversely, glutamine supplementation enhances macrophage phagocytic activity, helps maintain circulating T lymphocyte numbers, and normalizes lymphocyte function in models of severe sepsis. Predictably, glutamine supplementation of TPN solutions has been shown to reduce morbidity in some septic human patients *(Fuentes-Orozco et al, 2004)*.

When glutamine is supplemented orally, the form of glutamine that is administered is important. Glutamine utilization is significantly more efficient when glutamine is consumed as part of a polypeptide than when it is consumed as a free amino acid *(Boza et al, 2000)*.

GLUTAMINE ABSORPTION

Absorption and utilization of amino acids differs when they are fed as free amino acids or as part of intact polypeptides. A mixture of small peptides is of greater nutritive value than a mixture of free amino acids with a similar composition for both growth and recovery from malnutrition. When starved rats are re-fed, body weight gain is greater, and the plasma concentration of total amino acids -especially glutamine- is significantly higher in rats fed a whey protein hydrolysate-based diet compared with those fed an amino acid-based diet *(Boza et al, 2000)*.

In addition, energy conversion efficiency, protein efficiency ratio, and nitrogen retention are significantly higher in hydrolysate-fed rats. In humans, the glutamine concentration in the duodenal mucosa increases with the enteral supplementation of glutamine-rich proteins compared with a free glutamine solution, despite there being no difference in plasma glutamine concentrations

(Preiser et al, 2003). Potential explanations for these findings include poor solubility of certain free amino acids in the intestinal lumen, rapid absorption of free amino acids leading to an increase in hepatic oxidation, altered intestinal oxidation, and increased catabolism by intestinal flora of free amino acids over polypeptides.

Glutamine can be fed as a free amino acid supplement, as part of a polypeptide in a hydrolysed protein diet, or as part of an intact protein in a conventional food protein source. The combination of glutamine availability, digestibility, and reduced antigenicity may make moderately hydrolysed protein diets ideal for enteral feeding in severe inflammatory disease states.

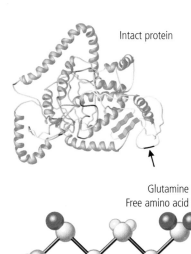

Intact protein

Glutamine
Free amino acid

Polypeptide

Glutamine

► Cell division

Other than essential amino acids and sufficient substrate for fuel, several vitamins are required for leukocyte function and replication (**Table 3**). During an immune response, this is particularly important for lymphocytes.

Deficiencies in any of the essential nutrients listed in **Table 2** will limit cell proliferation, and hence alter cell mediated and humoral immune responses.

Glutamine warrants special mention again, since its availability is often reduced in severe illness, and low plasma concentrations are correlated with morbidity in humans and experimental studies. The major use of glutamine by replicating lymphocytes is not simply as a fuel, but also for nucleotide synthesis (**Figure 8**), whereby low glutamine concentrations inhibit, and increased concentrations stimulate lymphocyte proliferation following stimulation. In addition, this effect of glutamine on replicating lymphocytes is enhanced by the amino acid arginine.

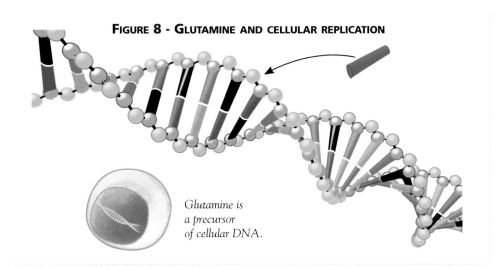

FIGURE 8 - GLUTAMINE AND CELLULAR REPLICATION

Glutamine is a precursor of cellular DNA.

TABLE 3 - KEY NUTRIENTS FOR LEUKOCYTE REPLICATION	
Vitamins	**Other compounds**
Biotin	Choline
Folic acid	Inositol
B$_{12}$	Para-amino benzoic acid
Pyridoxine	Glutamine
Riboflavin	
Thiamine	
Pantothenic acid	
Niacin	

487

FIGURE 9 - ANTIOXIDANTS: MODE OF ACTION

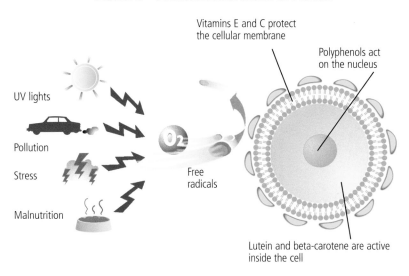

UV lights

Pollution

Stress

Malnutrition

Free radicals

Vitamins E and C protect the cellular membrane

Polyphenols act on the nucleus

Lutein and beta-carotene are active inside the cell

► Antioxidants

Generally speaking, dietary antioxidants fulfill two roles in immune responses. Firstly they protect leukocytes against endogenously derived free radical damage, and secondly they protect the host against bystander damage from the same free radicals (**Figure 9**). The requirement for increased intracellular antioxidant capacity in neutrophils and macrophages has been discussed above. This requirement is met by taurine, glutathione, ascorbate, and tocopherol. Glutathione plays a pivotal role as an antioxidant both through direct interaction with free radicals, but also as a substrate for the regeneration of ascorbate. Glutamine availability can limit glutathione production, and supplementation of glutamine can increase superoxide production by neutrophils.

In addition, several other dietary antioxidants have been shown to have an effect on immunity. Notable amongst them, are the carotenoids (**Figure 9**). Both β-carotene and lutein are incorporated into lymphocytes and neutrophils of both cats and dogs, especially mitochondrial membranes, where they probably function to protect the lipid membranes from endogenous free-radical damage (*Chew & Park, 2004*).

Extracellular (plasma) antioxidants are also important for limiting damage to whole tissues and the vascular endothelium during an immune response. Taurine, ascorbate, tocopherol, glutathione, and carotenoids, all contribute to whole organ defense against free radicals produced by activated phagocytes.

4-Effects of malnutrition on immunity

► Starvation

Starvation leads to atrophy of lymphoid organs, decreased numbers and function of circulating leukocytes, and physical and functional defects in the epithelial barriers (**Table 3**). The net result is an increase in susceptibility to infection from both endogenous sources such as skin and intestinal commensals, and exogenous sources such as nosocomially derived organisms.

In dogs, starvation results in decreased circulating lymphocyte numbers, decreased lymphocyte proliferation in response to stimulation, and impaired ability to generate antigen-specific T-lymphocyte and B-lymphocyte responses to exogenously administered antigens. Neutrophil chemotaxis, and hepatic production of acute phase proteins is reduced (*Dionigi et al, 1977*). Deficiencies of specific nutrients can produce various defects including vitamin E deficiency, which in dogs has been shown to reduce lymphocyte proliferation, an effect that is only partially restored by supplementation with other antioxidants (*Langweiler et al, 1983*). Although the effects of malnutrition on immunity have not been specifically evaluated in cats, it is unlikely to be significantly different from other species. Serum albumin concentration correlates strongly with body condition score in cats presenting to veterinary hospitals, and it is likely that immune-indices are likewise decreased (*Chandler & Gunn-Moore, 2004*).

▶ Leptin

Leptin receptors are expressed on many leukocytes including lymphocytes, monocytes, and neutrophils. Leptin has many influences on adaptive immunity, such as inducing a switch towards Th1-biased responses by increasing IFN-γ and TNF-α secretion, and by suppressing Th2-lymphocyte responses. Leptin promotes the generation, maturation and survival of thymic T cells, and it increases the proliferation of, and IL-2 secretion by, naive T cells. Thus during starvation or prolonged periods of weight loss, suppressed leptin secretion probably contributes to the immunosuppressive state, which can be corrected with either leptin administration or recovery of body fat mass (*Meyers et al, 2005*).

▶ Obesity

No studies have yet evaluated immune function in obese cats; It is expected that obesity in cats will result in similar alterations in immunocompetence as have been recognized in obese humans, and many studies of experimental obesity in rodents.

In species studied to date, reductions in lymphocyte responses to stimulation are seen in obesity and the normalization of these responses have been reported following weight reduction. Reduced NK cell function, altered CD8: CD4 lymphocyte ratios, and reduced respiratory burst activity by neutrophils have been described in obese humans and rodents.

Perhaps paradoxically, obesity in humans and experimental models is increasingly recognized as a state associated with chronic inflammation. Obesity is characterized by increased circulating inflammatory cytokine concentrations and increased acute phase protein production (*Tilg & Moschen, 2006*). The inflammatory cytokines are produced from activated macrophages within the excessive adipose tissue, but also from excessively full adipocytes themselves. The subclinical low-grade inflammation contributes to peripheral insulin resistance in humans, and may do so in obese cats as well.

5 - Effects of immune responses on nutritional status

Immune responses to infection, neoplasia, or as the result of immune-mediated disease, can affect the nutritional status of the patient (**Table 4**).

▶ Anorexia

An almost universal finding in significant inflammatory disease states is a disturbance in food intake that ranges from a suppressed appetite to complete anorexia. This loss of appetite is considered part of the acute phase response. Inflammatory cytokines are important mediators of the suppression of food intake, particularly IL-1, IL-6, and TNF-α (*Langhans, 2000*). The site of action of cytokines can be on central nuclei (hypothalamus) or on peripheral nerves that then produce ascending signals through sensory afferent pathways to central feeding centers.

The fact that anorexia of infection is an almost universal effect in all mammalian species, suggests that it might have a benefit. In support of this notion is the observation that force feeding of anorexic septic mice increases mortality, and in those that survive, the time

TABLE 4 - THE EFFECTS OF IMMUNE RESPONSES ON NUTRITIONAL STATUS

	Mechanisms	Sequelae or examples
Depressed food intake	IL-1, IL-6, TNF-α: CNS and peripheral effects	Weight loss, loss of lean body mass, loss of fat mass, nutrient deficiency
Impaired nutrient absorption	Villous atrophy, enteritis	Decreased fat soluble vitamin absorption, vitamin B$_{12}$ deficiency
Increased loss	Enteritis, increased glomerula permeability	Hypoproteinemia, vitamin A deficiency
Increased requirements	Fever, leukocyte replication, tissue repair	Increased glutamine, tocopherol, folic acid, vitamin A, energy requirements?
Altered metabolism and systemic transport		Insulin resistance and hyperglycemia, hyperlipidemia, decreased serum glutamine

TABLE 5 - SERUM ANALYTES THAT CHANGE DURING AN ACUTE PHASE RESPONSE (ACUTE PHASE REACTANTS)

Positive acute phase reactants in mammals	Negative acute phase reactants in mammals
TNF-α, IL-1, IL-6,	*Retinol binding protein*
Cortisol	Albumin
C-reactive protein, Serum amyloid A, fibrinogen, haptoglobulin, ceruloplasmin	Transferrin
Cu	Fe, Zn, Ca

to survival is increased (*Murray & Murray, 1979*). This deleterious effect of over-nutrition in sepsis and other systemic inflammatory responses has been confirmed in other species, including humans (see below).

These findings suggest that in seriously ill septic patients, consideration should be given to the risks of overfeeding, as well as what might constitute an ideal dietary composition. Thus although it is not suggested that starvation is preferable to supportive nutrition in severe infection, it is important that one considers how the evolved response of anorexia and the associated metabolic derangements might be instructive in formulating ideal diets for sepsis.

► The acute phase response

The acute phase response (APR) is a prominent systemic reaction of the organism to local or systemic disturbances in its homeostasis caused by infection, trauma or surgery, neoplasia, or immune mediated diseases. Cytokines activate receptors on different target cells leading to a systemic reaction resulting in activation of the hypothalamic-pituitary-adrenal axis, reduction of growth hormone secretion and a number of physical changes clinically characterized by fever, anorexia, negative nitrogen balance and catabolism of muscle cells (*Gruys et al, 2005*). Other effects on endocrine and nutritional parameters include a decrease in HDL and LDL, increased ACTH and glucocorticoids, decreased serum levels of calcium, zinc, iron, vitamin A and of α-tocopherol, and a change in concentration of several plasma proteins (**Table 5**) (*Gruys et al, 2005*).

The acute-phase response to injury or infection is associated with alteration in dynamics of many trace elements, particularly iron, zinc and copper. The fall in serum iron and zinc, and rise in serum copper, is brought about by changes in the concentration of specific tissue proteins controlled by cytokines, especially IL-1, TNF-α, and IL-6. These are generally believed to be beneficial aspects of the early acute phase response.

In addition to the decrease of serum zinc, iron and albumin, a decrease of transferrin, cortisol-binding globulin, transthyretin (TTR) and retinol-binding protein have been described. The resulting disturbance in vitamin A metabolism that occurs in chronic infestation and inflammatory states worsens the vitamin A deficiency that is seen in children and pregnant mothers in developing countries from malnutrition (*Stephensen, 2001*). Vitamin A deficiency has a well-known negative feedback effect on immunity, producing one of the best described immunosuppressive effects of malnutrition.

► Cachexia

Starvation (simple energy deprivation) is accompanied by metabolic adaptations to ensure essential nutrients are available for vital organs. Starvation results in decreased insulin secretion and a moderate increase in cortisol, leading to muscle catabolism and lipolysis. Lipolysis liberates fatty acids which are picked up by the liver, packaged into lipoproteins (VLDL), and exported back out into the circulation along with ketone bodies for utilization as fuel by the majority of cells in the body. Amino acids released from muscle are used by the liver for the synthesis of essential proteins (e.g. clotting proteins), and by the kidney and liver to synthesize glucose for those tissues dependant upon it (e.g. leukocytes, erythrocytes). As tissues (e.g. the brain) adapt to utilizing ketones in preference to glucose, the release of amino acids from muscle slows, and lean body mass is preserved. All of the metabolic adaptations can be reversed with feeding.

Severe inflammatory responses also induce a collection of metabolic derangements that result in accelerated lipolysis and muscle catabolism, producing wasting that is not explained solely by a decrease in food intake (**Table 6**). The defining difference between starvation and cachexia, is that in cachexia, forced feeding will not reverse the derangements, will not preserve the loss in lean body mass, and results only in fat accumulation. Cachexia has been shown to occur in association with sepsis, non-septic inflammatory disease, neoplasia, and cardiac failure. Cachexia accounts for 30-80% of cancer-related deaths in humans (diaphragmatic failure, edema, immune compromise) (*Kotler 2000*).

Inflammatory cytokines, particularly IL-6, TNF-α, and IL-1, are largely responsible for the derangements, and produce both local effects at the site of inflammation, but also endocrine effects (IL-6).

For instance, in severe infection, circulating TNF-α is an important inducer of accelerated lipolysis, and by up-regulating the ubiquitin-proteosome system, is largely responsible for the disproportionate muscle catabolism associated with cachexia (*Camps et al, 2006*). In addition to generalized muscle catabolism, the metabolism of individual amino acids can be deranged. In FIV infected cats, similar to human HIV-AIDS patients, the IFN-γ produced in response to the infection stimulates accelerated tryptophan catabolism and a decrease in serum tryptophan concentrations (*Kenny et al, 2007*). The exact consequences of this metabolic response are uncertain so far, although it does raise the possibility that supplementation with tryptophan metabolites such as niacin or melatonin might have some therapeutic benefit in FIV-infected cats.

Parameter	Starvation	Inflammation/Cachexia
Body weight	−	⇩ or no change
Body fat	⇩⇩⇩	⇩⇩
RER	⇩⇩⇩	⇧ or no change
MER	⇩⇩⇩	⇩
Protein synthesis	⇩⇩⇩	⇧ ou ⇩
Protein degradation	⇩⇩	⇧⇧⇧
Serum insulin	⇩⇩	⇧⇧⇧
Serum cortisol	No change	⇧⇧⇧
Serum glucose	No change	⇧⇧⇧
Serum lipids	⇧ VLDL, ⇧ fatty acids ⇧⇧⇧ ketones	⇧⇧ VLDL, ⇧⇧ fatty acids ⇩ ketones

TABLE 6 - METABOLIC DIFFERENCES BETWEEN SIMPLE STARVATION AND CACHEXIA

In inflammatory diseases, there is an exaggerated secretion of insulin in response to feeding, but most cells in the body (especially the liver) are resistant to the effects. This resistance prevents utilization of precious glucose and preserves blood glucose for essential tissues (brain, erythrocytes, leukocytes). There is a massive increase in cortisol which induces a large breakdown of fat and muscle, increasing the delivery of free fatty acids and amino acids to the liver, and greatly increasing muscle and visceral protein breakdown. Since the liver is resistant to insulin, feeding does little to prevent it from continuing to produce glucose, and hyperglycemia results (*Andersen et al, 2004*).

▶ Risks of over feeding and hyperglycemia

> Hyperglycemia – more than a number?

Therefore, any serious acute illness can result in:
- hyperglycemia
- insulin resistance
- increased hepatic glucose production.

This has been termed the "Diabetes of injury". Previously this insulin resistance and hyperglycemia was thought to be an adaptive response promoting glucose uptake by essential tissues and prevention of uptake by muscle. Thus moderate hyperglycemia has been tolerated by veterinary and medical clinicians.

In 2001, a study of 1548 human intensive care patients was instigated to determine if there was any benefit to tightly controlling blood glucose in severe illness (*van den Berghe et al, 2001*). Blood glucose was controlled with intensive insulin therapy to less than 6 mmol/L (110 mg/dL). Amazingly there was a 43% reduction in mortality in all patients, and even in "long stay"

FIGURE 10 - METABOLIC EFFECTS OF INSULIN ON THE CELLS

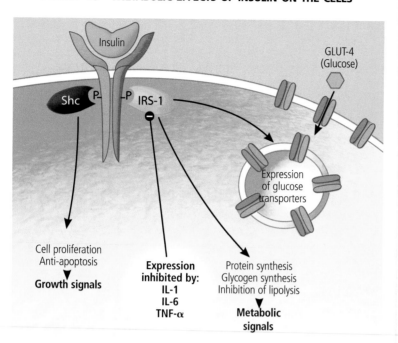

In systemic inflammatory states, cytokines reduce the expression of the insulin-receptor substrate (IRS-1), which prevents glucose transporter (GLUT-4) expression and produces peripheral insulin resistance. However, other signaling pathways that promote cellular proliferation and inhibit apoptosis still occur. The persistant hyperinsulinemia in response to the hyperglycemia leads to exaggerated signaling down growth pathways and cellular dysfunction.

TABLE 7 - RECOMMENDATIONS FOR FEEDING IN SEVERE INFLAMMATORY DISEASES

- Feed no more than RER until there is a demonstration of weight loss.
> BUT – ensure that the RER is being fed.
- Monitor for hyperglycemia and hyperlipidemia.
> If either are identified, reduce intake but keep feeding the gut
- Feed a high protein, high fat diet
> BUT consider the possibility of fat malabsorption
- Start with 25% RER for first 24 hours,
> then 50%, then 75%, then 100%.
- Weigh daily.

patients, mortality was reduced by 10.6%. In addition there was:
- shortened hospitalization
- reduced nosocomial infections
- reduced acute renal failure
- reduced anemia
- fewer cases of liver failure
- less multiple organ dysfunction
- reduced muscle weakness.

Although no similar studies have been performed in feline patients, a "stress-hyperglycemia" is a very common finding in seriously ill cats. In critically ill dogs, hyperglycemia is also common, and hyperglycemia at presentation is associated with increased duration of hospitalization, and the occurrence of sepsis was more frequent in hyperglycemia dogs than normoglycemic dogs (*Torre et al, 2007*). Finally, canine patients not surviving hospitalization had a higher median glucose concentration compared with those surviving to discharge (*Torre et al, 2007*).

> Is glucose toxic?

Hyperglycemia is not normally toxic in the short term. Normally, cells are relatively protected from hyperglycemia by down-regulation of glucose transporters. However, although the insulin secreted in inflammatory states does not result in reducing blood glucose, it does lead to other signaling effects within cells (**Figure 10**). Thus hyperglycemia stimulates continued insulin release which signals to many cell types to undergo metabolic changes associated with the post-prandial state, that are inappropriate in a diseased state. These alterations have been confirmed in canine sepsis.

In addition, although there is a relative insulin resistance, some glucose is forced into some cells leading to cellular glucose overload in neurons, endothelium, alveoli, vascular smooth muscle, and renal tubule cells.

This combination of exaggerated insulin signaling and glucose overload leads to:
- acute renal failure
- accelerated removal of erythrocytes and anemia
- polyneuropathy, brain edema, depression, seizures
- immunosuppression, decreased phagocytosis and killing
- increased sepsis
- increased vascular permeability, decreased responsiveness, activation, coagulation, disseminated intravascular coagulation.

> Recommendations for feeding in severe inflammatory diseases

Clearly feeding excessive carbohydrate will exacerbate hyperglycemia and increase morbidity, whilst feeding excessive fat exacerbates hepatic load and leads to fatty liver development and liver dysfunction. The recommendations for feeding in severe inflammatory diseases are presented in **Table 7**.

6-Immune response to dietary antigens (oral tolerance)

▶ Immunological basis for oral tolerance

Foreign dietary antigens interact with the intestinal immune system in such a way as to prevent unnecessary and detrimental immune reactions to them. In so doing, systemic immunity is rendered effectively unresponsive if the same antigen reaches the systemic circulation. This absence of reactivity to orally administered antigens is termed oral tolerance. Oral tolerance is generated in an antigen-specific and active manner that involves the induction of an atypical immune response.

Peyer's patches are the primary inductive area of the intestinal immune system. The specialized M-cells within the epithelium overlying the lymphoid follicles sample, unspecifically or by receptor-mediated uptake, particulate and insoluble antigens, and whole microorganisms (*Brandtzaeg, 2001*). Antigens and organisms are then transported to leukocytes that reside within basal membrane invaginations, namely B-cells, macrophages, and dendritic cells. In the normal intestine these antigen presenting cells (APCs) lack co-stimulatory molecules such as CD80 and CD86. Antigens processed by these "un-activated" APCs are then presented to naïve B and T cells within the follicle, which then proliferate poorly. This occurs within a local microenvironment that differs from other sites in the body and results in induction of hyporesponsive, Th3 or Th2 biased T cells (*Kellermann & McEvoy, 2001*). Activated cells then leave via lymphatics and pass via the mesenteric lymph nodes into the systemic circulation. They will then exit at mucosal sites via engagement of cell adhesion molecules (CAMs) specifically expressed by the high-endothelial venules of mucosal tissues. Thus activated or memory B and T lymphocytes enter the lamina propria to await a secondary encounter with their specific antigen **(Figure 11)**.

The activated cells may secrete cytokines, but full differentiation into effector T cells or plasma cells may not occur without secondary exposure. For both cell types to be re-exposed to antigen, intact antigens must reach the lamina propria. Intestinal epithelial cells are responsible for the absorption of antigen, release to professional APCs, and limited antigen presentation to cells within the mucosa on MHC class II. In the normal intes-

FIGURE 11 - ACTIVATION AND RE-HOMING OF INTESTINAL LYMPHOCYTES

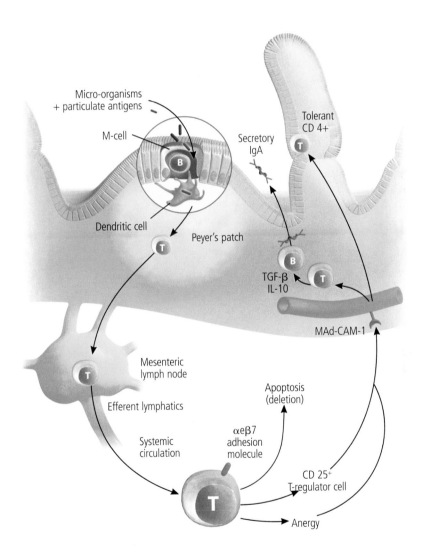

The Peyer's patches are the primary inductive sites of immune responses to intestinal luminal antigens. Dendritic cells in the Peyer's patch or mesenteric lymph nodes do not normally express co-stimulary molecules (e.g.CD 80 and CD 86) and induce either apoptosis, anergy, or a regulatory function in the T cell. Lymphocytes activated within the mucosa express a unique adhesion molecule (αeβ7) which binds to MadCAM-1 expressed by venules within mucosal tissues. Thus lymphocytes activated within mucosal tissues circulate, then exit as effector cells within mucosal tissues.

493

FIGURE 12 - THE GENERAL BASIS FOR IMMUNOLOGICAL TOLERANCE TO LUMINAL ANTIGENS

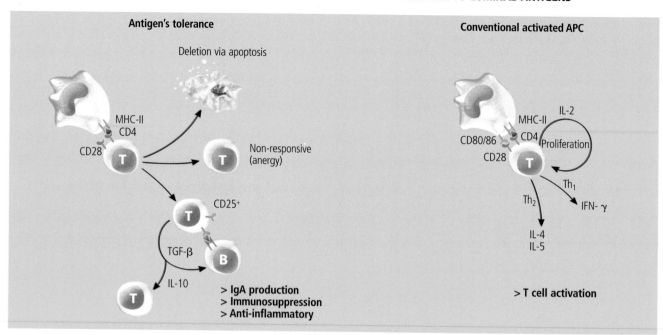

A: In the intestine, dendritic cells do not widely express co-stimulatory molecules such as CD 80 and CD 86. Antigen presentation leads to tolerance to the antigen through deletion, anergy, or induction of regulatory or suppressor effects in the T lymphocyte.
B: Conventional antigen presentation occurs with co-stimulatory molecule expression and results in T-lymphocyte activation as either Th1 or Th2.

tine, these secondary APCs will, like the primary presenters, lack co-stimulatory molecule expression and further add to the toleragenic environment. The effector T cell clones resident in the normal intestine secrete a bias towards Th2 and Th3 cytokines, in particular IL-10 and TGF-β, thus directing B-cell isotype switching to produce IgA-secreting plasma cells, whilst inhibiting the development of Th1 lymphocytes and IgG production.

It is important that the immune system reserves the ability to rapidly respond to pathogens. This ability to recognize pathogenicity is based on the engagement of PAMP receptors such as TLRs, producing "danger signals".

Predictably, expression of TLR-2 and TLR-4 is low to non-existent in the mucosal cells of the normal human intestine, but they can be rapidly expressed in response to inflammatory cytokines (Abreu et al, 2001). The absence of these "danger signals" results in relatively inefficient antigen processing by intestinal APCs, markedly reduced or absent TNF-α/IL-1/IL-12 production, and the absence of CD80/86 co-stimulatory molecule expression. T cells activated by such an APC, will divide less with most clones undergoing early deletion by apoptosis, whilst the surviving memory cells will tend to secrete IL-10, TGF-β, or no cytokines (Jenkins et al, 2001). This combination of apoptosis, functional defects in surviving clones, and T cells secreting the anti-inflammatory and IgA-supporting cytokines, is the general basis for immunological tolerance to luminal antigens (Figure 12).

Thus oral tolerance is composed of a delicate balance between induction of IgA, T cell deletion, anergy, and immunosuppression; and the retention of antigen-specific lymphocytes capable of responding to invasive pathogens though antibody isotype switching to IgM, IgE, or IgG, and the production of inflammatory cytokines such as IFN-γ, IL-12, and IL-6.

► Loss of tolerance to dietary antigens

Loss of tolerance to dietary antigens will produce a conventional but detrimental immune response against the dietary antigen. Such an inappropriate response may produce inflammation locally, or at another anatomical site. The response will be characterized by one or a combination of:

- Local cell mediated inflammation: the resulting chronic stimulus may lead to lymphocytic intestinal infiltrates characteristic of inflammatory bowel disease.
- Local antibody production of isotypes other than IgA: the production of IgE will lead to mast cell priming and intestinal hypersensitivity, i.e. food allergy with gastrointestinal signs (vomiting and/or diarrhea).
- Systemic antibody production: circulating IgE will lead to priming of mast cells at sites distal to the intestine such as dermal hypersensitivity, i.e. food allergy with pruritus as the clinical sign.

The initiating events that lead to loss of oral tolerance, or prevent it from developing have not been described in cats, and remain poorly understood in any species. Suggested mechanisms include:

- *increased mucosal permeability*: e.g. following mucosal injury, or the neonatal intestine
- *co-administration of a mucosal adjuvant*: that activates and changes the phenotype of intestinal dendritic cells e.g. bacterial enterotoxins
- *parasitism*: intestinal parasitism in cats leads to an exaggerated systemic humoral response that includes increased production of IgE (*Gilbert & Halliwell 2005*).

Currently, there is speculation as to the importance of infections that stimulate a Th-1-biased immune response in preventing Type-1 hypersensitivity reactions in people. This has been termed the "hygiene hypothesis", which states that a lack of maturation of the infant immune system from a Th-2 to a Th-1 type of immune response may be caused by less microbial stimulation in Western societies (*Romagnani, 2004*). It is proposed that bacterial and viral infections during early life promotes a net shift of the maturing immune system towards Th-1 biased responses, and reduce potentially allergenic Th-2 biased responses. The assumed reduction in the overall microbial burden is supposed to allow the natural Th-2 bias of neonates to persist and allow an increase in allergy.

The special role of parasites in modulating allergic responses to food and other allergens has been debated for half a century. Several older reports suggested that, similar to cats, parasitized humans are more likely to suffer from allergic diseases (*Warrell et al, 1975; Carswell et al, 1977; Kayhan et al, 1978*). In contrast to that is the higher incidence of allergic disease in Western populations, and the growing incidence of allergic disease in developing nations. Elevations of anti-inflammatory cytokines, such as interleukin-10, that occur during long-term helminth infections have been shown to be inversely correlated with allergy. It has recently been suggested that the host's response to the parasite determines their predisposition to develop allergic diseases, and that the induction of a robust anti-inflammatory regulatory response (e.g. IL-10) induced by persistent immune challenge offers a unifying explanation for the observed inverse association of many infections with allergic disorders (*Yazdanbakhsh et al, 2002*). In cats, the role parasitism and other infections that would fall within the hygiene hypothesis have yet to be defined in determining the development of food hypersensitivity. Since the immunological mechanism for the majority of food sensitivities may not be IgE-mediated, the story may be even more complicated.

► Food immunogenicity

Adverse reactions to food are surprisingly common in cats: they have been reported to be present in up to 29% of all cases of chronic gastrointestinal disease in cats (*Guilford et al, 2001*).

In addition, inflammatory bowel disease is the single most common cause of chronic gastrointestinal disease in cats, and novel antigen and hydrolysed protein diets are commonly reported to be effective in its management *(Guilford & Matz, 2003; Nelson et al, 1984)*. However, although the involvement of immunological mechanisms in a proportion of these adverse reactions is suspected, it is unproven. Indeed, the normal immunological response to ingested dietary antigens in cats has only recently been partially described *(Cave & Marks, 2004)*. Surprisingly, cats develop robust serum IgG and IgA responses to dietary proteins when fed as either aqueous suspensions or as part of canned diets.

The relatively short intestinal tract of the cat suggests that they may be poorly suited to poorly digestible diets *(Morris, 2002)*. It is well established that the commercial canning process decreases protein digestibility and that this has biologically significant effects in cats *(Kim et al, 1996)*.

In rodents and rabbits, intact particulate and insoluble antigens are preferentially absorbed across the intestine through M-cells overlying the Peyer's patches *(Frey et al, 1996)*. Classically, such antigens tend to invoke active immunity appropriate for microorganisms. In contrast, soluble antigens have been found to be associated with oral tolerance *(Wikingsson & Sjoholm, 2002)*. It has also been shown that oral tolerance can be abrogated when soluble proteins are fed in oil-in-water emulsions, resulting in robust systemic humoral responses *(Kaneko et al, 2000)*. This effect may also have relevance to the pet-food industry where interactions between dietary proteins and lipids in canned or extruded diets during the cooking and the manufacturing process could feasibly result in novel interactions not present in their native states.

In stark contrast to rodents is the intestinal response in chickens, where particulate antigens induce tolerance, whilst soluble antigens provoke active immunity *(Klipper et al, 2001)*. If the physical nature of the proteins within the natural diet of a species dictates how the intestinal immune system has evolved, this might have special relevance to species that are commonly fed diets different from their ancestors.

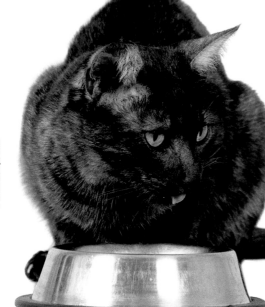

As obligate carnivores, felids have evolved on a highly digestible diet.

Commercial pet foods are subjected to significant heating during the manufacturing process. The effect of heat treatment on proteins is mostly to change the 3-dimensional conformation of the protein. Although this may disrupt some antigens, it may equally uncover previously hidden antigenic determinants, or create new ones. Other reactions occurring at high temperatures include the Maillard reactions, which involve the reactions between certain amino acids and reducing sugars to produce less digestible compounds called melanoidins, which give a characteristic brown color. Melanoidins tend to be less digestible, less soluble, and certain melanoidins have been shown to be more "allergenic" than the original uncooked protein *(Maleki et al, 2000; 2003)*.

The effect of heating during the canning process on the immunogenicity of dietary proteins has been evaluated in cats *(Cave & Marks 2004)*. Using soy and casein proteins, the canning process resulted in the creation of new antigens not present in the uncooked product. In addition, a product of heated casein induced a salivary IgA response that was not induced by the raw product. Thus commercial food processing can qualitatively and quantitatively alter the immunogenicity of food proteins. Although the significance of this finding is uncertain at present, it emphasizes the need for feeding highly digestible proteins sources, or perhaps even hydrolysed proteins, when enteritis is present.

FIGURE 13 - MECHANISMS FOR THE MODULATION OF IMMUNITY BY DIETARY POLYUNSATURATED FATTY ACIDS

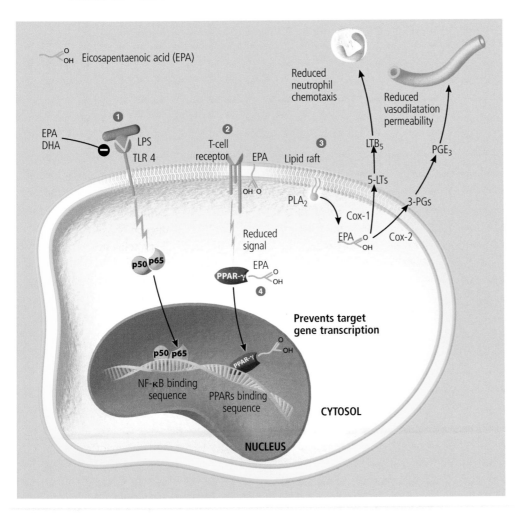

Polyunsaturated fatty acids can modulate immune responses through several mechanisms.

1. The n-3 PUFA EPA and DHA can directly inhibit signaling through TLR4 by LPS.
2. The 20 carbon PUFAs EPA and AA give rise to eicosanoids with differing biological actions.
3. Alterations in the physical properties of cell membrane lipid rafts leads to decreased signaling through the T-cell receptor.
4. EPA binds to the cytosolic protein PPAR-γ, which then diffuses to the nucleus where it binds to specific sequences and can inhibit gene transcription induced by NF-κB activation (e.g. following TLR signaling).

7 - Nutritional modulation of immunity

▶ Polyunsaturated fatty acids

Dietary polyunsaturated fatty acids (PUFA) can modulate immune responses through several mechanisms (**Figure 13**).

> Eicosanoid production

The dietary content of polyunsaturated fatty acids determines the proportions of the 20 carbon n-6 fatty acids arachidonic acid (ARA), dihomo-γ-linolenic acid (DGLA), and the n-3 fatty acid eicosapentaenoic acid (EPA) within the phospholipids cell membranes of leukocytes and other cell types. When ARA is used as the substrate, 2-series prostaglandins and thromboxane (e.g. PGE_2, and TXA_2), and 4-series leukotrienes (e.g. LTB_4) are produced. Those derived from EPA are the 3-series prostaglandins and thromboxane (e.g. PGE_3, and TXA_3), and the 5-series leukotrienes (e.g. LTB_5; **Figure 6**). EPA and ARA are competitive substrates for cycloxogenase (COX) and lipoxogenase (LOX). EPA is a less efficient substrate for COX, resulting in reduced prostaglandin production. In contrast, EPA is the preferred substrate for LOX, and when both ARA and EPA are available, the production of 5-series leukotrienes predominate.

Feeding diets that are enriched in the n-3 PUFA EPA can reduce ARA-derived eicosanoids by up to 75%. The conversion of the 18-carbon alpha linolenic acid (α-LA) into EPA does not occur to any significant degree in cats. Therefore the effect of enriching a diet in α-LA will likely have little effect on immunity in cats.

The EPA-derived thromboxane TXA_3 is a much less potent platelet aggregate and vasoconstrictor than TXA_2. In contrast, the efficacy of the prostacyclins PGI_2 and PGI_3 in inducing vasodilation and inhibiting platelet aggregation are equal. Thus diets enriched in n-3 PUFA will reduce thrombosis and improve microcirculation at sites of endothelial activation.

The EPA-derived leukotriene LTB_5 is a much less potent vasoconstrictor and neutrophil chemotaxin than the ARA-derived LTB_4. Similarly, PGE_3 is less biologically active than PGE_2, and is less effective in inducing fever, increasing vascular permeability, and vasodilation. However, PGE_2 and PGE_3 are similarly effective in decreasing Th1 cytokine production and shifting the Th1 - Th2 balance in favor of a Th2 response in human lymphocytes (*Dooper et al, 2002*).

Dietary EPA will therefore result in the production of eicosanoids that range from antagonistic to equipotent to those derived from ARA, and the overall effect of PUFA on immunity is not explained simply by the reduced efficacy of EPA-derived eicosanoids.

At present then, the effects and mechanisms of modulation of eicosanoids by dietary lipid is complex, and is very poorly described in cats, although there is some value to the generalization that diets enriched in n-3 PUFA will have an anti-inflammatory effect relative to diets enriched in n-6 PUFA. It is also not even known how significant alterations in eicosanoid production are in the modulation of immunity by n-3 PUFA, and it may be that other mechanisms are as, or even more important.

> Gene transcription

PUFA can directly affect gene transcription by interacting with nuclear receptors. The peroxisome proliferators-activated receptors (PPARs) are a family of cytosolic proteins that, once bound to an appropriate ligand, diffuse into the nucleus and either promote or inhibit gene transcription. PPARs are expressed by macrophages, T cells, B cells, dendritic cells, endothelial cells and other cell types (*Glass & Ogawa, 2006*). Both EPA and DHA are ligands for PPAR-α, PPAR-γ, and PPAR-δ (*Kliewer et al, 1997*). PPAR-α agonists have been shown to inhibit TNF-α, IL-6 and IL-1 production as well as inhibiting iNOS, matrix metalloprotease-9 and scavenger receptor expression by activated macrophages (*Kostadinova et al, 2005*). In T-lymphocytes, PPAR-·α agonists inhibit IL-2 production and hence indirectly depress lymphocyte proliferation (*Glass & Ogawa, 2006*).

Long chain n-3 PUFAs reduce expression of COX-2, 5-LOX and 5-LOX activating protein in chondrocytes. Thus, PUFAs alter eicosanoid synthesis at the level of gene expression, as well as by providing the substrates from which they are produced.

> Membrane structure (Figure 14)

Incorporation of EPA in place of ARA in phospholipid membranes alters the physical and structural properties of the cell membranes in lymphocytes. In particular, the assembly of lipid rafts, within which most cell surface receptors are localized, is altered. In T-lymphocytes in vitro, this has the effect of decreasing signal transduction through the T cell receptor and thus depresses T-lymphocyte activation (*Geyeregger et al, 2005*).

> Inhibition of LPS-signaling

Animals fed diets enriched in EPA and/or DHA produce decreased amounts of inflammatory cytokines, and experience less morbidity and mortality following challenge with gram negative sepsis or lipopolysaccharide. In addition, lipid emulsions administered to human patients with systemic sepsis results in reduced systemic inflammatory responses as a result of suppressing production of TNF-α, IL-1, IL-6, and IL-8 by LPS-stimulated macrophages (*Mayer et al, 2003*).

FIGURE 14 - MEMBRANE STRUCTURE

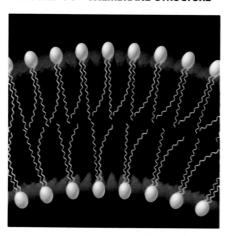

The basic biological membrane structure is always the same: it is a twin-lipid layer composed of two assembled rafts. The total thickness is 6-10 nm.

DHA and EPA, inhibit TLR4 agonist (LPS)-induced up-regulation of the costimulatory molecules, MHC class II, COX-2 induction, and cytokine production through suppression of NF-κB activation. In contrast, COX-2 expression by TLR2 or TLR4 agonists was increased by the saturated fatty acid, lauric acid (*Lee et al, 2004; Weatherill et al, 2005*).

> Dietary PUFA content, supplementation, and ratios

The complexity of eicosanoid production and effects is added to by the complexity of dietary fatty acid interactions and metabolism. The prediction of an effect of a given diet has to take into account all of the following:

- total fat content of the diet
- relative proportions of 18-carbon n-3 and n-6 fatty acids (ALA, GLA, and LA)
- relative proportions of 20 carbon n-3 and n-6 fatty acids (ARA, DGLA, and EPA)
- absolute amounts of all individual n-3 and n-6 fatty acids
- previous dietary history of the animal
- duration of exposure to the diet in question.

The reduction of the description of the fat content of a diet to a simple ratio of n-3 to n-6 fatty acids provides very limited and potentially misleading information.

In addition, it can be seen that supplementation of a diet with a source of n-3 fatty acids (e.g. marine fish oil) will have greatly varying effects depending on the nature of the basal diet and patient. Most commercial diets are highly concentrated in linoleic acid, and the addition of a small amount of n-3 fatty acids will achieve little.

> Recommendations

There is insufficient evidence to make firm recommendations for disease modulation in cats using dietary PUFA. Using a dietary fat content of approximately 70 g/kg DMB, Saker et al found that a total n-6 to n-3 ratio of 1.3:1 (using corn oil, animal fat, and menhaden fish oil) reduced platelet aggregation (*Saker et al, 1998*). Such a value provides a very rough estimate to the proportions required for modulating eicosanoid production, although the concentrations of EPA and ARA were not specifically assayed. In addition, the dietary concentrations required for the other effects of n-3 PUFA are unknown.

► Genistein

Genistein is an isoflavone compound principally found in plants of the family Leguminosae including soy, clover, and alfalfa (*Dixon & Ferreira, 2002*). Genistein is structurally similar to 17 , β-estradiol, as depicted in **Figure 15**.

Genistein has been confirmed as a phytoestrogen *in vivo* through its ability to increase uterine weight, mammary gland development, and stimulation of prolactin secretion in ovariectomized rats and function as an estrogen in some estrogen-dependant cell lines (*Santell et al, 1997; Morito et al, 2001*). However, due to the complexity of estrogen signaling in different tissues, in differing cells, perhaps even at varying times, genistein can have estrogenic activity, no activity, or anti-estrogenic activity (*Diel et al, 2001*).

> Tyrosine kinase and topoisomerase II inhibition

In addition to genistein's estrogenic activity is its ability to inhibit tyrosine kinases by competitively binding to their ATP-binding site and forming non-productive enzyme-substrate complexes (*Akiyama et al, 1987*). Inhibition of tyrosine kinases in turn inhibits numerous leukocyte signaling cascades involved in lymphocyte activation and proliferation, neutrophil activation and superoxide production, bacterial phagocytosis by macrophages, antibody responses, and delayed-type hypersensitivity responses (*Trevillyan et al, 1990; Atluru et al, 1991; Atluru & Atluru, 1991; Atluru & Gudapaty, 1993;*

FIGURE 15 - THE STRUCTURAL DIAGRAMS OF GENISTEIN AND 17 β-ESTRADIOL

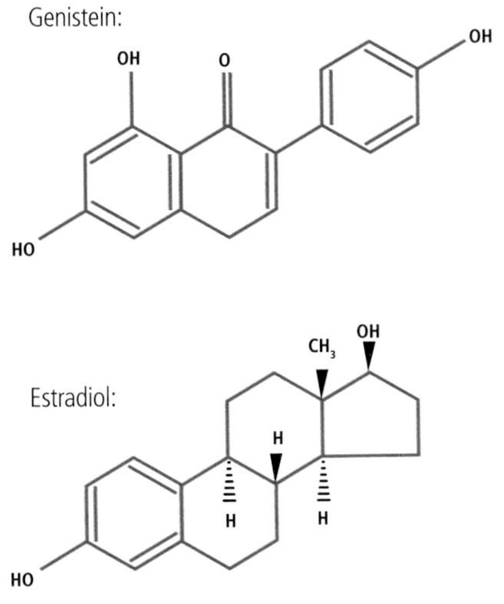

Genistein:

Estradiol:

Yellayi et al, 2002; 2003). Genistein has also been found to inhibit DNA topoisomerase II, resulting in double strand breaks in DNA, and has been linked to efficacy as a cancer chemotherapeutic, and as a disrupter of lymphocyte proliferation *(Markovits et al, 1989; Salti et al, 2000).*

> Genistein in cat food

Soy-based ingredients are common in commercial diets fed to cats; the soy plant provides a source of protein, fiber, and polyunsaturated oil. As a result, several commercial diets contain genistein concentrations that could be sufficient to affect immune responses in cats. The isoflavone content of several cat foods has been assayed and concentrations have been found that would result in a cat ingesting up to 8.13 mg/kg body weight *(Court & Freeman, 2002; Bell et al, 2006).*

Recently, it has been shown that once daily oral genistein treatment decreases circulating CD8+ cells, increases neutrophil respiratory burst, and decreases delayed-type hypersensitivity responses. Unexpected effects of genistein suggest that extrapolation from one species to other species may not be appropriate in regards to the effects of genistein on immunity.

► Carotenoids

Cats are capable of absorbing dietary carotenoids, including β-carotene and lutein **(Figure 16)**. Significant amounts of both compounds are incorporated into organelle membranes, especially in the mitochondria or lymphocytes *(Chew et al, 2000; Chew & Park, 2004).* It has been suggested that their efficiency in absorbing and stabilizing free radicals **(Figure 17)** and their ability to localize in the mitochondria combine to make them very effective antioxidants in protecting cells against endogenously derived oxidants. Their localization to organelle membranes makes them particularly effective in protecting mitochondrial proteins, lipid membranes, and DNA. In addition, since NF-κB can be activated in leukocytes in response to oxidative stress, antioxidants that concentrate in leukocytes might be expected to reduce NF-κB activation. One might question whether such effects would produce anti-inflammatory or even immunosuppressive effects, or whether simple cellular preservation through the antioxidant effect might enhance immunity.

In most studies performed to date, the supplementation of a diet with carotenoids with or without vitamin A activity (e.g. β-carotene vs. lutein) has produced enhanced responses in several different immunological assays *(Chew & Park 2004).*

The incorporation of lutein into the diet of cats has been shown to significantly affect immune responses *(Kim et al, 2000).* The DTH response to an intradermally administered vaccine was increased, as was the in vitro lymphocyte proliferation following activation. Finally, the total IgG response after vaccination was increased by lutein treatment *(Kim et al, 2000).* Overall then, carotenoids seem to enhance immunity independent of their vitamin-A activity. Whether this effect is solely, or even partially due to their ability to function as antioxidants is unsolved.

► Arginine

Arginine is an essential amino acid for cats because of their inability to synthesize sufficient

FIGURE 16 - THE STRUCTURE OF LUTEIN

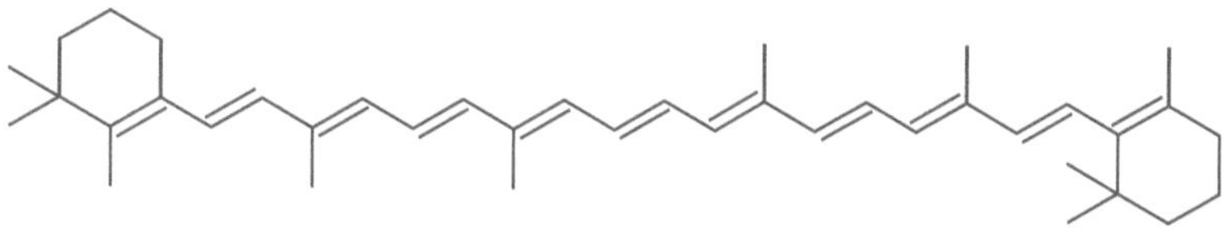

β-carotene

FIGURE 17 - LUTEIN EFFECTOR SITES

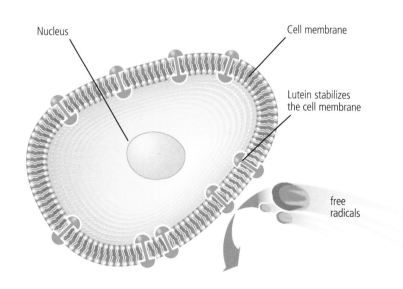

Nucleus

Cell membrane

Lutein stabilizes the cell membrane

free radicals

quantities in the fasting state. However, beyond its role as an essential intermediate in the ornithine cycle, dietary arginine has long been known to enhance certain aspects of immunity.

L-Arginine is oxidized to L-citrulline + •NO by nitric oxide synthetase (Figure 18). The inducible form within leukocytes (iNOS) produces much greater amounts of •NO than the constitutive endothelial (eNOS) or neuronal (nNOS) forms. The production of •NO after induction of iNOS in an activated phagocyte is limited mostly by the availability of free arginine. Therefore any increase in available arginine will increase the •NO produced by any given inflammatory stimulus (Eiserich et al, 1998).

Nitric oxide is a free radical. However, compared with other free radical species, in physiological conditions the molecule is relatively stable, reacting only with oxygen and its radical derivatives, transition metals, and other radicals. This low reactivity, combined with its lipophilicity, allows the molecule to diffuse away from its place of synthesis, and function as a signaling molecule on an intracellular, intercellular, and perhaps even systemic level.

Nitric oxide is required for normal intestinal epithelial maturation. It may be the principle inhibitory neurotransmitter in intestinal motility, and is essential for the maintenance of normal mucosal blood flow. In addition, •NO inhibits the expression of cellular adhesion molecules limiting unnecessary leukocyte entry, especially into the mucosal tissues. Nitric oxide inhibits T-cell proliferation, decreases NF-κB activation, and induces a Th-2 bias to local responses. However, in contrast to the paradigm that •NO inhibits the key pro-inflammatory transcription factor NF-κB, some studies have suggested that iNOS inhibition can increase pro-inflammatory cytokine production.

As mentioned, •NO is relatively unreactive with non-radical molecules. However, reaction with superoxide (O_2•⁻) to form peroxynitrite (ONOO⁻) is diffusion limited. Peroxynitrite is not a free radical, though it is a powerful oxidant, and has been shown to elicit a wide array of toxic effects ranging from lipid peroxidation, protein oxidation and nitration leading to inactivation of enzymes and ion channels, DNA damage, and inhibition of mitochondrial respiration (Virag et al, 2003). The cellular effect of ONOO⁻ oxidation is concentration dependant; for instance very low concentrations will be handled by protein and lipid turnover and DNA repair, higher concentrations induce apoptosis, whereas very high concentrations induce necrosis. Since both •NO and O_2•⁻ are produced in sites of inflammation, it is reasonable to propose that ONOO⁻ might be involved in the pathogenesis of many cases.

In light of differences in the radius of effect of both O_2•⁻ and NO, co-localization of both molecules within the same cell would be expected to lead to disease. In this context, the finding that iNOS is capable of generating O_2•⁻ in conditions when L-arginine is unavailable is significant. This has been demonstrated in macrophages, where limiting L-arginine availability resulted in the simultaneous production of functionally significant amounts of O_2•⁻ and NO, and the immediate intracellular formation of ONOO⁻ (Xia & Zweier 1997).

The large number of conflicting studies evaluating the role of •NO in inflammatory disease, has resulted in a polarization of view points between those that argue •NO is protective, and those that argue it contributes to the pathogenesis. This is unfortunate since both views are probably correct. The fate of any individual molecule of •NO is determined by multiple variables that determine its role in pathogenesis including:
- site of production

FIGURE 18 - ORIGIN OF NITRIC OXIDE

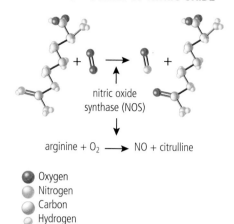

arginine + O_2 ⟶ NO + citrulline

● Oxygen
● Nitrogen
● Carbon
● Hydrogen

The reaction is catalyzed by the enzyme, nitric oxide synthase (NOS). There are three forms of NOS:
- *endothelial NOS (eNOS):*
  eNOS is required for maintenance
  of normal vascular tone and as a physiologic messenger
- *neuronal NOS (nNOS):*
  eNOS and nNOS are constitutive forms and are
  always produced in low levels
- *inducible NOS (iNOS): iNOS is inducible by a variety*
  of inflammatory mediators including the cytokines,
  tumor necrosis factor (TNF), and interleukin-1 (IL-1),
  and free radicals.

FIGURE 19 - INTEREST OF L-LYSINE SUPPLEMENTATION IN HERPES VIRUS INFECTION

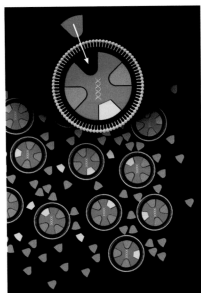

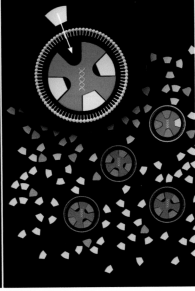

Figure 19A - Normal replication of the feline herpes virus when arginine is present.

Figure 19B - Inhibition of viral replication when L-lysine competes with arginine to enter the cells.

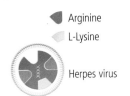

Arginine

L-Lysine

Herpes virus

Beyond a certain breakpoint, the addition of L-lysine tends to inhibit herpes virus replication in vivo *and* in vitro.

- timing within the local disease process that the molecule is produced
- amount of •NO produced
- redox status of the immediate environment
- chronicity of the disease.

Overall it appears that supplemental arginine, either parenterally or orally administered, enhances the depressed immune response of individuals suffering from trauma, surgery, malnutrition, or infection. This action is presumably through its ability to augment the production of •NO by iNOS in activated neutrophils and macrophages.

However, in cases of severe sepsis (i.e. infection accompanied by a systemic inflammatory response), augmentation of •NO production might be detrimental because of its effect as a negative cardiac ino- and chronotrope, its ability to inhibit coagulation and its potent venous and arterial dilator effects (*Suchner et al, 2002*).

Most commercial enteral nutritional formulas suitable for feeding to cats contain 1.5 to 2 times the minimum requirement of arginine for growth. However, supplementation of diets for intensive care nutrition has frequently been recommended, and is widely used in human medicine for enhancement of the immune system in critical care. Although clinical improvements in some studies have been reported, critically ill patients with SIRS, sepsis, or organ failure may actually deteriorate as the result of arginine supplementation (*Stechmiller et al, 2004*). Thus there may be cases where supplementation with arginine, beyond that provided by a conventional protein source may be beneficial, whilst in other cases it may be detrimental.

► Lysine

As indicated in **Figure 2**, the diet ingested by the host can directly affect the pathogen. The interaction between lysine and herpes viruses is an example of such an interaction, rather than an interaction between diet and immunity **(Figure 19)**.

The genome of the feline herpes virus (FHV-1) is similar to the genomes of other alpha-herpes viruses, and several different viral proteins have been described (*Mijnes et al, 1996*). All of the 20 common amino acids are utilized, including L-lysine (*Pellett et al, 1985*). However, when herpes viruses are grown in cell cultures in vitro, there is no requirement for lysine to be added to the culture media, thus what little lysine is required for viral replication is derived from the labile pool of free intracellular amino acids (*Maggs et al, 2000*). In contrast, the omission of arginine or histidine from the culture media profoundly inhibits viral replication more so that other amino acid omissions (*Tankersley, 1964*). The addition of lysine to the culture media actually inhibits viral replication, but the breakpoint at which replication is inhibited has not be clearly defined. Tankersley (1964) demonstrated that normal replication occurs at 70 μg/mL, but profound inhibition occurs at 180 μg/mL. It is worth noting that, when cats are fed a diet containing the adequate intake of lysine recommended by the NRC for gestating queens (i.e 1.1% in a 4000 kcal/kg diet), plasma concentrations of lysine are 14 ± 2.2 μg/mL (*Fascetti et al, 2004*).

It has been proposed that lysine may antagonize arginine availability in vitro by competing for arginine entry into cells **(Figure 19)** and in vivo by both competition, and by the induction of renal and hepatic arginase. However, Fascetti et al, have demonstrated that even very large dietary concentrations of lysine do not alter plasma arginine concentrations in cats within a two week period *(Fascetti et al, 2004)*.

- When 500 mg of L-lysine monochloride was given twice daily to cats as a bolus, starting 6 hours prior to inoculation with FHV-1, a mean plasma concentration of 97 µg/mL was achieved. Clinical signs associated with acute FHV-1 infection were reduced, but there was no reduction in viral shedding *(Stiles et al, 2002)*.
- A once daily bolus of 400 mg given to latently infected cats produced mean peak plasma concentrations of 65 µg/mL and reduced viral shedding, but had no significant effect on clinical signs *(Maggs et al, 2003)*.
- Finally, when a diet containing 5.1% lysine (as fed, in a 4000 kcal/kg diet) was fed to cats, a mean plasma concentration of 44 µg/mL was achieved. This diet was fed to groups of spontaneously latently infected cats, having recently experienced an epizootic upper respiratory disease, no effect was seen on clinical signs or herpes viral shedding *(Maggs et al, 2006)*. In fact, one group (the male cats) fed the lysine supplemented diet experienced worse clinical signs than any other, supplemented or not, and increased viral shedding. This observation was probably more due to stress or another pathogen (*Mycoplasma felis, Bordetella bronchiseptica*) than an effect of the diet, but did influence the results of the study.

Thus the efficacy of treatment with L-lysine on feline herpes viral infection remains to be challenged in cats with enzootic upper respiratory disease. To date, lysine supplementation has not show any toxic effects. Experimentally, the cat's dietary consumption is lower with a 13% lysine-diet (as fed, in a 4000 kcal/kg diet) but this level largely exceeds practical cat food formulation *(Fascetti et al, 2004)*.

8-Effect of route of nutrition

In addition to the composition and amount of diet fed, the route of feeding (enteral or parenteral) affects innate and adaptive aspects of immunity *(Kudsk, 2002)*. A lack of enteral stimulation leads to decreased intestinal and respiratory tract IgA production and established IgA-mediated antiviral and antibacterial immunity *(Renegar et al, 2001a)*. Increased mucosal permeability and bacterial translocation of luminal bacteria to the mesenteric lymph nodes, liver, and spleen are seen with parenteral nutrition *(Kudsk, 2003a)*. In healthy cats, parenteral nutrition (PN) administered for 2 weeks resulted in small intestinal villous atrophy and fusion, and increased numbers of inflammatory cells *(Lippert et al, 1989)*. These changes are reversed when enteral feeding is reinstated.

A lack of luminal nutrients results in an increased expression of proinflammatory adhesion molecules, especially ICAM-1. A lack of enteral feeding leads to infiltration of lymphocytes into the lamina propria and is associated with trapping of lymphocytes there, which is rapidly reversed with feeding *(Ikeda et al, 2003)*. In addition, neutrophils accumulate and are activated within the vasculature of the intestine during fasting *(Kudsk, 2002; 2003b)*.

The increased number of primed neutrophils adhering to the microvasculature throughout the intestinal tract are able to contribute to oxidative and enzymatic tissue damage following activation. Fasting or PN significantly increases ICAM-1 expression within the intestine and liver 3 hours after reperfusion compared with enteral feeding. Fasting or PN results in decreases in IL-4 and IL-10 that correlate with decreases in IgA and increases in ICAM-1. Lack of enteral feeding impairs the coordinated system of sensitization, distribution, and interaction of T and B cells important in the production of IgA, in the maintenance of normal gut cytokines, and in the regulation of endothelial inflammation. Thus the lack of luminal nutrients has been described as a "first hit", and increases the inflammatory response to a secondary insult in the GIT, but also the lungs, liver, and potentially other organs as well.

Perhaps the effect of enteral nutrition on intestinal integrity is best demonstrated in cases where there is a severe mucosal insult. In canine parvoviral enteritis, the early instigation of enteral nutrition decreases the time to normalization of demeanor, appetite, vomiting, and diarrhea (*Mohr et al, 2003*). In a model of methotrexate induced enteritis in cats, feeding a complex diet was superior to fasting or feeding a purified diet in normalizing clinical signs, maintaining intestinal integrity, and minimizing bacterial translocation (*Marks et al, 1997; 1999*).

Intestinal immunity can have a profound negative or positive influence in the development of the systemic inflammatory response to severe trauma, surgery, or infection. In human trauma patients, enteral feeding decreases the incidence of pneumonia compared with total parenteral nutrition or starvation. Enteral nutrition increases secretory IgA production at all mucosal sites and lack of enteral stimulation significantly impairs the generation of IgA-mediated mucosal immunity, including immunity against upper respiratory tract vial infections, hastening elimination of virus (*Renegar et al, 2001b; Johnson et al, 2003*). This has importance to feline medicine, where recovery from calici or herpes viral upper respiratory infection may be delayed in the absence of adequate enteral nutrition.

Intestinal integrity is compromised in the absence of enteral nutrients, and is accompanied by an increased rate of bacterial translocation, and increased risk of sepsis. These changes are seen with either complete fasting, or with parenteral nutrition. Thus oral fasting primes an animal for an exaggerated response to any subsequent or concurrent inflammatory insult and increases the bacterial challenge from enterically derived organisms. On the other hand, provision of enteral nutrition is one of the most important mechanisms by which systemic inflammatory responses can be reduced, and septicemia can be avoided. Compared to parenteral nutrition, enteral nutrition is beneficial in human critical patients. Patients without pre-existing septic shock who received enteral nutrition had fewer episodes of severe sepsis or septic shock, and the length of stay in ICU was shorter compared with those given PN (*Radrizzani et al, 2006*). This effect is so significant that it has lead some authors to recommend that parenteral nutrition be abandoned in cases of critical illness when enteral nutrition can be administered, even at an initial low caloric content.

Conclusion

The interaction between nutrition and immunity is complex, bi-directional, and incompletely understood. Nutrition can modify immunity by enhancing, suppressing, or changing the nature of an immune response. Immunity can be affected by diet in utero, and at the time of mounting a response. Nutrients of importance in this regard include glutamine, arginine, PUFA, carotenoids, and genistein. Nutrients can act as fuel, precursors for mediators, antioxidants, modifiers of gene transcription, and inhibitors of cellular functions. Defects in almost any essential nutrient can impair immunity, but also nutrient excess in obesity. Whether either suppression or enhancement is good or bad depends upon the specific disease state, and the individual patient.

Immune responses alter nutritional status through changes in usage, impaired uptake, increased loss, and altered metabolism. Sustained severe immune responses result in cachexia that cannot be reversed with feeding alone. The metabolic changes associated with systemic inflammatory responses leads to insulin resistance and hyperglycemia, and forced feeding can increase morbidity and mortality. Tight glucose control appears to be more important than meeting the resting energy requirements of critically ill patients. For optimal mucosal and systemic immunity, enteral nutrition is preferred to parenteral nutrition.

Diseases in which immunosuppression may be beneficial include chronic inflammatory diseases such as IBD, osteoarthritis, and immune-mediated diseases. It is less clear in which states enhancement of immunity is beneficial. Until more information is available, nutritional support should focus primarily on preventing nutritional deficiencies whilst avoiding overfeeding, rather than on immunomodulation.

Frequently asked questions concerning nutrition and immunity

Q	A
What is "immunonutrition"?	**Any aspect of nutrition that modulates the activity of the immune system in any way could be termed immunonutrition.** However, the term has been most commonly used to describe nutritional interventions that attempt to improve the clinical outcome in critically ill patients through modulation of immunity. There is an optimal diet for every animal in every disease state, and the optimal diets for different animals may differ widely, or be the same for very different diseases. The ambiguity of the term may well have contributed to the overly simplistic thinking about the role of diet in severe inflammatory diseases that has resulted in one-diet-for-all approaches (e.g. PN solutions supplemented with glutamine, arginine, and n-3 PUFA for all septic patients).
What does it mean to "boost immunity"?	For any given immune response, if that response is amplified, exaggerated, or made more efficient, it can be said to be "boosted". However, boosting immunity is not always of benefit to the animal. The normalization of cellular immune responses in malnourished animals with adequate nutrition can be said to be boosting the immune response from deficient to normal. However, in severe sepsis where widespread activation of macrophages and neutrophils contributes significantly to vital organ and vascular damage, increasing the activity of those cells can increase morbidity and mortality. The clearest example of that is with the supplementation of arginine to critically ill humans. At its most extreme, suppression of immunity may be of benefit to the animal if immune-mediated disease is present. **The most common reason for supplementing a diet with n-3 PUFA is to reduce inflammation.** Finally, it may be that boosting immunity is of neither benefit nor detriment.
Can feeding adversely affect immunity?	Feeding incomplete or imbalanced diets always has the potential to cause immune dysfunction. In addition, feeding in excess of the resting energy requirements of an animal in a systemic inflammatory response syndrome may lead to hyperglycemia and immune-dysfunction.
What is the ideal diet for severe sepsis?	The answer to this question is unknown and there is potential for harmful intervention. For hospitalized patients, the major goals of nutritional intervention are to meet the known requirements, and avoid over-nutrition and dehydration. In cases of severe sepsis, simply meeting the resting energy requirements with a complete and balanced diet via the enteral route when possible are reasonable goals. Whilst it has not been established what the ideal macronutrient proportions might be for severe sepsis, it is known that all three macronutrients (carbohydrate, protein, and fat) can be detrimental if fed in excess. For cats, carbohydrate might be especially poorly tolerated in severe sepsis, and low carbohydrate (< 20% of energy) high fat diets, fed to not exceed the resting energy requirements, may be ideal.

Q	A
How could anorexia in sepsis be beneficial?	A potential explanation is that **anorexia leads to muscle catabolism and the liberation of essential amino acids and glutamine for optimal leukocyte function**. In addition, the increased tissue catabolism increases immunosurveilance through increased presentation of self peptides on MHC-I molecules. Thus, feeding with an imbalanced formulation may impair leukocyte responses and decrease the efficiency of pathogen clearance. **However, when the infectious agent is being directly treated, and when supportive care is provided, nutritional intervention supersedes any slight benefit from anorexia.** Feeding a highly digestible, moderate to low carbohydrate diet, with adequate glutamine and arginine, supplemented with higher concentrations than required for maintenance of antioxidants (especially ascorbate and tocopherol), and avoidance of over-feeding, the outcome will be greatly improved.
How much fish oil should I supplement to produce immunosuppression in a cat?	As discussed above, there are too few studies on which to make any confident recommendations. In addition, **the required amount will depend on the type and severity of the disease, and the fat content of the cat's diet**. However it is likely that sufficient n-3 PUFA will need to be fed to produce a ratio of at most 1.3:1 (n-6:n-3).

Consider this example:
A typical adult maintenance dry cat food contains the following main ingredients: chicken, chicken by-product meal, corn grits, corn meal, chicken fat, dried egg product, fish meal, beat pulp. The total n-6 content of the diet is 2.6%, whilst the total n-3 content is 0.23%.

The diet has an energy density of 4 kcal/g (16.8 kJ/g), and a 4 kg cat, with a daily intake of 200 kcal (842 kJ) will consume a total of 50 g of food, which contains 1.3 g n-6 PUFA, and 0.115 g n-3 PUFA, or a ratio of 11.3 (n-6:n-3).

To reduce this ratio to less than 1.3, an additional 0.9 g n-3 PUFA needs to be added. Salmon oil contains approximately 34% n-3 PUFA, with the rest as saturated, monounsaturated, and a small amount of n-6 PUFA. Therefore, 2.6 g (2.9 mL) of salmon oil is needed to be added to the diet to reduce the ratio to 1.3. That supplement provides an additional 22 kcal (92 kJ), or 11% more than the required intake.

As stated above, it has not been determined what the most important variable for modulation of immunity is, though **the single most important ratio in the cat may be the ratio of ARA: EPA**. In the absence of evidence, the above calculation serves as an illustration of a starting point, where less than that amount is unlikely to have a significant effect. |

References

Abreu MT, Vora P, Faure E, et al. Decreased expression of Toll-like receptor-4 and MD-2 correlates with intestinal epithelial cell protection against dysregulated proinflammatory gene expression in response to bacterial lipopolysaccharide. J Immunol 2001; 167: 1609-1616.

Akira S. Mammalian Toll-like receptors. Curr Opin Immunol 2003; 15: 5-11.

Akiyama T, Ishida J, Nakagawa S, et al. Genistein, a specific inhibitor of tyrosine-specific protein kinases. J Biol Chem 1987; 262: 5592-5595.

Andersen SK, Gjedsted J, Christiansen C, et al. The roles of insulin and hyperglycemia in sepsis pathogenesis. J Leukoc Biol 2004; 75: 413-21.

Atluru D, Jackson TM, Atluru S. Genistein, a selective protein tyrosine kinase inhibitor, inhibits interleukin-2 and leukotriene B4 production from human mononuclear cells. Clin Immunol Immunopathol 1991; 59: 379-387.

Atluru D, Gudapaty S. Inhibition of bovine mononuclear cell proliferation, interleukin-2 synthesis, protein-tyrosine kinase and leukotriene B4 production by a protein-tyrosine kinase inhibitor, genistein. Vet Immunol Immunopathol 1993; 38: 113-122.

Atluru S, Atluru D. Evidence that genistein, a protein-tyrosine kinase inhibitor, inhibits CD28 monoclonal-antibody-stimulated human T cell proliferation. Transplantation 1991; 51: 448-450.

Bell KM, Rutherfurd SM, Hendriks WH. The isoflavone content of commercially-available feline diets in New Zealand. N Z Vet J 2006; 54: 103-138.

Boza JJ, Maire J-C, Bovetto L, et al. Plasma glutamine response to enteral administration of glutamine in human volunteers (free glutamine versus protein-bound glutamine). Nutrition 2000; 16: 1037-1042.

Brandtzaeg P. Nature and function of gastrointestinal antigen-presenting cells. Allergy 2001; 56 Supp 67: 16-20.

Camps C, Iranzo V, Bremnes RM, et al. Anorexia-Cachexia syndrome in cancer: implications of the ubiquitin-proteasome pathway. Support. Care Cancer. 2006; 14: 1173-83.

Carswell F, Merrett J, Merrett TG, et al. IgE, parasites and asthma in Tanzanian children. Clin. Allergy. 1977; 7: 445-53.

Cave NJ, Marks SL. Evaluation of the immunogenicity of dietary proteins in cats and the influence of the canning process. Am J Vet Res 2004; 65: 1427-33.

Chandler ML, Gunn-Moore DA. Nutritional status of canine and feline patients admitted to a referral veterinary internal medicine service. J Nutr 2004; 134: 2050S-2052S.

Chew BP, Park JS, Weng BC, et al. Dietary beta-carotene absorption by blood plasma and leukocytes in domestic cats. J Nutr 2000; 130: 2322-2325.

Chew BP, Park JS. Carotenoid action on the immune response. J Nutr 2004; 134: 257S-261S.

Court MH, Freeman LM. Identification and concentration of soy isoflavones in commercial cat foods. Am J Vet Res 2002; 63: 181-185.

Cunningham-Rundles S, McNeeley DF, Moon A. Mechanisms of nutrient modulation of the immune response. J. Allergy Clin Immunol 2005; 115: 1119-1128; quiz 1129.

DeLeo FR, Allen LA, Apicella M, et al. NADPH oxidase activation and assembly during phagocytosis. J Immunol 1999; 163: 6732-6740.

Diel P, Olff S, Schmidt S, et al. Molecular identification of potential selective estrogen receptor modulator (SERM) like properties of phytoestrogens in the human breast cancer cell line MCF-7. Planta Med 2001; 67: 510-514.

Dionigi R, Ariszonta, Dominioni L, et al. The effects of total parenteral nutrition on immunodepression due to malnutrition. Ann Surg 1977; 185: 467-474.

Dixon RA, Ferreira D. Genistein. Phytochemistry 2002; 60: 205-211.

Dooper MM, Wassink L, M'Rabet L, et al. The modulatory effects of prostaglandin-E on cytokine production by human peripheral blood mononuclear cells are independent of the prostaglandin subtype. Immunology 2002; 107: 152-159.

Eiserich JP, Patel RP, O'Donnell VB. Pathophysiology of nitric oxide and related species: free radical reactions and modification of biomolecules. Mol Aspects Med 1998; 19: 221-357.

Esper DH, Harb WA. The cancer cachexia syndrome: a review of metabolic and clinical manifestations. Nutr Clin Pract 2005; 20: 369-376.

Fascetti AJ, Maggs DJ, Kanchuk ML, et al. Excess dietary lysine does not cause lysine-arginine antagonism excess in adult cats. J Nutr 2004; 134: 2042S-2045S.

Frey A, Giannasca KT, Weltzin R, et al. Role of the glycocalyx in regulating access of microparticles to apical plasma membranes of intestinal epithelial cells: implications for microbial attachment and oral vaccine targeting. J Exp Med 1996; 184: 1045-1059.

Fuentes-Orozco C, Anaya-Prado R, Gonzalez-Ojeda A, et al. L-alanyl-L-glutamine-supplemented parenteral nutrition improves infectious morbidity in secondary peritonitis. Clin Nutr 2004; 23: 13-21.

Fukuda K, Hirai Y, Yoshida H, et al. Free amino acid content of lymphocytes nd granulocytes compared. Clin Chem 1982; 28: 1758-1761.

Geyeregger R, Zeyda M, Zlabinger GJ, et al. Polyunsaturated fatty acids interfere with formation of the immunological synapse. J Leukoc Biol 2005; 77: 680-688.

Gilbert S, Halliwell RE. The effects of endoparasitism on the immune response to orally administered antigen in cats. Vet Immunol Immunopathol 2005; 106: 113-120.

Glass CK, Ogawa S. Combinatorial roles of nuclear receptors in inflammation and immunity. Nat Rev Immunol 2006; 6: 44-55.

Gruys E, Toussaint MJ, Niewold TA, et al. Acute phase reaction and acute phase proteins. J Zhejiang Univ Sci B 2005; 6: 1045-1056.

Guilford WG, Jones BR, Markwell PJ, et al. Food sensitivity in cats with chronic idiopathic gastrointestinal problems. J Vet Intern Med 2001; 15: 7-13.

Guilford WG, Matz ME. The nutritional management of gastrointestinal tract disorders in companion animals. N Z Vet J 2003; 51: 284-291.

Harris SG, Padilla J, Koumas L, et al. Prostaglandins as modulators of immunity. Trends Immunol 2002; 23: 144-150.

Ikeda S, Kudsk KA, Fukatsu K, et al. Enteral feeding preserves mucosal immunity despite in vivo MAdCAM-1 blockade of lymphocyte homing. Ann Surg 2003; 237: 677-685.

Jenkins MK, Khoruts A, Ingulli E, et al. In vivo activation of antigen-specific CD4 T cells. Annu Rev Immunol 2001; 19:23-45: 23-45.

Johnson CD, Kudsk KA, Fukatsu K, et al. Route of nutrition influences generation of antibody-forming cells and initial defense to an active viral infection in the upper respiratory tract. Ann Surg 2003; 237: 565-573.

Kaneko T, Terasawa Y, Senoo Y, et al. Enhancing effect of dietary oil emulsions on immune responses to protein antigens fed to mice. Int Arch Allergy Immunol 2000; 121: 317-323.

Kayhan B, Telatar H, Karacadag S. Bronchial asthma associated with intestinal parasites. Am. J. Gastroenterol. 1978; 69: 605-6.

Kellermann SA, McEvoy LM. The Peyer's patch microenvironment suppresses T cell responses to chemokines and other stimuli. J Immunol 2001; 167: 682-690.

Kenny MJ, Baxter KJ, Avery NC, et al. Altered tryptophan metabolism in FIV-positive cats. In. Pp 539-541. 2007

Kim HW, Chew BP, Wong TS, et al. Modulation of humoral and cell-mediated immune responses by dietary lutein in cats. Vet Immunol Immunopathol 2000; 73: 331-341.

Kim SW, Rogers QR, Morris JG. Maillard reaction products in purified diets induce taurine depletion in cats which is reversed by antibiotics. J Nutr 1996; 126: 195-201.

Kitoh T, Asai S, Akiyama Y, et al. The inhibition of lymphocyte blastogenesis by asparaginase: critical role of glutamine in both T and B lymphocyte transformation. Acta Paediatr. Jpn 1992; 34: 579-583.

Kliewer SA, Sundseth SS, Jones SA, et al. Fatty acids and eicosanoids regulate gene expression through direct interactions with peroxisome proliferator-activated receptors alpha and gamma. Proc Natl Acad Sci USA 1997; 94: 4318-4323.

Klipper E, Sklan D, Friedman A. Response, tolerance and ignorance following oral exposure to a single dietary protein antigen in Gallus domesticus. Vaccine 2001; 19: 2890-2897.

Kostadinova R, Wahli W, Michalik L. PPARs in diseases: control mechanisms of inflammation. Curr Med Chem 2005; 12: 2995-3009.

Kotler DP. Cachexia. Ann Intern Med 2000; 133: 622-634.

Kudsk KA. Current aspects of mucosal immunology and its influence by nutrition. Am J Surg 2002; 183: 390-398.

Kudsk KA. Effect of route and type of nutrition on intestine-derived inflammatory responses. Am J Surg 2003a; 185: 16-21.

Kudsk KA. Effect of route and type of nutrition on intestine-derived inflammatory responses. Am J Surg 2003b; 185: 16-21.

Langhans W. Anorexia of infection: current prospects. Nutrition 2000; 16: 996-1005.

Langweiler M, Sheffy BE, Schultz RD. Effect of antioxidants on the proliferative response of canine lymphocytes in serum from dogs with vitamin E deficiency. Am J Vet Res 1983; 44: 5-7.

Lee JY, Zhao L, Youn HS, et al. Saturated fatty acid activates but polyunsaturated fatty acid inhibits Toll-like receptor 2 dimerized with Toll-like receptor 6 or 1. J Biol Chem 2004; 279: 16971-1699.

Lippert AC, Faulkner JE, Evans AT, et al. Total parenteral nutrition in clinically normal cats. J Am Vet Med Assoc 1989; 194: 669-676.

Maggs DJ, Collins BK, Thorne JG, et al. Effects of L-lysine and L-arginine on in vitro replication of feline herpesvirus type-1. Am J Vet Res 2000; 61: 1474-1478.

Maggs DJ, Nasisse MP, Kass PH. Efficacy of oral supplementation with L-lysine in cats latently infected with feline herpesvirus. Am J Vet Res 2003; 64: 37-42.

Maggs DJ, Sykes JE, Clarke HE, et al. Effects of dietary lysine supplementation in cats with enzootic upper respiratory disease. J Feline Med Surg 2007; 9: 97-108.

Maleki SJ, Chung SY, Champagne ET, et al. The effects of roasting on the allergenic properties of peanut proteins. J Allergy Clin Immunol 2000; 106: 763-768.

Maleki SJ, Viquez O, Jacks T, et al. The major peanut allergen, Ara h 2, functions as a trypsin inhibitor, and roasting enhances this function. J Allergy Clin Immunol 2003; 112: 190-195.

Markovits J, Linassier C, Fosse P, et al. Inhibitory effects of the tyrosine kinase inhibitor genistein on mammalian DNA topoisomerase II. Cancer Res 1989; 49: 5111-5117.

Marks SL, Cook AK, Griffey S, et al. Dietary modulation of methotrexate-induced enteritis in cats. Am. J. Vet. Res. 1997; 58: 989-96.

Marks SL, Cook AK, Reader R, et al. Effects of glutamine supplementation of an amino acid-based purified diet on intestinal mucosal integrity in cats with methotrexate-induced enteritis. Am J Vet Res 1999; 60: 755-763.

Mayer K, Meyer S, Reinholz-Muhly M, et al. Short-time infusion of fish oil-based lipid emulsions, approved for parenteral nutrition, reduces monocyte proinflammatory cytokine generation and adhesive interaction with endothelium in humans. J Immunol 2003; 171: 4837-4843.

Meyers JA, McTiernan A, Ulrich CM. Leptin and immune function: integrating the evidence. Nutr Res 2005; 25: 791-803.

Mijnes JDF, vanderHorst LM, vanAnken E, et al. Biosynthesis of glycoproteins E and I of feline herpesvirus: gE-gI interaction is required for intracellular transport. J Virol 1996; 70: 5466-5475.

Mohr AJ, Leisewitz AL, Jacobson LS, et al. Effect of early enteral nutrition on intestinal permeability, intestinal protein loss, and outcome in dogs with severe parvoviral enteritis. J Vet Intern Med 2003; 17: 791-8.

Morito K, Hirose T, Kinjo J, et al. Interaction of phytoestrogens with estrogen receptors alpha and beta. Biol Pharm Bull 2001; 24: 351-356.

Morris JG. Idiosyncratic nutrient requirements of cats appear to be diet-induced evolutionary adaptations. Nutr Res 2002; 15: 153-168.

Murray MJ, Murray AB. Anorexia of infection as a mechanism of host defense. Am J Clin Nutr 1979; 32: 593-596.

Nelson RW, Dimperio ME, Long GG. Lymphocytic-plasmacytic colitis in the cat. J Am Vet Med Assoc 1984; 184: 1133-1135.

Newsholme P, Gordon S, Newsholme EA. Rates of utilization and fates of glucose, glutamine, pyruvate, fatty acids and ketone bodies by mouse macrophages. Biochem J 1987; 242: 631-636.

Newsholme P, Newsholme EA. Rates of utilization of glucose, glutamine and oleate and formation of end-products by mouse peritoneal macrophages in culture. Biochem J 1989; 261: 211-218.

Oehler R, Roth E. Regulative capacity of glutamine. Curr Opin Clin Nutr Metab Care 2003; 6: 277-282.

Pellett PE, McKnight JLC, Jenkins FJ, et al. Nucleotide-sequence and predicted amino-acid sequence of a protein encoded in a small herpes-simplex virus-DNA fragment capable of trans-inducing alpha-genes. Proc Natl Acad Sci USA 1985; 82: 5870-5874.

Plantinga EA, Hovenier R, Beynen AC. Qualitative risk assessment of chronic renal failure development in healthy, female cats as based on the content of eicosapentaenoic acid in adipose tissue and that of arachidonic acid in plasma cholesteryl esters. Vet Res Commun 2005; 29: 281-286.

Preiser JC, Peres-Bota D, Eisendrath P, et al. Gut mucosal and plama concentrations of glutamine: a comparison between two enriched enteral feeding solutions in critically ill patients. Nutr J 2003; 2: 13.

Radrizzani D, Bertolini G, Facchini R, et al. Early enteral immunonutrition vs. parenteral nutrition in critically ill patients without severe sepsis: a randomized clinical trial. Intensive Care Med 2006; 32: 1191-2118.

Renegar KB, Johnson CD, Dewitt RC, et al. Impairment of mucosal immunity by total parenteral nutrition: requirement for IgA in murine nasotracheal anti-influenza immunity. J Immunol 2001a; 166: 819-825.

Renegar KB, Johnson CD, Dewitt RC, et al. Impairment of mucosal immunity by total parenteral nutrition: requirement for IgA in murine nasotracheal anti-influenza immunity. J Immunol 2001b; 166: 819-825.

Romagnani S. The increased prevalence of allergy and the hygiene hypothesis: missing immune deviation, reduced immune suppression, or both? Immunology. 2004; 112: 352-63.

Saker KE, Eddy AL, Thatcher CD, et al. Manipulation of dietary (n-6) and (n-3) fatty acids alters platelet function in cats. J Nutr 1998; 128: 2645S-2647S.

Salti GI, Grewal S, Mehta RR, et al. Genistein induces apoptosis and topoisomerase II-mediated DNA breakage in colon cancer cells. Eur J Cancer 2000; 36: 796-802.

Santell RC, Chang YC, Nair MG, et al. Dietary genistein exerts estrogenic effects upon the uterus, mammary gland and the hypothalamic/pituitary axis in rats. J Nutr 1997; 127: 263-269.

Schuller-Levis G, Mehta PD, Rudelli R, et al. Immunologic consequences of taurine deficiency in cats. J Leukoc Biol 1990; 47: 321-331.

Stechmiller JK, Childress B, Porter T. Arginine immunonutrition in critically ill patients: a clinical dilemma. Am J Crit Care 2004; 13: 17-23.

Stephensen CB. Vitamin A, infection, and immune function. Annu Rev Nutr 2001; 21: 167-192.

Stiles J, Townsend WM, Rogers QR, et al. Effect of oral administration of L-lysine on conjunctivitis caused by feline herpesvirus in cats. Am J Vet Res 2002; 63: 99-103.

Suchner U, Heyland DK, Peter K. Immune-modulatory actions of arginine in the critically ill. Br J Nutr 2002; 87 Suppl 1: S121-132.

Tankersley RV. Amino acid requirements of herpes simplex virus in human cells. J Bacteriol 1964; 87: 609.

Tilg H, Moschen AR. Adipocytokines: mediators linking adipose tissue, inflammation and immunity. Nat Rev Immunol 2006; 6: 772-783.

Torre DM, deLaforcade AM, Chan DL. Incidence and clinical relevance of hyperglycemia in critically ill dogs. In. Pp 971-975. 2007

Trevillyan JM, Lu YL, Atluru D, et al. Differential inhibition of T cell receptor signal transduction and early activation events by a selective inhibitor of protein-tyrosine kinase. J Immunol 1990; 145: 3223-3230.

Van den Berghe G, Wouters P, Weekers F, et al. Intensive insulin therapy in the critically ill patients. N Engl J Med 2001; 345: 1359-1367.

Virag L, Szabo E, Gergely P, et al. Peroxynitrite-induced cytotoxicity: mechanism and opportunities for intervention. Toxicol Lett 2003; 140-141: 113-124.

Weatherill AR, Lee JY, Zhao L, et al. Saturated and polyunsaturated fatty acids reciprocally modulate dendritic cell functions mediated through TLR4. J Immunol 2005; 174: 5390-5397.

Wikingsson L, Sjoholm I. Polyacryl starch microparticles as adjuvant in oral immunisation, inducing mucosal and systemic immune responses in mice. Vaccine. 2002; 20: 3355-3363.

Xia Y, Zweier JL. Superoxide and peroxynitrite generation from inducible nitric oxide synthase in macrophages. Proc Natl Acad Sci USA 1997; 94: 6954.

Yazdanbakhsh M, Kremsner PG, van Ree R. Allergy, parasites, and the hygiene hypothesis. Science. 2002; 296: 490-4.

Yellayi S, Naaz A, Szewczykowski MA, et al. The phytoestrogen genistein induces thymic and immune changes: a human health concern? Proc Natl Acad Sci 2002; 99: 7616-7621.

Yellayi S, Zakroczymski MA, Selvaraj V, et al. The phytoestrogen genistein suppresses cell-mediated immunity in mice. J Endocrinol 2003; 176: 267-274.

Immunity

Index

A

Adaptive immunity
chap 14: 481-482, 484, 486, 489

Adipose tissue
chap 1: 14-15, 19, 24, 27, 35, 41-42
chap 5: 190, 192-194
chap 6: 242, 245
chap 11: 389, 391-392
chap 12: 409
chap 14: 489, 509

Allergy
chap 2: 52, 60-61, 66, 68
chap 3: 89, 91, 114, 117-118, 128-129, 130, 133
chap 13: 461
chap 14: 495, 507-509

Alopecia
chap 1: 9
chap 2: 54, 57-58, 60-61, 64-65, 69, 71

Amylin
chap 1: 13
chap 5: 180, 186, 189, 191, 196-198, 205-206, 214-215

Anorexia
chap 2: 57
chap 3: 85, 101, 105-106, 110-111, 125
chap 4: 141, 144-147, 149, 153, 155-158, 160, 163-164, 166, 172, 176, 178-179
chap 5: 219-220
chap 7: 274, 276, 283
chap 8: 290
chap 9: 339, 343
chap 11: 386, 388, 393-394, 396-397, 400-402
chap 12: 406-407, 409-412, 415, 419, 423-424, 432-433, 435
chap 13: 443, 446, 458, 465-466, 472
chap 14: 489-490, 506, 508

Antioxidant
chap 1: 39
chap 2: 53
chap 3: 128
chap 4: 145-147, 150-152, 155-156, 158-159, 164-165, 173
chap 5: 210
chap 6: 241, 246
chap 7: 272, 283chap 9: 343-345, 348, 350, 352
chap 10: 383
chap 12: 408, 418-419, 436

chap 13: 476-477
chap 14: 481, 483, 488, 500, 504, 506, 508

Anxiety
chap 1: 8
chap 9: 328
chap 13: 460, 462-463, 465, 468-469

Appetite
chap 1: 7, 12-14, 24, 39-42
chap 3: 128, 135
chap 4: 147, 153, 154, 157, 159, 165, 167
chap 5: 221
chap 7: 266, 274-276, 279, 283
chap 10: 371
chap 11: 388, 391-392, 394-400
chap 12: 406-407, 410, 419-420, 424, 431-432, 435-436
chap 13: 441, 443, 457, 464-466, 474
chap 14: 489, 504

Arginine
chap 2: 54, 74
chap 3: 82, 128
chap 4: 149, 151, 157, 178
chap 5: 181, 185, 188, 196, 200, 203-204, 208-209, 211, 214-215, 217-218, 220-221
chap 7: 264, 272, 280
chap 8: 310
chap 9: 340, 346, 350
chap 11: 396, 401
chap 12: 408-409, 411, 416, 418-419, 433-434
chap 13: 442
chap 14: 481, 487, 500-506, 509

Aroma
chap 3: 131
chap 11: 395
chap 12: 420
chap 13: 454, 456, 476-477

Arterial hypertension
chap 7: 254, 263
chap 9: 325, 328-330, 334, 339, 346

Assisted feeding
chap 3: 95, 103
chap 4: 178
chap 11: 389, 392, 394-395
chap 12: 412, 414, 419, 426

Atherosclerosis
chap 1: 41, 43
chap 6: 226, 231-232, 234-235, 239-243
chap 9: 349

Aversion
chap 3: 129, 131
chap 4: 146, 153, 156, 159, 165, 169, 178
chap 11: 394-395, 397, 400
chap 12: 419
chap 13: 442, 447, 455, 458, 461, 465, 472, 474

Azotemia
chap 4: 158, 160
chap 5: 211
chap 7: 250-251, 254, 276, 281, 283
chap 8: 296, 301
chap 9: 327, 349-350
chap 12: 430

B

B vitamin
chap 4: 155
chap 9: 343

Bioelectrical impedance
chap 1: 15, 19, 41, 43
chap 7: 250
chap 8: 286
chap 12: 406

Body composition
chap 1: 14-16, 18-20, 27, 38, 41-43
chap 5: 207, 211
chap 11: 388-390
chap 12: 413
chap 13: 473

Body condition
chap 1: 3, 5-7, 9-10, 15-17, 20, 22, 28, 33, 40-43, 46-47
chap 3: 125-126
chap 4: 162, 169, 171
chap 5: 191, 203, 206, 217, 221
chap 6: 236, 240, 246
chap 7: 274, 276-277
chap 9: 339
chap 11: 385-387, 389-390, 392-394, 399, 401
chap 12: 412-413
chap 13: 464
chap 14: 488

Body score
chap 1: 30-31, 37, 46
chap 7: 277

Borage oil
chap 2: 72

C

Cachexia
chap 9: 339, 341, 345, 351
chap 11: 385, 389, 392-393, 396-398, 401-402
chap 12: 413
chap 14: 490-491, 504, 507-508

Calcium oxalate
chap 7: 280
chap 8: 287-288, 291-295, 297, 299-302, 304-309, 311-317, 321

Calcium phosphate
chap 8: 288, 294-295, 301-302, 308-310, 316

Cancer

chap 1: 11, 41, 43
chap 3: 102, 124
chap 9: 350-351
chap 11: 385-403
chap 13: 465
chap 14: 500, 507-509

Canine (tooth)

chap 3: 79
chap 10: 357-359, 366-367,373, 375, 379 383
chap 13: 453

Cardiac cachexia

chap 9: 339, 341

Carotenoids

chap 12: 418
chap 14: 481, 488, 500, 504

Catabolism

chap 1: 37chap 4: 146, 149-151, 154, 156
chap 5: 193
chap 6: 232-233, 240, 243
chap 7: 272, 276
chap 9: 336, 339, 341, 351, 353
chap 11: 389
chap 12: 409-410, 412, 436
chap 14: 486-487, 490-491, 506

Chemotherapy

chap 3: 107, 133
chap 4: 148
chap 11: 386-388, 392-394, 396, 398-402

Cholangitis/cholangiohepatitis

chap 4: 141, 144, 172

Cholestasis

chap 4: 142, 145-146, 150, 152-153, 158
chap 6: 229, 231-233, 239-240

Cholesterol

chap 1: 24, 29, 36
chap 2: 55
chap 4: 141, 148, 151, 176
chap 6: 223-228, 230-243, 246
chap 7: 270-271
chap 9: 337

Chronic renal failure (CRF)

chap 5: 214
chap 6: 240-243
chap 7: 250, 258, 280-281
chap 8: 301, 315
chap 9: 349-351
chap 14: 509

Chylomicron

chap 2: 65
chap 3: 82, 83
chap 6: 225-227, 229-231, 234-235, 239-242
chap 12: 427

Cobalamin (Vitamin B$_{12}$)

chap 3: 91, 129, 132
chap 4: 144, 146-147, 159-160, 164, 166-170, 172-175, 179
chap 9: 343
chap 11: 396, 402
chap 12: 402, 408, 418

Coenzyme Q10

chap 9: 345, 351

Colon

chap 1: 36
chap 3: 79, 81, 90-91, 113, 116, 119-125, 127-128, 133, 135
chap 9: 337
chap 12: 408
chap 14: 509

Congestive heart failure

chap 4: 142
chap 5: 198, 216
chap 7: 271
chap 9: 333-335, 338, 342, 346, 349-350
chap 12: 430
chap 13: 468

Constipation

chap 1: 4, 10, 36, 41
chap 3: 89, 108, 115, 119-121, 135-136
chap 4: 155, 157-158
chap 7: 274, 276
chap 11: 396

Creatinine

chap 5: 220
chap 7: 249-250, 252-255, 262, 266-269, 272, 274, 278, 281, 283
chap 8: 301
chap 9: 330

Critical care

chap 7: 274
chap 12: 405-437
chap 14: 502

Crystalluria

chap 4: 142, 148
chap 8: 291-292, 295, 308, 314

Cystine

chap 2: 54
chap 3: 95
chap 8: 288, 291-292, 294-295, 301-302, 310-313

D

Deglutition

chap 3: 79, 97-99
chap 12: 421

Dental calculus

chap 10: 362-363, 365, 374, 377

Dental formula

chap 10: 359

Dental plaque

chap 10: 363-366, 368, 372-377, 379-380, 382-383

Dentition

chap 3: 79
chap 10: 359, 374-375, 379

Diabetes mellitus

chap 1: 3-4, 8-9, 22, 28, 39, 43
chap 2: 64-65, 70-71
chap 4: 160, 164-165, 167-169, 176
chap 5: 180-187, 189-199, 201-203, 206-210, 212-217, 219-221
chap 6: 229, 231-232, 235-239, 243
chap 7: 271
chap 8: 288
chap 9: 325-327, 351
chap 10: 368, 372
chap 12: 406
chap 13: 462, 467, 469

Diarrhea

chap 1: 8, 10, 24, 36
chap 2: 58, 61
chap 3: 89-92, 94, 107-115, 117, 120-122, 124-127, 129-130, 133
chap 4: 141, 155, 157, 166-168, 171, 178
chap 5: 220
chap 7: 274
chap 11: 388, 393-394, 396
chap 12: 413-415, 421, 423, 435
chap 13: 467
chap 14: 485, 495, 504

Dietary allergy

chap 3: 89, 117-118, 129

Dietary antigen

chap 3: 84
chap 14: 495

Dietary hypersensitivity

chap 2: 57, 59-60, 71
chap 3: 95

Digestibility

chap 1: 24, 36-38, 41
chap 3: 81-82, 91-92, 108-109, 114, 118, 120, 123-124, 131-132
chap 4: 154, 158, 164, 169
chap 6: 240
chap 7: 276
chap 8: 298
chap 12: 408, 436
chap 13: 472
chap 14: 487, 496

Dilated cardiomyopathy (DCM)

chap 9: 323, 332-335, 337-338, 343-345, 347-350, 353-354
chap 12: 408

Diuresis

chap 7: 252
chap 8: 298-301, 303, 308, 312
chap 13: 467

Docosahexaenoic acid (DHA)

chap 1: 36
chap 2: 51, 56, 66
chap 6: 223, 237, 244-246
chap 7: 271, 283
chap 9: 340-341, 346
chap 12: 405, 408, 417, 419
chap 14: 497-499

DEXA (dual energy x-ray absorptiometry)

chap 1: 3, 15-17, 20, 22
chap 5: 214

Dysorexia

chap 3: 85, 98, 103-106, 112, 115
chap 4: 175
chap 11: 396

E

Eicosanoids

chap 2: 55
chap 7: 270
chap 9: 341
chap 12: 417
chap 14: 481, 484, 497-498, 508

Eicosapentanoic acid (EPA)

chap 1: 36
chap 2: 51, 56, 66
chap 6: 223, 237, 245-246
chap 7: 271, 283
chap 9: 340-341, 346, 351
chap 12: 405, 417, 419
chap 14: 479, 484, 497-499, 506

Electrophoresis

chap 6: 226-228, 230, 233

Elimination diet

chap 2: 61-64, 69
chap 3: 117, 124, 129

Energy balance

chap 1: 12, 30, 39
chap 4: 153, 156
chap 11: 391-392
chap 12: 410-411, 414, 419
chap 13: 452

Energy requirement

chap 1: 3, 28, 30-31, 40, 47
chap 5: 192, 194, 207
chap 9: 341
chap 11: 385, 390-391
chap 12: 405, 415-416, 424, 428-429, 437

Energy restriction

chap 1: 11, 13, 27-28, 30-31, 38-41
chap 9: 339

Enteral nutrition

chap 3: 95, 132
chap 4: 164-165, 173

chap 12: 405, 407, 414-415, 418, 420-426, 431, 433-434
chap 14: 504, 508

Esophagus

chap 3: 77, 79-80, 85, 96-103, 105, 108, 130, 132-133
chap 12: 415, 421, 423-424

Exocrine pancreas

chap 3: 133
chap 4: 140, 159, 166, 174

Exocrine pancreatic insufficiency

chap 3: 83, 89, 129, 133
chap 4: 139-140, 160, 164, 166-169, 172-174
chap 13: 459

F

Fasting

chap 1: 6, 11-12, 19, 44
chap 3: 99
chap 4: 142-143, 146, 151, 157, 167, 172, 176-177, 179
chap 5: 184, 190, 196, 202
chap 6: 224, 229, 239
chap 9: 338
chap 12: 409, 415, 435
chap 14: 500, 503-504

Fat free mass (lean mass)

chap 1: 3, 14, 15, 27, 48

Fat mass

chap 1: 3, 5, 15-16, 18-20, 34
chap 6: 234, 240
chap 14: 489

Fatty acid

chap 1: 3, 26, 35, 38-39, 42-44
chap 2: 51, 55, 65-73
chap 3: 77, 82, 133
chap 4: 151, 173, 176
chap 5: 181, 193-195, 198, 215-216
chap 6: 237, 240-244, 246
chap 7: 249, 270, 280, 282
chap 9: 334, 343, 348-350
chap 11: 402
chap 12: 405
chap 13: 476
chap 14: 484, 497, 499, 508

Feeding behavior

chap 1: 5, 8, 13, 26, 38
chap 3: 130
chap 10: 360-362
chap 13: 439-453, 458, 464, 470, 473

Feeding tubes

chap 3: 95, 131, 133
chap 12: 414-415, 420, 422, 425, 432-434, 436
chap 13: 466

Feline hepatic lipidosis

chap 4: 139, 143-144, 146, 149, 155, 172, 176, 179
chap 12: 405, 411, 433

Feline idiopathic cystitis

chap 8: 289, 295-296, 314-315

Feline trypsin-like immunoreactivity (TLI)

chap 3: 129
chap 4: 139, 160-161, 167, 174
chap 5: 220

Flavanols

chap 7: 272, 280

Food allergy

chap 2: 53, 57, 70-71
chap 3: 117-118, 133
chap 14: 495

Food aversion

chap 4: 146, 156, 159, 165, 178
chap 11: 394-395, 397, 400
chap 12: 419
chap 13: 447

Food intake

chap 1: 8, 12-13, 21, 24, 26-27, 32-33, 35-38, 41-43, 46, 48
chap 3: 130
chap 4: 153
chap 5: 182, 189-190, 192-194, 196, 215-216
chap 7: 274-276
chap 9: 339, 345
chap 11: 388-392, 394, 396-397, 399-400
chap 12: 412, 414, 420
chap 13: 443, 449-450, 452, 454, 456-458, 462-464, 466-468
chap 14: 489-490

Foreign body

chap 3: 85-88, 93, 97-99, 101-102, 105, 130
chap 12: 423

Fructosamine

chap 1: 22
chap 5: 202-203, 212, 214-217, 220-221

G

Gamma linolenic acid (GLA)
chap 2: 72-73
chap 9: 348
chap 14: 499

Gene transcription

chap 1: 42
chap 5: 187
chap 14: 497-498, 504

Gingival crevice

chap 10: 364-366

Gingivitis

chap 2: 64
chap 10: 362-363, 366-368, 370, 372-374, 377-379, 382
chap 13: 468

Glomerular filtration rate (GFR)

chap 7: 249, 252-254, 256-257, 262, 265, 269-271, 282-283
chap 8: 285, 301
chap 9: 331-332, 350

Glucagon

chap 1: 13
chap 4: 151
chap 5: 180-181, 189, 191, 196-197, 200, 203, 206, 214, 216, 218, 220
chap 12: 409-411

Glucagon-like peptide-1

chap 5: 180-181, 188

Glucosuria

chap 4: 160
chap 5: 195, 199-200, 202, 212, 220-221
chap 12: 430

Glucotoxicity

chap 5: 180, 186, 189, 191, 194-195, 199-200, 204, 207, 210, 218

Glutamine

chap 2: 54
chap 3: 94
chap 4: 152-153
chap 8: 305
chap 12: 405, 408, 417-419, 433
chap 14: 481, 486-489, 504-509

Glycated hemoglobin

chap 5: 202-203
chap 6: 230

H

Hair

chap 1: 6, 16, 29, 48
chap 2: 53-55, 60-61, 65, 67-68, 71, 73-75
chap 3: 89, 121, 136-137
chap 4: 166
chap 5: 191
chap 8: 306
chap 11: 387-389
chap 12: 413
chap 13: 453, 474

Healing

chap 2: 54, 56, 66, 71
chap 3: 99, 102
chap 11: 394, 401
chap 12: 409-410, 414, 418-419

Hepatic encephalopathy

chap 4: 139, 141, 143, 146-147, 150, 154-155, 157-158, 173, 178
chap 12: 416, 436

Hepatitis

chap 4: 144, 172-173

High Density Lipoprotein (HDL)

chap 1: 3, 29
chap 6: 223, 226-228, 230, 233, 239, 242
chap 14: 490

High protein diet

chap 1: 38
chap 4: 159
chap 5: 184-185, 188, 206-209, 211-213
chap 7: 270
chap 12: 425

High protein, low carbohydrate diet

chap 5: 180, 212

Hunger

chap 1: 12, 24, 45
chap 8: 318
chap 13: 447, 449, 451, 456-457, 464, 467, 472

Hydrolysed diet

chap 2: 63, 67
chap 3: 95

Hyperadrenocorticism

chap 1: 6, 8
chap 2: 64
chap 4: 162
chap 5: 219
chap 6: 229, 231-232, 238-239, 242
chap 9: 325-326
chap 13: 469

Hypercholesterolemia

chap 1: 29
chap 4: 151, 161
chap 6: 224, 231-232, 240, 243
chap 7: 270
chap 12: 430

Hyperchylomicronemia

chap 6: 230-231, 233-236, 238

Hyperglycemia

chap 3: 95
chap 4: 150-151, 154, 160-161, 178
chap 5: 184-185, 188-189, 191, 194-204, 206-208, 210, 212-215, 218-221
chap 6: 236
chap 12: 408-412, 416-417, 426, 430, 432, 43
chap 14: 489, 491-492, 504-505, 507, 509

Hyperlipidemia

chap 1: 8, 36
chap 5: 194
chap 6: 223-247

chap 12: 436
chap 14: 489, 492

Hyperlipoproteinemia

chap 2: 65
chap 6: 224, 242-243

Hyperphosphatemia

chap 7: 254, 257-259, 275-277, 283

Hypertriglyceridemia

chap 6: 224, 230, 232, 234, 241-243
chap 7: 270
chap 12: 412, 429-430

Hypervitaminosis

chap 2: 57
chap 9: 333

Hypoenergetic diet

chap 1: 27, 38

Hypokalemia

chap 4: 146, 155, 158, 160-161
chap 7: 264-267, 270, 274-275, 277, 280, 283
chap 9: 331-332, 342, 345-347
chap 12: 417, 430

I

Immune response

chap 2: 52, 56, 68
chap 3: 83-84
chap 4: 153, 164
chap 10: 363, 366
chap 14: 479, 481, 483, 487-488, 493-496, 502, 504-505, 507

Immune system

chap 2: 63, 66, 68
chap 3: 77, 83-84, 118
chap 9: 353
chap 10: 368, 372
chap 12: 418
chap 14: 479-481, 483-485, 493-496, 502, 505

Immunogenicity

chap 14: 495-496, 507

Immunological tolerance

chap 14: 494

Immunonutrition

chap 12: 433

Immunosuppression

chap 3: 111
chap 4: 164
chap 12: 410, 418-419, 424
chap 14: 481, 486, 492, 494, 504, 506

Incisor

chap 10: 357, 359, 379

Inflammatory bowel disease (IBD)

chap 1: 10
chap 3: 77, 84, 89, 91, 93, 103, 107, 115-117, 119, 122, 126, 131, 133, 134
chap 4: 144-146, 162, 164-165, 167-168, 170, 174
chap 11: 396
chap 14: 495, 504

Ingestion

chap 1: 12-13, 49
chap 3: 80, 85-86, 88, 98-102, 106, 111, 113, 120, 123
chap 4: 162
chap 5: 188
chap 6: 229
chap 7: 282
chap 9: 327, 331
chap 10: 361-362
chap 12: 435
chap 13: 439, 445, 452-453, 458-465

Innate immunity

chap 14: 481-482

Insulin resistance

chap 1: 8-9, 13, 31, 41, 48
chap 4: 150-151
chap 5: 180, 183, 186, 189-190, 192-193, 199, 207, 209-210, 216, 219-221
chap 6: 231, 235, 239-240
chap 9: 334
chap 12: 410
chap 14: 486, 489, 491-492, 504

Insulin secretion

chap 1: 39
chap 3: 130
chap 5: 180, 187-188, 191-195, 199, 207-208, 215-216, 218-219
chap 6: 235
chap 12: 409
chap 14: 490

Intensive care

chap 6: 240
chap 12: 405, 411, 432-434, 436
chap 14: 491, 502, 509

Intestinal microflora

chap 2: 70
chap 3: 78, 83, 94

J

Jaundice

chap 4: 141-143, 145, 150-151

K

Kidney

chap 1: 3, 11, 38, 42
chap 3: 86, 103
chap 4: 178

chap 5: 211
chap 6: 234, 240, 242-243
chap 7: 248-283
chap 8: 288, 291, 307, 313-316
chap 9: 323, 325-327, 331, 339, 346-347, 350
chap 10: 363, 368, 372
chap 12: 436
chap 13: 462, 468-469
chap 14: 490

L

L-carnitine

chap 1: 26, 38-39, 41, 44, 48
chap 4: 147, 151, 154, 157, 172
chap 5: 221
chap 9: 343, 349-350

Lean mass

chap 5: 221
chap 9: 341

Leptin

chap 1: 6, 12-13, 42
chap 5: 214-216
chap 13: 457, 472
chap 14: 481, 489, 508

Lipoprotein

chap 1: 3, 24, 29, 42-43
chap 2: 65, 70
chap 3: 82
chap 4: 141, 146, 152, 176
chap 5: 192-193, 215
chap 6: 223-235, 238-243
chap 7: 249, 270
chap 9: 344
chap 11: 401
chap 12: 409, 427
chap 14: 490

Lipotoxicity

chap 5: 194-196

Liver

chap 1: 22, 24, 36, 38, 44
chap 2: 54, 57, 59, 64-65, 73
chap 3: 82-83, 88, 107, 111, 115, 121, 128, 132
chap 4: 138-179
chap 5: 217
chap 6: 225, 227-228, 231-232, 234, 237, 240-244, 246
chap 8: 291, 309
chap 9: 335-337, 340, 343, 352
chap 10: 368, 372
chap 12: 407, 409, 427, 436
chap 13: 443, 469
chap 14: 486, 490-492, 503

L-lysine

chap 14: 502-503, 508-509

Low Density Lipoprotein (LDL)

chap 4: 176
chap 6: 223, 226-228, 230-233, 238, 240-243
chap 7: 249, 270
chap 9: 344
chap 14: 490

Low-fat diet

chap 2: 65
chap 3: 117
chap 6: 229, 236, 246

Lutein

chap 4: 156
chap 7: 272, 283
chap 14: 481, 488, 500, 508

Lymphoma

chap 1: 11
chap 2: 61
chap 3: 103, 105-107, 115, 125-127, 130, 133
chap 4: 143-144, 148
chap 9: 332
chap 11: 387-388, 393-394, 396-402

M

Magnesium

chap 1: 37
chap 7: 261
chap 8: 287, 297, 302-303, 306, 308, 311-312, 315-317, 319, 321
chap 9: 342-343, 349, 351
chap 12: 418, 426
chap 14: 485

Malnutrition

chap 1: 4, 26
chap 2: 54
chap 3: 116
chap 4: 141, 146, 149-150, 153, 159, 164, 168-169
chap 7: 269, 274, 276
chap 11: 388-389, 396
chap 12: 407, 409, 411-414, 418, 435
chap 14: 479, 481, 485, 487-488, 490, 502, 507

Megaesophagus

chap 3: 96-97, 99
chap 12: 423

Melanin

chap 2: 53, 66, 75

Metabolic acidosis

chap 7: 262, 265-266, 275, 277, 283
chap 8: 304-305, 308-309

Molar

chap 10: 357, 379

Motility

chap 3: 78, 80, 85-86, 92, 96, 98-100, 104, 106, 119-120, 128, 131-133, 137
chap 7: 274
chap 9: 353
chap 12: 411, 424
chap 14: 501

Muscle wasting

chap 4: 151
chap 9: 339
chap 11: 387, 389-390
chap 12: 425

N

Neophobia

chap 13: 447, 454, 460-461, 472, 474

Nephrotic syndrome

chap 6: 229, 231-232, 239-240, 242-243
chap 13: 468

Neutering

chap 1: 6, 13-14, 21, 34, 41-42, 47
chap 5: 183, 187, 194, 207, 214-216
chap 13: 462

Nitric oxide (NO)

chap 1: 7, 9, 11-14, 16-17, 24, 27, 29, 31, 33, 36-39, 42, 45
chap 2: 54, 58-60, 62-64, 66-67, 74
chap 3: 78, 81-82, 86, 90, 96, 98-99, 104-106, 108, 111, 115-117, 126, 129, 135-136
chap 4: 145-148, 161-162, 164-165, 167-168, 171, 176
chap 5: 183, 185, 191, 198, 200, 206-207, 209-213, 218, 220
chap 6: 229-230, 233-234, 236, 238, 241, 244
chap 7: 252, 255, 261, 263-264, 266-272, 275, 277-280
chap 8: 292, 294, 297, 301, 307, 310-311, 313
chap 9: 327-328, 331, 337-338, 340-341, 343-346, 350, 351, 354
chap 10: 359, 363, 373-375, 379-381, 383
chap 11: 395, 397-398, 400-401
chap 12: 407-408, 410, 412-413, 415, 417, 420-421, 423-424, 428, 431-432
chap 13: 441-443, 445, 447, 450-451, 453, 464, 467, 469-470, 475
chap 14: 479-483, 487, 489, 491-492, 494, 499, 501-503, 507, 509

Nutritional assessment

chap 11: 385-386, 388-391, 394
chap 12: 405, 412-415, 425, 433

Nutritional modulation

chap 9: 348
chap 14: 479, 481, 497-502, 505

Nutritional status

chap 4: 141
chap 11: 385-386, 388-389, 392-394, 398, 400-401
chap 12: 412, 414, 433
chap 14: 479, 489-492, 504, 507

Nutritional support

chap 2: 71
chap 3: 95
chap 4: 140-141, 144-145, 147, 153, 157, 163-164, 171-173, 178
chap 11: 388, 394, 399, 401
chap 12: 407, 411-416, 418, 420, 422, 424-426, 428, 430-433, 435
chap 14: 504

O

Obesity

chap 1: 2-49
chap 2: 54
chap 4: 149, 176
chap 5 : 180, 182-183, 185-186, 189-193, 200, 207, 212-215, 219-221
chap 6: 229, 231, 233, 236, 239, 241-242, 246
chap 8: 304
chap 9: 325-326, 339, 346, 350
chap 10: 358
chap 12: 411
chap 13: 450, 452, 456, 458, 462-463, 469
chap 14: 480, 489, 504

Odontoclastic resorptive lesion (FORL)

chap 10: 357, 366, 368-371, 382

Olfaction

chap 13: 442-443, 454, 465

Omega-3 fatty acids

chap 1: 36
chap 2: 55-56, 66
chap 6: 237, 244-246
chap 9: 340-342, 344-346, 349, 351
chap 12: 417-418

Oral disease

chap 10: 363, 376, 378

Oral tolerance

chap 2: 59, 70-71
chap 3: 84
chap 14: 479, 493-496

Oxidative stress

chap 1: 39
chap 4: 145-146, 152-153, 163, 165, 168, 172, 174
chap 5: 194, 210
chap 7: 272, 283
chap 9: 339, 343-344, 346, 348-349
chap 12: 436
chap 14: 500

P

Palatability

chap 1: 7, 24, 26, 35, 38, 40
chap 3: 83, 94, 125, 129, 134
chap 4: 154, 158-159, 164, 171
chap 7: 275, 277, 283
chap 10: 358, 360
chap 11: 395
chap 12: 420, 436
chap 13: 440, 442, 445, 447, 451-457, 462, 468, 474-477

Pancreatic amyloidosis

chap 5: 187, 197

Pancreatic enzymes

chap 4: 159, 163-164, 168-169, 171

Pancreatic lipase

chap 3: 83
chap 4: 139, 160-161, 172, 174
chap 6: 225, 235

Pancreatitis

chap 3: 86, 88, 115
chap 4: 139-140, 144-146, 156, 160-174
chap 5: 186
chap 6: 229, 231, 235, 237-241, 243
chap 12: 415, 418, 422, 426-427, 433, 436

Parenteral nutrition

chap 3: 77, 95, 130, 132
chap 4: 164-165, 171, 173
chap 11: 394-395
chap 12: 405, 411, 414-416, 425-434
chap 14: 503-504, 507-509

Periodontal disease

chap 10: 362-369, 371-378, 382-383

Periodontium

chap 10: 364-365, 372, 376

Phosphorus

chap 1: 37, 40
chap 7: 281-283
chap 8: 302, 304-305, 307-308, 314
chap 9: 343, 346
chap 12: 418, 427, 429
chap 13: 442

Pigmentation

chap 2: 53

Polydipsia

chap 4: 157
chap 5: 184, 199, 201, 204, 219
chap 7: 253
chap 13: 468-469

Polyphagia

chap 4: 166, 168
chap 5: 184, 201, 219
chap 13: 461-462

Polyphosphate

chap 10: 374-375, 379, 381, 383

Polyunsaturated fatty acid (PUFA)

chap 2: 51, 55, 66, 69
chap 5: 181, 210
chap 6: 240, 243-245
chap 7: 249, 270-271, 280, 282
chap 12: 405, 417
chap 13: 476
chap 14: 479, 481, 484, 497-499, 504-506, 508

Portosystemic shunt

chap 4: 143

Potassium

chap 1: 15, 37
chap 3: 114
chap 4: 146, 155, 163, 178
chap 7: 251-252, 263-267, 270, 273-275, 277, 279-281, 283
chap 8: 289, 297, 307-308, 310-312, 315, 318
chap 9: 331, 340, 342, 346-348
chap 12: 418, 426-427, 429-430

Prebiotic

chap 3: 93

Predation

chap 13: 443, 448, 450, 471, 473

Prehension

chap 10: 359-361, 364, 379
chap 13: 453-454, 475

Premolar

chap 3: 79
chap 10: 357, 359, 366-367, 373, 375
chap 13: 449

Probiotics

chap 2: 68, 70-71
chap 3: 83, 93, 117

Protein

chap 1: 3, 13, 15, 24-27, 35-38, 40-43, 45, 48-49
chap 2: 54, 56-57, 59, 62-65, 66-67, 74-75
chap 3: 80-81, 83, 91, 93, 95, 105, 109, 114, 117-119, 123-124, 128-130, 132, 134
chap 4: 141, 145-147, 149-159, 163-166, 168-172, 175, 177-179
chap 5: 180-182, 184-185, 187-188, 200, 202-204, 206-218, 221
chap 6: 223, 225-226, 228, 230, 232, 234, 236, 238, 240-242
chap 7: 249, 251-252, 254-255, 258, 266-271, 273-274, 276-277, 279-283
chap 8: 290, 302, 305, 308, 310-312, 317
chap 9: 330, 333, 335-336, 339, 345, 350-351
chap 11: 389, 392, 395, 401-402

chap 12: 407-417, 419-420, 425, 427-430, 433-434, 436
chap 13: 442, 455-458, 467, 469, 474, 477
chap 14: 482, 485, 487-492, 495-498, 500-502, 505, 507-509

Protein restriction

chap 4: 154, 156-158
chap 7: 269, 274, 279, 283

Proteinuria

chap 6: 232, 240-241, 243
chap 7: 254-255, 265, 267-271, 277-279, 281
chap 8: 291
chap 9: 330

Pruritus

chap 2: 57-58, 60-61, 64, 69
chap 3: 121
chap 14: 495

Psyllium

chap 1: 24
chap 3: 92, 120-121, 135, 137
chap 4: 155, 157
chap 5: 209, 221

R

Ration

chap 1: 26-27, 35, 40, 45-47, 49
chap 7: 259, 267
chap 9: 347
chap 10: 359
chap 12: 436
chap 13: 452, 466, 474

Refeeding

chap 4: 169
chap 12: 416, 418, 421, 424-427, 430, 433-434, 437

Refeeding syndrome

chap 12: 416, 418, 425-426, 430, 433-434

Relative supersaturation (RSS)

chap 8: 285, 296-297, 299-300, 302-308, 312, 315-317, 319, 321

Renal hyperparathyroidism

chap 7: 256-257, 259, 276, 280, 283

Renin-angiotensin system

chap 7: 254, 260
chap 9: 351

S

S-adenosyl methionine (SAMe)

chap 1: 11, 16, 22, 26, 33-35, 38, 40, 45-47
chap 2: 63, 72, 75
chap 3: 78, 96, 100, 105, 107, 114, 116, 118, 124, 126-127, 129
chap 4: 139, 145, 147, 152-153, 155-156
chap 5: 182-183, 190, 195, 203, 212

chap 6: 234, 244
chap 7: 252, 256, 260-261, 264, 269, 271, 276
chap 8: 288, 318
chap 9: 327, 330-333, 345
chap 10: 359, 374-375
chap 11: 388-389, 393, 395
chap 12: 413, 415, 432
chap 13: 440, 443-445, 447-448, 450, 452-453, 461-465, 467, 474, 477
chap 14: 488, 493, 498, 501, 505

Satiety

chap 1: 8, 12-13, 24, 26-27, 35-36, 40, 49
chap 11: 396
chap 12: 420
chap 13: 449, 457-458, 463, 472-474

Seborrhea

chap 2: 54, 72

Silica

chap 8: 288, 294-295, 308, 311

Skin

chap 1: 9, 18-19, 29, 35, 45, 48
chap 2: 52-58, 61, 64-75
chap 3: 92, 111, 123
chap 6: 234
chap 11: 387
chap 12: 413, 422-423
chap 13: 443, 460, 467
chap 14: 485, 488

Skin barrier

chap 2: 55, 57, 67-68

Small intestine

chap 1: 24
chap 3: 80-81, 83, 89, 91, 94, 105, 112-113, 115-116, 118, 122-123, 125-127, 133, 135
chap 4: 166, 168-169, 173
chap 6: 225, 241
chap 7: 256
chap 12: 408

Sodium

chap 1: 36
chap 3: 93, 98, 114, 119, 123
chap 4: 158
chap 6: 230
chap 7: 251-252, 256-258, 260-265, 271, 273-275, 277, 280-281
chap 8: 297-301, 303, 307-308, 310-312, 314-315, 317-318
chap 9: 324-327, 331-332, 337, 339, 341-342, 345-346, 348-351
chap 10: 374, 379, 381, 383
chap 12: 417-418, 430
chap 13: 457, 467, 474

Stenosis

chap 3: 85, 87-88, 96, 99-100, 122, 126
chap 12: 421, 423

Stomach

chap 1: 13, 24, 42, 49
chap 3: 77, 79-81, 85-88, 93-94, 99, 101-107, 115-116, 130-131, 135, 137
chap 4: 155, 166
chap 5: 209
chap 10: 381
chap 12: 415, 421-422
chap 13: 445, 450, 456, 458

Stomatitis

chap 2: 64
chap 5: 183-184, 199
chap 10: 363, 371-372, 376

Stress

chap 1: 12, 38-39
chap 3: 88, 108, 136
chap 4: 145-146, 152-153, 156, 163, 165, 168, 172, 174, 176
chap 5: 189, 194, 198, 202-203, 207, 210, 214-215, 220
chap 7: 272, 283
chap 8: 289, 295-296
chap 9: 326, 330, 339, 343-344, 346, 348-349, 351
chap 12: 410, 412, 419, 432, 436
chap 13: 446, 460, 465, 468, 472, 474
chap 14: 488, 500, 503

Stressed starvation

chap 12: 409

Struvite

chap 4: 148
chap 8: 287-289, 291-292, 294-295, 297, 300-305, 308-309, 311-317, 319-321

Systemic hypertension

chap 7: 255, 265, 268, 271, 281
chap 9: 323, 325-331, 348-351

Systolic blood pressure

chap 7: 262-263, 266, 268, 281
chap 8: 301
chap 9: 349, 351

T

Taste

chap 1: 37, 42
chap 3: 79, 129, 132, 135
chap 8: 298, 315
chap 11: 395
chap 13: 441-442, 447, 454-455, 461, 470, 472-473

Taurine

chap 1: 37, 40
chap 2: 62, 70
chap 3: 130
chap 4: 145, 149, 151-152, 155-158, 164, 173, 178
chap 5: 185, 214

chap 6: 225
chap 7: 272, 283
chap 9: 324-325, 332, 335-338, 340, 342, 344-345, 347-354
chap 12: 408, 411, 416, 418, 427, 436
chap 14: 483, 488, 508-509

Taurine deficiency cardiomyopathy

chap 9: 332, 335, 354

Texture

chap 10: 360, 373-376, 381, 383
chap 11: 395
chap 12: 436
chap 13: 446, 454-456, 461, 471

Tooth brushing

chap 10: 372-375, 377-379, 381, 383

Transient diabetes

chap 5: 180-181, 196, 199, 203, 212, 221

Trichobezoar

chap 3: 136

Tumor

chap 1: 11, 16, 43
chap 2: 53, 57, 61, 64-65, 70
chap 3: 77, 88-90, 93, 97, 100, 102-103, 105, 107, 122, 125-128, 131-132
chap 4: 148
chap 5: 181, 186, 193, 216
chap 6: 232
chap 8: 290-291, 293
chap 9: 325, 340
chap 10: 369
chap 11: 386-387, 389, 392-393, 395-401, 399, 402
chap 12: 405, 410, 413, 423
chap 13: 462, 465, 468
chap 14: 479, 481, 484, 501

Type 2 diabetes mellitus (2DM)

chap 1: 9
chap 5: 181-182, 185-186, 188-191, 193-198

Tyrosine

chap 2: 53, 66, 68-69, 71, 74-75
chap 3: 95
chap 5: 187
chap 13: 458
chap 14: 482, 499, 507-508

U

Urate

chap 4: 148
chap 8: 288, 291, 294-295, 301-302, 309-313, 315

Uremic syndrome

chap 7: 253, 256, 273-275

Urethral plug

chap 8: 287-290, 296, 298, 312, 315-316

Urinary pH

chap 8: 301, 305-306, 308, 312, 314, 317, 319
chap 13: 467, 472

Urinary saturation

chap 8: 310-312, 319

Urinary tract infection

chap 1: 11
chap 5: 214
chap 8: 287-288, 291, 302

Urine protein to creatinine ratio (UPC)

chap 7: 249, 254-255, 269-271, 277, 279
chap 9: 330

Urolithiasis

chap 1: 8, 11
chap 4: 147
chap 8: 287-288, 291-292, 296, 298, 301-317

V

Vitamin A

chap 1: 48
chap 2: 56-57
chap 4: 169
chap 12: 409
chap 14: 481, 485, 489-490, 500, 509

Vitamin B$_{12}$

chap 14: 489

Vomiting

chap 1: 24-25
chap 2: 58, 61
chap 3: 85-88, 90, 94-97, 99, 104-107, 110-111, 114-115, 120-121, 125, 129-130, 132-133, 136
chap 4: 141, 144-147, 153, 155, 157, 160, 163, 165-166, 171, 178
chap 5: 218-220
chap 7: 274-276
chap 8: 290
chap 9: 329
chap 11: 388, 393-400
chap 12: 411, 413-415, 420-424, 426, 435
chap 13: 454, 458, 467
chap 14: 495, 504

W

Water drinking

chap 13: 439, 466-468

Weight gain

chap 1: 12-13, 21-22, 27, 42, 47
chap 2: 64
chap 4: 146, 173
chap 5: 193, 207, 214-215
chap 6: 241
chap 11: 396-398
chap 12: 412, 416
chap 13: 462, 469
chap 14: 487

Weight loss

chap 1: 10, 13, 17-18, 20-33, 35-36, 38-49
chap 2: 54, 57-58, 64
chap 3: 90, 92, 101, 106-107, 111, 125-126, 135
chap 4: 141, 145-147, 150, 160, 166-169, 172-173, 179
chap 5: 193, 200, 207-209, 214-217, 219-221
chap 6: 229, 232-233, 236, 241, 246
chap 8: 321
chap 9: 329, 339, 350
chap 11: 386, 388-389, 392-394, 396-402
chap 12: 412, 416, 433, 436
chap 13: 451-452, 456, 462, 465
chap 14: 489, 492

Wool sucking

chap 13: 458-460

X

Xanthine

chap 8: 288, 291, 294-295, 310-312, 317

Z

Zinc

chap 1: 39, 48
chap 2: 54, 56, 64-66, 69
chap 3: 112, 128
chap 4: 141, 150, 152, 155-158, 178
chap 5: 205
chap 10: 383
chap 12: 418-419
chap 14: 481, 485, 490